SALEM HEALTH

INFECTIOUS DISEASES & CONDITIONS

SALEM HEALTH

INFECTIOUS DISEASES & CONDITIONS

Volume 1

Editor
H. Bradford Hawley
Wright State University

SALEM PRESS, INC.
Ipswich, Massachusetts   Hackensack, New Jersey

Note to Readers

The material presented in *Salem Health: Infectious Diseases and Conditions* is intended for broad informational and educational purposes. Readers who suspect that they or someone they know has any disorder, disease, or condition described in this set should contact a physician without delay. This set should not be used as a substitute for professional medical diagnosis. Readers who are undergoing or about to undergo any treatment or procedure described in this set should refer to their physicians and other health care providers for guidance concerning preparation and possible effects. This set is not to be considered definitive on the covered topics, and readers should remember that the field of health care is characterized by a diversity of medical opinions and constant expansion in knowledge and understanding.

Library of Congress Cataloging-in-Publication Data

Infectious diseases and conditions / editor, H. Bradford Hawley.
    p. ; cm. – (Salem health)
  Includes bibliographical references and indexes.
  ISBN 978-1-58765-776-4 (set : alk. paper) — ISBN 978-1-58765-777-1 (v. 1 : alk. paper) —
ISBN 978-1-58765-778-8 (v. 2 : alk. paper) — ISBN 978-1-58765-779-5 (v. 3 : alk. paper)
  1. Communicable diseases–Encyclopedias. I. Hawley, H. Bradford. II. Series: Salem health (Ipswich, Mass.)
  [DNLM: 1. Communicable Diseases–Encyclopedias–English. WC 13]
  RC112.I4577 2012
  616.003–dc23

2011020526

Contents

Contents

Publisher's Note

Salem Health: Infectious Diseases and Conditions presents essays on a variety of topics in infectious, or communicable, diseases. An infectious disease develops when a pathogen invades an organism (a host) and multiplies, followed by host symptomology and impairment. Pathogens–bacteria, viruses, fungi, protozoa, prions, and parasites–invade hosts with the help of biting vectors, such as mosquitoes and flies, and with the help of the hosts themselves, who ingest, inhale, or otherwise come in contact with the pathogen.

Despite decades of progress in identifying and controlling infectious diseases, humans remain vulnerable to an array of ever-evolving, resurgent, and stubborn organisms, such as those that cause human immunodeficiency virus (HIV) infection and acquired immunodeficiency syndrome (AIDS), staph infections, severe acute respiratory syndrome (SARS), seasonal influenza, and malaria. Emerging and reemerging diseases, especially prevalent in the developing world, continue to plague the poorest and most vulnerable people, including young children. Diseases that are spread through contaminated water, for example, are wide-ranging and include Escherichia coli infection, salmonellosis, cholera, dysentery, and giardiasis. More than 1 billion people worldwide do not have access to drinkable water, and 2.5 billion people live without basic sanitation. These diseases are endemic yet often preventable with proper sanitation, water treatment, and vector control.

Salem Health: Infectious Diseases and Conditions is an addition to the Salem Health series, which also includes both print and electronic versions of *Salem Health: Cancer* (2009), *Salem Health: Psychology and Mental Health* (2009), *Salem Health: Genetics and Inherited Conditions* (2010), and the core set *Magill's Medical Guide*, Sixth Edition (2011). All titles within the Salem Health series come with free online access with the purchase of the print set.

SCOPE AND COVERAGE

This A-Z encyclopedia arranges 610 essays covering all aspects of infectious diseases, including pathogens and pathogenicity, transmission, the immune system, vaccines, diagnosis, prevention, treatment, drug resistance, epidemiology, history, organizations, research, and social concerns such as aging, poverty and disease, children and disease, stress, quarantine, and bioterrorism. The essays were written for nonspecialists by medical professionals such as doctors, nurses, clinical practitioners, researchers, and therapists, as well as professors in science and medicine and professional medical writers. *Salem Health: Infectious Diseases and Conditions* will interest science and premedical students, students of epidemiology and public health, students of global and tropical medicine, public library patrons, and librarians building collections in science and medicine.

Salem Health: Infectious Diseases and Conditions surveys infectious disease from a variety of perspectives, offering historical and technical (disease-specific) background with a balanced discussion of discoveries, developments, and prognoses. Essays on specific diseases and conditions constitute the core coverage and range from discussions of the common, such as acne and influenza, to the rare, such as prion diseases and necrotizing fasciitis, or flesh-eating bacteria. Essays also provide overviews of disease prevention, diagnosis, and treatment; outline specific disease-causing agents, such as bacteria, viruses, fungi, parasites, prions, and protozoa; examine pathogen types and structures, modes of transmission, clinical significance, and susceptibility to drugs; and address the social significance of infectious diseases.

The set also includes essays reflecting the global reach of infectious disease, exploring topics such as emerging and reemerging infectious diseases, developing countries, epidemics and pandemics, endemic diseases, tropical medicine, globalization, neglected tropical diseases, water quality and treatment, sanitation, and travel. Prominent in the set is discussion of the work of the World Health Organization and other such global health agencies.

ORGANIZATION AND FORMAT

Essays vary in length from one to five pages. Every essay begins with ready-reference top matter:
- CATEGORY lists the focus of the essay:
  Diagnosis
  Diseases and conditions
  Epidemiology
  Immune response
   Pathogen

Prevention
Transmission
Treatment

- ALSO KNOWN AS provides alternative names used, where applicable.
- TRANSMISSION ROUTE (such as blood, direct contact, ingestion, and inhalation) is listed for pathogen essays.
- ANATOMY OR SYSTEM AFFECTED, which appears for diseases and conditions, lists areas of the body affected.
- DEFINITION introduces, defines, and describes the essay topic.

Essays on diseases and conditions provide information in the following text subsections:
- CAUSES identifies the known cause or causes of the disease or condition.
- RISK FACTORS identifies the major factors involved and the population affected.
- SYMPTOMS lists the main symptoms associated with the disease or condition.
- SCREENING AND DIAGNOSIS identifies the procedures used to screen for and diagnose the disease or condition; diagnosis includes physical examination and various types of testing.
- TREATMENT AND THERAPY identifies the treatment and therapy regimens, if any.
- PREVENTION AND OUTCOMES identifies any behaviors that can catch the infection early, mitigate its effect, or prevent its occurrence, as well as typical short-term and long-range outcomes.

Pathogen essays include the following three text subsections:
- NATURAL HABITAT AND FEATURES discusses where the pathogen is commonly found and describes its structure and composition.
- PATHOGENICITY AND CLINICAL SIGNIFICANCE outlines the significance of the pathogen to human disease and how this pathology is maintained through transmission.
- DRUG SUSCEPTIBILITY focuses on drug treatments that may or may not be effective against the pathogen.

Pathogen essays also feature a sidebar providing the pathogen's taxonomic classification, listing information on genus and species (namely those affecting humans), among other ranks.

The main text of essays covering diagnosis, epidemiology, immune response, prevention, and treatment offer the following subsections:
- Topical subheads, chosen by the author, divide the text and guide readers through the essay.
- IMPACT outlines the effects of the topic on areas such as public health, epidemiology, the practice of medicine, medical research, and pharmacology and treatment.

All essays conclude with the following material:
- The contributor's byline notes the specialist who wrote the essay and his or her advanced degrees and other credentials.
- FURTHER READING lists sources for further study, often with annotations, and includes the latest relevant works and full citation data for easy library access.
- WEB SITES OF INTEREST provides a list of authoritative Web sites. This section, which appears at the end of every essay, lists U.S. governmental agencies such as the Centers for Disease Control and Prevention and the National Center for Emerging and Zoonotic Infectious Diseases; nongovernmental organizations such as the World Health Organization, the Alliance for the Prudent Use of Antibiotics, and the Clean Hands Coalition; professional and academic societies such as the American Academy of Pediatrics; online texts such as Microbiology and Immunology On-line; and health consumer sites such as MedlinePlus (National Library of Medicine and National Institutes of Health) and WebMD.
- SEE ALSO lists cross-references to related essays within the set.

Many essays in the encyclopedia include sidebars featuring key terms, key facts, newsworthy topics, questions to ask one's health care provider, and other topics. Other essays feature tables with statistics and other data on infection rates, pathogen types, disease trends, and affected populations.

SPECIAL FEATURES

The articles in *Salem Health: Infectious Diseases and Conditions* are arranged alphabetically by title; a Complete List of Contents appears at the beginning of each volume. More than 200 photographs illustrate the text.

In addition, nine appendixes appear at the end of volume 3. In the section "Reference Tools," the Glossary provides hundreds of definitions of commonly used scientific and medical terms and concepts, especially as they apply to infectious diseases, along with definitions of dozens of common medical prefixes and suffixes. The Bibliography offers citations for both classic and recently published sources for additional research. The Resources appendix provides a list of organizations and support groups. The importance of the Internet to general education in infectious diseases is reflected in the annotated Web Sites appendix. Other appendixes include Medical Journals, which lists professional journals commonly encountered in any study of infectious diseases, and a Pharmaceutical List, categorized by type of drug (antibiotic, antiviral, antifungal, antimalarial, antimycobacterial, and antiparasitic).

In the section "Historical Resources," the Time Line offers a chronological overview of major developments in infectious disease from 1700 B.C.E. to the present. The Biographical Dictionary of Scientists in Infectious Disease features 144 scientists who had an impact on the science of infectious diseases. Nobel Prizes for Discoveries in Infectious Diseases lists Nobel laureates who made significant contributions to areas related to that field.

Three indexes appear at the end of volume 3 including Entries by Anatomy or System Affected, a Category Index, and a comprehensive subject index that directs readers to related topics throughout the set.

ACKNOWLEDGMENTS

The editors of Salem Press wish to thank the many medical professionals, scholars, and writers who contributed to this set; their names, degrees and other credentials, and academic and other affiliations appear in the list of contributors that follows. Special mention must be made of consulting editor H. Bradford Hawley, M.D., an infectious disease specialist who applied his broad medical knowledge to shaping this set's contents.

***

ABOUT THE EDITOR

H. Bradford Hawley, M.D. is an Emeritus Professor of Medicine and former Chief of Infectious Diseases at the Boonshoft School of Medicine, Wright State University. He has been elected to fellowship in the American College of Physicians, American College of Chest Physicians, Society for Healthcare Epidemiologists, and Infectious Diseases Society of America. Dr. Hawley is a former member of the Board of Directors of the Certification Board of Infection Control and past President of the Infectious Diseases Society of Ohio. He has made more than one hundred contributions to the medical literature and currently serves as a manuscript reviewer for several medical journals, including the *Annals of Internal Medicine* and *Clinical Infectious Diseases*. He is a frequent contributor to Salem Press publications and is a medical editor of *Magill's Medical Guide*, Sixth Edition (2011).

Editor's Introduction

The struggle for life is a never-ending quest for precious and necessary resources. The food chain begins with the plant kingdom, able to transform the mixture of earth, air, and sunlight into life-forms. From this beginning, the food chain changes to a system in which one living thing consumes another living thing. This is a shortcut to obtaining the basic ingredients of life. Big things eat small things: Cats eat mice and whales eat krill. Still another side exists in the battle for life; it is a David and Goliath story in which the small–the microbes–assume the throne by causing infectious diseases in the big, in this case humans.

Humans and microbes have evolved together, each seeking an advantage over the other. Microorganisms have developed metabolic pathways, complex cell membranes and cell walls, toxins, and rapid evolutionary changes to stay ahead of human defenses. Humans have countered with a highly developed immune system that can ward off and cope with the attacks of most microbes. Still, history has shown that the microbes have often won, sometimes in dramatic fashion. Worldwide epidemics of plague, smallpox, typhus, cholera, poliomyelitis, and influenza have killed millions over the centuries. When the human immune system fails, the mind works to find ways to control disease. In understanding pathogens and the infectious diseases they cause, humans have been able to tip the scales in their own favor.

Long before causative microbes were identified, humans already could appreciate some of the basics about the transmission of infectious diseases. As early as 1403, Venetians employed quarantine to protect against infections being introduced by travelers. Not all ideas about disease transmission have proven correct. As recent as about one hundred years ago, epidemiologists believed that most infectious diseases were spread through the air. Such thinking was the logical consequence of seeing the malodorous process of putrefaction and wound infection. This oversimplification of disease transmission led to much misunderstanding.

Malaria derives its name from the Italian words meaning "bad air," as many malaria cases occurred near foul-smelling swamp lands in Italy. City air, made unclean by coal-burning industrial plants and homes, combined with poor sanitation facilities, could easily be blamed for ill health. In the summer of 1854, a cholera epidemic struck the densely populated city of London. John Snow countered the experts of the day, who professed bad air as the problem, and demonstrated that contaminated drinking water was the culprit. Snow's removal of the handle to the Broad Street water pump prevented residents from consuming the contaminated water and quelled the epidemic. His studies serve as the foundation for modern epidemiology.

Robert Koch and Louis Pasteur shed new light on the etiology of many of the most serious and lethal infections of humans. Indeed, the then-new field of bacteriology seemed to be the answer to infectious diseases. We now know this time marked only the beginning of our understanding of disease-causing microbes.

Some disease-causing organisms, or pathogens, are large and easily seen with the naked eye. For example, three-foot-long female guinea worms emerge through the skin of their human hosts. Other microbes can be observed only by employing the magnifying optics of a microscope. Grapelike clusters of staphylococci are visible in stained material from infected wounds. Even smaller infecting organisms can be seen only through a powerful electron microscope. The tiny, 27-nanometer, icosahedral poliovirus, for example, is visible using this technology.

The human mind has allowed for the development of methods for growing microorganisms in both non-human animal hosts and artificial media. The cultivation of microbes in the laboratory has made it possible to understand the structure and function of the organisms and to develop defensive strategies, such as vaccines and antibiotics. In fact, most antibiotics are derived from chemicals manufactured by microbes to protect themselves from other microbes. Microbes grown on artificial media may be tested, in vitro, for their susceptibility to various antibiotics, thereby increasing the likelihood of success of treatment by selection of the most effective antimicrobial agent.

More recently, molecular microbiology has allowed us to probe the inner workings of infectious organisms as never before. We can study microbic genomes to elucidate their evolution and genetic origins, refining relationships and classification schemes. Unique genetic sequences can be targeted by gene probes to provide rapid and accurate disease diagnosis. In the future, alteration of genes important for microbe virulence may allow us to control the infection of humans by certain organisms. Regulator genes, which turn on and off genes that are responsible for the production of virulence factors, can be targeted by drugs that prevent the production of these disease-enabling proteins.

By understanding microbes and the diseases they cause, humans can overcome the advantage of millions of years of evolution and rapid adaptation of infectious microbes. The increasing human population has led to our expansion into new habitats, increasing exposure to new pathogens such as the human immunodeficiency virus (HIV). In the case of HIV, this exposure, along with some unwise human behavior, has led to a worldwide epidemic. In other cases, such as Ebola, localized outbreaks have occurred but no widespread epidemics.

Global travel and immigration have provided new avenues for the spread of infectious disease. Climate change is already altering the range of many endemic infectious diseases. Organisms are stepping up the pace of antibiotic resistance, spurred on by the overuse and misuse of antibiotics.

Despite a century of rapid scientific development, new pathogens and diseases are still being discovered. Some old diseases, such as peptic ulcer disease, first thought to be understood, have only recently been found to be caused by infectious microbes, requiring a different approach to diagnosis and treatment. All these challenges, and more, make it necessary to expand our knowledge of infectious diseases.

Salem Health: Infectious Diseases and Conditions is designed to be a step in expanding this knowledge. As an encyclopedia enhanced with many extra features, this text provides not only an introduction but also a basic understanding of most infectious diseases. It is not a textbook for a course in infectious diseases, but rather a quick and useful reference for specific infectious diseases and their associated conditions. For some readers, this is all that is required; for others wishing to delve deeper, each essay concludes with suggestions for further reading; to further assist the reader, an appendix in volume 3 lists medical and science journals and their special areas of coverage. It is hoped that the design of this encyclopedic set will provide easy and quick access to current information on infectious diseases and that it will inspire the mind as well.

M. Bradford Hawley, M.D., FACP, FCCP, FIDSA,
Boonshoft School of Medicine, Wright State University

Contributors

Shara Aaron, M.S., RD
Nutrition Communications LLC

Christine Adamec, M.B.A.
Southern New Hampshire
    University

Richard Adler, Ph.D.
University of Michigan, Dearborn

Rick Alan
Medical writer and editor

Brian S. Alper, M.D., M.S.P.H.
DynaMed, EBSCO Publishing

Wendell Anderson, B.A.
American Medical Writers
    Association

Jeff Andrews, M.D., FRCSC,
    FACOG
Vanderbilt University Medical
    Center

Deborah A. Appello, M.S.
Brick, New Jersey

Mihaela Avramut, M.D., Ph.D.
Verlan Medical Communications

Michelle Badash, M.S.
Wakefield, Massachusetts

Amanda Barrett, M.A.
Health Library, EBSCO Publish-
    ing

Allison C. Bennett, Pharm.D.
Duke University Hospital

Alvin K. Benson, Ph.D.
Utah Valley University

Janet Ober Berman, M.S., CGC
Temple University School of
    Medicine

R. L. Bernstein, Ph.D.
New Mexico State University

Dawn M. Bielawski, Ph.D.
Wayne State University

Anna Binda, Ph.D.
American Medical Writers
    Association

Jennifer Birkhauser, M.D.
University of California, Irvine

Adriane Bishko, M.A.
Cambridge, Massachusetts

Stephanie McCallum Blake,
    M.S.N.
Duke University Medical Center

Maria Borowski, M.A.
Medical writer

Wanda Bradshaw, M.S.N., R.N.,
    NNP-BC, PNP, CCRN
Duke University School of
    Nursing

Michael A. Buratovich, Ph.D.
Spring Arbor University

Steven D. Burdette, M.D.
Wright State University

David Caldwell, Ph.D.
Indianapolis, Indiana

Mary Calvagna, M.S.
Medical writer

Carita Caple, M.S.H.S., R.N.
Wilmington, Delaware

Richard P. Capriccioso, M.D.
University of Phoenix

Adrienne Carmack, M.D.
Brenham, Texas

Christine M. Carroll, R.N.
American Medical Writers
    Association

Rosalyn Carson-DeWitt, M.D.
Durham, North Carolina

Judy Chang, M.D., FAASM
University of Pittsburgh Physi-
    cians

Paul J. Chara, Jr., Ph.D.
Northwestern College

Richard W. Cheney, Jr., Ph.D.
Christopher Newport University

Christopher Cheyer, M.D.
Wayne State University School of
    Medicine

Rose Ciulla-Bohling, Ph.D.
Lansdale, Pennsylvania

Christine Colpitts, M.A., CRT
Medical writer

Julie Y. Crider, Ph.D.
Collaborative Medical Writing

L. Lee Culvert, B.S., CLS
Bartonville, Texas

Luke Curtis, M.D.
Cincinnati, Ohio

Arun S. Dabholkar, Ph.D.
Northwestern University

Amanda Dameron, M.A.
Blue Cross Blue Shield of
Massachusetts

Cynthia L. De Vine, B.A.
American Medical Writers
Association

Shawkat Dhanani, M.D., M.P.H.
VA, Greater Los Angeles Healthcare System

Stephanie Eckenrode, B.A.
New York, New York

Patricia Stanfill Edens, R.N.,
Ph.D., FACHE
The Oncology Group

Renée Euchner, R.N.
American Medical Writers
Association

Merrill Evans, M.A.
Tucson, Arizona

David M. Faguy, Ph.D.
Doc-write

Adi R. Ferrara, B.S., ELS
Bellevue, Washington

Rebecca J. Frey, Ph.D.
Yale University

Cathy Frisinger, M.P.H.
Arlington, Texas

Susan Gifford, M.S.
West Newbury, Massachusetts

Margaret Ring Gillock, M.S.
Libertyville, Illinois

Lenela Glass-Godwin, M.S.
Texas A&M University
Auburn University

Katherine Hauswirth, M.S.N.,
R.N.
Hauswirth Writing Solutions

H. Bradford Hawley, M.D.
Boonshoft School of Medicine,
Wright State University

Jennifer Hellwig, M.S., RD
Medical writer

Julie Henry, R.N., M.P.A.
Myrtle Beach, South Carolina

Jenna Hollenstein, M.S., RD
Genzyme

David L. Horn, M.D., FACP
Medical writer

Brian Hoyle, Ph.D.
Square Rainbow

Mary Hurd, M.A.
East Tennessee State University

David Hutto, Ph.D.
Tetrascribe

Christopher Iliades, M.D.
Centerville, Massachusetts

April Ingram, B.S.
Kelowna, British Columbia

Cheryl Pokalo Jones
Townsend, Delaware

Clair Kaplan, M.S.N., M.H.S.,
R.N., MT(ASCP), APRN,
WHNP
Planned Parenthood of Southern
New England

Karen Schroeder Kassel, M.S.,
RD, M.Ed.
Fallon Clinic

Kari Kassir, M.D.
Orange, California

John C. Keel, M.D.
Medical writer

Gerald W. Keister, M.A.
American Medical Writers
Association

Patricia Griffin Kellicker, B.S.N.
Upton, Massachusetts

Camillia King, M.P.H.
Huntsville, Alabama

Sid Kirchheimer
Medical writer

M. Barbara Klyde, PA
House Call Physicians

Jeffrey A. Knight, Ph.D.
Mount Holyoke College

Marylane Wade Koch, M.S.N.,
R.N.
University of Memphis, Loewen-
berg School of Nursing

Ernest Kohlmetz, M.A.
Millbrook, New York

Diana Kohnle
Platte Valley Medical Center

Diep Koly, M.D.
Media, Pennsylvania

Anita P. Kuan, Ph.D.
Lyme, Connecticut

Steven A. Kuhl, Ph.D.
V & R Consulting

Contributors

Jeanne L. Kuhler, Ph.D.
Benedictine University

Jill D. Landis, M.D.
Rye, New York

Dawn Laney, M.S.
Emory University

Kathleen LaPoint, M.S.
Greensboro, North Carolina

Laurie LaRusso, M.S., ELS
University School of Nutrition
    Science and Policy

Joan Y. Letizia, Ph.D.
Medical and Scientific Writing
    Services

Jennifer Lewy, M.S.W.
Medical writer

Lisa M. Lines, M.P.H.
University of Massachusetts
    Medical School

Nicky Lowney, M.A.
Groton, Massachusetts

Julie Rackliffe Lucey, M.S.
Medical writer

Rimas Lukas, M.D.
University of Chicago

Krisha McCoy, M.S.
American Medical Writers
    Association

Marianne M. Madsen, M.S.
University of Utah

Daus Mahnke, M.D.
Gastroenterology of the Rockies

Judy Majewski, M.S.
Geneva, Illinois

Katia Marazova, M.D., Ph.D.
Paris, France

Lindsey Marcellin, M.D., M.P.H.
Purcellville, Virginia

Mary E. Markland, M.A.
Argosy University

Julie J. Martin, M.S.
Medical writer

J. Thomas Megerian, M.D., Ph.D.,
    FAAP
Neurometrix
North Shore Children's Hospital
Children's Hospital, Boston

Ralph R. Meyer, Ph.D.
University of Cincinnati

Cynthia L. Mills, D.V.M.
Portland, Oregon

Beatriz Manzor Mitrzyk,
    Pharm.D.
Mitrzyk Medical Communications

Linda J. Miwa, M.P.H.
Burke, Virginia

Marjorie M. Montemayor, M.A.
Medical writer

Marvin L. Morris, M.P.A.
American Medical Writers
    Association

Laura Morris-Olson, D.M.D.
Medical writer

Micki Pflug Mounce, B.A.
Mundelein, Illinois

Karen M. Nagel, Ph.D.
Midwestern University

Kimberly A. Napoli, M.S.
KanCom Biomedical
    Communications

Ronald Nath, M.D.
Medical writer

Olalekan E. Odeleye, Ph.D.
Phillipsburg, New Jersey

David A. Olle, M.S.
Eastshire Communications

Colm A. O'Morain, M.D., D.Sc.
Medical writer

Oladayo Oyelola, Ph.D.,
    SC(ASCP)
American Medical Writers
    Association

Ravinder Pandher, M.D.
University of Calgary

Robert J. Paradowski, Ph.D.
Rochester Institute of Technology

Kathryn Pierno, M.S.
American Medical Writers
    Association

Laura J. Pinchot, B.A.
Clarion University of Pennsylvania

Ricker Polsdorfer, M.D.
Medical writer

Marie President, M.D.
Sequoia Medical Associates

Ganson Purcell, Jr., M.D.,
    FACOG, FACPE
Medical writer

Igor Puzanov, M.D.
Vanderbilt University

Cynthia F. Racer, M.P.H., M.A.
New York Academy of Sciences

Elie Edmond Rebeiz, M.D., FACS
Tufts-New England Medical
    Center
Tufts University School of
    Medicine

Andrew J. Reinhart, M.S.
University of Hawaii, Hilo

Julie Riley, M.S., RD
Tufts University School of
    Medicine

Ana Maria Rodriguez-Rojas, M.S.
GXP Medical Writing

Alayne Ronnenberg, Sc.D.
Harvard School of Public Health
Tufts University School of
    Nutrition

Laurie Rosenblum, M.P.H.
Education Development Center,
    Massachusetts

Claudia Daileader Ruland, M.A.
Johns Hopkins University

Jen Rymaruk
Medical writer

Diane Safer, Ph.D.
Medical writer

Tina M. St. John, M.D.
St. John Health Communications
    & Consulting

David A. Saunders, M.D.
Wright State University

Diane Savitsky
Medical writer

Elizabeth D. Schafer, Ph.D.
Loachapoka, Alabama

Amy Scholten, M.P.H.
Inner Medicine Publishing

Skye Schulte, M.S., M.P.H.

David L. Horn, M.D., FACP
Medical writer

Miriam E. Schwartz, M.D., Ph.D.
University of California, Los
    Angeles

Lynda A. Seminara, B.A.
American Medical Writers
    Association

Sibani Sengupta, Ph.D.
American Medical Writers
    Association

Diane W. Shannon, M.D., M.P.H.
Medical writer

Martha A. Sherwood, Ph.D.
Kent Anderson Law Office

Jill Shuman, M.S., RD, ELS
Tufts University

R. Baird Shuman, Ph.D.
University of Illinois,
    Urbana-Champaign

Vonne Sieve, M.A.
American Medical Writers
    Association

Bridget Sinnott, M.D., FACE
Medical writer

David N. Smith, M.D.
Medical writer

Nathalie Smith, M.S.N., R.N.
Lincoln, Nebraska

Rebecca Stadolnik
Stow, Massachusetts

Rebecca J. Stahl, M.A.
Medical writer

Diane Stresing
Kent, Ohio

Annie Stuart
Pacifica, California

Carol Ann Suda, B.S., MT(ASCP)
    SM
Holy Cross Hospital, Clinical
    Laboratory

John M. Theilmann, Ph.D.
Converse College

Bethany Thivierge, M.P.H.
Technicality Resources

Susan E. Thomas, M.L.S.
Indiana University, South Bend

Nicole M. Van Hoey, Pharm.D.
Arlington, Virginia

Oluseyi A. Vanderpuye, Ph.D.
Albany State University

Charles L. Vigue, Ph.D.
University of New Haven

Beth Walsh, M.A.
Health Imaging & IT magazine

C. J. Walsh, Ph.D.
Mote Marine Laboratory

Melissa Walsh
Powerplay Communications

Brandy Weidow, M.S.
Nashville, Tennessee

Judith Weinblatt, M.S., M.A.
New York, New York

Contributors

Alicia Williams, M.A.
Columbia University Medical
    Center

S. M. Willis, M.S., M.A.
Huntington Beach, California

Barbara Woldin, B.S.
American Medical Writers
    Association

Debra Wood, R.N.
Brewster, Massachusetts

Robin Wulffson, M.D., FACOG
American Medical Writers
    Association

Rachel Zahn, M.D.
Angels Foster Family Network

Ross Zeltser, M.D., FAAD
Westchester Dermatology and
    Mohs Surgery Center

Susan M. Zneimer, Ph.D.,
    FACMG
US Labs

Complete List of Contents

Volume 1

Volume 2

Volume 3

SALEM HEALTH

INFECTIOUS DISEASES
& CONDITIONS

A

Abscesses

CATEGORY: Diseases and conditions
ANATOMY OR SYSTEM AFFECTED: All
ALSO KNOWN AS: Boils, carbuncles, cysts, fistulas, pustules, whiteheads

DEFINITION

An abscess is an encapsulated accumulation of pus that can form during the body's response to infections from bacteria, viruses, or parasites. Abscesses can form in any part of the body, including the liver, brain, abdomen, skin, muscle, and bones, and in the tissues of the mouth, teeth, uterus, and ovaries.

CAUSES

In general, an abscess forms when the body responds to bacteria, viruses, parasites, and other foreign objects. When tissue is damaged, the cells die, leaving a space where infected cells and fluid can accumulate. White blood cells move into the infected area to fight the infection. As these cells die, they accumulate as pus. The pus pushes against the surrounding tissue, and the surrounding tissue eventually grows around the infected area, encapsulating the pus and thus forming an abscess.

Depending on the location, the causes of abscesses vary. Liver abscesses are predominantly (80 percent) caused by polymicrobial infections, but can also be caused by parasitic (amebic) or fungal (*Candida*) infections. The most common bacterium isolated from liver abscesses is *Escherichia coli*. Another bacterium associated with liver abscesses is *Staphylococcus aureus*. These abscesses usually result from distant infections.

Dental abscesses are found in the mouth, face, jaw, throat, or tooth. They are caused by the bacteria in a cavity or by the bacteria that accumulate within pockets formed in supportive bone in periodontal disease. Poor dental health and a lack of proper dental care that leads to cavities or gum disease can lead to the formation of dental abscesses.

Skin abscesses are caused by clogged oil ducts or sweat glands that become infected. Skin abscesses also are caused by bacteria entering through pores, hair follicles, or minor cuts.

A ruptured appendix is one of the common causes of an abdominal abscess. Brain abscesses are caused by bacteria or fungi infecting the brain. Although brain abscesses are rare (because the blood-brain barrier protects the brain), some conditions, such as heart disease and some congenital diseases (especially in children), allow infections from other parts of the body to reach the brain. Ovarian abscesses are usually caused by bacterial infections from the genital tract. There are cases in which abscesses can form within the ovary from *Salmonella* infections remote from the site.

RISK FACTORS

For liver abscesses, some risk factors include biliary tract disease, in which the obstruction of bile flow allows bacteria to grow. Risk factors for liver and other abdominal abscesses include appendicitis (if the appendix ruptures and releases bacteria), inflammatory bowel disease, and trauma. A urinary tract infection can cause pelvic or kidney abscesses.

There is also evidence that persons with a prior injury (for example, a history of benign ovarian cysts) that leaves a scar or cavity at the injury site may be more susceptible to abscesses of the ovaries or uterus. One case involved the formation of a uterine abscess at the site where an intrauterine device was removed years earlier. *Salmonella* infections from other sources can lead to abscess formation in the ovaries weeks to years after the original infection.

Poor dental hygiene and periodontal gum disease, which lead to bacteria accumulation in the mouth, are risk factors for dental abscesses. Also, in general, underlying autoimmune disorders or conditions that weaken the immune system increase the risk for abscess formation because of the body's decreased ability to fight infections. The use of some medications, such as corticosteroids and chemotherapy, which weaken the immune system, are also risk factors.

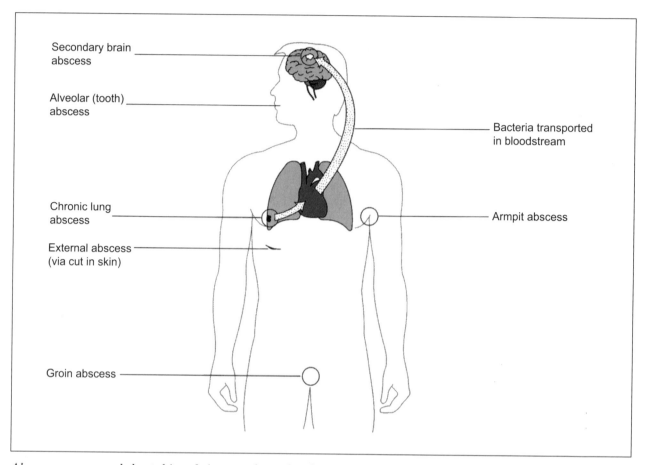

- Secondary brain abscess
- Alveolar (tooth) abscess
- Chronic lung abscess
- External abscess (via cut in skin)
- Groin abscess
- Bacteria transported in bloodstream
- Armpit abscess

Abscesses are commonly located in soft tissues and near lymph nodes but may appear in internal organs and may cause other abscesses through bacterial migration.

SYMPTOMS

Symptoms of an abscess vary depending on the location of the abscess, on whether it interferes with the function of the specific organ, and on whether it affects the nerves. In general, tenderness, pain, swelling, and redness are early signs of superficial abscesses. Deeper abscesses, which may go undiagnosed for some time, may also be accompanied by pain, tenderness, nausea, vomiting, fever, and chills.

SCREENING AND DIAGNOSIS

Skin abscesses appear as bumps or inflamed areas that may be tender to the touch. Deeper skin abscesses usually display the foregoing symptoms. An X ray, computed tomography (CT) scan, magnetic resonance imaging (MRI) scan, or ultrasound can be used to diagnose suspected deeper abscesses.

TREATMENT AND THERAPY

Antibiotics alone cannot cure an abscess because the medication cannot enter the skin encapsulating the pus. Abscesses need to be drained by a medical provider, who will insert a sterile needle into the abscess and then aspirate (drain) the contents. For deep abscesses, the procedure is guided by MRI or CT scans. Then, antibiotic therapy is used to prevent reinfection and to treat the underlying infection. The antibiotic used depends on the location of the abscess and on the microorganism causing the infection. Sometimes, abscesses drain on their own. Incomplete drainage can cause the abscess to reform.

PREVENTION AND OUTCOMES

Bacteria are everywhere. The prevention of dental abscesses and superficial skin abscesses can be accomplished by good dental and general hygiene. The treatment of other infections and the control of associated risk factors may also help prevent the formation of deeper abscesses in other parts of the body.

Joan Y. Letizia, Ph.D.

FURTHER READING

"Abscess." In *Ferri's Clinical Advisor 2011: Instant Diagnosis and Treatment*, edited by Fred F. Ferri. Philadelphia: Mosby/Elsevier, 2011.

"Abscesses." In *The Merck Manual Home Health Handbook*, edited by Robert S. Porter et al. 3d ed. Whitehouse Station, N.J.: Merck Research Laboratories, 2009.

Langlais, Robert P., and Craig S. Miller. *Color Atlas of Common Oral Diseases.* 4th ed. Philadelphia: Lippincott Williams & Wilkins, 2009.

Parkham, Peter. *The Immune System.* 2d ed. New York: Garland Science, 2005.

Peralta, Ruben, et al. "Liver Abscess." Available at http://emedicine.medscape.com/article/188802-overview.

Weedon, David. *Skin Pathology.* 3d ed. New York: Churchill Livingstone/Elsevier, 2010.

WEB SITES OF INTEREST

American Academy of Dermatology
http://www.aad.org

American Dental Association
http://www.ada.org

See also: Actinomycosis; Anal abscess; Boils; Cold sores; *Eikenella* infections; Empyema; Hygiene; Infection; Inflammation; Mastitis; Mouth infections; Mycetoma; Oral transmission; Pilonidal cyst; Skin infections; Tooth abscess.

Acanthamoeba infections

CATEGORY: Diseases and conditions
ANATOMY OR SYSTEM AFFECTED: Brain, central nervous system, eyes, skin, vision
ALSO KNOWN AS: Acanthamoeba encephalitis, acanthamoeba keratitis, cutaneous acanthamebiasis, granulomatous amebic encephalitis

DEFINITION

An acanthamoeba infection is an infection of the eye, skin, and brain, as a rare form of encephalitis.

CAUSES

Acanthamoeba is a genus of single-celled protozoa found in soil and in contaminated water. Acanthamoeba infections can occur when the organism enters the body through corneal abrasions, lesions in the skin, upper-respiratory-tract olfactory epithelium, or through inhalation of airborne cysts.

RISK FACTORS

One common risk factor for acanthamoeba keratitis (eye infection) is wearing contact lenses. Persons who wear soft contact lenses appear to be at a higher risk than persons who wear rigid lenses. Poor compliance with prescribed contact lens hygiene is another factor that increases the likelihood of developing acanthamoeba keratitis. Orthokeratology, a procedure that uses a rigid contact lens to modify the shape of the cornea, also leads to an increased risk of infection.

Other risk factors include swimming while wearing contact lenses, a lack of adequate lens disinfection, corneal trauma, and contaminated water exposure. Human immunodeficiency virus (HIV) infection, acquired immunodeficiency syndrome (AIDS), and the use of immunosuppressive drugs are risk factors for cutaneous (skin) acanthamoeba infections.

SYMPTOMS

Symptoms of acanthamoeba keratitis include blurred vision, conjunctival hyperemia, a corneal ring, a foreign-body sensation in the eye, pain, perineural infiltrates, photophobia, redness, and tearing. Symptoms of granulomatous amebic encephalitis (GAE), which affects the brain, include anorexia, confusion, hallucinations, headache, irritability, loss of balance, nausea, seizures, sleep disturbances, stiff neck, and vomiting. Skin lesions are hallmarks of cutaneous acanthamoeba infections.

SCREENING AND DIAGNOSIS

The initial diagnosis of acanthamoeba infection is typically based on a person's medical history. Corneal scrapings stained with such agents as acridine orange or calcofluor white, or a Giemsa stain, may reveal the cyst and trophozoite forms of the organism. Corneal culturing on non-nutrient agar plates seeded with bacteria such as *Escherichia coli* is frequently performed. Confocal microscopy can be used as a noninvasive diagnostic tool. Useful aids in obtaining an acute diagnosis for the GAE and cutaneous forms include a biopsy, indirect immunofluorescence, a culture, and the polymerase chain reaction technique.

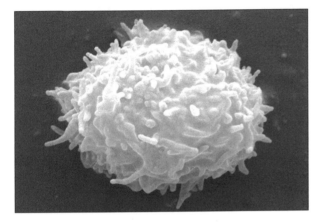

A *micrograph of* Acanthamoeba polyphaga, *a common protozoan parasite that causes several types of infections in humans.* (CDC)

TREATMENT AND THERAPY

Because of the resistance of the cystic form of *Acanthamoeba*, treatment can be problematic. For keratitis, aggressive treatment with agents such as 0.1 percent propamidine isethionate, 0.02 to 0.04 percent chlorhexidine, and 0.02 percent PHMB is standard practice. A corneal transplant may be required for some cases. Medications such as amphotericin B, azithromycin, chlorhexidine, clindamycin, fluconazole, fluorocytosine, itraconazole, ketoconazole, metrometronidazole, pentamidine, sulfamethoxazole, and trimethoprim have been used to treat other forms of acanthamoeba infection. The mortality rate for these infections can be quite high. For persons with HIV infection or AIDS, the mortality rate for cutaneous acanthamebiasis without central nervous system involvement is thought to be about 75 percent.

PREVENTION AND OUTCOMES

To minimize the risk of acanthamoeba infection, persons should avoid swimming or bathing in contaminated water, should practice good contact-lens hygiene, and should maintain a healthy immune system.

Julie Y. Crider, Ph.D.

FURTHER READING

Awwad, Shady T., et al. "Updates in Acanthamoeba Keratitis." *Eye and Contact Lens* 33 (2007): 1-8.

Cassel, Gary H., Michael D. Billig, and Harry G. Randall. *The Eye Book: A Complete Guide to Eye Disorders and Health.* Baltimore: Johns Hopkins University Press, 2001.

Hammersmith, Kristin M. "Diagnosis and Management of Acanthamoeba Keratitis." *Current Opinion in Ophthalmology* 4 (2006): 327-331.

Marciano-Cabral, Francine, and Guy Cabral. "*Acanthamoeba* spp. as Agents of Disease in Humans." *Clinical Microbiology Reviews* 16, no. 2 (2003): 273-307.

Paltiel, Michael, et al. "Disseminated Cutaneous Acanthamebiasis: A Case Report and Review of the Literature." *Cutis* 73 (2004): 241-248.

Sutton, Amy L., ed. *Eye Care Sourcebook: Basic Consumer Health Information About Eye Care and Eye Disorders.* 3d ed. Detroit: Omnigraphics, 2008.

Weedon, David. *Skin Pathology.* 3d ed. New York: Churchill Livingstone/Elsevier, 2010.

Wiederholt, Wigbert C. *Neurology for Non-neurologists.* 4th ed. Philadelphia: W. B. Saunders, 2000.

WEB SITES OF INTEREST

American Academy of Dermatology
http://www.aad.org

American Academy of Ophthalmology
http://www.aao.org

Encephalitis Society
http://www.encephalitis.info

National Institute of Neurological Disorders and Stroke
http://www.ninds.nih.gov

Public Health Agency of Canada
http://www.phac-aspc.gc.ca

See also: Bacterial infections; Bacterial meningitis; Conjunctivitis; Encephalitis; *Escherichia*; Eye infections; Impetigo; Keratitis; Skin infections; Soilborne illness and disease; Waterborne illness and disease.

Acariasis

CATEGORY: Diseases and conditions
ANATOMY OR SYSTEM AFFECTED: Gastrointestinal system, skin, urinary system
ALSO KNOWN AS: Acaridiasis, acarinosis, scabies

DEFINITION

Acariasis is both an infestation of mites and a disease caused by mites.

CAUSES

Mites are a vast and diverse species of tiny parasitic and free-living arthropods that can infect the skin, gastrointestinal tract, lungs, urinary tract, and other areas of the body. Cutaneous infestation is one of the most common forms of acariasis and occurs when mites, such as *Sarcoptes scabiei* var. *hominis* (human scabies), burrow into the skin or hair follicles and deposit proteins that produce an allergic cutaneous dermatitis. The remains of dead dust mites and their fecal matter are also a major source of allergens. These allergens mediate a type 1 hypersensitivity reaction in atopic persons. In addition to causing cutaneous dermatitis and producing allergens, mites can cause illness by acting as vectors for parasitic diseases. For example, the larvae of trombiculid mites, the chigger mite (*Trombicula*), transmits scrub typhus (tsutsugamushi disease) and other rickettsial agents.

RISK FACTORS

Mites often thrive and multiply in warm moist areas and feed on dead skin from humans and animals. Some mites are also highly contagious. Thus, environmental factors such as overcrowding and poor hygiene are important risk factors for acariasis. Other risk factors include delayed treatment of primary cases, which can foster the spread of acariasis, and a lack of public awareness. Some persons may also have a genetic predisposition for developing hypersensitive reactions to mites.

SYMPTOMS

The symptoms of acariasis vary depending on the type of infestation. The inflammation and skin lesions of cutaneous acariasis are often accompanied by severe itching. Infestation of the gastrointestinal tract can present with symptoms such as abdominal pain and diarrhea. Pulmonary acariasis can cause respiratory symptoms such as a runny nose, coughing, sneezing, and wheezing. Acariasis of the urinary tract can result in symptoms of urinary frequency, urinary urgency, and hematuria.

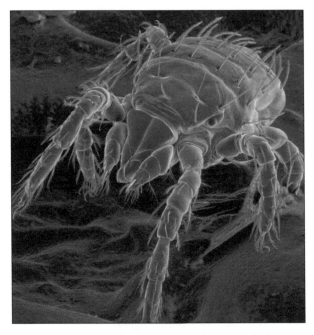

A micrograph of the chigger mite Trombicula, *which causes acariasis.*

SCREENING AND DIAGNOSIS

The diagnosis of acariasis differs depending on the organ affected. Cutaneous acariasis is diagnosed by the presence of mites and mite eggs in microscopic analysis of skin scrapings. Gastrointestinal acariasis is diagnosed by detection of mites in stools. Pulmonary acariasis is diagnosed by isolating and identifying mites using physical or chemical methods of sputum liquefaction. The presence of mites in microscopic analysis of the urine is helpful in the diagnosis of acariasis of the urinary tract. In addition, blood examination for eosinophils and specific antibodies, and radiographic studies of the affected organs, may be useful in diagnosing acariasis.

TREATMENT AND THERAPY

A number of effective topical, oral, and systemic therapies, and avoidance and containment strategies, are available for the treatment of acariasis. The specific treatment plan depends on the type of acariasis being treated. For example, treatment of allergic rhinitis and asthma symptoms in people who are allergic to dust mites includes reducing exposure; taking medications such as antihistamines, decongestants, and topical nasal steroids; and getting allergy shots.

PREVENTION AND OUTCOMES

Acariasis can be prevented by addressing the risk factors. Preventive measures include reducing overcrowding, improving hygiene, promptly and adequately treating the illness to stop further disease spread, and promoting public awareness of the disease.

Diep Koly, M.D.

FURTHER READING

Diaz, J. H. "Endemic Mite-Transmitted Dermatoses and Infectious Diseases in the South." *Journal of the Louisiana State Medical Society* 162 (2010): 140-145, 147-149.

Goddard, Jerome. *Physician's Guide to Arthropods of Medical Importance.* 4th ed. Boca Raton, Fla.: CRC Press, 2002.

Service, M. W., ed. *Encyclopedia of Arthropod-Transmitted Infections.* New York: CABI, 2001.

Shakespeare, Martin. *Zoonoses.* 2d ed. London: Pharmaceutical Press, 2009.

WEB SITES OF INTEREST

Centers for Disease Control and Prevention, Division of Vector Borne Infectious Diseases
http://www.cdc.gov//ncidod/dvbid

Microbiology and Immunology On-line: Parasitology
http://pathmicro.med.sc.edu/book/parasit-sta.htm

National Center for Emerging and Zoonotic Infectious Diseases
http://www.cdc.gov/ncezid

See also: Arthropod-borne illness and disease; Body lice; Crab lice; Fleas and infectious disease; Flies and infectious disease; Head lice; Insect-borne illness and disease; Mites and chiggers and infectious disease; Mosquitoes and infectious disease; Parasitic diseases; Scabies; Ticks and infectious disease; Vectors and vector control.

Acid-fastness

CATEGORY: Diagnosis

DEFINITION

Acid-fastness is a physical property attributed to a type of bacterium with an unusually high concentration of lipids in its cell walls, which allows the bacterium to resist acid decolorization during diagnostic staining.

Acid-fast bacilli. Bacteria are referred to as acid-fast bacilli (AFB). The most clinically relevant AFB are mycobacteria, especially *Mycobacterium tuberculosis* (the causative agent of tuberculosis) and *M. leprae* (the causative agent of leprosy). Mycobacteria are not the only group with this unique characteristic. Other acid-fast organisms include members of the genus *Nocardia* and parasites of the genus *Cryptosporidium.* Other species may be partially acid-fast depending on their cell-wall lipid content.

AFB stain principle. Acid-fast staining is a differential staining method used to differentiate AFB from non-AFB. Acid-fastness is a characteristic that differs from most bacterial species. Acid-fast bacilli, such as mycobacteria, possess cell walls that contain mycolic acids, a type of long-chain fatty acid. Attachment of these fatty acids to the bacterial cell wall (also known as the peptidoglycan or murein layer) results in a hydrophobic cell surface. This cell-wall structure makes the AFB difficult to characterize using standard Gram-staining techniques. Acid-fast stains strongly adhere to this lipid composition and are especially important in the detection of *M. tuberculosis* for the presumptive diagnosis of tuberculosis.

AFB stain techniques. The acid-fast staining techniques employed for the rapid detection and visualization of acid-fast bacilli includes fluorochrome staining, the Ziehl-Neelsen method, and the Kinyoun method. The fluorochrome staining procedure uses an auramine-rhodamine dye followed by specimen examination under a microscope. The Ziehl-Neelsen or hot method uses carbolfuchsin as the primary dye and heat to enhance penetration. The Kinyoun or cold method uses higher concentrations of fuchsin and phenol without heat. Staining is followed by a wash with an acid-alcohol decolorizing agent. Most bacteria are decolorized and are labeled as non-acid-fast while acid-fast bacilli retain the original stain color.

Although the identification of acid-fast bacilli are

indicative of tuberculosis, other organisms can cause a false positive. For a definitive diagnosis, an acid-fast culture analysis is performed. This process includes the cultivation, isolation, identification, and drug susceptibility testing of the bacilli under investigation.

IMPACT

Globally, tuberculosis is a leading public health issue. It is one of the world's deadliest infectious diseases, affecting one-third of the human population. The prompt detection of tuberculosis-causing mycobacteria is essential for successful treatment and management of the disease. Because acid-fastness is a distinctive feature of mycobacteria, it is crucial in the detection of tuberculosis.

Rose Ciulla-Bohling, Ph.D.

FURTHER READING

Ferri, Fred F. *Ferri's Differential Diagnosis: A Practical Guide to the Differential Diagnosis of Symptoms, Signs, and Clinical Disorders.* Philadelphia: Mosby/Elsevier, 2006.

Forbes, Betty A., Daniel F. Sahm, and Alice S. Weissfeld. *Bailey and Scott's Diagnostic Microbiology.* 12th ed. St. Louis, Mo.: Mosby/Elsevier, 2007.

Pagana, Kathleen Deska, and Timothy J. Pagana. *Mosby's Manual of Diagnostic and Laboratory Tests.* 3d ed. St. Louis, Mo.: Mosby/Elsevier, 2006.

Phillips, Pamela A. "Acid-Fast Culture." In *The Gale Encyclopedia of Nursing and Allied Health*, edited by Jacqueline L. Longe. 2d ed. Vol. 1. Detroit: Gale, 2006.

Sackheim, George I., and Dennis D. Lehman. *Chemistry for the Health Sciences.* Upper Saddle River, N.J.: Pearson/Prentice Hall, 2009.

Voet, Donald, and Judith G. Voet. *Biochemistry.* 3d ed. Hoboken, N.J.: John Wiley & Sons, 2004.

WEB SITES OF INTEREST

Centers for Disease Control and Prevention
http://www.cdc.gov

National Institutes of Health
http://www.nih.gov

Todar's Online Textbook of Bacteriology
http://www.textbookofbacteriology.net

See also: Bacteria: Classification and types; Biochemical tests; Cryptosporidiosis; Diagnosis of bacterial infections; Gram staining; Immunoassay; Microbiology; Microscopy; *Mycobacterium*; Pulsed-field gel electrophoresis; Serology.

Acne

CATEGORY: Diseases and conditions
ANATOMY OR SYSTEM AFFECTED: Skin
ALSO KNOWN AS: Acne vulgaris, blackheads, pimples, whiteheads

DEFINITION

Acne is a skin condition that occurs when the pores of the skin become clogged, inflamed, and sometimes infected. These clogged pores can lead to the formation of blackheads, whiteheads, or pimples. Acne is more prevalent in teenagers but also occurs in adults.

CAUSES

The main causes of acne include changes in levels of male hormones called androgens, increased sebum production, changes inside the hair follicle, and bacteria. Acne starts in the skin's sebaceous glands. These glands secrete an oily substance called sebum. The sebum normally travels through a tiny hair follicle from the gland to the skin's surface. Sometimes the sebum becomes trapped, mixing with dead skin cells and bacteria. This causes clogged pores called comedones.

Blackheads are comedones that reach the skin's surface. Whiteheads are comedones that stay beneath the surface of the skin. Small red bumps, pimples, and cysts may also develop.

RISK FACTORS

Risk factors for acne include an age range of twelve to twenty-four years; Caucasian; changes in hormone levels, such as during puberty and pregnancy and before a menstrual period; stress; certain medicines (for example, androgens, lithium, and barbiturates); and certain cosmetic products.

SYMPTOMS

Acne symptoms vary from person to person and can range from mild to severe. They include excess oil in the skin, blackheads, whiteheads, papules (small pink bumps that may be tender to the touch), pimples (inflamed, pus-filled bumps that may be red at

U.S. Government Registry for Women Using Accutane

On March 1, 2006, the U.S. Food and Drug Administration (FDA) started iPledge, a mandatory registry designed to control use of the powerful acne medicine isotretinoin, sold under the brand name Accutane and also under the trade names Amnestreem, Claravis, and Sotret. The registry had been recommended by FDA advisory committees in 2000 and 2004 to help prevent birth defects and disorders in children born to women using isotretinoin and to collect information on the incidence of suicide among users.

The manufacturer of Accutane, Roche Pharmaceuticals, had always strongly warned women of the dangers posed to developing fetuses by the use of Accutane during pregnancy. Even so, Roche reported that between 1982, when the FDA first approved the sale of isotretinoin, and 2000 there had been 383 live births among women taking the drug; 162 of the infants (42 percent) were born with brain or heart defects or mental retardation.

Women who plan to become pregnant and who seek a prescription for isotretinoin must register with iPledge and must submit two negative pregnancy tests before receiving a prescription; they also must be tested before each monthly refill, and they must agree to take two forms of birth control while using the drug–or else promise to abstain from sex for one month before treatment, while under treatment, and for one month afterward. Women have to sign a document acknowledging that they understand isotretinoin increases the risk of birth defects, depression, and suicide. Men desiring the drug are required to sign the document as well, to ensure that they know why they should not share pills with women. Physicians prescribing isotretinoin and wholesalers and pharmacists who distribute it are also required to register with iPledge and to agree to enforce the restrictions.

Many dermatologists and other doctors are uncomfortable with the iPledge regulations. Although aware of the drug's dangers, they consider isotretinoin indispensable in treating severe cases of acne that are resistant to less powerful medications, and they fear that onerous conditions for access to the drug might discourage persons from obtaining the medication they really need.

Milton Berman, Ph.D.

the base; also called pustules), nodules (large, painful, solid lumps that are lodged deep within the skin), and cysts (deep, inflamed, pus-filled lumps that can cause pain and scarring).

SCREENING AND DIAGNOSIS

A health care provider will examine areas of skin with the most sebaceous glands, such as the face, neck, back, chest, and shoulders. If the acne is severe, the patient may be referred to a dermatologist, or skin specialist.

TREATMENT AND THERAPY

Acne may require a combination of treatments, but most acne does not require surgery. Some treatments may take several weeks to work, and the skin may actually appear to get worse before it gets better.

Over-the-counter topical medicines (for example, cleansers, creams, lotions, and gels) reduce the amount of oil or bacteria, or both, in the pores. These medicines may contain benzoyl peroxide, salicylic acid, sulfur, and resorcinol.

Prescription topical medicine includes cleansers, creams, lotions, and gels to reduce the amount of oil or bacteria, or both, in the pores. These prescription medicines include antibiotics such as clindamycin (Cleocin T), erythromycin, tretinoin (Retin-A, Avita), adapalene (Differin), azelaic acid (Azelex), tazarotene (Tazorac), and dapsone (Aczone). Oral antibiotics, aimed at controlling the amount of bacteria in pores, include doxycycline, minocycline, tetracycline, erythromycin, clindamycin, amoxicillin, cephalosporins, sulfamethoxazole, and trimethoprim.

Oral medicines, aimed at controlling androgen levels, include birth control pills (pills that have a combination of hormones, such as estrogen and progestin, may be the most effective in improving acne); spironolactone; oral retinoids, aimed at reducing the size and secretions of sebaceous glands and used only for severe cases of cystic acne; and isotretinoin (Accutane), which must not be taken by women who are pregnant or who may become pregnant because of the risks of serious birth disorders.

There are a number of procedures to treat acne. These procedures, some of which have risks, such as scarring and infection, include the injection of corticosteroid directly into the cyst (mostly used for large, cystic acne lesions); acne surgery, in which specialized extractors are used to open, drain, and remove contents of acne lesions; and acne scar revision to minimize acne scars, which includes chemical peels (consisting of glycolic acid and other chemical agents to loosen blackheads and decrease acne papules) and dermabrasion (which smooths the skin by "sandpapering" it). Other procedures to treat acne include scar excision (a tiny punch tool or a scalpel is used to remove scars), collagen fillers (the pits of scars are filled with a collagen substance), laser resurfacing (scars are removed and underlying skin is tightened), and phototherapy (skin is exposed to an ultraviolet light source for a set time).

PREVENTION AND OUTCOMES

It can be difficult to prevent acne. This is because it can be difficult to control the factors that cause it. However, there are some things one can do to keep acne from getting worse, such as gently washing one's face with mild soap and warm water twice a day (no more than twice) to remove excess oil. Scrubbing or washing too often can make acne worse. When washing one's face, one should use his or her hands rather than a washcloth, use mild soap, and allow the face to dry before applying any lotion. One should not pick at or squeeze blemishes. Also, one should use lotions, soaps, and cosmetics labeled noncomedogenic, which keeps these products from clogging pores. Topical acne treatments should be used only as directed; using them more often could worsen the condition. One should wear sunscreen year-round. This is especially important when using medicine that can make skin more sensitive to the sun. Also helpful is recognizing and limiting emotional stress.

Jennifer Hellwig, M.S., RD;
reviewed by Ross Zeltser, M.D., FAAD

FURTHER READING

Arowojolu, A., et al. "Combined Oral Contraceptive Pills for Treatment of Acne." *Cochrane Database of Systematic Reviews* (2009): CD004425. Available through *EBSCO DynaMed Systematic Literature Surveillance* at http://www.ebscohost.com/dynamed.

EBSCO Publishing. *Health Library: Phototherapy.* Available through http://www.ebscohost.com.

National Institute of Arthritis and Musculoskeletal and Skin Diseases. "Questions and Answers About Acne." Available at http://www.niams.nih.gov/health_info/acne.

WEB SITE OF INTEREST

American Academy of Dermatology
http://www.aad.org

See also: Abscesses; Boils; Chickenpox; Children and infectious disease; Impetigo; Infection; Pilonidal cyst; Pityriasis rosea; Rubella; Scabies; Skin infections.

Acquired immunodeficiency syndrome. *See* AIDS

Actinomycosis

CATEGORY: Diseases and conditions
ANATOMY OR SYSTEM AFFECTED: Abdomen, gastrointestinal system, jaw, lungs, mouth, respiratory system

DEFINITION

Actinomycosis is a treatable bacterial infection that results in abscesses (collections of pus) in the abdominal cavity, jaw (cervicofacial), lungs (thoracic), or throughout the body (generalized actinomycosis).

CAUSES

Actinomycosis is most often caused by infection by the bacterium *Actinomyces israelii*, which is present in the gums, teeth, and tonsils.

RISK FACTORS

The risk factors that increase the chance of developing actinomycosis include dental disease, trauma, and aspiration (that is, when liquids or solids are sucked into the lungs).

SYMPTOMS

The symptoms of actinomycosis include pain; fever; vomiting; diarrhea; constipation; weight loss; sputum-producing cough; drainage of pus through the skin; and small, flat, hard, and sometimes painful swellings around the mouth, neck, or jaw, which may or may not discharge pus.

SCREENING AND DIAGNOSIS

Screening for actinomycosis includes a full medical history, questions about symptoms, and a physical exam. Tests may include analyses of pus, sputum, or tissue, and could include X rays.

TREATMENT AND THERAPY

Treatment options include medications (high doses of antibiotics) and the drainage of abscesses.

PREVENTION AND OUTCOMES

The best way to reduce the chance of developing actinomycosis is to prevent dental disease by practicing good dental hygiene and by regularly visiting a dentist for cleaning and an examination.

Krisha McCoy, M.S.;
reviewed by David L. Horn, M.D., FACP

FURTHER READING

EBSCO Publishing. *DynaMed: Actinomycosis.* Available through http://www.ebscohost.com/dynamed.

Gorbach, Sherwood L., John G. Bartlett, and Neil R. Blacklow, eds. *Infectious Diseases.* 3d ed. Philadelphia: W. B. Saunders, 2004.

Langlais, Robert P., and Craig S. Miller. *Color Atlas of Common Oral Diseases.* 4th ed. Philadelphia: Lippincott Williams & Wilkins, 2009.

The Merck Manuals, Online Medical Library. "Actinomycosis." Available at http://www.merck.com/mmhe.

Sutton, Amy L., ed. *Dental Care and Oral Health Sourcebook.* 3d ed. Detroit: Omnigraphics, 2008.

WEB SITES OF INTEREST

American Dental Association
http://www.ada.org

Canadian Dental Association
http://www.cda-adc.ca

National Institutes of Health
http://www.nih.gov

See also: Abscesses; Bacterial infections; Intestinal and stomach infections; Mouth infections; Tooth abscess.

Acute cerebellar ataxia

CATEGORY: Diseases and conditions
ANATOMY OR SYSTEM AFFECTED: Brain, muscles, nervous system
ALSO KNOWN AS: Cerebellitis

DEFINITION

Acute cerebellar ataxia is a disorder of the nervous system marked by the sudden onset of a disturbance in muscle coordination, especially in the trunk, arms, and legs. The cerebellum, the part of the brain that controls balance and coordination, does not function properly in the case of cerebellar ataxia. Although the abnormality of the limbs is most often noticed, the disorder also can cause abnormal eye movements. Nausea and vomiting may also occur as part of the disorder.

While it can occur at any age, acute cerebellar ataxia is most common in young children. It can occur several weeks after a viral infection, such as chickenpox. Most cases disappear without treatment in a matter of months. However, recurrent or chronic progressive cerebellar ataxia does occur.

CAUSES

Causes of acute cerebellar ataxia include viral infections such as chickenpox, coxsackie disease, Epstein-Barr virus, *Mycoplasma* pneumonia, human immunodeficiency virus (HIV), and Lyme disease; exposure to insecticides called organophosphates and exposure to certain toxins, such as lead, mercury, thallium, and alcohol; cerebellar hemorrhage; abscess; blood clot; and obstruction of an artery. Causes of recurrent or chronic acute ataxia include stroke malformation of the cerebellum, multiple sclerosis, migraine or vertigo, genetic or metabolic disorders, brain tumor, alcoholism, and seizures.

RISK FACTORS

Several factors increase the chance of developing acute cerebellar ataxia. These factors include viral infections, recent vaccination, and exposure to certain insecticides, drugs, or toxins. Children three years of age or younger are especially at higher risk.

SYMPTOMS

Symptoms of acute cerebellar ataxia include uncoordinated movements of the limbs or trunk; clumsiness with daily activities; difficulty walking (unsteadiness); speech disturbances, including slurred speech and changes in tone, pitch, and volume; visual complaints; and abnormal eye movements. Accompanying symptoms may include headache, dizziness, changes in mental state (such as personality or behavioral changes), chaotic eye movement, and clumsy speech pattern.

SCREENING AND DIAGNOSIS

A doctor will observe limb coordination to assess the degree and nature of the ataxia. Further tests may include examination of cerebrospinal fluid, a magnetic resonance imaging (MRI) scan (a scan that uses radio waves and a powerful magnet to produce detailed computer images), a computed tomography (CT) scan (a detailed X-ray picture that identifies abnormalities of fine tissue structure), metabolic blood tests, ultrasound (a test that uses sound waves to examine the head), and urine analysis.

Tests to detect other possible diseases that are causing the symptoms include a nerve conduction study (measures the speed and degree of electrical activity in a nerve to determine if it is functioning normally) and electromyography (EMG; measures and records the electrical activity that muscles generate at rest and in response to muscle contraction).

TREATMENT AND THERAPY

There is no treatment for acute cerebellar ataxia. Ataxia usually disappears within a few months without treatment. For cases in which an underlying cause is identified, a health care provider will treat that cause. In extremely rare cases, the patient may have continuing and disabling symptoms. Treatment includes corticosteroids, intravenous immunoglobulin, and plasma exchange therapy. Drug treatment to improve muscle coordination has a low success rate. However, the following drugs may be prescribed: clonazepam (such as Klonopin), amantadine (such as Symmetrel), gabapentin (such as Neurontin), and buspirone (such as BuSpar). Occupational or physical therapy might also alleviate a lack of coordination, as might diet changes and nutritional supplements.

PREVENTION AND OUTCOMES

Acute cerebellar ataxia cannot be prevented. However, children can receive vaccines against the viral infections that increase the risk of getting acute cerebellar ataxia.

Amanda Barrett, M.A.;
reviewed by J. Thomas Megerian, M.D., Ph.D., FAAP

FURTHER READING

Berman, P. "Ataxia in Children." *International Pediatrics* 14 (1999): 44-47.

Bradley, Walter G., et al., eds. *Neurology in Clinical Practice.* 5th ed. Philadelphia: Butterworth Heinemann/ Elsevier, 2007.

MedLink. "Acute Cerebellar Ataxia in Children." Available at http://www.medlink.com.

The Merck Manuals, Online Medical Library. "Cerebellar Disorders." Available at http://www.merck.com/mmhe.

National Institute of Neurological Disorders and Stroke. "Encephalopathy." Available at http://www.ninds.nih.gov.

Ropper, A. H., and R. H. Brown. *Adams and Victor's Principles of Neurology.* 8th ed. New York: McGraw-Hill Medical, 2005.

Stumpf, D. A. "Acute Ataxia." *Pediatrics in Review* 8 (1987): 303-306.

WEB SITES OF INTEREST

National Ataxia Foundation
http://www.ataxia.org

National Institute of Neurological Disorders and Stroke
http://www.ninds.nih.gov

See also: Bell's palsy; Chickenpox; Children and infectious disease; Epstein-Barr virus infection; Guillain-Barré syndrome; HIV; Progressive multifocal leukoencephalopathy; Viral infections.

Acute cystitis

CATEGORY: Diseases and conditions
ANATOMY OR SYSTEM AFFECTED: Bladder, urinary system
ALSO KNOWN AS: Bladder infection

DEFINITION

The urinary tract normally contains no microorganisms. However, sometimes bacteria or yeast from the lower gastrointestinal tract or rectal area enter the urinary tract, usually through the urethra (the tube that allows urine to pass from the bladder). If bacteria or yeast cling to the urethra, they can multiply and infect the urethra. They then travel up and infect the bladder with a condition called acute cystitis.

CAUSES

Most cases of cystitis are caused by bacteria from the rectal area. In women, the rectum and urethra are fairly close to each other. This makes it relatively easy for bacteria to make their way into the urethra. Some women develop cystitis after a period of frequent sexual intercourse. This happens because bacteria enter the urethra during sex and cause infection.

RISK FACTORS

Risk factors for acute cystitis include being sexually active; using a diaphragm for birth control; condom use (this may also increase infection rates in women, especially when Nonoxynol-9-coated condoms are used); menopause; abnormalities of the urinary system, including vesicoureteral reflux or polycystic kidneys; paraplegia and other neurologic conditions; sickle-cell disease; history of kidney transplant; diabetes type 1 and type 2; kidney stones; enlarged prostate; weak immune system; bladder catheter in place or recent instrumentation of the urinary system; tight underwear and clothing; and chemicals in soaps, douches, and lubricants. Women are at higher risk for acute cystitis.

SYMPTOMS

The symptoms of cystitis, which vary from person to person and can range from mild to severe, include frequent and urgent need to urinate; passing only small amounts of urine; pain in the abdomen or pelvic area, or in the low back; burning sensation during urination; leaking urine; increased need to get up at night to urinate; cloudy, bad-smelling urine; blood in the urine; low-grade fever; and fatigue.

SCREENING AND DIAGNOSIS

A health care provider will ask about symptoms and medical history, perform a physical exam, and test the urine for blood, pus, and bacteria. If bacteria are present in the urine, it is likely that cystitis will be diagnosed. Children and men who develop cystitis may require additional testing. In these cases, a cystoscope is used to check for structural abnormalities of the urinary system that predispose a person to infection.

TREATMENT AND THERAPY

Bacterial cystitis is treated with antibiotic drugs. Antibiotics (usually trimethoprim/sulfamethoxazole, nitrofurantoin, or fluoroquinolones) will be prescribed for at least two to three days and perhaps for as long as several weeks. The length of the treatment depends on the severity of the infection and the patient's personal history. Symptoms should subside in about one or two days. To ensure that the infection has disappeared, the health care provider will again test the patient's urine.

Recurrent infections might be treated with stronger antibiotics or over more time. Low-dose antibiotics, which are prescribed as a preventive measure, might be prescribed either for daily use or for use after sexual intercourse. Patients with recurrent infections could be referred to a specialist.

Phenazopyridine (Pyridium) is a medicine that decreases pain and bladder spasms. Taking phenazopyridine will turn urine and sometimes sweat an orange color. This medication is generally available without a prescription and can relieve symptoms effectively while the patient waits for medical treatment to work.

PREVENTION AND OUTCOMES

The chance of having cystitis can be lessened by preventing bacteria from entering the urinary tract. Of the following logical and commonly recommended steps, only the use of cranberry juice has been clearly shown to be of value in reducing infection risk. One should drink large amounts of liquids; urinate when having the urge; empty the bladder and then drink a full glass of water after having sexual intercourse; wash the genital area daily; wipe from front to back (for women) after having a bowel movement; avoid using douches and feminine hygiene sprays; drink cranberry juice (which may help prevent and relieve cystitis); and avoid wearing tight underwear or clothing.

The foregoing prevention recommendations apply largely to healthy young women at risk for bladder infections. Those with some of the unusual risk factors, or women for whom the foregoing suggestions do not reduce recurrence, might find that other medically recommended prevention techniques help.

Julie Riley, M.S., R.D.;
reviewed by Adrienne Carmack, M.D.

FURTHER READING

Kahn, B. S., et al. "Management of Patients with Interstitial Cystitis or Chronic Pelvic Pain of Bladder Origin: A Consensus Report." *Current Medical Research and Opinion* 21, no. 4 (2005): 509-516.

Katchman, E. A., et al. "Three-Day Versus Longer Duration of Antibiotic Treatment for Cystitis in Women: Systematic Review and Meta-Analysis." *American Journal of Medicine* 118, no. 11 (2005): 1196-1207.

Parsons, M., and P. Toozs-Hobson. "The Investigation and Management of Interstitial Cystitis." *Journal of the British Menopause Society* 11, no. 4 (2005): 132-139.

Phatak, S., and H. E. Foster, Jr. "The Management of Interstitial Cystitis: An Update." *Nature: Clinical Practice in Urology* 3 (2006): 45-53.

Schrier, Robert W., ed. *Diseases of the Kidney and Urinary Tract.* 8th ed. Philadelphia: Wolters Kluwer Health/Lippincott Williams & Wilkins, 2007.

WEB SITES OF INTEREST

Kidney Foundation of Canada
http://www.kidney.ab.ca

National Institute of Diabetes and Digestive and Kidney Diseases
http://www.niddk.nih.gov

National Kidney Foundation
http://www.kidney.org

UrologyHealth.org
http://www.urologyhealth.org

See also: Bacterial infections; *Enterococcus*; Kidney infection; Pelvic inflammatory disease; Prostatitis; Sexually transmitted diseases (STDs); Urethritis; Urinary tract infections; Women and infectious disease.

Acute interstitial nephritis

CATEGORY: Diseases and conditions
ANATOMY OR SYSTEM AFFECTED: Kidneys, urinary system

DEFINITION

Acute interstitial nephritis is a kidney disorder in which the kidneys cannot properly filter waste materials and fluid. This is a potentially serious condition that requires medical attention.

CAUSES

Acute interstitial nephritis can be caused by infections such as *Streptococcus* infection, herpes, mumps, hepatitis C, syphilis, and human immunodeficiency virus (HIV). It can also be caused by particular medications, including certain antibiotics, antiulcer drugs, nonsteroidal anti-inflammatory drugs, certain diuretics, and conditions that affect the immune system (such as lupus).

RISK FACTORS

The risk factors that increase the chance of developing acute interstitial nephritis include drug and medication use in adults and infection in children.

SYMPTOMS

Symptoms of acute interstitial nephritis include a decrease in urine output, blood in urine, nausea, vomiting, loss of appetite, weakness, aching joints, fever, and rash.

SCREENING AND DIAGNOSIS

Screening for acute interstitial nephritis may include blood tests for levels of BUN (blood urea nitrogen), creatinine, electrolytes, phosphorus, uric acid, and calcium; urine tests; a kidney ultrasound; and, in severe cases, a kidney biopsy.

TREATMENT AND THERAPY

If medications are the cause of the interstitial nephritis, a doctor may cease the patient's medications or prescribe different ones. Antibiotics are used to treat an infection, and drugs such as corticosteroid or cyclophosphamide medications may also be used to help treat interstitial nephritis. A kidney biopsy is often done to confirm the diagnosis before starting corticosteroid or cyclophosphamide. Some people with interstitial nephritis need dialysis, in which a machine does the work of the kidneys to purge waste.

PREVENTION AND OUTCOMES

To help reduce the chance of developing acute interstitial nephritis, a doctor may suggest avoiding certain medications, such as penicillin or nonsteroidal anti-inflammatories.

Krisha McCoy, M.S.;
reviewed by Adrienne Carmack, M.D.

FURTHER READING

Kodner, C. M., and A. Kudrimoti. "Diagnosis and Management of Acute Interstitial Nephritis." Available at http://www.aafp.org/afp/20030615/2527.html.

Plakoglannis, R., and A. Nogid. "Acute Interstitial Nephritis Associated with Coadministration of Vancomycin and Ceftriaxone: Case Series and Review of the Literature." *Pharmacotherapy* 27 (2007): 1456-1461.

Schrier, Robert W., ed. *Diseases of the Kidney and Urinary Tract.* 8th ed. Philadelphia: Wolters Kluwer Health/Lippincott Williams & Wilkins, 2007.

Sierra, F., et al. "Systematic Review: Proton Pump Inhibitor-Associated Acute Interstitial Nephritis." *Alimentary Pharmacology and Therapeutics* 26 (2007): 545-553.

WEB SITES OF INTEREST

American Academy of Family Physicians
http://familydoctor.org

Kidney Foundation of Canada
http://www.kidney.ab.ca

National Kidney Foundation
http://www.kidney.org

National Kidney and Urologic Diseases Information Clearinghouse
http://kidney.niddk.nih.gov

See also: Acute cystitis; Hepatitis C; Herpesvirus infections; HIV; Kidney infection; Mumps; *Streptococcus*; Viral infections.

Acute necrotizing ulcerative gingivitis

CATEGORY: Diseases and conditions
ANATOMY OR SYSTEM AFFECTED: Gums, mouth, tissue
ALSO KNOWN AS: Trench mouth, Vincent's angina, Vincent's stomatitis

DEFINITION

Acute necrotizing ulcerative gingivitis (ANUG) is a serious infection of the gums that causes ulcers, swelling, and dead tissues in the mouth. Although a painful condition, it can be healed with treatment.

CAUSES

Acute necrotizing ulcerative gingivitis is typically caused by excess bacteria in the mouth. Too much bacteria can form in the mouth from smoking, stress, a lack of dental care, a virus, and a poor diet.

RISK FACTORS

Risk factors for ANUG include lack of dental care and overall poor dental hygiene; a poor diet; vitamin deficiencies; infections in the throat, teeth, or mouth; a compromised immune system; smoking; stress; and age thirty-five years or younger.

SYMPTOMS

Symptoms of ANUG include pain in the gums, gums that bleed easily, bad taste in the mouth, extremely bad breath, red and swollen gums, gray residue on the gums, large ulcers or loss of gum tissue between teeth, fever, and swollen lymph nodes.

SCREENING AND DIAGNOSIS

The dental examination will include a search for inflammation of the gums, destroyed gum tissue, and crater-like ulcers in the gums that may harbor plaque and debris from food. The exam might also include dental and facial X rays.

TREATMENT AND THERAPY

Treatment options for ANUG include antibiotics to clear up the infection, dental surgery, an improved diet and diet changes, and regular dental cleanings.

PREVENTION AND OUTCOMES

To help reduce the chance of getting ANUG, one should maintain a balanced, nutritional diet and should take proper care of teeth and gums, which includes regular dentist visits.

Diana Kohnle;
reviewed by Laura Morris-Olson, D.M.D.

FURTHER READING

Contreras, A., et al. "Human Herpesviridae in Acute Necrotizing Ulcerative Gingivitis in Children in Nigeria." *Oral Microbiology and Immunology* 12 (1997): 259-265.

Langlais, Robert P., and Craig S. Miller. *Color Atlas of*

Common Oral Diseases. 4th ed. Philadelphia: Lippincott Williams & Wilkins, 2009.

The Merck Manuals, Online Medical Library. "Actinomycosis." Available at http://www.merck.com/
mmhe.

Schreiner C., and F. B. Quinn. "Stomatitis." University
of Texas, Medical Branch. Available at http://www.
utmb.edu/otoref/grnds/stomatitis.htm.

Sutton, Amy L., ed. *Dental Care and Oral Health Sourcebook.* 3d ed. Detroit: Omnigraphics, 2008.

WEB SITES OF INTEREST

American Academy of Periodontology
http://www.perio.org

American Dental Association
http://www.ada.org

Canadian Dental Association
http://www.cda-adc.ca

See also: Abscesses; Bacterial infections; Gangrene;
Gingivitis; Mouth infections; Tooth abscess; Vincent's
angina; Viral infections.

Adenoviridae

CATEGORY: Pathogen
TRANSMISSION ROUTE: Direct contact

DEFINITION

Adenoviridae is a family of adenoviruses that cause
various diseases and asymptomatic infections in vertebrate animals, including humans.

NATURAL HABITAT AND FEATURES

Adenoviruses are thought to be distributed worldwide. Different types of adenovirus have different
prevalence rates and geographic distributions that
vary with time. Adenoviruses infect all classes of vertebrate animals examined, are found in some
amebas, and remain infectious for weeks on common
surfaces.

An adenovirus virion is a symmetrical nonenveloped particle having a diameter of 80 to 110 nanometers (nm). It comprises an external capsid (protein
shell), a core, and some of the enzymes needed for

Taxonomic Classification for Adenoviridae

Order: Unassigned
Family: Adenoviridae
Genera: *Atadenovirus, Aviadenovirus, Ichtadenovirus,
   Mastadenovirus, Siadenovirus*
Species: *M. human adenoviruses B, C, E,* and *F*

---

viral replication. The virion capsid has twenty sides
made of hexon capsomeres, and has twelve vertices
made of penton capsomeres that join the sides and
are joined to one or two fibers having a terminal knob.
Particular fiber lengths of 9 to 77.5 nm are characteristic of the different types of adenovirus. The virion
core contains one linear double-stranded molecule of
genomic deoxyribonucleic acid (DNA), containing
from 33,000 to 45,000 nucleotide base pairs, associated with proteins. This DNA itself is infectious. The
ends of the DNA molecule contain repeated sequences
of nucleotide base pairs. The five-prime end of each
DNA strand is attached to one molecule of terminal
protein that primes DNA replication.

Different types of adenovirus within each species
share an overall pattern of traits, such as calculated
degree of evolutionary relatedness, DNA structure,
kinds of animals they infect, kinds of diseases they
cause, growth characteristics, ability to cause erythrocytes to clump, and ability of fiber and hexon to bind
to particular antibodies. The ability of fiber and
hexon to bind to particular antibodies also defines
the different types of adenovirus within each species.
Molecular diagnostic methods such as polymerase
chain reaction (PCR), restriction analysis, and DNA
sequencing can be used to rapidly identify the species
or type of an adenovirus.

PATHOGENICITY AND CLINICAL SIGNIFICANCE

At least fifty-two different types of human adenovirus cause different diseases, in part because their
type-specific fibers and penton capsomeres specify the
infection of different cell types. Human adenoviruses
most frequently infect epithelial cells, specifically
those of the respiratory or gastrointestinal tracts, of
lymphatic tissue, of the kidney or bladder, or of the
eye conjunctiva. Infection can be lytic, whereby disease symptoms result from the destruction of the host

cell, caused by the production and release of newly formed viruses; or infection can be asymptomatic, whereby those symptoms and processes can be delayed or greatly diminished for years. People without symptoms may shed infectious virus for years after infection. More than one type of adenovirus can co-infect a cell, facilitating genetic recombination that creates new types of adenovirus.

Nearly all adults have been infected by adenoviruses at some time in their lives and have serum antibodies to several types of adenovirus. Immunocompromised persons (such as those receiving tissue or organ transplants or those with acquired immunodeficiency syndrome), babies and young children, and military recruits are at greatest risk for severe, and sometimes fatal, disease. Crowded conditions (such as in day-care centers, hospitals, military housing, shipyards, and summer camps) increase the risk of infection.

Reported clinical illnesses caused by, or associated with, adenovirus infection include intussusception in babies; acute febrile pharyngitis, acute hemorrhagic cystitis, diarrhea, pertussis-like syndrome, and pneumonia in babies and young children; adenopharyngoconjunctival fever in school-age children; acute respiratory disease with pneumonia in military recruits; epidemic keratoconjunctivitis in adults; severe disseminated disease in immunocompromised people; cardiomyopathy; encephalitis; follicular conjunctivitis; gastroenteritis; meningitis; obesity; and skin rash. The most prevalent human adenoviruses causing clinical illness are species B types 3 and 7; species C types 1, 2, and 5; species E type 4; and species F types 40 and 41.

DRUG SUSCEPTIBILITY

No drugs or therapies generally available to the public specifically prevent or treat human adenoviral infections. Because most adenovirus infections of previously healthy people are self-limited and mild, caregivers usually treat only the symptoms and provide supportive care.

The spread of adenovirus can be decreased through the use of masks and gloves by caregivers and by chlorination of water used for drinking and swimming. Routine washing of hands with soap and water does not prevent spread of the virus.

An enteric live oral vaccine directed against human adenovirus types 4 and 7, available only to the U.S.

military, has been used to effectively prevent respiratory disease among recruits. Development of adenovirus-specific T cell vaccines for immunocompromised people is also underway.

Severe infections, which can result in death, have been treated with general virus inhibitors such as ribavirin, cidofovir, ganciclovir, leukocyte transfusions, or intravenous immunoglobulin. The safety and efficacy of such treatments remains to be established.

David Caldwell, Ph.D.

FURTHER READING

Centers for Disease Control and Prevention. "Adenoviruses." Available at http://www.cdc.gov/ncidod/dvrd/revb/respiratory/eadfeat.htm.

Echavarria, Marcela. "Adenoviruses." In *Principles and Practice of Clinical Virology*, edited by Arie J. Zuckerman et al. 6th ed. Hoboken, N.J.: John Wiley & Sons, 2009.

Foy, H. M. "Adenoviruses." In *Viral Infections in Humans: Epidemiology and Control*, edited by A. Evans and R. Kaslow. 4th ed. New York: Plenum, 1997.

Gray, G. C. "Adenovirus Transmission—Worthy of Our Attention." *Journal of Infectious Diseases* 194 (July, 2006): 871-873.

Horwitz, M. S. "Adenoviruses." In *Fields' Virology*, edited by David M. Knipe and Peter M. Howley. Philadelphia: Wolters Kluwer Health/Lippincott Williams & Wilkins, 2007.

WEB SITES OF INTEREST

About Kids Health
http://www.aboutkidshealth.ca

Centers for Disease Control and Prevention
http://www.cdc.gov

See also: Adenovirus infections; Adenovirus vaccine; Contagious diseases; Infection; Mutation of pathogens; Pathogens; Viral infections; Viruses: Types.

Adenovirus infections

CATEGORY: Diseases and conditions

ANATOMY OR SYSTEM AFFECTED: Eyes, gastrointestinal system, intestines, lungs, respiratory system, urinary system

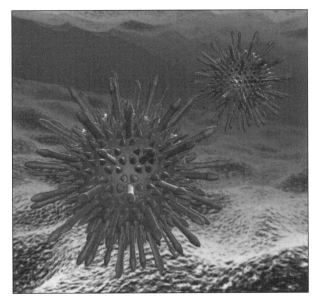

An illustration of an adenovirus. (©Dreamstime.com)

DEFINITION

Adenovirus infections are highly contagious infections caused by a virus. The infections can happen in the respiratory tract, the eyes, the intestines, and the urinary tract.

CAUSES

Adenoviruses, which often are the cause of the common cold, also cause a number of other types of infections. Adenoviruses can be spread through exposure to a sneeze or cough of an infected person, exposure to fecal contamination (for example, water supplies and poor hygiene), eating food contaminated by houseflies, person-to-person contact, handling an object that was exposed to an infected person, and swimming in contaminated lakes and pools.

RISK FACTORS

Children, especially young children, are at special risk of developing an adenovirus infection.

SYMPTOMS

Symptoms of adenovirus infection depend on where the infection occurs and may include fever, flulike symptoms, sore throat, runny nose, cough, swollen lymph nodes, middle-ear infection, lower respiratory problems, diarrhea, vomiting, headache, abdominal cramps, frequent urination, conjunctivitis, red eyes,

---

In the News: Adenovirus Mutation Responsible for Fatalities

In 2007, an adenovirus that caused fatal respiratory infection was identified at U.S. military bases in Texas, Washington State, Oregon, South Carolina, and New York, according to the Centers for Disease Control and Prevention (CDC). Although adenoviruses of various types have been causing numerous illnesses since being identified in the 1950's, they have typically not caused deaths so quickly. Most adenoviruses cause pneumonia, conjunctivitis, and gastrointestinal disease as a result of insufficient use of disinfectants. Only a small percentage of cases has required hospitalization, and deaths have been rare.

However, adenovirus serotype 14 (Ad14), one of the first adenovirus strains to be identified in 1955, has developed a mutation that causes it to be much more lethal. Seven of the thirty hospitalized persons died within days of the first symptoms. Infectious disease expert David N. Gilbert discovered this mutated Ad14. Samples from all five states were analyzed and found to have exactly the same sequence data of genes, and each had the same mutation, according to polymerase chain reaction and immunofluorescence studies.

According to Oregon health investigators, for example, Ad14 has increased dramatically from rarely occurring to causing more than 50 percent of all adenovirus infections in Oregon. This Ad14 can survive on surfaces for weeks, thus making it even more crucial for people to adhere to good handwashing habits and to seek medical treatment at the occurrence of escalating flulike symptoms to prevent the development of pneumonia.

Jeanne L. Kuhler, Ph.D.

---

keratoconjunctivitis (corneal inflammation), and burning, pain, or blood in the urine.

SCREENING AND DIAGNOSIS

Depending on the type of infection that is suspected, samples may be taken from the patient and then sent to a lab. The samples may be mucus, stool, blood, or urine.

TREATMENT AND THERAPY

Treatment options include the management of symptoms. The infection will usually end on its own.

Steps that might help relieve these symptoms include getting extra rest, drinking increased amounts of fluids, using a humidifier, and taking acetaminophen or other over-the-counter medications. For conjunctivitis, the doctor might recommend using warm compresses, or the doctor could recommend eye ointments or drops. For severe diarrhea or vomiting, fluids may need to be given by IV. This will prevent dehydration.

A compromised or weak immune system can lead to a more serious infection. In this case, a doctor may need to administer certain medicines.

PREVENTION AND OUTCOMES

The best way to prevent adenovirus infection is to avoid contact with infected persons; to practice good hygiene, including frequent handwashing and cleaning of surfaces (such as toys and counter tops); and to keep swimming pools adequately chlorinated, which will help prevent outbreaks of adenovirus infection associated with swimming pools.

Krisha McCoy, M.S.; reviewed by David L. Horn, M.D., FACP

FURTHER READING

Centers for Disease Control and Prevention. "Adenoviruses." Available at http://www.cdc.gov/ncidod/dvrd/revb/respiratory/eadfeat.htm.

Foy, H. M. "Adenoviruses." In *Viral Infections in Humans: Epidemiology and Control*, edited by A. Evans and R. Kaslow. 4th ed. New York: Plenum, 1997.

Gray, G. C. "Adenovirus Transmission—Worthy of Our Attention." *Journal of Infectious Diseases* 194 (July, 2006): 871-873.

Horwitz, M. S. "Adenoviruses." In *Fields' Virology*, edited by David M. Knipe and Peter M. Howley. Philadelphia: Wolters Kluwer Health/Lippincott Williams & Wilkins, 2007.

Nemours Foundation. "Infections: Adenovirus." Available at http://kidshealth.org/parent/infections/lung/adenovirus.html.

Pickering, Larry K., et al., eds. *Red Book: 2009 Report of the Committee on Infectious Diseases.* 28th ed. Elk Grove Village, Ill.: American Academy of Pediatrics, 2009.

WEB SITES OF INTEREST

About Kids Health
http://www.aboutkidshealth.ca

American Academy of Pediatrics
http://www.healthychildren.org

Centers for Disease Control and Prevention
http://www.cdc.gov

See also: Adenoviridae; Adenovirus vaccine; Bronchiolitis; Bronchitis; Children and infectious disease; Common cold; Conjunctivitis; Croup; Enteritis; Infection; Influenza; Norovirus infection; Pneumonia; Respiratory syncytial virus infections; Rotavirus infection; Travelers' diarrhea; Viral infections.

Adenovirus vaccine

CATEGORY: Prevention

DEFINITION

An adenovirus vaccine is a nonpathogenic form of an adenovirus or its antigens. The vaccine is given to animals, including humans, to stimulate the formation of a memory immune response to adenovirus infection.

B cell vaccine. Adenovirus B cell vaccines stimulate B cells to differentiate into long-lived plasma cells. Upon subsequent contact with adenovirus, these plasma cells secrete antibodies that specifically neutralize adenovirus.

From 1971 to 1996, the U.S. military routinely administered to recruits an enteric-coated live oral vaccine against human adenovirus types 4 and 7, which frequently cause acute respiratory disease and pneumonia in that population. The vaccine induced a strong immune response because it presented B cells with strong antigens in their natural shape. Infection of epithelial cells in the small intestine allowed viral replication but was asymptomatic. The vaccine was not available to civilians because most adenovirus infections are mild and self-limiting.

T cell vaccine. Many people carry adenovirus without symptoms. Immunodeficiency, induced so that a person can receive a tissue or organ transplant, allows the virus to spread in the infected person and cause severe and potentially lethal disseminated infection. An adenovirus T cell vaccine gives those persons cytotoxic T cells (or killer T cells), which recognize and destroy cells infected by adenovirus, or gives them helper T cells, which help cytotoxic T cells perform those functions.

A vaccine can be prepared by selecting and growing donated helper T cells that naturally recognize antigenic fragments of the adenovirus capsid hexon protein. Or, a vaccine can be prepared by using donated monocytes to train donated naïve cytotoxic T cells to recognize antigenic fragments of all adenovirus capsid proteins. The monocytes are modified by infection with recombinant adenovirus to produce the antigenic fragments, and they present the antigenic fragments to the cytotoxic T cells.

Recombinant vaccine. The antigens of many viruses (such as hepatitis C virus or human immunodeficiency virus) stimulate only weak production of antibodies by B cells. However, recombinant adenoviruses linking those antigens to the adenovirus capsid proteins can greatly increase production of antibodies to the antigens.

Most people have been infected by adenovirus and have associated antibodies. Those antibodies weaken the vaccine by neutralizing the recombinant adenovirus. Attempts to overcome this problem include changing the adenovirus capsid hexon or fiber to a form less recognizable by the immune system, and administering vaccines by a mucosal, rather than by an intramuscular or subcutaneous, route.

IMPACT

The B cell vaccine previously used against human adenovirus types 4 and 7 decreased adenovirus respiratory disease in military recruits by 82 to 95 percent. The economic value of that health benefit is estimated to be worth $22 million annually.

Clinical trials suggest that T cell vaccines may decrease the significant risk of illness or death caused by severe disseminated adenovirus infection. Clinical trials will determine if recombinant vaccines can be made suitable for the clinic.

David Caldwell, Ph.D.

FURTHER READING

Chatziandreou, Ilenia, et al. "Capture and Generation of Adenovirus Specific T Cells for Adoptive Immunotherapy." *British Journal of Haematology* 132 (2006): 117-126.

Foy, H. M. "Adenoviruses." In *Viral Infections in Humans: Epidemiology and Control*, edited by A. Evans and R. Kaslow. 4th ed. New York: Plenum, 1997.

Grandi, Guido, ed. *Genomics, Proteomics, and Vaccines.* Hoboken, N.J.: John Wiley & Sons, 2004.

Heymann, David L., ed. *Control of Communicable Diseases Manual.* 19th ed. Washington, D.C.: American Public Health Association, 2008.

Horwitz, M. S. "Adenoviruses." In *Fields' Virology*, edited by David M. Knipe and Peter M. Howley. Philadelphia: Wolters Kluwer Health/Lippincott Williams & Wilkins, 2007.

Plotkin, Stanley A., and Walter A. Orenstein, eds. *Vaccines.* 5th ed. Philadelphia: Saunders/Elsevier, 2008.

Russell, Kevin L., et al. "Vaccine-Preventable Adenoviral Respiratory Illness in U.S. Military Recruits, 1999-2004." *Vaccine* 24 (2006): 2835-2842.

Stern, Alexandra Minna, and Howard Markel. "The History Of Vaccines and Immunization: Familiar Patterns, New Challenges." *Health Affairs* 24, no. 3 (2005): 611-621.

WEB SITES OF INTEREST

Centers for Disease Control and Prevention
http://www.cdc.gov

International Committee on Taxonomy of Viruses
http://www.ictvonline.org

U.S. Food and Drug Administration: Vaccines, Blood, and Biologics
http://www.fda.gov/biologicsbloodvaccines

See also: Adenoviridae; Adenovirus infections; Antibodies; Contagious diseases; Immunity; Immunization; Infection; Mutation of pathogens; Pathogens; Vaccines: Types; Viral infections.

African sleeping sickness

CATEGORY: Diseases and conditions
ANATOMY OR SYSTEM AFFECTED: Brain, central nervous system, lymphatic system
ALSO KNOWN AS: African trypanosomiasis, East African trypanosomiasis, West African trypanosomiasis

DEFINITION

African sleeping sickness, also known as African trypanosomiasis, is a parasitic disease involving parasites belonging to the *Trypanosoma* genus of protozoa. The disease is usually transmitted by infected tsetse flies, which are found in sub-Saharan Africa. These flies live in vegetation by rivers, lakes, and forests. There are two types of African sleeping sickness, East African trypanosomiasis, which is caused by *T. brucei rhodesiense*, and West African trypanosomiasis, caused by *T. brucei gambiense.*

Causes

African sleeping sickness develops from an infection with protozoa. It is not transmitted from person to person through direct contact. In very rare cases, an infected pregnant woman can pass the disease to her fetus. An infected person donating blood can also pass it into a blood bank, risking infection for recipients in blood transfusions. When the protozoa reach the central nervous system, they can cause behavioral and neurological changes leading to coma and eventually death.

Risk Factors

A tsetse fly bite is the biggest risk for contracting African sleeping sickness. Therefore, for Westerners, travel to Africa, the natural habitat of these flies, creates the opportunity for transmission.

Symptoms

The initial symptom is a red swollen sore, called a chancre, at the site of the tsetse fly bite. The disease then starts to spread into the bloodstream, which causes fever, headache, lymphedema, and sweating. As the parasitic infection reaches the nervous system, extreme tiredness results. As African sleeping sickness progresses, irreversible neurological damage occurs. Other symptoms that may occur include rash, tremors, painful joints, swollen lymph glands, and muscle weakness. If the infection enters the brain, seizures, irritability, and confusion are some of the symptoms that may develop. Untreated, the disease may progress over months or years, finally leading to coma and death.

Screening and Diagnosis

Diagnosis in the early stages of the disease can be made with a thick blood smear. The blood needs to be fresh to allow for good visualization of the protozoa. A number of sensitive techniques can be used to detect the parasite in the bloodstream; for example, the card agglutination trypanosomiasis test is used to screen for *T. b. gambiense*. Also, a spinal tap is performed and a sample of fluid taken from a swollen lymph gland.

Treatment and Therapy

The treatment of African sleeping sickness is dependent upon on the stage of the disease when first diagnosed. When the disease is recently acquired, less toxic drugs can be used to eradicate it. The earlier the disease is detected, the more probable the cure. When the disease is in the second stage of development, however, the medication must be able to cross the blood-brain barrier. Hospitalization is necessary, and periodical checkups are needed for two years. Late-stage disease may be untreatable.

Prevention and Outcomes

The only method of preventing African sleeping sickness is avoiding insect bites, which involves insect control programs and wearing protective clothing.

Some research shows that injections of the medication pentamidine show favorable results in treating the early stages of *T. b. gambiense* infection, while suramin is more effective against *T. b. rhodesiense*. Eflornithine is used to treat second-stage *T. b. gambiense* disease and resistant disease.

Marvin L. Morris, M.P.A.

Further Reading

Bonomo, Robert A., and Robert A. Salata. "African Trypanosomiasis (Sleeping Sickness; *Trypanosoma brucei* Complex)." In *Nelson Textbook of Pediatrics*, edited by Richard E. Behrman, Robert M. Kliegman, and Hal B. Jenson. 18th ed. Philadelphia: Saunders/Elsevier, 2007.

Braakman, H. M., et al. "Lethal African Trypanosomiasis in Travelers: MRI and Neuropathology." *Neurology* 66 (2006): 1094-1096.

Centers for Disease Control and Prevention. "Parasites: African Trypanosomiasis." Available at http://www.cdc.gov/parasites/sleepingsickness.

Maudlin, I., P. H. Holmes, and M. A. Miles, eds. *The Trypanosomiases.* Cambridge, Mass.: CABI, 2004.

Web Sites of Interest

American Society of Tropical Medicine and Hygiene
http://www.astmh.org

Centers for Disease Control and Prevention
http://www.cdc.gov/parasites

World Health Organization
http://www.who.int

See also: Antiparasitic drugs: Types; Developing countries and infectious disease; Diagnosis of protozoan diseases; Flies and infectious disease; Parasitic diseases; Prevention of protozoan diseases; Protozoa: Classification and types; Protozoan diseases; Sleeping sickness; Treatment of protozoan diseases; Tropical medicine; *Trypanosoma*; Trypanosomiasis; Trypanosomiasis vaccine.

Agammaglobulinemia

CATEGORY: Diseases and conditions
ANATOMY OR SYSTEM AFFECTED: Blood, immune system
ALSO KNOWN AS: Bruton syndrome, Bruton's agammaglobulinemia, congenital agammaglobulinemia, sex-linked agammaglobulinemia, X-linked agammaglobulinemia

DEFINITION

Agammaglobulinemia is an inherited disorder in which the levels of antibodies (immunoglobulins) in the blood are abnormally low. Without these protective antibodies, persons with agammaglobulinemia are at high risk for infection.

Agammaglobulinemia is a primary immunodeficiency syndrome (in which a part of the immune system is missing or not working correctly). Primary immunodeficiencies are inherited, so the cause of the immune deficiency is considered primary, that is, it is not caused by drug treatment, another disease, or environmental exposure to toxins.

CAUSES

Agammaglobulinemia is usually inherited on the X chromosome (X-linked); thus, mostly males are affected. The gene called Bruton's tyrosine kinase (Btk) is responsible for this condition. When Btk is abnormal or mutated, the B cells (or B lymphocytes) do not develop normally and do not mature. B cells are the immune cells that are responsible for making antibodies. Antibodies play a critical role in recovery from certain infections and also protect against getting these infections again. In the past, agammaglobulinemia was often mistaken for a more severe deficiency of the immune system—severe combined immunodeficiency (SCID), popularly known as bubble-boy syndrome—in which both B and T cells are affected.

Agammaglobulinemia can also be inherited on autosomal chromosomes (non-sex chromosome). These forms of agammaglobulinemia are usually referred to as autosomal recessive agammaglobulinemia. The clinical presentation of these disorders is the same as X-linked agammaglobulinemia. The autosomal recessive agammaglobulinemias are a rare group of disorders, caused by various defects in the development of mature B cells, including defects in the following genes (and the proteins for which they encode): CD79A (Ig alpha), IGHM (C), VpreB/ 5 (pseudolight chain), and BLNK (B cell linker, a protein associated with Btk).

RISK FACTORS

Because agammaglobulinemia is an inherited disorder, there are no risk factors.

SYMPTOMS

Typical symptoms of agammaglobulinemia include frequent bouts of bronchitis, chronic diarrhea, conjunctivitis (eye infection), otitis media (middle-ear infection), pneumonia, sinusitis, skin infection, and upper respiratory tract infection. Infections usually begin early in life (by the age of four years). Additional symptoms include bronchiectasis (damage or enlargement of the small air sacs in the lungs) and unexplained asthma.

SCREENING AND DIAGNOSIS

A diagnosis is usually made based on a person's history of repeated infections of the respiratory tract and most typically throughout childhood. The most commonly reported bacterial infections are pneumococcal (*Streptococcus pneumoniae*), *Staphylococcus*, and *Haemophilus influenzae.*

A lack of, or a deficiency in, B cells or antibodies in the blood is a strong indicator of agammaglobulinemia. A Western blot test can determine the lack of the Btk protein, another indicator of X-linked agammaglobulinemia. To confirm a diagnosis, a genetic blood test can be performed to identify the specific Btk mutation.

TREATMENT AND THERAPY

Because there is no cure for agammaglobulinemia, the main goal of therapy is to reduce the frequency and severity of infections. However, persons can be given the antibodies they are lacking. This treatment, called intravenous immunoglobulin (IVIg), helps boost the immune system. Regular treatment with IVIg, generally every three to four weeks for life, can increase the person's life span and quality of life.

Additionally, antibiotics are often given to treat bacterial infections. If long-term treatment is needed, local antibiotics (such as lotions and drops) are used whenever possible before systemic antibiotics (in pill form) are prescribed.

People are now diagnosed earlier in life. Early diagnosis generally leads to early treatment. This, with the advent of IVIg and improvements in the treatment of infection, allows more people to avoid long-term pulmonary (lung) insufficiency and to live a relatively healthy life.

A possible treatment of the future may be gene therapy, which has the potential to cure agammaglobulinemia. However, this technology is in its early stages and not ready to be applied to agammaglobulinemia therapy.

Affected persons should not receive live vaccines (such as measles, mumps, rubella vaccine, or MMR), polio vaccine, varicella (chickenpox) vaccine, or the intranasal influenza vaccine (FluMist). Treatment with IVIg is usually a necessity; without treatment, most severe infections are fatal.

PREVENTION AND OUTCOMES

If a person has a relative with X-linked agammaglobulinemia and plans to have children, genetic counseling before pregnancy is recommended. The impact of early recognition and effective treatments on life span and quality of life (and on health care costs) can affect public health interventions. To improve health outcomes of primary immunodeficiency diseases such as agammaglobulinemia, the Centers for Disease Control and Prevention developed a population-based public health framework. Initial findings indicate that routine newborn screening for agammaglobulinemia, IVIg therapy, and improved antibiotics appear to reduce the burden of the disease.

Anita P. Kuan, Ph.D.

FURTHER READING

Abbas, Abul K., and Andrew H. Lichtman. *Basic Immunology: Functions and Disorders of the Immune System.* 2d ed. Philadelphia: Saunders/Elsevier, 2006.

Kumar, A., et al. "Current Perspectives on Primary Immunodeficiency Diseases." *Clinical and Developmental Immunology* 13 (June-December, 2006): 223-259.

Moreau, T., et al. "Potential Application of Gene Therapy to X-linked Agammaglobulinemia." *Current Gene Therapy* 7, no. 4 (August, 2007): 284-294.

National Library of Medicine. "Agammaglobulinemia." Available at http://www.nlm.nih.gov/medlineplus/ency/article/001307.htm.

Winkelstein, J. A., et al. "Status of Adults with X-Linked Agammaglobulinemia: Impact of Disease on Daily Lives, Quality of Life, Educational and Socioeconomic Status, Knowledge of Inheritance, and Reproductive Attitudes." *Medicine* (Baltimore) 87, no. 5 (September, 2008): 253-258.

WEB SITES OF INTEREST

Centers for Disease Control and Prevention
http://www.cdc.gov/genomics

Genetic and Rare Diseases Information Center
http://rarediseases.info.nih.gov/gard

Immune Deficiency Foundation
http://www.primaryimmune.org

National Center for Biotechnology Information
http://www.genetests.org

Primary Immunodeficiency Association
http://www.pia.org.uk

Microbiology and Immunology On-line
http://pathmicro.med.sc.edu/book/welcome.htm

See also: Antibiotics: Types; Antibodies; Autoimmune disorders; Idiopathic thrombocytopenic purpura; Immunity; Immunoassay; Immunodeficiency; Inflammation; Neutropenia; Seroconversion.

Aging and infectious disease

CATEGORY: Epidemiology

DEFINITION

The elderly population, which includes persons who are sixty-five years of age or older, makes up about 13 percent of the total population of the United States and is expected to grow to about 20 percent of all Americans by the year 2030. Infectious diseases are the cause of one-third of all deaths in the elderly. The most common infectious diseases among older people can be categorized as follows: urinary tract infections (UTIs), respiratory tract infections (RTIs), skin and soft tissue infections (SSTIs), and gastrointestinal tract infections (GTIs).

RISK FACTORS, ETIOLOGY, AND PATHOGENESIS

As a person ages, his or her immune system weakens and becomes less effective (immunosenescence). Studies have shown that increasing age is associated with a decline in the number of (or with functional alterations in) CD8+ cells, naive T cells, and B cells, all of which are involved in fighting infections. Other causes may include the impact of other diseases (comorbidities) and a decline in bodily functions. Malnutrition may also play a role, as approximately 10 to 25 percent of elderly persons have nutritional deficiencies and up to 50 percent of the elderly who are hospitalized have some kind of caloric or micronutrient deficiency. Malnutrition is a risk factor for infection, and infection can lead to malnutrition, particularly in the geriatric population.

UTIs are the most common infection in the elderly. Although urine is normally sterile, older persons are more likely to have bacteria in their urine (bacteriuria), with a prevalence of 15 to 30 percent in men and 25 to 50 percent in women. Factors contributing to this increased bacterial colonization include reduction in bladder capacity, decreased urinary flow, incomplete voiding, prostatic disease in men, and prolapsed bladder and lower estrogen levels in women.

An indwelling urinary catheter, common among institutionalized and elderly persons, is another risk factor for UTIs, as catheters contain stagnant urine in a warm environment, which promotes the growth of microorganisms. Thinning of the urinary epithelium also contributes to increased bacterial colonization, particularly in women, as does a higher vaginal pH and deficiencies in vaginal and periurethral antibodies that occur with age. Regular urination and strong urinary flow are protective against infectious bacteria, but the aging bladder is less able to sense the need to void. Urinary flow rates are slower in the elderly, and the elderly are more likely to experience incomplete bladder emptying.

Escherichia coli is the main pathogen responsible for UTIs in women, but about one-third of elderly persons have polymicrobial infections, which are rarely seen in younger persons. Infection with multiple organisms is more common in catheterized persons.

RTIs such as pneumonia and influenza are the second-most common infections in the elderly. Older people are at increased risk relative to younger people because they frequently have deficiencies in protective airway reflexes (such as coughing) and mucus clearance. Decreased elasticity of the alveoli (air sacs in the lung), poorer lung capacity, smoking, and pre-existing conditions such as chronic obstructive pulmonary disease (COPD) and congestive heart failure are also common risk factors for lung infections. The elderly are also more prone to active tuberculosis (TB) infections. Latent (inactive) TB is prevalent in all ages, but decreasing immune function with age can lead to the infection becoming active.

The epithelial cells of the skin, bladder, bronchus, and digestive system form a physical barrier to bacteria, fungi, and viruses that may become compromised with age. For example, the skin becomes thinner, dryer, and more easily breached, leading to a higher risk of skin infections. Skin also loses collagen over time, affecting the ability to resist trauma. Epidermal renewal time (the time it takes the body to make all new skin cells) increases from twenty days in younger adults to thirty days in older people, delaying wound healing and making wounds more likely to be colonized by microorganisms. Cellulitis, a bacterial infection often seen in the legs, is much more common in the elderly, especially those with diabetes. Shingles are caused by the reactivation of the varicella zoster virus (chickenpox), which is dormant after the initial infection (usually in childhood) but can flare up in old age.

GTIs, including gastroenteritis and colitis, are also more common in older adults. Predisposing factors include pH changes in the stomach, decreased intestinal movement, and changes in the composition of the gut bacteria. The risk of gastrointestinal infections is also affected by the presence of *Helicobacter pylori*, which is found in 40 to 70 percent of elderly people. *H. pylori* causes chronic gastritis in about one-third of those infected, which can lead to lower acid levels in the stomach and a higher risk of infections from other pathogens. Treatment with antibiotics and proton pump inhibitors can change the composition of the stomach's normal bacteria, which can lead to susceptibility to infectious organisms such as *Clostridium difficile*.

Other factors that increase the risk of infectious diseases among the elderly include a higher likelihood of being bedridden, which increases the risk of pressure ulcers and subsequent skin infections, and more frequent institutionalization and hospitalization, which increase the risk of nosocomial (hospital-acquired) infections and higher exposure to pathogens in confined settings. In addition, older people are more likely to have comorbid conditions such as diabetes, cancer, and heart disease; both the diseases and their treatments (for example, chemotherapy) can weaken the immune system and lead to a higher risk for infections.

SYMPTOMS

Older people often do not have the same symptoms associated with infections that younger people do. For example, the classic symptoms of infection include fever, inflammation, pain, chills, and vomiting. However, elderly people with infections often have nonspecific symptoms such as delirium, confusion, fatigue, loss of appetite, decline in function, mental status changes, incontinence, falls, or subnormal temperature. This atypical presentation can potentially lead to a delay in diagnosis and treatment, especially because the same symptoms are also present in noninfectious diseases in the elderly. The average body temperature for older adults is often lower too, meaning that if a baseline temperature is unknown, a fever may be missed. In an institutional setting, cognitive comorbidities increase the risk of a missed infection. For example, about one-half of nursing home residents have dementia and are unable to describe symptoms at all.

UTIs generally cause symptoms such as an urgent need to urinate, increased frequency of urination, and pain. Fever may also be present. However, these symptoms may be hidden by preexisting incontinence. In some cases, delirium, confusion, and rapid functional decline are the main symptoms of a UTI, and these infections may even manifest with respiratory symptoms such as cough or shortness of breath. Diagnosis relies on symptoms, urinalysis, and urine culture, although elderly persons with symptomatic UTIs may have lower bacterial counts than younger persons: Although 105 or more colony-forming units (CFU) per milliliter (mL) of urine is the standard definition, bacterial counts in the elderly may be only 102 to 103 CFU/mL.

RTIs can affect the nose, throat, airways, and lungs and are typically associated with cough, fever, weakness, sore throat, irritability, difficulty breathing, and aches and pains. Often, any type of RTI is attributed to the flu, because the different types of infections are difficult to distinguish; other types of infections have not been studied as thoroughly. In persons with COPD, even a simple cold can cause an acute exacerbation, leading to hospitalization and even death.

SSTIs such as cellulitis generally present with redness, warmth, and swelling. The primary symptom associated with shingles is pain, and even after the infection clears, persons frequently experience postherpetic neuralgia, or nerve pain, which can last up to one year or longer.

GTIs are typically associated with gastrointestinal pain, diarrhea, fever, cramping, nausea, and vomiting. Diarrhea may be bloody in the case of *E. coli* infections but typically is not bloody among persons infected with *C. difficile*. As with other infectious diseases, GTIs may be hard to distinguish from other conditions in the elderly, including incontinence, irritable bowel, or medication-induced diarrhea. Initial infection with *H. pylori* is associated with nausea, upper abdominal pain, vomiting, and fever lasting anywhere from three days to two weeks; after the original infection subsides, the bacteria tend to colonize the gastrointestinal tract, triggering subsequent gastritis episodes, unless treated.

PREVENTION AND TREATMENT

UTIs may be prevented through personal hygiene, avoidance of catheterization wherever possible, and possibly certain nutritional approaches such as cranberry juice. Although asymptomatic bacteriuria is very common, the guidelines of the Infectious Diseases Society of America do not recommend screening for or treating the condition because of a lack of proof that doing so prevents future UTIs or reduces morbidity; in addition, overtreatment for asymptomatic infections may contribute to antibiotic resistance. In persons with symptomatic UTIs, existing catheters are removed and the infection is treated with an oral antibiotic specific to the pathogen involved. If the infection is serious, intravenous antibiotic therapy may be required. Polymicrobial infections may require a broad-spectrum antibiotic.

The most reliable ways to prevent RTIs include smoking cessation and vaccination. In addition, vigilance on the part of health care providers and caregivers is required, because symptoms can be subtle, particularly for TB. Vaccines for both pneumonia and influenza are available and recommended for all adults age sixty years and older. The United States has one of the highest rates of influenza and pneumonia vaccination in elderly persons in the world, at about 80 percent for flu and 70 percent for pneumonia, although the rate is still less than the government target of 90 percent.

Although the preventive efficacy of the influenza and pneumonia vaccines is lower in older persons, vaccination has been shown to reduce the severity of cases in terms of length of hospital stays and in terms of mortality, when they do occur. Some health care institutions are now instituting standing orders for vaccinations for the elderly, a strategy that takes the physician out of the equation and allows pharmacists, nurses, and physician assistants to provide routine vaccinations after a simple screening. Treatment for RTIs varies from simple bed rest to complex antiviral or antibiotic regimens lasting weeks.

SSTIs are best prevented through awareness and through good hygiene by both older people and their caregivers. Pressure ulcers may be prevented through regular repositioning of persons restricted to their bed, using supportive devices and surfaces, and keeping skin hydrated. Diabetics and people with poor circulation, who are at higher risk of cellulitis, can wear supportive stockings and keep the lower extremities elevated whenever possible to prevent swelling. A vaccine is approved for herpes zoster, indicated for all adults age sixty years and older, regardless of their history of zoster infection. The vaccine has been shown to be both effective and cost-effective in the elderly.

GTIs are best prevented through scrupulous personal hygiene, proper food-safety measures, and avoidance of antibiotics and proton pump inhibitors unless necessary. Institutional settings should ensure against transmission from infected persons, including visitors and staff, to healthy residents. Risk-based food-safety programs and ongoing food safety education for staff are necessary. Treatment for GTIs includes hydration and supportive care and the discontinuation of any antibiotic that may have caused the problem. Treatment with antidiarrheal agents is not recommended in infections related to *C. difficile* or *E. coli.* Oral metronidazole or vancomycin may be used to treat *C. difficile* infections. Alcohol-based hand sanitizers are not effective at killing *C. difficile,* so soap and water should be used if that is the infectious agent. Treatment regimens for *H. pylori* infections may include proton pump inhibitors, amoxicillin, clarithromycin, and metronidazole.

IMPACT

Infectious diseases are major causes of death, disability, morbidity, cost, and health-services utilization in the elderly. The infectious disease hospitalization rate in the United States increased by about 12 percent from 1998 to 2006 and is about four times higher among the elderly than among younger adults.

UTIs led to about seven million outpatient visits and one million emergency room visits in 1997. Among institutionalized elderly persons, prevalence ranges from 0.1 to 2.4 cases per 1,000 resident days, and 12 to 30 percent of residents have a minimum of one UTI every year.

RTIs such as pneumonia, influenza, and chronic bronchitis are the fourth-leading cause of death in this age group, after heart disease, cancer, and stroke. In 2008, the elderly accounted for 35 percent of all inpatient stays in the United States (with nearly fourteen million discharges), totaling more than $157 billion in costs. Pneumonia was the second-most common reason for admission in this age group (after congestive heart failure). Among those age sixty-five years and older, there were nearly 600,000 discharges costing more than $5 billion for influenza and pneumonia in 2008. COPD, which is an umbrella diagnosis that includes chronic bronchitis and emphysema and is generally related to smoking, is found in approximately 10 percent of all adults and is more common in older persons. In 2000 in the United States, COPD was the cause of 1.5 million emergency department visits, 726,000 hospitalizations, and 119,000 deaths. Most were a result of acute exacerbations of the disease, which are caused by viral, bacterial, or fungal infections in about two-thirds of cases. People age sixty-five years and older make up more than 50 percent of cases of active TB in the United States, and nursing home residents have higher infection rates than do community-dwelling older people.

Bacterial, viral, and fungal SSTIs that are common in the elderly include shingles (herpes zoster), cellulitis, pressure ulcers, scabies, and chronic fungal infections of the nails (onychomycosis). Other SSTIs that have a higher incidence in older people include necrotizing fasciitis, methicillin-resistant *Staphylococcus aureus* infections of the skin, and surgical site infections. The incidence of herpes zoster is 3.2 per 1,000 person years, while the prevalence of pressure ulcers is about 17 to 28 percent; approximately two-thirds of people age seventy years and older have a minimum of one skin problem.

GTIs caused by *H. pylori* are common in elderly persons, and if left untreated, chronic infection with *H. pylori* can lead to gastritis, gastric ulcers, and even stomach cancer, which is the second-most frequent cause of cancer-related death worldwide. The incidence and severity of *C. difficile*-associated diarrhea has increased since the 1970's, when it was first identified, so that it is now endemic to hospitals and long-term care facilities. An antibiotic-resistant strain has been identified and is associated with a high rate of recurrent infection.

Lisa M. Lines, M.P.H.

FURTHER READING

Castle, Steven C., et al. "Host Resistance and Immune Responses in Advanced Age." *Clinics in Geriatric Medicine* 23 (2007): 463-479. Focuses on immunosenescence in elderly people.

Gavazzi, Gaetan, and Karl-Heinz Krause. "Ageing and Infection." *The Lancet: Infectious Diseases* 2 (2002): 659-666. Reviews risk factors, epidemiology, clinical aspects, diagnosis, and treatment of infections.

High, Kevin. "Immunizations in Older Adults." *Clinics in Geriatric Medicine* 23 (2007): 669-685. Discusses the reasons for decreased vaccine efficacy and poor uptake of vaccination for influenza, pneumonia, and herpes zoster.

Htwe, Tin Han, et al. "Infection in the Elderly." *Infectious Disease Clinics of North America* 21 (2007): 711-743. Discusses epidemiology, clinical features, diagnosis, and treatment of infection, including skin infections, UTIs, RTIs, and GTIs.

Liang, Stephen Y., and Philip A. Mackowiak. "Infections in the Elderly." *Clinics in Geriatric Medicine* 23 (2007): 441-456. Provides an overview of the etiology, symptoms, diagnosis, and treatment of pneumonia, UTIs, and skin infections.

Mouton, Charles P., et al. "Common Infections in Older Adults." *American Family Physician* 63 (2001): 257-268. Primarily focuses on assessment, diagnosis, and treatment of pneumonia, influenza, UTIs, and skin infections.

Yoshikawa, Thomas T. "Epidemiology and Unique Aspects of Aging and Infectious Diseases." *Clinical Infectious Diseases* 30 (2000): 931-933. Brief article providing insight into unique aspects of infections in the elderly, including altered clinical manifestations and diverse microbial causes of infections.

WEB SITES OF INTEREST

American Geriatrics Society Foundation for Health in Aging
http://www.healthinaging.org

Infectious Diseases Society of America
http://www.idsociety.org

National Center for Preparedness, Detection, and Control of Infectious Diseases
http://www.cdc.gov/ncpdcid

See also: Cancer and infectious disease; Cellulitis; Epidemiology; Men and infectious disease; Osteomyelitis; Pacemaker infections; Postherpetic neuralgia; Prostatitis; Prosthetic joint infections; Psychological effects of infectious disease; Public health; Shingles; Social effects of infectious disease; Women and infectious disease.

AIDS

CATEGORY: Diseases and conditions
ANATOMY OR SYSTEM AFFECTED: All
ALSO KNOWN AS: Acquired immunodeficiency syndrome

DEFINITION

AIDS, an immunodeficiency disorder, is a disease of the immune system caused by infection with the human immunodeficiency virus (HIV). The disease leads to a progressive deterioration of the immune system and is characterized by the development of opportunistic infections and cancers.

CAUSES

Before a person develops AIDS, the HIV in his or her body attacks white blood cells called helper T cells (CD4). These cells are part of the immune system, and they fight infections and disease.

HIV infection occurs through contact with HIV-infected blood or other body fluids, including semen, vaginal fluid, and breast milk. HIV is spread through sexual contact with an HIV-infected person, especially by having vaginal intercourse or anal sex; through transfer of HIV from a woman to a fetus during pregnancy and from a woman to a child during birth; through breast-feeding; through an HIV-contaminated needle; and through a transfusion of HIV-infected blood (now rare because all donated blood, since 1985, is tested for HIV).

Rarely, HIV can be spread by infected blood getting into the open wound of an uninfected person, by being bitten by someone infected with HIV, and by sharing personal hygiene items (such as razors or toothbrushes) with an HIV-infected person.

An HIV infection leaves a person vulnerable to severe illnesses, compromising that person's immunity. AIDS develops when T cells are destroyed by HIV infection.

RISK FACTORS

Certain behaviors, including having unprotected sex and injecting illegal drugs, greatly increase the risk of HIV infection. Most people become infected with HIV through sexual activity. A person can be infected by not using a condom when having sexual relations with a person infected with HIV. Not using condoms properly can also increase the risk of HIV infection. During sex, the vagina, vulva, penis, rectum, and mouth can provide entry points for the virus. Other risky behaviors include having sex without knowing a partner's HIV status, having more than one sex partner, having sex with someone who has more than one sexual partner, and having anal intercourse.

Injecting illegal drugs, too, increases the risk of HIV infection. Using a needle or syringe that contains even a small amount of infected blood can transmit HIV.

Certain medical conditions, such as sexually transmitted diseases (STDs) and vaginal infections caused by bacteria, tend to increase the risk of HIV transmission during sex with an HIV-infected partner. Examples of STDs include syphilis, genital herpes, chlamydia, and gonorrhea. Also, uncircumcised men are more at risk for HIV infection.

Blood products, tissue and organ transplantation, and "artificial" insemination increase the risk of HIV infection and AIDS. Even though blood products are screened for HIV, there is still some degree of risk because tests cannot detect HIV immediately after transmission. Before 1985, blood transfusions and the like increased the risk of HIV infection and AIDS. Before blood banks began testing donated blood for HIV in 1985, there was no way of knowing if donated blood was contaminated with HIV; recipients risked becoming infected through transfusions. Health care workers, too, are at higher risk for developing HIV infection because they are often exposed to contaminated blood and needles.

SYMPTOMS

HIV infection may not cause symptoms for a number of years or may cause a person to experience some early symptoms within six to eight weeks of becoming infected. During this acute HIV infection, the virus is rapidly reproducing, and the body's immune system is mounting a defense. The virus can easily be passed to other people during this period.

Initial symptoms of acute HIV infection include fever; extreme, unexplained fatigue; swollen lymph nodes in the armpits, neck, or groin; headache; dry cough; night sweats; rash; sore throat; and joint pain. After these initial symptoms are gone, there may be no symptoms for months to years, depending on the person's health status and lifestyle choices. It may be ten years or longer before a person with HIV develops symptoms. Some infected people have had the virus for even longer without developing symptoms. Even in persons without symptoms, the virus is multiplying and damaging the immune system and can be passed to someone else.

Once the virus sufficiently weakens the immune system, the following symptoms may occur over the course of one to three years: swollen lymph glands all over the body; fatigue; fungal infections of the mouth, fingernails, or toes; repeated vaginal infections (such as yeast infection and trichomoniasis); development

Children Younger than Age Thirteen Living with AIDS, by Year of Diagnosis and Race/Ethnicity, U.S. Estimates (2003-2007 and Cumulative)

Race/ethnicity	Year of Diagnosis					Cumulative[a]
	2003	2004	2005	2006	2007	
American Indian/Alaska Native	0	1	0	0	0	32
Asian[b]	0	0	1	1	0	47
Black/African American	49	34	39	29	21	5,699
Hispanic/Latino[c]	10	9	9	4	2	1,757
Native Hawaiian/Other Pacific Islander	0	1	0	0	0	7
White	12	8	4	3	5	1,602
Total[d]	73	55	54	38	28	9,209[e]

Note. These numbers do not represent reported case counts. Rather, these numbers are point estimates, which result from adjustments of reported case counts. The reported case counts have been adjusted for reporting delays, but not for incomplete reporting.

a. From the beginning of the epidemic through 2007.
b. Includes Asian/Pacific Islander legacy cases (see Technical Notes).
c. Hispanics/Latinos can be of any race.
d. Includes children of unknown race or multiple races. Because column totals were calculated independently of the values for the subpopulations, the values in each column may not sum to the column total.
e. Includes 64 children of unknown race or multiple races.

Source: HIV/AIDS Surveillance Report (2007), Centers for Disease Control and Prevention

of many warts; exacerbations of prior conditions such as eczema, psoriasis, and herpes infection; shingles; fever; night sweats; weight loss; chronic diarrhea; and memory loss.

If HIV has progressed to AIDS, the immune system has become weakened and prone to opportunistic infections, that is, infections that people with a normal immune system do not usually get. These infections occur in people with AIDS because the immune system cannot fight infection. Examples of opportunistic infections and other complications of AIDS include thrush (an overgrowth of yeast); pneumonia (particularly pneumocystis pneumonia); invasive fungal infections (resulting in brain and/or lung infections); toxoplasmosis infection; tuberculosis; viral brain infection; Kaposi's sarcoma; lymphoma; cervical cancer; eye disease caused by cytomegalovirus infection; intestinal infections, especially from *Shigella, Salmonella,* and *Campylobacter*; severe weight loss (known as wasting

syndrome); severe skin rashes; reactions to medications; and psychiatric problems, including depression and dementia.

Symptoms of these conditions (opportunistic infections and other complications of AIDS) include shortness of breath, coughing with blood-tinged sputum, swallowing problems, confusion and forgetfulness, severe diarrhea, nausea and vomiting, vision loss, severe headaches, coma (but only in severe cases of viral brain infection or terminal cases), and reddish, brownish, or purple spots on the mouth or skin.

SCREENING AND DIAGNOSIS

The purpose of screening is early diagnosis and treatment. Screening tests are usually administered to people without current symptoms, but who may be at high risk for certain diseases or conditions. Also, potential blood donors are tested for HIV.

Persons who are at increased risk of HIV infection

may be screened for the virus through testing. These tests include ELISA (enzyme-linked immunoabsorbent assay). This test is used to detect HIV infection. If an ELISA test is positive, the Western blot test is usually performed to confirm the diagnosis. The ELISA test may be negative if a person was recently infected with HIV. Many people with HIV (95 percent) will have a positive test within three months of the time they became infected. Most people with HIV (99 percent) will have a positive test within six months.

The Western blot test is specific to identifying HIV. It is used to confirm a positive ELISA test result. The OraQuick rapid HIV-1 antibody is a preliminary test using saliva and should be confirmed by an ELISA test. A CD4+T cell count is a blood test used to evaluate the status of the immune system. The viral load test measures the amount of HIV in the blood.

The general population is not screened for HIV infection. Counseling and testing for HIV is recommended by the Centers for Disease Control and Prevention (CDC) for anyone who has engaged in risky behavior or who has a work-related exposure. Local health departments and other organizations often provide anonymous HIV testing.

The CDC recommends that gay and bisexual men at high risk for HIV infection be screened annually for STDs, including HIV infection. Others who should be offered counseling and testing for HIV include persons who are being treated for other STDs; males who have had sex with other males since 1975; persons who are injecting drugs or who have done so in the past; sex workers (prostitutes); women and men who are or have been in sexual relationships with partners who are HIV-positive, homosexual or bisexual, use injectable drugs, had blood transfusions between 1978 and 1985, or are pregnant; and infants of women who are HIV-positive, who have AIDS, or who have risk factors for HIV infection or AIDS. Also, all pregnant women should be offered counseling and testing for HIV.

TREATMENT AND THERAPY

Treatment aims to decrease the amount of HIV in the body and to keep the immune system as healthy as possible to prevent infections and cancers. Treatment for HIV infection may involve medications, lifestyle changes, alternative and complementary medicine, and surgical procedures, which are sometimes combined with medical therapy for the treatment of various

Speaking with a Health Care Provider About AIDS

QUESTIONS TO ASK ABOUT AIDS
How is my immune system functioning?
What is my viral load and CD4+ T cell count?
How quickly will my condition worsen?

QUESTIONS ABOUT THE RISK OF DEVELOPING AIDS
Am I at risk for other infections besides HIV infection and AIDS?
Do I need to be tested for these other infections?
What can I do to lessen my chance of progressing to AIDS?

QUESTIONS ABOUT TREATMENT OPTIONS
What is my best treatment option?
What other options are there?
What are the risks and benefits associated with each treatment option?
What medications are available to help me?
What are the benefits and side effects of these medications?
When should I start taking them?
Will these medications interact with other medications, over-thecounter products, or dietary and herbal supplements?
How long will I have to take these medications?
What should I do if I miss a dose?
What can I do to prevent other infections?

QUESTIONS ABOUT LIFESTYLE CHANGES
What will I need to change in my daily routine?
How long can I expect to continue working at my present job, or caring for myself?
Should I exercise?
What type of exercise is best?
How much should I be exercising?
How do I get started with an exercise program?
Are there dietary changes I should make? How do I go about it?
Should I stop drinking alcohol?
How can I find help to quit smoking?
What can I do to prevent complications?
How can I avoid giving this disease to someone I love and to other people?

QUESTIONS ABOUT OUTLOOK
What are my risks for developing complications?
Will I still be able to have children?
Will I put my future children at risk for this disease?
Will I be able to live a normal life?
What is the likelihood I will be totally disabled or need help with personal care?
Am I likely to die soon? Do I need to put my affairs in order?

opportunistic infections and cancers associated with HIV and AIDS.

PREVENTION AND OUTCOMES

There are several ways one can reduce the risk of developing HIV/AIDS. One should use protection during sex because sexual activity is the most likely way to become infected with HIV. People infected with HIV may not look sick, so often there is no way to tell if one's partner has HIV without having been tested. One should take precautions when engaging in intercourse or any other sexual act that results in an exchange of body fluids.

To lower the risk of HIV infection, one should abstain from sex or should, if having sex, use a latex condom and water-based lubricants, limit the number of sexual partners, learn the HIV status and HIV risk-factors of potential sexual partners, learn if potential sexual partners have had any STDs, and avoid sexual relationships with people who are HIV-positive or who are using injected drugs. In addition, circumcised males are less at risk for HIV infection.

One should not share needles or syringes. Using a needle or syringe contaminated with HIV-infected blood can lead to infection. Health care workers and caregivers should use appropriate safety precautions. When caring for patients, one should wear gloves and facial masks during all procedures or when handling bodily fluids. Also, providers should carefully handle and properly dispose of needles, carefully follow universal precautions, and cover all cuts and sores (both of the provider and of the HIV-infected person) with bandages.

One should donate his or her own blood for elective surgical procedures. Blood products are screened for HIV, but there is still a small risk because tests cannot detect HIV immediately after transmission. The risk of contracting HIV through blood products can be minimized by donating one's own blood for future elective surgical procedures.

Debra Wood, R.N.;
reviewed by David L. Horn, M.D., FACP

FURTHER READING

Bartlett, John G. *The Johns Hopkins Hospital 2005-6 Guide to Medical Care of Patients with HIV Infection.* 12th ed. Philadelphia: Lippincott Williams & Wilkins, 2005. An informative resource for clinicians caring for person with HIV infections.

Centers for Disease Control and Prevention. *Quality Assurance Guidelines for Testing Using the OraQuick Rapid HIV-1 Antibody Test.* Atlanta: Department of Health and Human Services, 2003. CDC guidelines for laboratory clinicians working on HIV antibody testing.

Cichocki, Mark. *Living with HIV: A Patient's Guide.* Jefferson, N.C.: McFarland, 2009. A good resource for general readers and other persons with HIV infection.

Clark, Rebecca A., Robert T. Maupin, Jr., and Jill Hayes Hammer. *A Woman's Guide to Living with HIV Infection.* Baltimore: Johns Hopkins University Press, 2004. A good resource on HIV infection, written especially for women.

Fan, Hung Y., Ross F. Conner, and Luis P. Villarreal. *AIDS: Science and Society.* 5th ed. Sudbury, Mass.: Jones and Bartlett, 2007. Examines the perspectives of science and society on HIV infection and AIDS.

St. Georgiev, Vassil. *Opportunistic Infections: Treatment and Prophylaxis.* Totowa, N.J.: Humana Press, 2003. Examines HIV infection as an opportunistic infection. Covers prevention and treatment.

Stine, Gerald J. *AIDS Update 2010.* New York: McGraw-Hill Higher Education, 2010. A thorough examination of the HIV and AIDS pandemics as they affected world populations in 2009-2010.

WEB SITES OF INTEREST

AIDSinfo
http://aidsinfo.nih.gov

AIDS.org
http://www.aids.org

National Pediatric AIDS Network
http://www.npan.org

See also: Blood-borne illness and disease; Breast milk and infectious disease; Contagious diseases; Epidemics and pandemics: History; HIV; HIV vaccine; Immunoassay; Incubation period; Integrase inhibitors; Kaposi's sarcoma; Maturation inhibitors; Opportunistic infections; Oral transmission; *Pneumocystis*; Pneumocystis pneumonia; Protease inhibitors; Reverse transcriptase inhibitors; Saliva and infectious disease; Sexually transmitted diseases (STDs); Viral infections.

Airborne illness and disease

Category: Transmission

Definition

Airborne diseases are those diseases transmitted by contaminated droplets in the air. Common types of airborne disease include the common cold, the flu (influenza), chickenpox (varicella), and tuberculosis.

Exposure

Cold and flu. Both the common cold and the flu are highly contagious. They can be spread from person to person when an infected person coughs or sneezes. People can also catch a common cold or the flu by touching an contaminated object (a fomite) that contains the live virus and by then touching their eyes, nose, or their mouth. Other methods of transmission include kissing and sharing food or drinks.

There are certain risk factors that may cause a person to be more susceptible to a cold or flu. Those risk factors include age (young children and adults age sixty-five years and older are more susceptible), a compromised immune system caused by illness or treatment of an illness (such as human immunodeficiency virus [HIV] infection or chemotherapy), living in a residential care facility, or working in health care.

Chickenpox. Chickenpox is also highly contagious and can be spread from person to person when an infected person coughs or sneezes. One of the main symptoms of chickenpox is a rash that eventually blisters. Touching an open blister that is leaking fluid can also lead to the spread of the disease.

As with the cold or flu, there are certain risk factors that may cause a person to be more susceptible to chickenpox. Risk factors for increased susceptibility to chickenpox include not having had chickenpox in the past, not being given the chickenpox vaccine, and spending a lot of time around children.

Tuberculosis. Although tuberculosis is a contagious disease, it does not spread as easily as the common cold, the flu, or chickenpox. It can still be spread from person to person when an infected person coughs or sneezes, but it is most commonly spread when people spend a lot of time together in close quarters, such the home or office. Tuberculosis is not spread by handshaking, kissing, or sharing food or drinks.

In addition to living with or working with someone who has tuberculosis, there are other risk factors that may make someone more susceptible to contracting the disease, including the following: having a compromised immunity, living in a region where there are high rates of tuberculosis, age (sixty-five years and older), long-term drug or alcohol use, living in a residential care facility, and working in health care.

People who are at high risk for contracting tuberculosis, or those who think they may have been exposed to the disease, should be tested for tuberculosis. The following persons should be periodically tested for tuberculosis infection: health care workers, people with HIV or other immune system disorders, people who live in areas with high rates of infection, people who live in residential care facilities, persons who have symptoms of active tuberculosis, people who live or work in correctional facilities, injection-drug users, and persons who have lived with or who have spent much time with someone who has active tuberculosis.

Prevention

Cold. There is currently no vaccination for the prevention of the common cold. The best method of preventing the common cold is frequent handwashing, particularly before eating or preparing food.

Another way to help prevent the common cold is to periodically clean with antibacterial wipes all shared surfaces, such as telephones, computer keyboards, refrigerator handles, doorknobs, and toys. A third method for preventing the common cold is to teach children to drink from their own drinking glass, rather than sharing. A fourth method of common cold prevention is to avoid close contact with people who have a cold or other respiratory tract infection.

Flu. The best way to prevent the flu is to get a flu shot (influenza vaccination). In the fall of 2010, the flu vaccine began protecting against the most common types of flu viruses, seasonal influenza and the H1N1 virus (swine flu). The Centers for Disease Control and Prevention (CDC) recommends that all persons age six months and older be vaccinated, although there are some exceptions. The following people should not get a flu vaccine without consulting a physician: persons who are allergic to eggs, who have had a previous allergic reaction to the flu vaccine, who have Guillain-Barré syndrome, or who are already sick and who have a fever. Vaccination is recommended after illness, however.

In addition to vaccination, there are other steps to

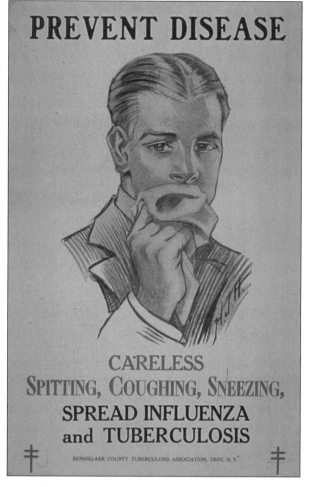

An early twentieth century poster urges people to avoid "careless spitting, coughing,[and] sneezing" to prevent the spread of influenza and tuberculosis. (CDC)

help prevent the spread of influenza, including frequent handwashing, using a tissue to cover the nose or mouth when coughing or sneezing, periodically cleaning shared surfaces, avoiding close contact with people who have symptoms of a cold or flu, not sharing drinking glasses, and not going to work when sick.

Chickenpox. The best method for preventing chickenpox is the varicella (chickenpox) vaccine. The CDC recommends that all children and adults who do not have evidence of immunity to varicella be vaccinated. Evidence of immunity, according to the CDC, includes documentation of either of the following: two doses of varicella vaccine, blood tests that show immu-

nity, laboratory confirmation of prior varicella disease, a diagnosis of chickenpox or verification of a history of chickenpox from a qualified health care provider, or a diagnosis of herpes zoster (shingles) or verification of a history of herpes zoster (shingles) from a qualified health care provider.

Some people are given the chickenpox vaccine after exposure to help prevent them from contracting the disease. According to the CDC, the chickenpox vaccine is not recommended for the following people: those allergic to gelatin, those who have a moderate or serious illness, pregnant women, persons with compromised immune systems because of illness or treatment of illness, persons who have received blood or blood products three to eleven months before considering vaccination, and persons with a family history of immune deficiency.

Tuberculosis. Although a vaccine has been developed for the prevention of tuberculosis, that vaccine is not commonly used in the United States. The tuberculosis vaccine, which is known as the Bacille Calmette-Guérin vaccine, does not always protect against tuberculosis and could cause a false-positive result in people who are later tested for tuberculosis.

Preventing the spread of tuberculosis is still possible without the vaccine. For example, persons who are infected with tuberculosis can be treated before their disease becomes active. This involves regular testing of people who may be at risk. For persons who test positive for tuberculosis infection, medications that can be prescribed by doctors to help prevent active disease. Other methods of preventing the spread of tuberculosis include covering the nose and mouth with a tissue when coughing or sneezing, opening windows to ventilate rooms if the weather permits, avoiding the workplace when sick, wearing a mask around others, and avoiding close contact with family members for the first few weeks of treatment.

SYMPTOMS

Cold. Symptoms of the common cold begin from one and three days after exposure, and may include runny or stuffy nose, coughing, sneezing, congestion, sore throat, fatigue, and a general feeling of being unwell.

Flu. Flu symptoms are much like symptoms of the common cold, but are more severe. In addition to cold symptoms, persons who have the flu will also experience fever and chills, headache or body aches;

other persons, particularly children, also may experience nausea and vomiting. There are potential complications that are related to the common cold or flu. Complications may include ear infection (particularly in small children), sinus infection, bronchitis, and pneumonia.

Chickenpox. The main symptom of chickenpox is a skin rash, mostly on the face, scalp, chest, and back. The rash eventually blisters, then dries up and crusts over. Some people may also experience fever, headache, sore throat, and a general feeling of being unwell.

As with the cold and flu, some people do experience complications that are related to chickenpox. Complications may include pneumonia, skin infection, and, in rare cases, encephalitis (infection of the brain). Another complication of chickenpox may occur many years after a person has the disease. This complication is shingles, an infection that is characterized by a painful rash. It is usually seen in older adults and is caused by the same virus that causes chickenpox.

Tuberculosis. Many people who contract tuberculosis have no symptoms. Persons who are asymptomatic have latent TB (tuberculosis) infection and cannot spread the disease to others unless their disease becomes active.

When tuberculosis bacteria begin actively multiplying in the body, the person who is infected is said to have active TB disease. Symptoms of active TB include a persistent cough (sometimes coughing up blood), chest pain when breathing or coughing, fever, chills, night sweats, fatigue, loss of appetite, and weight loss. People with active TB are contagious and can spread the disease to others.

Complications from tuberculosis can be serious or even fatal. Tuberculosis complications may include lung damage, joint damage, damage to other organs, meningitis, and death.

TREATMENT

Cold. There is no cure for the common cold. Cold "treatments" are designed not to cure the cold but to relieve symptoms. Over-the-counter (OTC) drugs that can help to relieve cold symptoms include nasal sprays, decongestants, and cough medicines. These medications are not recommended for children under the age of two years unless okayed by a physician. People who have the common cold should rest and drink plenty of fluids.

Flu. As with the common cold, the "cure" for the flu is rest, liquids, and symptom relief. OTC decongestants and cough syrups can be used to relieve nasal congestion and cough. OTC pain relievers, such as Tylenol or Advil, can help to relieve headache, body aches, and sore throat.

Some fever can be beneficial because it helps the body fight the virus, so many doctors recommend that fever not be treated unless it is above 102° Fahrenheit, although an exception can be made if the fever is causing a great deal of discomfort. Fever in infants under three months of age can be a sign of a serious infection, so one should seek immediate medical attention.

In some cases, a physician may prescribe antiviral medications, which are also used for symptom reduction rather than as a cure for the flu. Antiviral medications are generally only given to people who are at increased risk of flu complications, such as young children, the elderly, pregnant women, people who are in the hospital, and people who suffer from certain chronic medical conditions.

Antibiotics will not cure the common cold or the flu. They also will not relieve cold or flu symptoms because antibiotics are used to treat bacterial infections, and both the common cold and the flu are viruses.

Chickenpox. Most healthy people do not require medical treatment for chickenpox, but some doctors may prescribe an antihistamine to help relieve itching. Oatmeal baths or calamine lotion can also help to prevent itching.

People who have other health problems or who may be considered at high risk for complications of chickenpox, may be given antiviral medications or immunoglobulin treatment. These treatments are intended to lessen the severity of the disease and, therefore, to prevent complications. OTC pain medications, such as Tylenol or Advil, can be given to reduce fever, but people with chickenpox should not be given aspirin because aspirin can cause a serious medical condition called Reye's syndrome.

Tuberculosis. Prescribed medication can prevent TB from becoming active. It can also help cure active TB.

IMPACT

According to the National Institutes of Health, the United States experiences more than 1 billion cases of the common cold each year. The World Health Organization (WHO) estimates that there are between

3 and 5 million cases of severe influenza illness each year during seasonal epidemics, resulting in between 250,000 and 500,000 deaths. CDC statistics show that during an average flu season, 5 to 20 percent of the U.S. population will get the flu and more than 200,000 will be hospitalized because of complications of the flu. Since the last decades of the twentieth century, deaths from influenza in the United States have ranged from a low of 3,000 to a high of 49,000 persons.

According to the CDC, before the varicella vaccine was developed in 1995, around 4 million cases of chickenpox were reported each year in the United States. Also, there was an average of 10,600 hospitalizations and 100 to 150 deaths. From 1995 to 2005, the incidence of chickenpox declined 90 percent overall. In 2002, hospitalizations from chickenpox had decreased 88 percent from the years 1994 and 1995. Death rates dropped 66 percent between 1990 and 2001.

WHO estimates that one-third of the world's population is infected with tuberculosis at any given time, and that 5 to 10 percent of those who are infected will develop active TB. In 2009, about 1.7 million people died from tuberculosis.

Julie Henry, R.N., M.P.A.

FURTHER READING

Centers for Disease Control and Prevention. "Basic TB Facts." Available at http://www.cdc.gov/tb/topic/basics. A tuberculosis fact sheet that includes information about how tuberculosis is spread and discusses the difference between latent TB and TB disease.

_____. "Seasonal Flu: What to Do if You Get Sick." Available at http://www.cdc.gov/flu/whattodo.htm. Discusses influenza diagnosis, symptoms, medical treatment, recovery, and emergency warning signs.

Mason, Robert J., et al., eds. *Murray and Nadel's Textbook of Respiratory Medicine.* 5th ed. Philadelphia: Saunders/Elsevier, 2010. Details basic anatomy, physiology, pharmacology, pathology, and immunology of the lungs.

Mayo Foundation for Medical Education and Research. "Chickenpox." Available at http://www.mayoclinic.com/health/chickenpox/DS00053. A detailed description of chickenpox that includes a definition of chickenpox, symptoms, risk factors, complications, prevention, and treatment.

_____. "Common Cold." Available at http://www.mayoclinic.com/health/common-cold/DS00056. A detailed description of the common cold that includes a definition of the common cold, symptoms, risk factors, complications, prevention, and treatment.

_____. "Tuberculosis." Available at http://www.mayoclinic.com/health/tuberculosis/DS00372. A detailed description of tuberculosis that includes a definition of tuberculosis, symptoms, risk factors, complications, prevention, and treatment.

MedlinePlus. "Chickenpox." Available at http://www.nlm.nih.gov/medlineplus/ency/article/001592.htm. An overview of chickenpox, including causes, symptoms, diagnosis, treatment, prevention, prognosis, and possible complications.

U.S. Department of Health and Human Services. "Tuberculosis: Getting Healthy, Staying Healthy." Available at http://www.niaid.nih.gov/topics/tuberculosis/understanding/documents/tb.pdf. An overview of tuberculosis, including how the disease is spread, how it is diagnosed, and treatment options.

WEB SITES OF INTEREST

American Academy of Family Physicians
http://familydoctor.org

Centers for Disease Control and Prevention
http://www.cdc.gov

Flu.gov
http://www.flu.gov

WebMD: Chickenpox
http://www.webmd.com/a-to-z-guides/chickenpox-varicella-topic-overview

WebMD: Cold Guide
http://www.webmd.com/cold-and-flu/cold-guide

World Health Organization
http://www.who.int

See also: Chickenpox; Common cold; Contagious diseases; Influenza; Over-the-counter (OTC) drugs; Public health; Transmission routes; Tuberculosis (TB); Vaccines: Types.

Allergic bronchopulmonary aspergillosis

CATEGORY: Diseases and conditions
ANATOMY OR SYSTEM AFFECTED: Lungs, respiratory system

DEFINITION

Allergic bronchopulmonary aspergillosis (ABPA) is an allergic lung disorder. It is related to the fungus Aspergillus fumigatus (AF). ABPA also can occur as a lung infection that spreads to other parts of the body (more common in persons with suppressed immune systems) and as a fungal growth (aspergilloma) in a lung cavity that has healed from a previous lung disease or infection.

CAUSES

ABPA is caused by an allergic reaction to inhaled AF, which is a common fungus. AF grows and flourishes in decaying vegetation and in soil, certain foods, dust, and water. The allergic reaction worsens respiratory symptoms in people with asthma or cystic fibrosis. The inhaled AF colonizes mucus in the lungs, causing sensitization to AF, recurring allergic inflammation of the lungs, and packing of the alveoli (tiny air sacs in the lungs) with eosinophils (a type of white blood cell involved in certain allergic reactions and infections with parasites).

RISK FACTORS

Risk factors for ABPA include asthma; cystic fibrosis; tuberculosis; sarcoidosis; human immunodeficiency virus (HIV); acquired immunodeficiency syndrome (AIDS); lowered immune resistance, as occurs with certain cancers or chemotherapy, or after organ transplants; use of steroid or antimicrobial medications; and hospitalization.

SYMPTOMS

Symptoms of ABPA are usually those of progressive asthma. These include shortness of breath, wheezing, weakness, malaise, unintended weight loss, and chest pain. As ABPA progresses, other symptoms may occur, including the production of thick, brownish, or bloody sputum and a low-grade fever. In severe, long-term cases, ABPA can cause bronchiectasis, the widening of areas of the bronchus usually caused by inflammation, and scarring of the lungs.

SCREENING AND DIAGNOSIS

Screening includes a chest X ray to check the lungs; sputum tests to check sputum for the presence of AF and for high levels of eosinophils; blood tests for high levels of eosinophils and for antibodies suggesting an allergic reaction to AF; skin prick tests for allergic sensitivity by placing small amounts of AF in the skin; a biopsy of lung or sinus tissue; and pulmonary function tests to monitor the breathing capacity of the lungs.

Because ABPA can appear similar to non-ABPA-induced asthma, it is often difficult to determine to what extent ABPA is contributing to symptoms. Therefore, ABPA is typically diagnosed after several repeat tests for ABPA are positive over a number of months or years.

TREATMENT AND THERAPY

The goals of treatment include suppressing the allergic reaction to AF, minimizing lung inflammation, and preventing AF from colonizing the lungs. ABPA is usually treated with two medications: prednisone (an oral corticosteroid medication) and antifungal drugs, such as itraconazole (Sporanox), amphotericin B, or voriconazole.

PREVENTION AND OUTCOMES

Avoiding exposure to AF is the best way to prevent ABPA. However, this is difficult, because AF is so prevalent in the environment. Guidelines to help prevent exposure to AF include avoiding areas with decaying vegetation and standing water; keeping the home as dust-free as possible; and remaining in air-filtered, air-conditioned environments whenever possible. Measures to avoid symptoms and prevent permanent lung damage caused by ABPA include ongoing testing and monitoring of ABPA and early and continuing medical treatment for the disease.

Rick Alan; reviewed by Christine Colpitts, M.A., CRT

FURTHER READING

Barnes, Penelope D., and Kieren A. Marr. "Aspergillosis: Spectrum of Disease, Diagnosis, and Treatment." *Infectious Disease Clinics of North America* 20 (2006): 545-561.

Ferri, Fred F., ed. *Ferri's Clinical Advisor 2011: Instant*

Diagnosis and Treatment. Philadelphia: Mosby/Elsevier, 2011.

Patterson, Thomas F. "*Aspergillus* Species." In *Mandell, Douglas, and Bennett's Principles and Practice of Infectious Diseases*, edited by Gerald L. Mandell, John F. Bennett, and Raphael Dolin. 7th ed. New York: Churchill Livingstone/Elsevier, 2010.

Porter, Robert S., et al., eds. *The Merck Manual Home Health Handbook.* 3d ed. Whitehouse Station, N.J.: Merck Research Laboratories, 2009.

Richardson, Malcolm D., and Elizabeth M. Johnson. *Pocket Guide to Fungal Infection.* 2d ed. Malden, Mass.: Blackwell, 2006.

WEB SITES OF INTEREST

American Lung Association
http://www.lungusa.org

Canadian Lung Association
http://www.lung.ca

Centers for Disease Control and Prevention
http://www.cdc.gov

See also: Airborne illness and disease; Aspergillosis; *Aspergillus*; Atypical pneumonia; Bronchiolitis; Bronchitis; Coccidiosis; Cryptococcosis; Diagnosis of fungal infections; Fungal infections; Fungi: Classification and types; Histoplasmosis; Legionnaires' disease; Mucormycosis; Paracoccidioidomycosis; Respiratory route of transmission; Soilborne illness and disease; Tuberculosis (TB); Waterborne illness and disease; Zygomycosis.

Alliance for the Prudent Use of Antibiotics

CATEGORY: Epidemiology

DEFINITION

The Alliance for the Prudent Use of Antibiotics (APUA), a nonprofit organization that seeks to improve the treatment of infectious diseases worldwide, advocates for the wise use of antibiotics and for combating the causes of antibiotic resistance. APUA was founded in 1981 by Stuart B. Levy, a professor of medicine, molecular medicine, and microbiology and director of the Center for Adaptation Genetics and Drug Resistance at Tufts University in Boston. APUA promotes education, research, surveillance, and public health policy regarding antibiotic use and resistance. APUA's work is made possible by membership contributions, private donations, government grants, and unrestricted grants from several pharmaceutical and related companies, consumer groups, and charitable foundations. APUA has members in more than one hundred countries worldwide and has affiliated chapters in sixty countries.

RESEARCH ACTIVITIES

Examples of APUA projects include the Global Advisory on Antibiotic Resistance Data project, which collects international data to provide a comprehensive overview of antibiotic-resistance patterns worldwide; the International Surveillance of Reservoirs of Resistance, which aims to analyze antibiotic resistance patterns worldwide to assist in national defense against bioterrorism; and the Antibiotic Situation and Needs Assessment project based in Uganda and Zambia, which analyzes antibiotic use and resistance in these countries to decrease mortality from pneumonia and diarrheal diseases.

PUBLIC POLICY AND EDUCATIONAL ACTIVITIES

APUA monitors and comments upon actions affecting antibiotic use by federal agencies such as the U.S. Food and Drug Administration and the U.S. Environmental Protection Agency, and by the U.S. Congress.

APUA hosts meetings, such as the EU Ban on Use of Antibiotics for Growth Promotion in Agriculture: Review of Scientific Evidence and Implications for Public Health, which was held in Paris in 2010. The APUA also provides educational materials for consumers and practitioners.

IMPACT

The scientific community has concluded that if the world community does not take notice of the growing threat of antibiotic-resistance posed to human health, more people will die from bacterial infections that cannot be treated. Routine medical procedures to simple scrapes in the school yard will carry a higher risk for serious illness and death as antibiotic-resistant bacteria, or superbugs, become more widespread not only in hospitals and other health care facilities but also in the community at large.

Since 1981, APUA has been focused on the critical importance of antibiotic resistance. In conjunction with other infectious disease and public health organizations, APUA continues to work to educate the public, health care workers, and policy makers.

Linda J. Miwa, M.P.H.

FURTHER READING

Arias, Cesar A., and Barbara E. Murray. "Antibiotic-Resistant Bugs in the Twenty-first Century: A Clinical Super-Challenge." *New England Journal of Medicine* 360 (2009): 439.

Clemmitt, Marcia. "Fighting Superbugs: Are Disease-Resistant Bacteria Becoming Unstoppable?" *CQ Researcher* 17, no. 29 (August 24, 2007): 673-696.

Groopman, Jerome. "Superbugs: The New Generation of Resistant Infections Is Almost Impossible to Treat." *The New Yorker*, August 11, 2008.

Koenig, Ellen. "The Birth of the Alliance for the Prudent Use of Antibiotics (APUA)." In *Frontiers in Antimicrobial Resistance: A Tribute to Stuart B. Levy*, edited by David G. White et al. Washington, D.C.: ASM Press, 2005.

Levy, Stuart B. *The Antibiotic Paradox: How the Misuse of Antibiotics Destroys Their Curative Powers.* Cambridge, Mass.: Perseus, 2001.

Rosenblatt-Farrell, Noah. "The Landscape of Antibiotic Resistance" *Environmental Health Perspectives* 117, no. 6 (2009): 244-250.

Science 321, no. 5887 (July 18, 2008). Special issue on antibiotic resistance.

Spellberg, Brad. *Rising Plague: The Global Threat from Deadly Bacteria and Our Dwindling Arsenal to Fight Them.* Amherst, N.Y.: Prometheus Books, 2009.

Walsh, Christopher. *Antibiotics: Actions, Origins, Resistance.* Washington, D.C.: ASM Press, 2003.

WEB SITES OF INTEREST

Alliance for the Prudent Use of Antibiotics
http://www.tufts.edu/med/apua

Centers for Disease Control and Prevention
http://www.cdc.gov/drugresistance

Keep Antibiotics Working
http://www.keepantibioticsworking.com

National Institute of Allergy and Infectious Diseases
http://www.niaid.nih.gov/topics/antimicrobialresistance

See also: Alternative therapies; Antibiotics: Experimental; Antibiotics: Types; Antifungal drugs: Types; Antiparasitic drugs: Types; Bacterial infections; Cephalosporin antibiotics; Home remedies; Hospitals and infectious disease; Iatrogenic infections; Infection; Microbiology; Mutation of pathogens; Over-the-counter (OTC) drugs; Parasitic diseases; Pathogenicity; Pathogens; Public health; Secondary infection; Superbacteria; Treatment of bacterial infections.

Alternative therapies

CATEGORY: Treatment

DEFINITION

The National Center for Complementary and Alternative Medicine (NCCAM) defines "complementary and alternative medicine," or CAM, as a group of diverse medical and health care systems, products, and practices not considered part of conventional medicine. Alternative medicine, or therapy, replaces conventional medicine. Conventional medicine includes osteopathic medicine (practiced by a doctor of osteopathy or D.O.) and allopathic medicine (practiced by a medical doctor or M.D.). Alternative therapy, for example, uses products such as echinacea, zinc, and vitamin C to decrease common cold symptoms.

Complementary medicine, or therapy, differs from alternative medicine in that it is used with, not in place of, conventional medicine; it "complements" conventional therapy. Complementary medicine combines alternative therapy with the care of medical doctors, osteopaths, and associated conventional health professionals such as psychologists, nurses, and radiologists. Complementary therapy includes, for example, using massage or aromatherapy to lessen discomfort associated with the complications and discomfort of an infectious disease treated earlier with antibiotics and surgical wound debridement.

Tested CAM therapy, which has quality scientific support, and mainstream (conventional) treatment, is known as integrative medicine. Integrative medicine combines the best of CAM and conventional medicine to optimize health and well being. An example would be the use of cranberry products to avoid repeated urinary tract infection after successful treatment of a urinary tract infection with antibiotics.

MAJOR TYPES OF CAM

Five major CAM categories, defined by the National Institutes of Health (NIH), provide a helpful outline for different complementary and alternative options. The five categories are alternative medical systems, biological based systems, manipulative and body-based systems, mind-body interventions, and energy therapies. These categories organize alternative and complementary approaches, and this organization guides study and approaches to CAM therapies.

Alternative medical systems. Complete systems of theory and practice and central philosophies define alternative medical systems, such as traditional Chinese medicine (TCM) and Ayurvedic medicine. Multiculturalism and ancient heritage provided by medical systems outside Western conventional care provide attractive alternatives for many people seeking to optimize their health and well being. TCM and Ayurvedic medicine (in India) are integral to local heritage and culture. TCM and Ayurvedic medicine are mainstream in China and India because of thousands of years of practice in those countries; the practices now coexist with conventional medicine.

The NIH, through NCCAM, analyzes and funds studies of alternative medical systems and procedures to best determine what health care approaches have benefit. The NIH has determined that scientific evidence supports needle acupuncture to treat nausea and vomiting associated with chemotherapy and postoperatively. Some infectious disease treatments, such as surgical wound debridement, result in pain and discomfort; these types of problems could be alleviated with acupuncture techniques. More follow-up study can help to develop the effective range of acupuncture as adjunct to conventional medicine in the treatment of infectious diseases.

Western cultures have developed alternative medical systems that include homeopathic and naturopathic medicine. Homeopathy began in Germany in the late eighteenth century with the work of Samuel Christian Hahnemann, and naturopathy started in Europe in the nineteenth century. Naturopathy's healing system shares many principles with conventional medicine, including the principles of first doing no harm, and the identification and treatment of disease origins. Major naturopathic tenets involve belief in nature's healing power, teaching, and disease prevention.

Hahnemann founded homeopathy by selecting therapies based on how closely symptoms produced by remedies matched the symptoms of the disease. He named this the principle of similars. A similar procedure is used in modern vaccine development. Homeopathic practice includes careful examinations of the mental, emotional, and physical aspects of a person's health and the analysis of distinctive personality and physical traits.

Homeopathy uses dilute liquid and pills. Minute or nonexistent amounts of the original molecules remain after vigorous shaking and multiple dilutions. The contention is that the "memory" of the original molecule impacts surrounding water molecules, and that this essence confers therapeutic properties to the solutions. Most scientific study finds little evidence supporting homeopathy. Skepticism exists in part because nonexistent or minuscule doses are used in homeopathic remedies. Although most analyses do not support homeopathy, NCCAM has identified some studies, laboratory research, and clinical trials supporting homeopathic remedies.

Biologically based therapies. Biologically based treatments are natural compounds that include herbs, food supplements, and vitamins. Many find the natural aspect of these therapies alluring, but natural products interact with prescription drugs and have side effects, some quite serious. The difference between the regulation of prescription medications and the regulation of herbs, food supplements, and vitamins is important to understand. The approval and marketing of prescription medications require extensive clinical testing and clinical trials. Regulation of dietary supplements resembles the regulation of salt and pepper production more than it resembles the regulation of prescription drugs. Regulation of supplements, and production oversight, varies greatly from the regulation of prescription drugs.

Aromatherapy studies provide scientific evidence supporting beneficial effects. Infections caused by bacteria, viruses, or fungi have been shown to respond positively to various aromatherapies. Fragrant essences, found in plants such as geranium, roman chamomile, lavender, lemon, and cedar wood, are extracted as essential oils from plants in natural ways.

Aromatherapy includes inhalation or skin application of these oils. Studies consistently show that pleasant odors improve mood and reduce anxiety. Aromatherapies offer a sense of well being, calm, and energy.

Many studies document antibacterial effects with the application of the essential oils on skin. Antifungal activity against some vaginal and mouth fungus infections has been demonstrated. Some essential oils have been shown to alleviate problems associated with infections caused by the herpes simplex virus.

Stressed rats in laboratory experiments developed enhanced immune responses when exposed to certain aromas. Aromatherapy is usually thought of as a positive adjustment of the central nervous system, but one study showed that markers of the fragrant aromas are found in the blood. This could mean that aromatherapy agents act like drugs or medications, rather than as adjusters of brain perception. Side effects of aromatherapy include dermatitis and allergies.

Milk thistle seeds are used to treat liver diseases. A strong antioxidant, silymarin, provides the active ingredient for milk thistle. Silymarin regenerates liver tissue and may aid treatments of hepatitis and may work as adjunctive liver cancer therapy, helping chemotherapeutic agents. More study will help isolate therapeutic benefits of silymarin.

Cranberries, a fruit, may help prevent urinary tract infections (UTIs) and reduce *Helicobacter pylori* stomach infections that cause ulcers. Although some evidence supports using cranberries for UTI prevention, cranberries are not effective treatments for existing UTIs. Cranberries may keep bacteria such as *Escherichia coli and H. pylori* from adhering to cell wells in the urinary tract and in stomach linings, thus preventing UTIs and stomach ulcers.

Cranberries are found in juices and dietary supplements. Tablets or capsules of cranberry extracts are available as well. The excessive use of cranberry juice extracts or beverages can result in diarrhea or gastrointestinal upset. Although cranberry products may help prevent UTIs, the diagnosis and treatment of UTIs should be done by qualified health care personnel. Cranberries may interact with medications affecting the liver or with blood thinning drugs.

Echinacea is thought to kindle the immune system and prevent or treat colds, the flu, or other infections. NCCAM funded studies that did not support the use of echinacea for colds, but other studies showed that echinacea may be beneficial for both the treatment and the prevention of colds. Echinacea is used as a tea, a pill extract, or as juice. Allergic reactions can occur, particularly among those who have asthma, genetic tendencies to allergic reactions, or allergies to ragweed, marigold, chrysanthemum, and daisy. Echinacea comes from plants in the daisy family.

Goldenseal is a plant used for respiratory tract infections and colds. Some cold preparations combine goldenseal with echinacea. Native Americans traditionally use goldenseal for a variety of ailments, including gonorrhea and ulcers. Goldenseal is also used for gastrointestinal infections, vaginal infections, and eye infections. Sore throats and canker sores are treated with goldenseal too. Little scientific evidence supports the use of goldenseal for any of these infections, but more study may show that an active goldenseal ingredient, berberine, can help with some infections, like those causing diarrhea.

Vitamin C and zinc preparations are often used to treat colds. A primary goal of vitamin C and zinc use is to decrease the duration and perhaps the severity of the illness. No cure exists for colds in either conventional or alternative medicine. Studies indicate that zinc doses higher than 70 milligrams daily reduce cold duration, and other studies support vitamin C use for cold-symptom reduction.

Different viruses cause colds and influenza. No vaccine or conventional antibiotic exists to treat or prevent these viral infections. Many vitamins, minerals, herbs, and other compounds, such as honey, peppermint, selenium, or ginseng, are used in an attempt to fill in this treatment and prevention gap. Elderberries and elder flowers are used for flu, colds, sinus infections, and fevers. With the possible exception of echinacea, zinc, and vitamin C, the various other remedies do not have much scientific support for their use, particularly in children. Handwashing prevents the spread of cold and flu viruses, and frequent handwashing, particularly in cold and flu seasons, provides a reasonable approach to cold and flu prevention.

Manipulative and body-based methods. Manipulation or movement of body parts characterizes these therapeutic techniques. Massage therapy is helpful for stress relief and the discomfort experienced with many chronic conditions, including acquired immunodeficiency syndrome (AIDS) and recurrent hepatitis. Trager bodywork, Rolfing, reflexology, the Alexander and Bowen techniques, the Feldenkrais method, and chiropractic or osteopathic manipulations are some of the therapies and techniques in this category. Popular in the United States, chiropractic and massage therapy appointments represent one-half of all visits to CAM practitioners in the United States.

Bones, joints, and muscles, and the circulatory and lymphatic systems, are often the focus of these body-based therapies. An emphasis on the interdependence of body parts, body self-regulation, and the "laying on of hands" are desirable methods for people seeking relief from health problems and for those trying to optimize individual health.

Mind-body interventions. A variety of processes in this category, such as meditation, prayer, group support, and self-hypnosis, enhance overall well being. Creative channels tapped in music, art, dance, and writing, improve interaction between the mind and physical symptoms.

Self-hypnosis is a mind-body intervention that improves self-confidence and fosters positive attitudes. Self-hypnotic positive attitudes and autosuggestions can enhance pain relief, help manage stress, improve immune response, and improve diseases like asthma and arthritis. Focused concentration and a willingness to follow one's own instructions are important parts

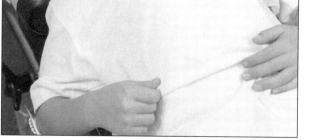

A boy receives chiropractic care, a type of alternative therapy. (PhotoDisc)

of successful self-hypnosis. A personal mantra, such as "My confidence grows daily because I am getting better," can help focus one's thoughts.

Energy therapies. Energy therapies claim that manipulating energy fields enhances well being. Scientific proof of these energy fields is lacking, and these energy fields have not been sufficiently measured in controlled scientific studies. Biofield therapies, such as therapeutic touch and Reiki, purportedly change energy fields surrounding the body to enhance wellness and health. Practitioners of these types of therapies claim that biofields change by applying forces on, in, or through these energy fields. Bioelectromagnetic therapies use electromagnetic fields, including direct-current and alternating-current fields. Pulsed and magnetic electromagnetic fields also are used in these alternative therapies.

Steps for Self-Hypnosis

Step 1. This relaxation phase requires about thirty minutes in a comfortable setting with no disturbances. Tension release can be accomplished with deep breathing exercises or the progressive relaxation of muscle groups. One should visualize tightness and tension lightening from the toes to the top of the head.

Step 2. Induction occurs by imagining oneself on a pleasant journey, such as a walk along a beach, a stroll along a wooded path, or descending a long spiral staircase. The idea is to bring one's mind to another place.

Step 3. One should repeat his or her positive mantra many times and should use positive affirmations to help achieve a goal.

Step 4. After about thirty minutes, come back from the journey; walk back along the beach, wooded path, spiral staircase, or other path taken.

IMPACT

Sick persons want to optimize their health and get better, and persons who are well want to stay healthy. To do so, one should consult conventional health care providers, including allopathic and osteopathic providers, about individual health care issues. No substitute exists for the advice and medical expertise of primary care providers, and decisions about treatment or care options should be discussed with these providers.

Conventional health care is an important part of any health care plan, but people who seek out and use CAM therapies want to maintain health and optimize disease defense mechanisms. Most CAM users do not reject conventional health care; they simply want to enhance their overall well being. Typical CAM users are inquisitive and educate themselves on the various aspects of illness or disease prevention. CAM users are often health enthusiasts, in much the same way that exercisers study various options for optimal physical fitness.

Critical thinking skills are important when using alternative therapies for infectious disease. CAM therapies should be discussed with one's conventional health care provider. Critical thinking helps decipher the many options available and helps discern whether a therapy is helpful or harmful. Integrative medicine incorporates the best CAM with indicated alternative or complementary treatments. Some scientific studies have been completed on CAM treatments, but more scientific studies are needed to uncover potentially helpful alternative treatments.

Optimal wellness techniques meld scientific-based medical care with the best of CAM. Integrative medical systems often involve more personal responsibility for individual wellness. More responsibility engenders a healthier lifestyle, enabling better choices. CAM users have many options available. The challenge is sorting out what is best for an individual and how to best develop a healthy lifestyle. More study and knowledge of healthy mechanisms enables successful health preservation and the ability to prevent and treat infectious disease processes when they occur.

Richard P. Capriccioso, M.D.

FURTHER READING

"Complementary and Alternative Medicine." In *Current Medical Diagnosis and Treatment 2011*, edited by Stephen J. McPhee and Maxine A. Papadakis. 50th ed. New York: McGraw-Hill Medical, 2011.

Fontaine, K. L. *Complementary and Alternative Therapies for Nursing Practice*. 2d ed. Upper Saddle River, N.J.: Prentice Hall, 2005. Well organized and informative, this work includes sections that integrate CAM and nursing practices.

Linde, K., et al. "Echinacea for Preventing and Treating the Common Cold." *Cochrane Database of Systematic Reviews* (2006): CD000530. Available through *EBSCO DynaMed Systematic Literature Surveillance* at http://www.ebscohost.com/dynamed.

Peters, David, and Anne Woodham. *Encyclopedia of Natural Healing*. London: DK, 2000. A well-illustrated compendium of CAM therapies, with information on CAM practitioners and organizations.

WEB SITES OF INTEREST

Clean Hands Coalition
http://www.cleanhandscoalition.org

Mayo Clinic, Complementary and Alternative Medicine
http://mayoclinic.com/health/alternative-medicine/pn00001

National Center for Complementary and Alternative Medicine
http://nccam.nih.gov

See also: Common cold; Home remedies; Hyperbaric oxygen; Infection; Influenza; Over-the-counter (OTC) drugs; Stress and infectious disease; Treatment of bacterial infections; Treatment of fungal infections; Treatment of viral infections.

Amebic dysentery

CATEGORY: Diseases and conditions
ANATOMY OR SYSTEM AFFECTED: Gastrointestinal system, intestines, stomach
ALSO KNOWN AS: Amebiasis

DEFINITION

Amebic dysentery is a treatable intestinal illness associated with stomach pain, bloody stools, and fever.

<table>
<tr><td>

Key Terms

- *Colitis.* Inflammation of the large intestine (colon), which usually is associated with bloody diarrhea and fever

- *Diarrhea.* Loose or watery stools, usually a decrease in consistency or increase in frequency from an individual baseline

- *Intestines.* The tube connecting the stomach and anus in which nutrients are absorbed from food; divided into the small intestine and the colon, or large intestine

- *Mucosa.* The semipermeable layers of cells lining the gut, through which fluid and nutrients are absorbed

- *Peristalsis.* The wavelike muscular contractions that move food and waste products through the intestines; problems with peristalsis are called motility disorders

- *Stool.* The waste products expelled from the body through the anus during defecation; feces

</td></tr>
</table>

CAUSES

Amebic dysentery is caused by the parasitic protozoan *Entamoeba histolytica.* A person can develop amebic dysentery by placing something in his or her mouth that has touched the stool of a person infected with *E. histolytica,* by swallowing water or food that has been contaminated with *E. histolytica,* and by touching cysts (eggs) from *E. histolytica*-contaminated surfaces and bringing those cysts to the mouth.

RISK FACTORS

The risk factors that increase the chance of developing amebic dysentery include living in or traveling to developing countries, places that have poor sanitary conditions, or tropical or subtropical areas; living in institutions; and having anal intercourse.

SYMPTOMS

The symptoms of amebic dysentery include loose stools, nausea, weight loss, stomach pain, stomach cramping, bloody stools, fever, and (rarely) liver abscesses.

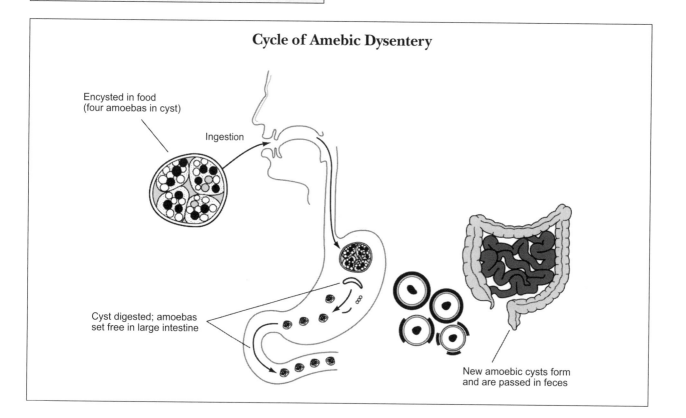

Cycle of Amebic Dysentery

Encysted in food
(four amoebas in cyst)

Ingestion

Cyst digested; amoebas
set free in large intestine

New amoebic cysts form
and are passed in feces

SCREENING AND DIAGNOSIS

Tests for amebic dysentery include stool samples and blood tests.

TREATMENT AND THERAPY

Several antibiotics are available to treat amebic dysentery.

PREVENTION AND OUTCOMES

To help reduce the chance of getting amebic dysentery, one should take the following steps when traveling to a country that has poor sanitation: Drink only bottled water or water that has been boiled for a minimum of one minute; avoid eating fresh fruit or vegetables that have been peeled by another person; avoid eating or drinking unpasteurized milk, cheese, or dairy products; and avoid eating or drinking items sold by street vendors.

Krisha McCoy, M.S.;
reviewed by David L. Horn, M.D., FACP

FURTHER READING

Centers for Disease Control and Prevention. "Amebiasis." Available at http://www.cdc.gov.

DuPont, Herbert L., and Charles D. Ericsson. "Drug Therapy: Prevention and Treatment of Travelers' Diarrhea." *New England Journal of Medicine* 328 (June 24, 1993): 1821-1826.

EBSCO Publishing. *DynaMed: Amoebic Dysentery.* Available through http://www.ebscohost.com/dynamed.

"Infectious Diarrheal Diseases and Bacterial Food Poisoning." In *Harrison's Principles of Internal Medicine,* edited by Joan Butterton. 17th ed. New York: McGraw-Hill, 2008.

Johnson, Leonard R., ed. *Gastrointestinal Physiology.* 7th ed. Philadelphia: Mosby/Elsevier, 2007.

WEB SITES OF INTEREST

American College of Gastroenterology
http://www.acg.gi.org

American Society of Tropical Medicine and Hygiene
http://www.astmh.org

Centers for Disease Control and Prevention
http://www.cdc.gov/parasites

National Center for Emerging and Zoonotic Infectious Diseases
http://www.cdc.gov/ncezid

National Institute of Allergy and Infectious Diseases
http://www.niaid.nih.gov

See also: Antibiotic-associated colitis; Ascariasis; *Campylobacter*; Cholera; Cryptosporidiosis; Developing countries and infectious disease; Diverticulitis; Enteritis; Fecal-oral route of transmission; Food-borne illness and disease; Giardiasis; Hookworms; Intestinal and stomach infections; Norovirus infection; Parasitic diseases; Parasitology; Protozoan diseases; Travelers' diarrhea; Tropical medicine; Typhoid fever; Waterborne illness and disease.

Aminoglycoside antibiotics

CATEGORY: Treatment

DEFINITION

Aminoglycoside is an antibacterial drug class that consists of six-membered rings with amino (NH2) and glycoside groups, derived from or related to the soil bacteria *Streptomyces*, which block bacterial ribosomal functions.

DISEASES TREATED

Aminoglycosides, such as neomycin, kanamycin, tobramycin, and daptomycin, are active primarily against aerobic, gram-negative bacilli. The first aminoglycoside, named streptomycin for its origin in *Streptomyces* soil bacteria, was discovered in 1943 and was used to treat tuberculosis caused by *Mycobacterium tuberculosis*. All aminoglycoside antibiotics are naturally or synthetically derived from either *Streptomyces* or *Micromonospora* soil bacteria and treat similar types of bacterial infections. Aminoglycosides are active against *Neisseria gonorrhoeae* and *Pseudomonas aeruginosa* and against more common gram-negative pathogens. They are used topically for eye and ear infections and for skin infections resulting from burns or ulcers. These antibiotics also may successfully treat serious infections such as sepsis, meningitis, and enterococcal endocarditis.

ADMINISTRATION

Drugs in the aminoglycoside class generally have a short half-life of two to three hours and have poor oral absorption. Neomycin in particular is used frequently in topical creams or ointments for minor infections and in topical liquid preparations for eye and ear infections. Aminoglycosides are administered parenterally (by injection into a muscle or vein) in cases of complicated infection to achieve high enough drug levels for antibacterial action. Aminoglycosides also are given by oral inhalation to treat lung infections such as pneumonia and as topical irrigations to treat skin infections locally.

MECHANISM OF ACTION

Aminoglycosides disrupt bacterial cell-wall permeability to a degree proportional to the antibiotic concentration in bacterial cells. Specifically, aminoglycosides reversibly bind to mRNA (messenger ribonucleic acid) nucleotides at the 30S subunits of prokaryotic ribosomes. This binding causes conformational changes in the bacterial cell adenines, which blocks translation of mRNA in the cell. The ribosomal binding reduces protein synthesis in the cell wall. Resistance to aminoglycosides is rare but focuses on A-to-G mutations and on changes in the subunit that decrease binding of the drugs.

SIDE EFFECTS

The primary side effects of aminoglycosides are nephrotoxicity, ototoxicity, and increased neuromuscular block. Nephrotoxicity may be reversible and proportional to dose, whereas ototoxicity is possibly irreversible. Persons who receive aminoglycosides, especially for more than two weeks, should be observed carefully for any early signs of ear and hearing damage. Neuromuscular block alone is infrequent but is more likely when aminoglycosides are given concomitantly with drugs that inhibit acetylcholine, such as pancuronium. Side effects of aminoglycosides are more likely to occur in older persons, and they can be reduced by using shorter treatment courses and dosing regimens designed to minimize toxicity.

IMPACT

Aminoglycosides were developed from natural sources in the 1940's, leading to increased resistance and high toxicity and contributing to its reduced use. In the early twenty-first century, medical treatments often combine beta-lactams with cephalosporins instead of aminoglycosides for these reasons. However,

aminoglycosides are still used for serious infections and they retain usefulness in remote areas of the world. As resistance develops to agents in the beta-lactam class, aminoglycosides may again prove necessary in more populated areas of the world.

Nicole M. Van Hoey, Pharm.D.

FURTHER READING

Durante-Mangoni, E., et al. "Do We Still Need the Aminoglycosides?" *International Journal of Antimicrobial Agents* 33, no. 3 (2009): 201-205.

Gilbert, David N., and James E. Leggett. "Aminoglycosides." In *Mandell, Douglas, and Bennett's Principles and Practice of Infectious Diseases*, edited by Gerald L. Mandell, John F. Bennett, and Raphael Dolin. 7th ed. New York: Churchill Livingstone/Elsevier, 2010.

Leibovici, L., L. Vidal, and M. Paul. "Aminoglycoside Drugs in Clinical Practice: An Evidence-Based Approach." *Journal of Antimicrobial Chemotherapy* 62, no. 2 (2009): 246-251.

The Merck Manuals, Online Medical Library. "Aminoglycosides." Available at http://www.merck.com/mmpe.

Murray, Patrick R., Ken S. Rosenthal, and Michael A. Pfaller. "Antibacterial Agents." In *Medical Microbiology*. 6th ed. Philadelphia: Mosby/Elsevier, 2009.

Sanford, Jay P., et al. *The Sanford Guide to Antimicrobial Therapy*. 18th ed. Sperryville, Va.: Antimicrobial Therapy, 2010.

Wilson, Michael, Brian Henderson, and Rod McNab. *Bacterial Disease Mechanisms: An Introduction to Cellular Microbiology*. New York: Cambridge University Press, 2002.

WEB SITES OF INTEREST

The Merck Manuals, Online Medical Library
http://www.merck.com/mmpe

Todar's Online Textbook of Bacteriology
http://www.textbookofbacteriology.net

See also: Antibiotics: Types; Bacterial infections; Cephalosporin antibiotics; Kidney infection; *Mycobacterium*; Neisserial infections; Penicillin antibiotics; *Pseudomonas*; *Pseudomonas* infections; Soilborne illness and disease.

Anal abscess

CATEGORY: Diseases and conditions
ANATOMY OR SYSTEM AFFECTED: Anus, gastrointestinal system, glands, rectum, skin
ALSO KNOWN AS: Anal fistula, anal rectal abscess, anal rectal fistula, anorectal abscess, anorectal fistula

DEFINITION

An anal abscess is a pus-filled glandular cavity near the anus, either deep in the rectum or close to the opening of the anus. Between eight and nine of every ten thousand persons will experience this condition.

CAUSES

An anal abscess results when bacteria infect a mucus-secreting gland in the anus or rectum, causing blockage and damage to surrounding intramuscular tissue. It is unknown why the infection occurs because, normally, this area is free from infection.

RISK FACTORS

The chance of developing an anal abscess increases for males and for persons with colitis or other inflammatory bowel disease, such as Crohn's disease.

SYMPTOMS

In the case of an abscess near the surface of the skin on the buttocks, the symptoms will include pain and tenderness radiating from the location of the abscess, visible redness and swelling, and fever. In the case of an abscess located deeper within the rectum, the symptoms will include pain in the lower abdomen, swelling in the rectum that can be seen during examination of the rectum, and fever. Furthermore, anal abscesses may be accompanied by pain with stool or stool incontinence (inability to restrain stools), or both.

SCREENING AND DIAGNOSIS

Although a doctor will be able to see an abscess near the surface of the skin, he or she also may need to examine the rectum with a gloved finger to determine the presence of a deeper abscess.

TREATMENT AND THERAPY

Treatment normally consists of draining the abscess, which is done by making an incision through the skin near the anus into the abscess. For this, a local anesthesia is administered. In rare cases, admittance to a hospital is required, and the patient might receive a general anesthesia. Antibiotics may be given to reduce fever or under other special circumstances.

Following drainage (or natural rupture) of an abscess, more than one-half the cases will develop into anal fistulas (usually occurring weeks but sometimes years later). In this condition, a permanent abnormal channel is formed from the site of the original abscess to the surface of the skin near the anus. This channel (fistula) allows for the continuous drainage of the abscesses' puslike fluid. In the case of a fistula, surgery to remove and close the channel is normally recommended. Recurrence of a fistula is common, and stool incontinence may occur, after surgery.

PREVENTION AND OUTCOMES

There are no known ways to prevent anal abscesses or subsequent fistulas because the cause of the original infection of the anal glands is unknown.

Amanda Barrett, M.A.; reviewed by David L. Horn, M.D., FACP

FURTHER READING

"Abscess." In *Ferri's Clinical Advisor 2011: Instant Diagnosis and Treatment*, edited by Fred F. Ferri. Philadelphia: Mosby/Elsevier, 2011.

"Abscesses." In *The Merck Manual Home Health Handbook*, edited by Robert S. Porter et al. 3d ed. Whitehouse Station, N.J.: Merck Research Laboratories, 2009.

American College of Gastroenterology. "Common Gastrointestinal Problems: Rectal Complaints." Available at http://www.acg.gi.org/patients/cgp/cgpvol3.asp#rectal.

EBSCO Publishing. *DynaMed: Fistual-in-Ano*. Available through http://www.ebscohost.com/dynamed.

WEB SITES OF INTEREST

American College of Gastroenterology
http://www.acg.gi.org

American Society of Colon and Rectal Surgeons
http://www.fascrs.org

See also: Abscesses; Bacterial infections; Boils; Men and infectious disease; Pilonidal cyst; Skin infections.

Anaplasmosis

CATEGORY: Diseases and conditions
ANATOMY OR SYSTEM AFFECTED: All
ALSO KNOWN AS: Human granulocytic anaplasmosis,
human granulocytic ehrlichiosis

DEFINITION

Anaplasmosis is an infection caused by the bite of a tick infected with the bacterium *Anaplasma phagocytophilum*.

CAUSES

A. phagocytophilum is transmitted by black-legged ticks (*Ixodes* (tick) *scapularis*) and Pacific black-legged ticks (*I. pacificus*) in North America, by the common tick (*I. ricinus*) in Europe, and by the Taiga tick (*I. persulcatus*) in Asia. Common reservoirs for ixodid ticks include deer and the white-footed mouse (*Peromyscus leucopus*) and other small mammals.

RISK FACTORS

People who frequent tick-infested environments are at risk of being bitten by an infected tick and of contracting anaplasmosis. Immunocompromised persons are at greater risk of complications if not treated promptly.

SYMPTOMS

The symptoms of anaplasmosis typically occur within three weeks of exposure to a tick bite and include fever, headache, chills, muscle aches, vomiting, and malaise. The nonspecific nature of symptoms can make it difficult to diagnose anaplasmosis, but expedient treatment is important to reduce the chance of complications from the disease, particularly in immunocompromised persons.

SCREENING AND DIAGNOSIS

Anaplasmosis may be suspected based on a person's symptoms and a history of recent tick exposure. Infection can be confirmed by identifying the bacterium in blood samples by polymerase chain reaction and by testing blood serum for antibodies by indirect fluorescent antibody assay. Blood samples may also indicate infection by the characteristic clustering of bacteria in infected cells.

TREATMENT AND THERAPY

Tetracycline antibiotics, particularly doxycycline, are prescribed for the treatment of anaplasmosis. Ten to fourteen days is the typical course of treatment.

PREVENTION AND OUTCOMES

The best way to prevent anaplasmosis is to avoid habitats where ticks are likely to be found; these habitats include wooded areas and tall grasses. Because avoidance of these habitats is not always possible or preferable, one can take measures to limit exposure to ticks, such as by wearing light-colored clothing to increase the visibility of ticks, by applying repellents containing permethrin or NN-diethyl metatoluamide (DEET), and by thoroughly checking one's body for ticks, particularly around the hairline.

Susan Gifford, M.S.

FURTHER READING

Bakken, J. S., and J. S. Dumler. "Clinical Diagnosis and Treatment of Human Granulocytotropic Anaplasmosis." *Annals of the New York Academy of Sciences* 1078 (October, 2006): 236-247.

Bratton, R. L., and G. R. Corey. "Tick-Borne Disease." *American Family Physician* 71 (2005): 2323.

Chapman, Alice S., et al. "Diagnosis and Management of Tickborne Rickettsial Diseases: Rocky Mountain Spotted Fever, Ehrlichioses, and Anaplasmosis—United States." *Morbidity and Mortality Weekly Report* 55, RR-4 (March 31, 2006).

Demma, Linda J., et al. "Epidemiology of Human Ehrlichiosis and Anaplasmosis in the United States, 2001-2002." *American Journal of Tropical Medicine and Hygiene* 73, no. 2 (2005): 400-409.

Wormser, Gary P. "The Clinical Assessment, Treatment, and Prevention of Lyme Disease, Human Granulocytic Anaplasmosis, and Babesiosis: Clinical Practice Guidelines by the Infectious Diseases Society of America." *IDSA Guidelines*, November 1, 2006, p. 43.

WEB SITES OF INTEREST

American Lyme Disease Foundation
http://www.aldf.com/anaplasmosis

Centers for Disease Control and Prevention
http://www.cdc.gov/ticks/diseases/anaplasmosis

Infectious Diseases Society of America
http://www.idsociety.org

See also: Acariasis; Arthropod-borne illness and disease; Bacterial infections; Blood-borne illness and disease; Colorado tick fever; Ehrlichiosis; Encephalitis; Hemorrhagic fever viral infections; Lyme disease; Mediterranean spotted fever; Mites and chiggers and infectious disease; *Rickettsia*; Rocky Mountain spotted fever; Ticks and infectious disease; Transmission routes; Vectors and vector control.

Aneurysm. *See* Mycotic aneurysm.

Anthrax

CATEGORY: Diseases and conditions
ANATOMY OR SYSTEM AFFECTED: All

DEFINITION

Anthrax is an infection caused by bacteria that can be life-threatening. The disease is more common in hoofed animals, such as cattle and goats. In rare cases, people can contract anthrax infection from infected animals or anthrax spores. The bacteria produce spores that can survive in the environment for decades.

There are three forms of human anthrax, and they are identified according to where the spores enter the body. These forms are inhalation anthrax (about 5 percent of cases), caused by breathing airborne spores into the lungs; cutaneous or skin anthrax (about 95 percent of cases), caused by spores entering a cut or break in the skin; and gastrointestinal anthrax (extremely rare), caused by ingesting spores in raw or undercooked food.

CAUSES

The bacterium *Bacillus anthracis* causes anthrax. Anthrax occurs after exposure to infected animals, infected animal products, and bacterial spores. Once in the body, the spores germinate, meaning that the spores change to the active bacteria. They multiply and release toxins, leading to swelling, bleeding, and tissue death. All forms of anthrax can cause death. Only 10 to 20 percent of untreated cutaneous cases, however, are lethal. Inhalation anthrax is highly lethal

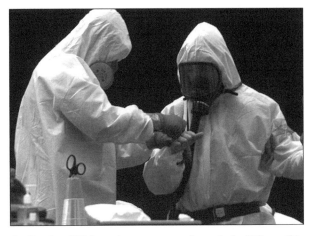

In October, 2001, anthrax was sent through the U.S. mail in an act of bioterrorism. Here, a firefighter decontaminates a federal law enforcement officer after they leave a building where an envelope with anthrax was found. (AP/Wide World Photos)

once symptoms develop, and death can occur within a few days.

RISK FACTORS

Risk factors for anthrax include working in a laboratory with *B. anthracis*, working with anthrax-infected animals (such as on a farm or at a leather tannery, woolery, or veterinary clinic) or animal products, and exposure to acts of biological terrorism or other criminal acts that involve anthrax.

SYMPTOMS

The symptoms usually start within a few days of exposure, and they vary depending on the type of disease. Inhalation anthrax symptoms occur in stages over several days and include cold or flu symptoms such as cough, fatigue, weakness, fever, chills, headache, and muscle aches. There is sometimes a brief period of seeming recovery, followed by rapid onset of severe difficulty in breathing, chest pain, sweating, shock, delirium, and death.

Cutaneous or skin symptoms occur in the following stages: raised bump, like an insect bite, that is itchy and round; the raised area opens, forming an ulcer with a black area in the center and producing drainage of clear or pinkish fluid; swelling around the wound; and swollen, painful lymph nodes.

Gastrointestinal lesions can occur in the mouth and throat. Symptoms include sores in the mouth or esophagus, swelling in the throat, swollen lymph nodes, and sore throat. Lesions can occur in the intestines too, with symptoms including nausea, vomiting, fever, abdominal pain, and bloody diarrhea.

SCREENING AND DIAGNOSIS

A doctor or other health care provider will look for a possible source of exposure and also perform a physical examination of the patient. Tests may include a chest X ray for inhalation anthrax; cultures of wounds, mucous membranes, and body fluids to check for bacteria; and a blood test to detect antibodies to anthrax.

TREATMENT AND THERAPY

Infected persons should start antibiotics early, as any delay greatly increases the risk of death in cases of inhalation anthrax. Treatment, begun intravenously, includes oral antibiotics for several weeks. Skin lesions are carefully cleaned and dressed with bandages. The patient might be prescribed ciprofloxacin (Cipro), penicillin, or doxycycline.

Finding the source of the anthrax is critical. Public health officials will check the patient's home and place of work. Contaminated surfaces should be disinfected. Other people who may have been exposed will be tested, and they might be given antibiotics.

PREVENTION AND OUTCOMES

It is difficult to know if one has been exposed to anthrax because it is colorless and has no smell or taste. One case could lead to fears that others in the same environment might have encountered the spores. Antibiotics may be able to prevent infection following exposure, but a vaccine exists to help prevent anthrax in the first place. The vaccination requires multiple injections and is only partially effective. The vaccine is not recommended for the general population but is routinely given to certain military personnel. Strategies to prevent exposure to anthrax include avoiding contact with infected animals or animal products and avoiding fluid that is draining from an anthrax wound.

Debra Wood, R.N.;
reviewed by David L. Horn, M.D., FACP

FURTHER READING

Andreoli, Thomas E., et al., eds. *Andreoli and Carpenter's Cecil Essentials of Medicine.* 8th ed. Philadelphia: Saunders/Elsevier, 2010.

Centers for Disease Control and Prevention. "Bioterrorism-Related Anthrax." *Emerging Infectious Diseases* 8 (October, 2002): 1013-1183.

_____. "Use of Anthrax Vaccine in the United States: Recommendations of the Advisory Committee on Immunization Practices." *Morbidity and Mortality Weekly Report* 49 (2000): 1-20.

Dixon, Terry C., et al. "Anthrax." *New England Journal of Medicine* 341 (September 9, 1999): 815-826.

EBSCO Publishing. *DynaMed: Anthrax.* Available through http://www.ebscohost.com/dynamed.

Kyrincou, Demetrios N., Alys Adamski, and Nanci Khardori. "Anthrax: From Antiquity and Obscurity to a Front-Runner in Bioterrorism." *Infectious Disease Clinics of North America* 20 (2006): 227-251.

Mandell, Gerald L., John E. Bennett, and Raphael Dolin, eds. *Mandell, Douglas, and Bennett's Principles and Practice of Infectious Diseases.* 7th ed. New York: Churchill Livingstone/Elsevier, 2010.

WEB SITES OF INTEREST

Center for Biosecurity
http://www.upmc-biosecurity.org

Centers for Disease Control and Prevention, Emergency Preparedness and Response
http://emergency.cdc.gov

U.S. Department of Health and Human Services
http://www.hhs.gov

U.S. Surgeon General's Office: Anthrax Vaccine Information Program
http://www.anthrax.osd.mil

See also: Airborne illness and disease; Anthrax vaccine; Atypical pneumonia; Bacterial infections; Biological weapons; Bioterrorism; Botulinum toxin infection; Botulism; Bubonic plague; *Clostridium*; Food-borne illness and disease; Glanders; Melioidosis; Plague; Respiratory route of transmission; SARS; Smallpox; Soilborne illness and disease; Tularemia; Zoonotic diseases.

Anthrax vaccine

CATEGORY: Prevention

DEFINITION

The anthrax vaccine is used to prevent infection with anthrax, a serious and sometimes fatal disease caused by the bacterium *Bacillus anthracis*. The vaccine protects against cutaneous anthrax (the most common form) and inhalation anthrax.

HISTORY AND DEVELOPMENT

The anthrax vaccine was licensed in 1970 in the United States after a successful clinical trial of a precursor formulation in mills that processed imported animal hair. Based on this research, experts estimate that the vaccine is 92.5 percent effective. Only one anthrax vaccine is licensed for use in the United States (Anthrax Vaccine Adsorbed, or BioThrax), but new vaccine formulations have been in development.

RECOMMENDATIONS

The Centers for Disease Control and Prevention recommends vaccination against anthrax for persons between the age of eighteen and sixty-five years who could be exposed to large amounts of *B. anthracis* as part of their jobs; these jobs include certain types of laboratory or remediation work, work with animals or animal products, and work in specific U.S. Department of Defense-designated occupations (including certain military and associated personnel).

Women who are nursing can safely receive the vaccine, and it may be recommended to pregnant women who have been exposed to inhalation anthrax. However, persons with a history of a severe allergic reaction to the vaccine or any other vaccine or vaccine component should not get the vaccine; health care providers may recommend against vaccination in sick persons and in persons with Guillain-Barré syndrome.

ADMINISTRATION

The vaccine is administered in the muscle in a recommended five doses (each 0.5 milliliter [mL]) the first when the risk for exposure is identified. The four follow-up doses are scheduled for week four and months six, twelve, and eighteen after the first dose. Annual booster vaccinations are recommended to preserve immunity.

The vaccine also can be given to people who already have been exposed to anthrax. In these cases the vaccine is given under the skin and in a recommended three doses only, each at 0.5 mL (after first exposure, then two and four weeks after the first dose).

SIDE EFFECTS

An extremely small risk of serious harm comes with the anthrax vaccine. Serious allergic reactions are very rare, and when they occur, they appear within the first hour of administration. Signs of a serious reaction that require immediate medical attention include trouble breathing, wheezing, rapid heartbeat, swelling, hives, hoarseness, dizziness, weakness, and paleness. Other potential problems are mild and include tenderness, redness, itching, or a lump or bruise at the injection site; muscle aches or limited movability of the arm following injection; headaches; and fatigue.

IMPACT

The use of the anthrax vaccine in persons at risk for anthrax infection is likely to prevent fatalities, which would otherwise be expected in up to 20 percent of cutaneous anthrax cases and in the large majority of cases of inhalation anthrax.

Katherine Hauswirth, M.S.N., R.N.

FURTHER READING

Centers for Disease Control and Prevention. "Bioterrorism-Related Anthrax." *Emerging Infectious Diseases* 8 (October, 2002): 1013-1183.

_____. "Use of Anthrax Vaccine in the United States: Recommendations of the Advisory Committee on Immunization Practices." *Morbidity and Mortality Weekly Report* 49 (2000): 1-20.

Dixon, Terry C., et al. "Anthrax." *New England Journal of Medicine* 341 (September 9, 1999): 815-826.

Friedlander, A. M., and S. F. Little. "Advances in the Development of Next-Generation Anthrax Vaccines." *Vaccine* 27, suppl. 4 (November 5, 2009): D61-64.

Institute of Medicine. *An Assessment of the CDC Anthrax Vaccine Safety and Efficacy Research Program.* Washington, D.C.: National Academy Press, 2003.

Plotkin, Stanley A., Walter A. Orenstein, and Paul A. Offit. *Vaccines.* 5th ed. Philadelphia: Saunders/Elsevier, 2008.

WEB SITES OF INTEREST

BioThrax
http://www.biothrax.com

Centers for Disease Control and Prevention
http://www.bt.cdc.gov/agent/anthrax/vaccination

U.S. Food and Drug Administration: Vaccines, Blood, and Biologics
http://www.fda.gov/biologicsbloodvaccines/vaccines/ucm061751.htm

U.S. Surgeon General's Office: Anthrax Vaccine Information Program
http://www.anthrax.osd.mil

Vaccine Research Center
http://www.niaid.nih.gov/about/organization/vrc

See also: Airborne illness and disease; Anthrax; Bacteria: Classification and types; Bacterial infections; Biological weapons; Bioterrorism; Botulinum toxin infection; Botulism; Immunity; Immunization; Outbreaks; Public health; Respiratory route of transmission; SARS; U.S. Army Medical Research Institute of Infectious Diseases; Vaccines: History; Vaccines: Types.

Antibiotic-associated colitis

CATEGORY: Diseases and conditions
ANATOMY OR SYSTEM AFFECTED: Abdomen, colon, gastrointestinal system, intestines, stomach
ALSO KNOWN AS: Antibiotic-associated diarrhea, *Clostridium difficile*-induced colitis, *Clostridium difficile* infection

DEFINITION

Antibiotic-associated colitis occurs when the colon (the large intestine) becomes inflamed because of an infection. The infected person might have diarrhea and abdominal cramping, and the infection is often serious.

CAUSES

The colon is normally full of good bacteria. Antibiotics, however, often kill all the good bacteria in the intestine, creating a perfect environment for the bacterium *Clostridium difficile*, which is not killed by the antibiotics, to grow out of control. The overgrowth of *C. difficile* leads to inflammation and irritation.

RISK FACTORS

Risk factors that increase a person's chances of having this condition include the use of antibiotics.

Other possible risk factors include enteral feeding (tube feeding), taking medicine to decrease the amount of acid the stomach makes, gastrointestinal surgery (stomach or intestine surgery), chemotherapy, and bone marrow transplant. Persons at higher risk include the elderly, persons who are or have been hospitalized, and persons with a severe illness.

SYMPTOMS

Having the following symptoms does not always mean that a person has antibiotic-associated colitis. These symptoms may be caused by other, less serious health conditions. If the following symptoms do appear, one should see a doctor: loose stools, watery diarrhea or diarrhea with mucus, abdominal pain, fever, nausea and vomiting, dehydration, and low blood pressure.

SCREENING AND DIAGNOSIS

A doctor will ask about symptoms and medical history and will do a physical exam. Tests may include stool samples (to identify the toxins made by the bacteria), a computed tomography (CT) scan (a detailed X ray that identifies abnormalities of fine tissue structure), and a colonoscopy (a thin, lighted tube inserted through the rectum and into the colon to examine the lining of the colon).

TREATMENT AND THERAPY

If diagnosed with this condition, one should follow the doctor's instructions and consult him or her about the best treatment plan. Treatment options include fluid replacement, in which the first step is to stop taking the antibiotic and to replace lost fluids. However, one should consult the doctor before stopping the antibiotic. The colitis usually disappears within two weeks of stopping the antibiotic.

Another treatment option is medication, such as antibiotics that kill *C. difficile*. Also useful are probiotics (good bacteria), which help to replace normal bacteria in the colon. Furthermore, one should not use antidiarrheal drugs such as loperamide and opiates.

In rare cases the infected person may need surgery, during which a surgeon would connect the small intestine to an opening in the abdomen. This will divert stool from the large intestine and rectum. This surgery is called an ileostomy. Alternatively, the surgeon could remove the large intestine. This surgery is called a colectomy.

Prevention and Outcomes

The best way to prevent this condition is to reduce the use of antibiotics. One should use antibiotics only when a doctor has confirmed a bacterial infection. Persons who are prescribed antibiotics should consult the doctor about also taking a probiotic, which may help protect the normal bacterial growth in the intestines.

Krisha McCoy, M.S.; reviewed by Daus Mahnke, M.D.

Further Reading

Bäckhed, Fredrik, et al. "Host-Bacterial Mutualism in the Human Intestine." *Science* 307 (March 25, 2005): 1915-1920.

DynaMed: Antibiotic-Associated Diarrhea. Available through http://www.ebscohost.com/dynamed.

EBSCO Publishing. *DynaMed: "Clostridium difficile" colitis.* Available through http://www.ebscohost.com/dynamed.

Feldman, Mark, Lawrence S. Friedman, and Lawrence J. Brandt, eds. *Sleisenger and Fordtran's Gastrointestinal and Liver Disease: Pathophysiology, Diagnosis, Management.* New ed. 2 vols. Philadelphia: Saunders/Elsevier, 2010.

Peikin, Steven R. *Gastrointestinal Health.* Rev. ed. New York: Quill, 2001.

"Use of Gastric Acid-Suppressive Agents and the Risk of Community-Acquired *Clostridium difficile*-Associated Disease." *Journal of the American Medical Association* 294, no. 23 (December 21, 2005): 2989-2995.

Web Sites of Interest

American College of Gastroenterology
http://www.acg.gi.org

Canadian Association of Gastroenterology
http://www.cag-acg.org

Canadian Digestive Health Foundation
http://www.cdhf.ca

Crohn's and Colitis Foundation of America
http://www.ccfa.org

National Digestive Diseases Information Clearinghouse
http://digestive.niddk.nih.gov

See also: Alliance for the Prudent Use of Antibiotics; Amebic dysentery; Antibiotic resistance; Antibiotics: Types; Bacterial infections; *Clostridium*; *Clostridium difficile* infection; Diverticulitis; Drug resistance; Hookworms; Iatrogenic infections; Intestinal and stomach infections; Norovirus infection; Viral gastroenteritis.

Antibiotic resistance

Category: Treatment
Also known as: Antimicrobial resistance, bacterial resistance, drug resistance

Definition

Microbes, typically bacteria, change and resist the activity of antibiotic medications, which attempt to slow bacterial growth or kill bacterial cells. This resistance is called antibiotic resistance.

Common Bacteria Resistant to Antibiotics, with Associated Infections

- *Bacillus anthracis* (anthrax)
- *Enteroccoci* (vancomycinresistant enterococci infections)
- Group B *Streptococcus* (group B strep)
- *Klebsiella pneumoniae* (klebsiella infections)
- *Mycobacterium tuberculosis* (tuberculosis)
- *Neisseria gonorrhoeae* (gonorrhea)
- *Neisseria meningitidis* (bacterial meningitis)
- *Salmonella typhi* (typhoid fever)
- *Shigella* (shigellosis)
- *Staphylococcus aureus* (Methicillinresistant staph infections)
- *Streptococcus pneumoniae* (various infections)

Development History

The first antibiotics, penicillin and the aminoglycoside streptomycin, were identified in the 1940's, and bacteria adapted quickly to block the drugs' effects. Resistance to beta-lactam antibiotics was noted in 1944 and accounted for more than three-quarters of hospital acquired infections in 1950. The long-term risk of resistance was acknowledged as early as 1956.

Excitement about the treatment potential of these early antibiotics, which were introduced in the 1940's and 1950's, contributed to the drugs' rapid, widespread use. Antibiotic use became more promoted and more commonplace in the 1950's and 1960's and was often prescribed empirically and inappropriately, without regard to long-term resistance effects such as increased virulence and multiple resistance mechanisms.

By the 1960's, methicillin-resistant *Staphylococcus aureus* (MRSA) was identified, and MRSA rates continued to increase in the United States into the twenty-first century, from just greater than 2 percent in 1975 to nearly 60 percent in 2003. As MRSA spread through hospital populations and even into animal and community groups, the last-resort glycopeptide antibiotic vancomycin was used more frequently. In September, 2007, vancomycin-resistant and vancomycin-intermediate *S. aureus* were identified in the United States. Bacteria have developed physical methods and genetic mutations to prevent, reduce, or inactivate antibiotic activity against them.

MECHANISMS OF RESISTANCE

Microbes have eight identified major mechanisms of drug resistance that are typically based on an attack of the drug structure, drug-bacteria interaction, or drug quantity around the bacterial cell. More than one mechanism can be used at a time to develop widespread resistance, and different mechanisms are more effective for different antibiotic classes. Once the bacteria develop resistance to an antibiotic, the benefit is passed on to others in the same drug class through genetic mutations in the infectious deoxyribonucleic acid (DNA). Thus, the mutations and resistance spread among people as the bacterial disease is spread. This concept of antibiotic-resistant bacteria in people who have not been directly exposed to the antibiotic supports the urgency of counteracting resistance throughout the human population.

Bacterial resistance develops because of changes to enzymes, target sites, or cell-wall components. Examples of enzyme-mediated resistance are the development of beta-lactamase, which targets beta-lactam antibiotics for inactivation, and the development of a new enzyme that is not affected by antibiotics. Reduced bacterial cell-wall permeability, particularly with gram-negative bacteria, is also a common resis-

tance method; drug efflux, which occurs when bacteria pump antibiotics from the bacterial cell, is most common with tetracycline antibiotics. Changes to the target site on the bacteria, in which antibiotics cannot recognize the binding site and attack bacteria, are less common with beta-lactams and more common with quinolones and macrolides. In some cases, bacteria may otherwise block the target site to prevent antibiotic binding; this occurs against tetracycline antibiotics in particular. Bacteria may increase the amount of binding sites on the wall too, so that antibiotics cannot achieve sufficient proportional concentrations for activity, especially with sulfonamide treatment and with glycopeptides such as vancomycin.

Cellular adaptations that help bacteria avoid any interaction with antibiotics and binding of antibiotics elsewhere on the bacteria to prevent action on the bacterial cell target also incur drug resistance; the latter method is specific to glycopeptides like vancomycin.

METHODS TO REDUCE RESISTANCE

Early attempts to decrease resistance started in the 1980's, when hospitals began instituting guidelines to cycle, or rotate, antibiotic use for certain diseases. Cyclic administration of antibiotics consists of restricting the prescribing of the most commonly used antibiotic and favoring an alternative antibiotic treatment instead.

Research in the late twentieth and early twenty-first centuries has identified no real evidence of success at minimizing resistance with cycling, and many factors about resistance and efficacy are still unknown. However, restricted antibiotic use in the Netherlands and in Scandinavia resulted in decreased hospital occurrences of MRSA, which supports closely monitored antibiotic prescribing as a means to reduce resistance buildup.

A clear correlation between occurrence of resistance and empiric use of antibiotics, reported in the May, 2010, issue of the *British Medical Journal*, has supported the longstanding belief that nonempiric treatment (treatment that is identified on the basis of factual data that shows efficacy, such as a sensitivity analysis) will reduce the likelihood of increasing antibiotic resistance because of ineffective antibiotic use. Although occurrence reductions have not been proven, the rate of resistance development is likely to be lower when antibiotics are used properly.

The prohibition of the use of human antibiotics in animals is debated among health experts. The use of antibiotics in animal husbandry to prevent infections in livestock, such as cattle, pigs, and chickens, can increase the rate of resistant bacteria development by introducing primary antibiotics before they even infect humans. Although animal use of antibiotics began in the 1950's to improve the health and quantity of livestock for food use, the practice is now banned in the European Union and in countries around the world. However, the United States has not banned antibiotic use in animals; the U.S. Food and Drug Administration, though, has emphasized the importance of reducing antibiotics in meat consumed by humans to reduce drug resistance for treatment of human infections.

Impact

Drastic changes to bacteria can occur in a relatively short time (often within one decade) to reduce antibiotic efficacy, and much needs to be done in identifying the means to long-term resistance. To preserve the effectiveness of antibiotics, doctors must prescribe them with more care and attention. Sensitivity analyses, which identify the antibiotics that retain activity against specific microbes in a particular patient, are increasingly used in hospital settings to determine initial antibiotic therapy and to monitor continued antibiotic use and infection response.

Beginning in 1996, antimicrobial stewardship identified the connection of bacterial resistance with widespread antibiotic use even in persons who had not received the particular resistance-antibiotic treatment. Fewer antibiotics are being developed in the twenty-first century, in part because of the high cost of development. These high costs, fewer successful treatment options, and increased resistance mutations (including multidrug or multimechanism patterns) have increased the urgency to improve antibiotic use and to find nontraditional methods to suppress bacterial infections.

Nicole M. Van Hoey, Pharm.D.

Further Reading

Arias, Cesar A., and Barbara E. Murray. "Antibiotic-Resistant Bugs in the Twenty-first Century: A Clinical Super-Challenge." *New England Journal of Medicine* 360, no. 5 (2009): 439-443. Reviews the mechanisms and history of bacterial resistance to antibiotics. The discussion covers types, ranges, and examples of resistance, and includes the use of case study examples and diagrams for clear explanations.

Polk, Ronald E., and Neil O. Fishman. "Antimicrobial Stewardship." In *Mandell, Douglas, and Bennett's Principles and Practice of Infectious Diseases*, edited by Gerald L. Mandell, John F. Bennett, and Raphael Dolin. 7th ed. New York: Churchill Livingstone/Elsevier, 2010. Describes the beginning of antibiotic resistance awareness and the definition of "stewardship." Discusses techniques being used in hospitals to reduce resistance and improve antibiotic longevity.

Rosenblatt-Farrell, Noah. "The Landscape of Antibiotic Resistance" *Environmental Health Perspectives* 117, no. 6 (2009): 244-250. A detailed article examining the issue of antibiotic resistance and the future of existing antibiotic therapies.

Schmitz, Franz-Josef, and Ad C. Fluit. "Mechanisms of Antibacterial Resistance." In *Cohen and Powderly Infectious Diseases*, edited by Jonathan Cohen, Steven M. Opal, and William G. Powderly. 3d ed. Philadelphia: Mosby/Elsevier, 2010. Describes connections between bacterial resistance levels and treatment outcomes; lists and details eight methods by which bacteria develop resistance to antibiotics alone or as multiple-resistance mechanisms. Discusses bacteria susceptibility to different antibiotics and the impact of antibiotic use in animals on the treatment of human diseases.

Science 321, no. 5887 (July 18, 2008). A special issue devoted to problems of antibiotic resistance, highlighting some particularly difficult infections and discussing issues pertaining to the genetics of antibiotic resistance.

Walsh, Christopher. *Antibiotics: Actions, Origins, Resistance.* Washington, D.C.: ASM Press, 2003. Examines such topics as how antibiotics block specific proteins, how the molecular structure of drugs enables such activity, the development of bacterial resistance, and the molecular logic of antibiotic biosynthesis.

Web Sites of Interest

Centers for Disease Control and Prevention
http://www.cdc.gov/drugresistance

National Institute of Allergy and Infectious Diseases
http://www.niaid.nih.gov/topics/
antimicrobialresistance

Todar's Online Textbook of Bacteriology
http://www.textbookofbacteriology.net

World Health Organization
http://www.who.int/drugresistance

See also: Alliance for the Prudent Use of Antibiotics; Antibiotics: Experimental; Antibiotics: Types; Bacterial infections; Chemical germicides; Drug resistance; Glycopeptide antibiotics; Hospitals and infectious disease; Iatrogenic infections; Ketolide antibiotics; Macrolide antibiotics; Methicillin-resistant staph infection; Microbiology; Public health; Quinolone antibiotics; Reinfection; Secondary infection; Superbacteria; Treatment of bacterial infections; Vancomycin-resistant enterococci infection.

Antibiotics: Experimental

CATEGORY: Treatment

DEFINITION

Experimental antibiotics are antibiotics under study in clinical trials, antibiotics awaiting U.S. Food and Drug Administration (FDA) approval, and antibiotics that have been approved by the FDA but are not available to the public.

CEFTAROLINE AND CEFTOBIPROLE

Two new cephalosporin antibiotics comprise what is termed "fifth-generation cephalosporins": ceftobiprole and ceftaroline. Ceftobiprole is fifth-generation broad-spectrum cephalosporin awaiting FDA approval. In studies, ceftobiprole has shown broad coverage of gram-positive and gram-negative bacteria (both aerobes and anaerobes), including activity against methicillin-resistant *Staphylococcus aureus* (MRSA) and *Pseudomonas*. Its mechanism of action is similar to other cephalosporins.

Because of the broad-spectrum nature of ceftobiprole, many experts believe it may be utilized as empirical treatment in hospital settings in cases when antibiotic treatment needs to be started before culture and sensitivity results are complete. Two phase-three studies looked at ceftobiprole for the treatment of skin and complicated skin-structure infections. In these two published phase-three clinical trials, study subjects re-

ceived a 500 milligram (mg) dose intravenously, every eight hours or every twelve hours; this dosage was compared with a 1 gram (g) dose of vancomycin given every twelve hours (with or without ceftazidime at 1 g every eight hours). Combined, more than fifteen hundred study subjects were enrolled in the trials. In both trials, ceftobiprole was found to be noninferior to the comparator with a similar adverse-effect profile.

Additional phase-three trials were conducted for the indication of hospital- and community-acquired pneumonia and in persons with fever and neutropenia after chemotherapy. Adverse events were similar between treatment groups in both trials. Additionally, ceftobiprole has been studied for endocarditis, orthopedic infections, and pneumonia. The most common adverse events reported in clinical trials, most classified as mild to moderate, include gastrointestinal upset and headache. The FDA has not approved ceftobiprole, and it has requested additional clinical trials be completed by the manufacturer.

Ceftaroline is a broad-spectrum cephalosporin with a mechanism of action similar to other beta-lactams. It provides coverage of gram-positive, gram-negative, and anaerobic bacteria. Importantly, it displays gram-positive activity against most pathogens, including MRSA. Ceftaroline has been approved for two indications: acute bacterial skin and skin-structure infections and community-acquired bacterial pneumonia (CABP).

Two phase-three trials were conducted to investigate ceftaroline for the indication of moderate to severe CABP requiring treatment with intravenous antibiotics. Two additional phase-three trials investigated ceftaroline for the treatment of complicated skin and skin-structure infections. In clinical trials, the most common adverse events (reported in less than 2 percent of study subjects) were diarrhea, nausea, and rash. Overall, the medication was well tolerated and had adverse-event rates similar to comparator treatments.

FIDAXOMICIN

Fidaxomicin is a novel, narrow-spectrum macrocyclic antibiotic that targets bacterial RNA (ribonucleic acid) polymerase studied in clinical trials for *Clostridium difficile* infection. Fidaxomicin has been studied in phase-three clinical trials in adults with *C. difficile* infection. The two compounds most often, and almost exclusively, used for the treatment of *C.*

difficile infection are oral metronidazole and oral vancomycin. Study subjects were randomized to receive either fidaxomicin 200 milligrams (mg) twice daily or standard therapy with oral vancomycin 125 mg four times daily. More than six hundred persons were enrolled, and the study found fidaxomicin to be noninferior to treatment with vancomycin.

One of the proposed benefits of this therapy is its minimal systemic absorption; also, it does not affect most normal gut flora. Additionally, its spectrum of action (no gram-negative coverage and some gram-positive coverage) means it is highly specific for *C. difficile*. In two phase-three trials, fidaxomicin was given orally at 200 mg every twelve hours for ten days and was found to be noninferior in terms of clinical cure rates.

IMPACT

Antibiotic resistance results in longer times to eradicate pathogens, more frequent clinical failures, and a heavy burden on the health care system. The importance of using targeted antibiotics and of decreasing unwarranted widespread use of antibiotics is critical to curbing antibiotic resistance and to maintaining the efficacy of available therapies.

Experimental antibiotics can be designed to target a broad spectrum of bacteria, such as the newer fifth-generation cephalosporins, or they can be niche antibiotics with a narrow spectrum, such as fidaxomicin for *C. difficile* infection. The significance of these and other antibiotics undergoing clinical trials will be fully analyzable once they are widely available.

Allison C. Bennett, Pharm.D.

FURTHER READING

Dauner, Daniel G., Robert E. Nelson, and Donna C. Taketa. "Ceftobiprole: A Novel, Broad-Spectrum Cephalosporin with Activity Against Methicillin-Resistant *Staphylococcus aureus*." *American Journal of Health-System Pharmacy* 67, no. 12 (2010): 983-993.

Louie, Thomas J., et al. "Fidaxomicin Versus Vancomycin for *Clostridium difficile* Infection." *New England Journal of Medicine* 364 (2011): 422-431.

Noel, G. J., et al. "A Randomized, Double-Blind Trial Comparing Ceftobiprole Medocaril with Vancomycin plus Ceftazidime for the Treatment of Patients with Complicated Skin and Skin-Structure Infections." *Clinical Infectious Diseases* 46, no. 5 (2008): 647-655.

Sanford, Jay P., et al. *The Sanford Guide to Antimicrobial Therapy*. 18th ed. Sperryville, Va.: Antimicrobial Therapy, 2010.

Steed, Molly E., and Michael J. Rybak. "Ceftaroline: A New Cephalosporin with Activity Against Resistant Gram-Positive Pathogens." *Pharmacotherapy* 30, no. 4 (2010): 375-389.

WEB SITES OF INTEREST

ClinicalTrials.gov
http://www.clinicaltrials.gov

eMedicineHealth: Antibiotics
http://www.emedicinehealth.com/antibiotics

Todar's Online Textbook of Bacteriology
http://www.textbookofbacteriology.net

See also: Alliance for the Prudent Use of Antibiotics; Antibiotic resistance; Antibiotics: Types; Bacteria: Classification and types; Bacterial infections; Bacteriology; Cephalosporin antibiotics; *Clostridium difficile* infection; Diagnosis of bacterial infections; Methicillin-resistant staph infection; Microbiology; Prevention of bacterial infections; *Pseudomonas* infections; Treatment of bacterial infections; Vaccines: Experimental; Vancomycin-resistant enterococci infection.

Antibiotics: Types

CATEGORY: Treatment

DEFINITION

Antibiotics are grouped by type, or class, to identify groups of similar antibiotics that act on specific bacteria types (such as gram-negative bacilli) and in the same manner (such as to kill cells or slow growth). The most common method of separating antibiotics by class is according to the type of chemical drug structure.

BETA-LACTAMS

Penicillins and cephalosporins are two subclasses of beta-lactam antibiotics, as they share a five- or six-membered ring structure. All beta-lactams are bactericidal and work at the bacterial cell-wall level. Beta-lactams irreversibly bind as a false substrate to an active site on the enzyme that is responsible for cell-wall peptide cross-linking; by preventing the cross-linking, beta-lactams prevent the completion of the bacterial cell wall.

Penicillin, the first beta-lactam, was identified as a mold spore, *Penicillium notatum* (now called *P. chrysogenum*), in 1928 by bacteriologist Alexander Fleming; the antibiotic itself was derived from *P. chrysogenum* in 1941 and was active against strains of the *Staphylococcus* bacterium. Although penicillin had only a narrow, gram-positive spectrum, later penicillin-related antibiotics, such as methicillin and ampicillin, provided expanded activity by avoiding bacterial resistance or by acting against select gram-negative organisms, respectively. Penicillins generally are used to treat skin, ear, respiratory, and urinary tract infections for which bacteria remain sensitive.

Cephalosporins provide much broader-spectrum coverage within the beta-lactam class compared with penicillins. Although their mechanism of action is like that of penicillin, they have varied spectrums of activity because of structural alterations. Cephalosporins are typically used to treat otitis media (ear), skin, and urinary tract infections, but are also used in surgical prophylaxis and to treat bone infections and pneumonia.

The activity of cephalosporins can be defined by four subtypes, or generations, to provide wide bacterial coverage. First-generation drugs, such as cephalexin and cefazolin, provide primarily gram-positive activity; second-generation cephalosporins, such as cefuroxime and cefaclor, provide gram-negative and gram-positive activity but have a range of sensitivities. Third-generation examples include ceftriaxone, cefixime, and ceftibuten; these drugs provide wide gram-negative coverage but lose much of the class gram-positive coverage. Fourth-generation drugs cefepime and cefquinone have similar gram-positive activity as early cephalosporins but have better activity against beta-lactamase-resistant bacteria, and they cross the blood-brain barrier to treat meningitis and encephalitis.

All beta-lactams are well tolerated and are associated with the mild side effects of nausea and diarrhea. However, allergy to drugs in the beta-lactam class is not uncommon and may develop with both penicillin and cephalosporin use.

MACROLIDES

Unlike penicillins and cephalosporins, which act on the bacterial cell-wall, macrolides interact with bacteria at protein synthesis, and they are typically bacteriostatic but may become bactericidal, depending on their concentrations and the bacteria types attacked. Macrolides such as erythromycin, clarithromycin, and azithromycin bind to the 50S section of the ribosome during bacterial protein development to change the ribosome and prevent peptide bonding. Erythromycin additionally may prevent formation of the 50S subunit itself.

Macrolides are composed of a macrocyclic lactone and are derived from the bacterium *Streptomyces*. Erythromycin, the first-in-class macrolide, has similar activity to penicillin; conversely, the two newer macrolides have their best activity in lung diseases, and clarithromycin is particularly effective against *Helicobacter pylori*, which often causes stomach ulcers. Macrolides are used against *Staphylococcus*, *Streptococcus*, and *Mycoplasma* infections, and they are used to treat Legionnaires' disease, which is caused by the *Legionella* bacterium. Side effects include mild nausea, diarrhea, and stomach upset.

TETRACYCLINES

Like macrolides, tetracyclines are derived from *Streptomyces*; they are made of four connected rings. Tetracyclines block the beginning of protein synthesis by binding the ribosome and preventing the addition of aminoacyl tRNA (transfer ribonucleic acid) building blocks. In addition, tetracyclines may change the ribosome itself to prevent successful protein synthesis. Tetracyclines provide bacteriostatic activity against a broader spectrum of bacteria than do penicillins.

Tetracycline, minocycline, and doxycycline are common examples of drugs in this class. They have unique activity against *Rickettsia* and some amebic parasites; they can treat sinus, middle ear, urinary tract, and intestinal infections. However, a common use of drugs in this class is to treat skin conditions such as rosacea or moderate acne. Tetracyclines have a greater risk of side effects, especially with prolonged use. Photosensitivity, cramps, diarrhea, and possible bone and tooth changes may occur with tetracycline use.

FLUOROQUINOLONES

Fluoroquinolones, unlike beta-lactams, are synthetic rather than derived directly from a bacterial source. They are well absorbed, are distributed into bone, and can be given by mouth or intravenously. They consist of a dual ring and a fluor group that increases the antibiotic activity.

The Action of Antibiotics

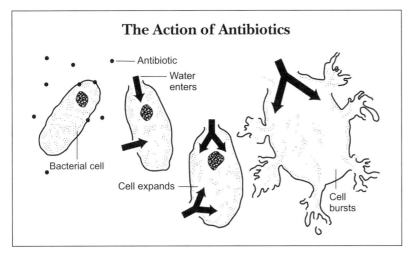

An antibiotic destroys a bacterium by causing its cell walls to deteriorate. Water then enters the bacterium unchecked until it bursts.

Fluoroquinolones are bactericidal against a broad spectrum of bacteria. Fluoroquinolones act by blocking deoxyribonucleic acid (DNA) building within the bacteria to prevent multiplication. Early examples, such as ciprofloxacin, are primarily active against gram-negative bacteria; newer agents, including levofloxacin, keep gram-negative activity and add activity against gram-positive bacteria such as the pneumococcus (*Streptococcus pneumoniae*). They are often used to treat urinary tract and skin infections and respiratory infections such as bronchitis and bacterial pneumonia. Moxifloxacin, one of the newest of the fluoroquinolones, has additional activity against anaerobic bacteria.

GLYCOPEPTIDES

Vancomycin and teicoplanin are the two most common glycopeptide antibiotics, the newest class of antibiotics. Because their chemical makeup is so large and because these drugs cannot cross a cell membrane, they affect only gram-positive bacteria outside the cell. Each glycopeptide is made of two sugars and one aglycone moiety with a heptapeptide core that provides antibiotic action. Glycopeptides block the end of cell-wall peptidoglycan synthesis so that the cell wall cannot be completed and the bacteria cannot survive. Vancomycin is useful in the treatment of methicillin-resistant *Staphylococcus aureus* (MRSA) in hospital settings; however, bacteria are also developing intermediate to full resistance to vancomycin.

OTHER ANTIBIOTICS

Aminoglycoside antibiotics, discovered in 1944, contain an amino and some sugar groups. They provide limited-spectrum coverage against gram-negative and gram-positive agents. Aminoglycosides insert themselves incorrectly into proteins during synthesis by binding to the ribosome. They are particularly active against *Pseudomonas aeriginosa*.

Lincosamides, such as clindamycin, have greater activity against anaerobes, such as those causing intestinal or gastric infections, and they are also used to treat gram-positive *Staphylococcus* skin infections, including moderate acne. Lincosamides are bacteriostatic and act by inhibiting protein synthesis by the bacterial ribosome.

IMPACT

With the development of bacterial resistance shortly after penicillin's introduction in the 1940's, antibiotic drug development has greatly expanded within the beta-lactam class and beyond. However, bacterial resistance appears to be developing faster than new antibiotics are being discovered or developed in laboratories, so that infections from common bacteria are once again complicated to treat. Research continues to identify the best use of antibiotics within and among classes and to find the safest combination therapies against specific bacteria.

Nicole M. Van Hoey, Pharm.D.

FURTHER READING

Mandell, Gerald L., John E. Bennett, and Raphael Dolin, eds. *Mandell, Douglas, and Bennett's Principles and Practice of Infectious Diseases.* 7th ed. New York: Churchill Livingstone/Elsevier, 2010. This thorough, two-volume textbook provides background and detailed information about all types of microbes and infectious sources. Section E in particular discusses antibiotic and other anti-infective therapies. Chapters in this section discuss efficacy, sensitivity, and pharmacologic activities of antimicrobial agents. In addition, chapters address each antibiotic type singly with specific details about mechanisms, spectrums, dosages, and combination therapies.

Murray, Patrick R., Ken S. Rosenthal, and Michael A. Pfaller. *Medical Microbiology*. 6th ed. Philadelphia: Mosby/Elsevier, 2009. Primarily describes bacteria and other infectious microbes. Later discussion presents diseases by site of infection.

Sanford, Jay P., et al. *The Sanford Guide to Antimicrobial Therapy*. 18th ed. Sperryville, Va.: Antimicrobial Therapy, 2010. A premier guide to antibiotic use with descriptions of agents in each class and their antibacterial activity. Text and tables document treatment options, antiresistance treatment options, drug-drug interactions, and treatment dosages and regimens.

Van Bambeke, Françoise, et al. "Antibiotics That Act on the Cell Wall." In *Cohen and Powderly Infectious Diseases*, edited by Jonathan Cohen, Steven M. Opal, and William G. Powderly. 3d ed. Philadelphia: Mosby/Elsevier, 2010. Describes the mechanisms of action of antibiotics that block or kill bacteria by interacting with the bacterial cell wall. Focuses on beta-lactam and glycopeptide antibiotics. Also discusses bacterial cell-wall development, beta-lactamase-resistance development, and the latest developments in beta-lactam use. The glycopeptides discussion expands from mechanisms to treatment of vancomycin-resistant bacteria.

Walsh, Christopher. *Antibiotics: Actions, Origins, Resistance*. Washington, D.C.: ASM Press, 2003. Examines such topics as how antibiotics block specific proteins, how the molecular structure of drugs enables such activity, the development of bacterial resistance, and the molecular logic of antibiotic biosynthesis.

WEB SITES OF INTEREST

eMedicineHealth: Antibiotics
http://www.emedicinehealth.com/antibiotics

National Institute of Allergy and Infectious Diseases
http://www.niaid.nih.gov/topics/antimicrobialresistance

Todar's Online Textbook of Bacteriology
http://www.textbookofbacteriology.net

See also: Alliance for the Prudent Use of Antibiotics; Aminoglycoside antibiotics; Antibiotic resistance; Antibiotic-associated colitis; Antibiotics: Experimental; Bacteria: Classification and types; Bacteria: Structure and growth; Bacteriology; Cephalosporin antibiotics; Drug resistance; Glycopeptide antibiotics; Ketolide antibiotics; Lipopeptide antibiotics; Macrolide antibiotics; Methicillin-resistant staph infection; Microbiology; Oxazolidinone antibiotics; Penicillin antibiotics; Prevention of bacterial infections; Quinolone antibiotics; Reinfection; Secondary infection; Superbacteria; Tetracycline antibiotics; Treatment of bacterial infections; Vancomycin-resistant enterococci infection; Virulence.

Antibodies

CATEGORY: Immune response
ALSO KNOWN AS: Gammaglobulins, immunoglobulins

DEFINITION

Antibodies are proteins produced by the B lymphocyte (white blood) cells of the immune system of human and nonhuman animals in response to the introduction of foreign material such as viruses, bacteria, or parasites and their molecules. A particular B lymphocyte (or B cell) and its progeny cells (clones) produces a singular antibody molecule that binds specifically to a structural determinant on a specific foreign molecule (antigen). A given antigen may elicit different antibodies from a number of genetically distinct B lymphocytes, each of which produces a single type of antibody that binds to a select part of the foreign molecule. Such diverse antibody production is called polyclonal response and the products are called polyclonal antibodies.

The antibody synthesized by a particular B lymphocyte and its clones is called a monoclonal antibody. Production of such antibodies is extremely useful and widely applied in medicine and science.

The basic unit of an antibody molecule is a structure comprising four polypeptides: two identical "heavy" chains and two identical "light" chains. Five classes of heavy chain lead to five classes of antibody: IgG, IgD, IgE, IgA, and IgM (the letters *Ig* mean "immunoglobulin").

Proteins in the antibody classes IgG, IgD, and IgE, and serum IgA, have the four polypeptide chain structure. IgA molecules in external secretions of the body

Key Terms

- *Antibody*. A molecule of the immune system, produced by B cells and targeted toward eliminating a specific antigen

- *Antigen*. Foreign material that stimulates the host organism to produce antibodies specific to that material

- *Autoantibody*. An antibody that binds to a protein that is a normal part of the human body from which it originates (as opposed to part of a *bacteria*, virus, or another human being)

- *Heavy chain*. The larger subunits of an antibody

- *Immune system*. The cells and organs of the body that fight infection; destruction of these cells leaves the body vulnerable to numerous diseases

- *Immunoglobulin (Ig)*. A protein activated by the immune system

- *Isotypes*. The different classes of antibodies

- *Light chain*. The smaller subunits of an antibody

- *Lymphocytes*. White blood cells that specifically target a foreign organism for destruction; the two classes of lymphocytes are B cells, which produce antibodies, and T cells, which kill infected cells

have two or more of the basic four polypeptide antibody unit in combination with J-chain and secretory component polypeptides. IgM consists of five of the basic four-polypeptide antibody unit in combination with a J-chain polypeptide.

The basic four-chain unit of antibodies is further subdivided by proteolytic fragmentation into regions (domains) called Fab and Fc. The Fab region consists of the N-terminal parts of a heavy and light chain and binds to antigen, thus each four-chain unit of antibodies contains two binding sites for antigens. The Fc region consists of the C-terminal parts of two heavy chains and modulates interactions of antibodies with other molecular and cellular components of the immune system. The Fc regions of different antibody classes differ in the effects that they mediate. Upon binding antigen—for example, on a bacteria or virus—the Fc regions of IgG and IgM undergo a change in shape and activate another group of proteins that belong to the complement system. Other antibody classes do not do this. The different complement proteins are deposited on the surface of the microorganisms to which the IgG or IgM antibodies are bound with certain consequences. White blood cells such as macrophages and neutrophils can bind to complement proteins; through this attachment, the white blood cells engulf the foreign bodies, in a process called phagocytosis, and destroy them. Other

Classes, Locations, and Functions of Antibodies

Class	Location	Functions
IgG	Blood plasma, tissue fluid, fetuses	Produces primary and secondary immune responses; protects against bacteria, viruses, and toxins; passes through the placenta and enters fetal bloodstream, thus providing protection to fetuses.
IgM	Blood plasma	Acts as a B-cell surface receptor for antigens; fights bacteria in primary immune response; powerful agglutinating agent; includes anti-A and anti-B antibodies.
IgD	Surface of B cells	Prompts B cells to make antibodies (especially in infants).
IgA	Saliva, milk, urine, tears, respiratory and digestive systems	Protects surface linings of epithelial cells, digestive, respiratory, and urinary systems.
IgE	In secretion with IgA, skin, tonsils, respiratory and digestive systems	Acts as receptor for antigens causing mast cells (often found in connective tissues surrounding blood vessels), to secrete allergy mediators; excessive production causes allergic reactions (including hay fever and asthma).

Five Classes of Antibodies

IgM is produced first in a response to foreign antigen, but its concentration declines rapidly. With five Y-shaped monomer subunits forming a pentamer structure, IgM is very effective in binding many copies of the same antigen and agglutinating them, but is too big to cross the placenta.

IgG is the most abundant class of antibodies in circulating blood, a monomer capable of passing through vessel walls to protect cells and tissues. In some species, including humans, it crosses the placenta to pass on the woman's immune protection to the fetus. Produced after IgM in an immune response, it is much more effective against bacteria, viruses, and toxins.

IgA is secreted as a dimer (two subunits) into milk, sweat, saliva, and tears. It is especially important in colostrum, the secretion before milk production begins that is the only way some newborn animals receive their mother's antibodies. IgA prevents bacteria and viruses from binding to epithelial cell surfaces, especially in the digestive tract.

IgE antibodies bind to the surfaces of mast cells and basophils with the arms of the Y-shaped monomer extended. Foreign antigens bind to the ends of the Y arms and trigger these cells to release histamine and other chemicals that cause the inflammation of allergy. IgE is also the antibody that attacks parasites inside the body, such as worms.

IgD molecules are monomers located mainly on the surfaces of B cells, apparently acting as receptors for the antigen that is recognized by each B cell and triggers its activation.

complement proteins create holes in bacteria, which leads to their death.

White blood cells also use some of their cell surface proteins, called Fc-gamma receptors, to bind to IgG antibodies that are attached to foreign infectious bodies; this also leads to phagocytosis, or the release of killing molecules from the white blood cells.

The Fc region of IgG is essential to the transplacental transfer of passive immunity from a pregnant woman (or girl) to her fetus. Placental Fc-gamma receptors bind the IgG molecules to allow their uptake and subsequent transfer across placental cells to fetal blood, thus providing months of antibody-mediated immunity to the newborn. In hoofed animals such as cows, goats, and sheep, immunoglobulins are transferred from a special form of mother's milk called colostrum across the calf's small intestine. This form of antibody transport does not occur in humans. However, IgA antibodies in human milk are believed to be beneficial in reducing the chance of intestinal infections in infants.

VIRAL AND MICROBIAL DISEASES

Vaccines or immune responses to natural viral infection may elicit the production of antibodies that neutralize the infective agent. Such antibodies are important in the cases of influenza, hepatitis B, human papilloma virus, respiratory syncytial virus, measles, mumps, vaccinia, varicella zoster viruses, and poliovirus. In the case of dengue virus infection, antibodies can prevent infection with a previously encountered strain or exacerbate effects of infection if infection occurs with a different strain of the virus.

Antibodies also feature prominently in immunity or therapy directed against bacterial infection. Tetanus treatment includes the use of passive immunization with human antitetanus antibodies, which neutralize the toxin produced by the bacterium *Clostridium tetani*. Widespread childhood vaccinations include those against bacteria causing diphtheria, tetanus, and pertussis (DTP).

METHODS AND DIAGNOSTICS

Antibodies are used in various techniques for research studies of infectious diseases. These techniques include enzyme-linked immunoabsorbent assay (ELISA), immunofluorescence, Western blotting, immunoprecipitation, and flow cytometry.

One newer avenue of research aims at isolating B lymphocytes that make protective antibody to influenza from vaccinated people; the antibodies would be used to provide passive immunity to influenza.

IMPACT

Antibody technology is prevalent in diagnostic testing for infectious diseases and is widely applied in biomedical research at a global level. Antibodies are used not only in research involving humans but also in animal diagnostic tests, both for farm animals and for household pets. Many companies around the world produce monoclonal and polyclonal antibodies from various animals, including mice, rats, rabbits, sheep, goats, donkeys, camels, sharks, chickens, ducks, and guinea pigs. Other companies produce instruments such as microplate readers, flow cytometers, fluorescence microscopes, electrophoresis equipment, and microarray readers, all of which are used in techniques involving antibodies.

Oluseyi A. Vanderpuye, Ph.D.

FURTHER READING

Abbas, Abul K., and Andrew H. Lichtman. *Basic Immunology: Functions and Disorders of the Immune System.* 2d ed. Philadelphia: Saunders/Elsevier, 2006. An easy-to-read introduction to the human immune system. Includes excellent figures and a thorough glossary.

Coico, Richard. *Immunology: A Short Course.* 6th ed. Hoboken, N.J.: Wiley-Blackwell, 2009. An understandable treatment of the immune response and the different components of the immune system.

Parham, Peter. *The Immune System.* 3d ed. New York: Garland Science, 2009. Provides extensive coverage of mechanisms, concepts, and components of the immune system and self-assessment exercises to promote understanding of the material.

Parslow, Tristram G., et al., eds. *Medical Immunology.* 10th ed. New York: Lange Medical Books/McGraw-Hill, 2001. This book discusses the synthesis, structure, and functions of antibodies and their roles in clinical tests and different diseases, organ by organ.

Salyers, Abigail A., and Dixie D. Whitt. *Microbiology, Diversity, Disease, and the Environment.* Bethesda, Md.: Fitzgerald Science Press, 2001. This work places antibodies in the context of the rest of the immune system and of viral, bacterial, and other microbial diseases.

Sompayrac, Lauren M. *How the Immune System Works.* 3d ed. Hoboken, N.J.: Wiley-Blackwell, 2008. The author provides a concise description and explanation of the immune system and the role of antibodies.

WEB SITES OF INTEREST

Microbiology and Immunology On-line
http://pathmicro.med.sc.edu/book/welcome.htm

National Institutes of Health
http://www.nih.gov

See also: Agammaglobulinemia; AIDS; Autoimmune disorders; Bacterial infections; Drug resistance; HIV; Idiopathic thrombocytopenic purpura; Immune response to bacterial infections; Immune response to parasitic diseases; Immune response to viral infections; Immunity; Immunoassay; Immunodeficiency; Incubation period; Microbiology; Neutropenia; Parasitic diseases; Seroconversion; T lymphocytes; Viral infections; Virulence.

Antifungal drugs: Mechanisms of action

CATEGORY: Treatment

DEFINITION

Antifungal drugs are used to prevent the growth and reproduction of fungi that are harmful to the human body. The components of fungal cell walls are different from those in bacterial cell walls and are composed primarily of chitin, a polysaccharide. The differences in cell-wall composition have enabled researchers to target antifungals to components and building blocks specific to fungal cells.

ALLYLAMINES AND BENZYLAMINES

Allylamines are inhibitors of squalene 2,3-epoxidase, the enzyme responsible for the conversion of squalene to squalene oxide. Squalene oxide is an intermediate and marks a beginning step in the production of ergosterol, one of the key fungal cell-wall components.

Inhibiting the conversion of squalene to squalene oxide results in two important downstream results, which lead to cell death. The two resulting consequences are a decrease in the amount of ergosterol available and, more critical, the increased concentration of squalene within the fungal cell. Examples of commercially available allylamines are naftine and terbinafine. They are often used for topical and nail fungal infections.

The mechanism of action of benzylamines is similar to that of allylamines. Benzylamines inhibit squalene epoxidase, leading to the same dual mechanism of fungal cell death seen with allylamines: a decrease in the amount of ergosterol and the accumulation of squalene. Butenafine, the only commercially available benzylamine, is an over-the-counter medication for topical fungal infections such as ringworm.

AZOLES

Azole antifungals include imidazoles and triazoles. Azoles are some of the most commonly used antifungals. Some are available over-the-counter and others require a prescription. They are used for both topical and systemic infections.

Imidazoles contain two nitrogen atoms in the core azole ring, whereas triazoles contain three nitrogen atoms. However, their mechanisms of action do not differ substantially. Azoles are fungistatic, although they may be fungicidal at much higher than normal concentrations.

Azoles inhibit the lanosterol 14-alpha demethylase, the enzyme responsible for converting lanosterol to ergosterol, a key component of the fungal cell membrane. Decreasing the concentration of ergosterol results in increased permeability and rigidity and a decrease in replication and growth of the of the fungal cells. Examples of commercially available azoles include clotrimazole, econazole, fluconazole, itraconazole, ketoconazole, miconazole, oxiconazole, and voriconazole.

POLYENES

Polyenes bind irreversibly to ergosterol, a sterol component of the fungal cell-wall membrane. This interaction creates pores within the fungal cell membrane, facilitating the release of intracellular components and eventual fungal cell death. Examples of commercially available polyenes include nystatin and amphotericin B. Amphotericin B is generally reserved for intravenous use for systemic fungal infections, whereas nystatin can be used for either systemic or oral fungal infections.

OTHER ANTIFUNGALS

Echinocandins are lipopeptides that exert fungicidal activity against some fungal species through noncompetitive inhibition of (1,3)beta-glucan synthase. This decreases the glucan, a cell-wall component specific to fungal cells, and decreases the amount of ergosterol and lanosterol. Commercially available echinocandins include caspofungin, micafungin, and anidulafungin.

Flucytosine is an antimetabolite that disrupts protein synthesis and disrupts ribonucleic acid (RNA), deoxyribonucleic acid (DNA), and pyrimidine metabolism; it is used for severe fungal infections. After entering the fungal cell, flucytosine undergoes a series of deamination and phosphorylation reactions and is eventually incorporated into RNA. Ciclopirox olamine, the only commercially available hydroxypyridone, has a mechanism of action distinct from other antifungals. Ciclopirox creates a polyvalent cation through chelation reactions with trivalent cations. This large polyvalent cation disrupts enzyme function, electron transport, cellular uptake mechanisms, and energy production. Griseofulvin is a fungistatic compound with a mechanism of action not completely understood. It is thought to potentially bind to alpha and beta tubulin, leading to the disruption of mitosis and nucleic acid synthesis.

IMPACT

Fungal infections can range from the relatively harmless tinea pedis (athlete's foot) to more serious systemic fungal infections, such as histoplasmosis and aspergillosis, in immunocompromised persons. As with bacterial resistance to antibiotics, fungal resistance has developed against some commonly used, older antifungals. Understanding the mechanism and spectrum of action of antifungals can help guide the clinician to more targeted, successful therapy. The improper use of antifungals puts at risk the health of the infected person and, ultimately, the public.

Allison C. Bennett, Pharm.D.

FURTHER READING

Baran, Robert, Rod Hay, and Javier Garduno. "Review of Antifungal Therapy, Part II: Treatment Rationale, Including Specific Patient Populations." *Journal of Dermatological Treatment* 19 (2008): 168-175. Review article with emphasis on treating fungal infections in adolescents, pregnant girls and women, immunocompromised persons, and the elderly.

Ghannoum, Mahmoud, and Louis Rice. "Antifungal Agents: Mode of Action, Mechanism of Resistance, and Correlation of These Mechanisms with Bacterial Resistance." *Clinical Microbiology Reviews* 12 (1999): 501-517. A detailed article, including chemical structures and models, where applicable, of multiple antifungals. Also includes information on mechanisms of resistance and prevention of resistance.

Ruiz-Herrera, Jose. *Fungal Cell Wall: Structure, Synthesis, and Assembly.* Boca Raton, Fla.: CRC Press, 1992. Comprehensive textbook on fungal cell walls. Includes information on cell-wall structure, chitin and chitosan, and cell-wall growth and assembly.

Thompson, George, Jose Cadena, and Thomas Patterson. "Overview of Antifungal Agents." *Clinics in Chest Medicine* 30 (2009): 203-215. Summary of triazole, echinocandins, polyenes, and antimetabolites. Includes a diagram of effectiveness of individual agents against common molds and yeasts. Includes information on clinical use and antifungals for which therapeutic drug monitoring is recommended.

Zhang, Alexandra, William Camp, and Boni Elewski. "Advances in Topical and Systemic Antifungals." *Dermatologic Clinics* 25 (2007): 165-183. Review of most antifungals that includes a table of various drugs within each class and their classifications as fungicidal or fungistatic. Includes brief sections on clinical use, kinetics, and available dosage forms.

WEB SITES OF INTEREST

British Mycological Society
http://fungionline.org.uk

Centers for Disease Control and Prevention, Division of Foodborne, Bacterial, and Mycotic Diseases
http://www.cdc.gov/nczved/divisions/dfbmd

DoctorFungus
http://www.doctorfungus.org/thedrugs/antif_pharm.htm

Microbiology and Immunology On-line: Mycology
http://pathmicro.med.sc.edu/book/mycol-sta.htm

See also: Antifungal drugs: Types; Diagnosis of fungal infections; Echinocandin antifungals; Fungal infections; Fungi; Fungi: Classification and types; Imidazole antifungals; Immune response to fungal infections; Infection; Mycoses; Polyene antifungals; Prevention of fungal infections; Thiazole antifungals; Treatment of fungal infections; Triazole antifungals.

Antifungal drugs: Types

CATEGORY: Treatment

DEFINITION

Many fungi live in the human body, usually without causing illness. Fungi that do cause human illness affect the skin; nails; body hair; internal organs, such as the lungs; and body systems, such as the nervous system. Antifungal medications are used to prevent the growth and reproduction of harmful fungi.

The treatment of a fungal infection depends on the type and location of infection. Superficial infections that affect the skin, hair, and nails can be treated with a topical cream or ointment. Systemic infections that affect the internal organs require aggressive treatment with either oral or intravenous drugs. Three classes of drugs typically are used to treat fungal infections: polyenes, azoles, and echinocandins.

POLYENES

Polyenes are drugs that work by attaching to the sterol component found in the fungal membrane, injuring the plasma membrane of fungi. This action causes the cells to become porous and then die. The two polyenes most commonly used are nystatin (Mycostatin) and amphotericin B (Fungizone).

Nystatin is often used as a topical agent to treat superficial infections, or it is taken orally to treat such candidal infections as oral or esophageal candidiasis. Nystatin is prescribed in oral, topical, and vaginal formulations for the treatment of fungal infections of the gastrointestinal tract, skin, and vagina, respectively.

Amphotericin B was the first antifungal drug to be approved, and it is still standard therapy for the most severe systemic fungal infections. Fungizone intravenous is specifically intended to treat potentially life-threatening fungal infections such as aspergillosis, cryptococcosis, blastomycosis, systemic candidiasis, coccidioidomycosis, histoplasmosis, and zygomycosis. This potent drug should not be used to treat noninvasive fungal infections such as oral thrush, vaginal candidiasis, and esophageal candidiasis. Several new types of amphotericin B (Abelcet, Amphotec, and AmBisome) have been introduced. These drugs cause fewer side effects than traditional amphotericin B, but they are more expensive.

AZOLES

Azoles stop fungal growth by preventing the production of the essential membranes that surround the fungal cell-wall. Ketoconazole (Nizoral) has been used since the 1970's. It is slightly more toxic than the other azoles and does not work for aspergillosis and many candidiasis infections.

This broad-spectrum antifungal medication is most often used to treat fungal infections that can spread to different parts of the body through the bloodstream. These infections include yeast infections of the mouth, skin, urinary tract, and certain infections that begin on the skin or in the lungs. Ketoconazole is also used to treat fungal infections of the skin or nails that cannot be treated with other medications. Topical ketoconazole is used for treating ringworm, jock itch, athlete's foot, dandruff, and tinea versicolor (a noninflammatory infection of the skin, especially of the trunk, that is caused by a lipophilic fungus).

Fluconazole (Diflucan) is used for treating vaginal, oral, and esophageal fungal infections caused by *Candida*. It is effective in treating urinary tract infections, peritonitis, pneumonia, cryptococcal meningitis, and disseminated infections caused by *Candida*. Although fluconazole is effective against both superficial and systemic candidiasis, some strains of this fungus have now become resistant to the drug.

Itraconazole (Sporanox) is effective against a range of fungal infections. Unlike ketoconazole or fluconazole, itraconazole can be used to treat aspergillosis. Itraconazole capsules are used to treat infections that begin in the lungs and can spread through the body; the drug is also used to treat fungal infections of the fingernails and toenails (onychomycosis). Itraconazole oral solution is used to treat yeast infections of the mouth and throat. It is active against fungal infections such as blastomycosis, histoplasmosis, and candidiasis. Because of its low toxicity profile, this agent can be used for the long-term maintenance treatment of chronic fungal infections.

Voriconazole (Vfend) is used to treat serious fungal infections such as invasive aspergillosis (a fungal infection that begins in the lungs and spreads through the bloodstream to other organs) and esophageal candidiasis (infection by a yeastlike fungus that may cause white patching in the mouth and throat). It acts as an enzyme inhibitor blocking the synthesis of ergosterol, a constituent of fungal membranes, thereby preventing the growth of the microorganism.

Clotrimazole (Lotrimin) is a broad-spectrum antifungal medication used to treat yeast infections of the vagina, mouth, and skin, including athlete's foot, jock itch, and body ringworm. It can also be used to prevent oral thrush in certain persons. Clotrimazole is available as a cream, lotion, powder, and solution to apply to the skin; lozenges to dissolve in the mouth; and vaginal tablets and cream to be inserted into the vagina.

Sulconazole nitrate (Exelderm) is a broad-spec-
trum topical antifungal agent. Exelderm solution has antifungal and antiyeast activity. Sulconazole nitrate solution 1.0 percent is indicated for the treatment of jock itch, ringworm, and tinea versicolor. Effectiveness has not been proven in athlete's foot.

Miconazole (Micatin and Monistat) is an antifungal medication used topically to treat vaginal infections caused by *C. albicans* and several fungal infections of the skin, including tinea versicolor, athlete's foot, jock itch, and ringworm. Miconazole vaginal cream and suppositories are for use only in the vagina. For fungal skin infections, the topical cream is applied as a thin layer to cover the affected skin and surrounding area. These products are not to be taken by mouth.

ECHINOCANDINS

Echinocandins make up a newer class of antifungal drugs that work by disrupting the wall that surrounds fungal cells. They are fungicidal against yeast such as *Candida* species and fungistatic against *Aspergillus* species. Their limited toxicity profile and minimal drug-to-drug interactions make them an attractive option for treating invasive fungal infections.

Three echinocandins are available on the market: caspofungin, micafungin, and anidulafungin. Caspofungin (Cancidas) is an effective treatment for severe systemic fungal infections and is given to persons who do not respond to other therapies. Micafungin is effective in treating aspergillosis in persons with leukemia. Anidulafungin is used to treat candidemia and other forms of invasive candida infections, specifically abscesses in the abdomen and peritonitis, and candida infection of the esophagus.

Gerald W. Keister, M.A.

FURTHER READING

Bennett, John E. "Diagnosis and Treatment of Fungal Infections." In *Harrison's Principles of Internal Medicine*, edited by Joan Butterton. 17th ed. New York: McGraw-Hill, 2008.

Gubbins, Paul O., and Elias J. Anaissie. "Antifungal Therapy." In *Clinical Mycology*, edited by Elias J. Anaissie, Michael R. McGinnis, and Michael A. Pfaller. 2d ed. New York: Churchill Livingstone/Elsevier, 2009.

Murray, Patrick R., Ken S. Rosenthal, and Michael A. Pfaller. "Antifungal Agents." In *Medical Microbiology*. 6th ed. Philadelphia: Mosby/Elsevier, 2009.

Rex, John H., and David A. Stevens. "Systemic Antifungal Agents." In *Mandell, Douglas, and Bennett's Principles and Practice of Infectious Diseases*, edited by Gerald L. Mandell, John E. Bennett, and Raphael Dolin. 7th ed. New York: Churchill Livingstone/Elsevier, 2010.

WEB SITES OF INTEREST

British Mycological Society
http://fungionline.org.uk

Centers for Disease Control and Prevention, Division of Foodborne, Bacterial, and Mycotic Diseases
http://www.cdc.gov/nczved/divisions/dfbmd

DoctorFungus
http://www.doctorfungus.org/thedrugs/antif_pharm.htm

Microbiology and Immunology On-line: Mycology
http://pathmicro.med.sc.edu/book/mycol-sta.htm

See also: Antifungal drugs: Mechanisms of action; Diagnosis of fungal infections; Echinocandin antifungals; Fungal infections; Fungi: Classification and types; Imidazole antifungals; Immune response to fungal infections; Infection; Mycoses; Polyene antifungals; Prevention of fungal infections; Thiazole antifungals; Treatment of fungal infections; Triazole antifungals.

Antiparasitic drugs: Mechanisms of action

CATEGORY: Treatment

DEFINITION

Antiparasitic drugs, or antiparasitics, are used to prevent parasites (harmful organisms) from multiplying in and colonizing the human body.

PARASITES AND PARASITIC DISEASES

Parasites are organisms that live at the expense of another organism, or host. Pathogenic parasites cause diseases such as malaria, trypanosomiasis (sleeping sickness), leishmaniasis, schistosomiasis, and filariasis, all of which affect millions of people around the world each year. These diseases are a significant public health problem in tropical developing countries and lead to blindness, impaired physical and intellectual development, organ failure, disfiguration, and death. Children are especially at risk in endemic areas.

Most pathogenic parasites fit into one of the following three categories: protozoa, helminths, and ectoparasites. Protozoa are single-celled organisms that replicate rapidly in the infected host, often in the gastrointestinal tract. Helminths are complex multicellular organisms such as tapeworms, roundworms, and flukes. Ectoparasites live on the outer surface of the body and include lice, scabies, and ticks.

DISEASE CONTROL

Local and international efforts to control parasitic diseases have had some success by educating people about the spread of parasites. In addition, vaccine and vector control have had beneficial effects. However, effective drugs against these pathogens remain essential to reduce the burden of these diseases. Antiparasitic agents act through a variety of different mechanisms, including inhibition of the neuromuscular system, inhibition of the neuronal system, inhibition of energy metabolism, damage of the membrane, and interference with reproduction.

Inhibition of the neuromuscular system. Inhibiting the neuromuscular system of a parasite results in paralysis, which enables the host body to expel it naturally. This inhibition can be achieved by blocking the transmission of nerve impulses to the muscle fiber at the neuromuscular junction. Drugs that are competitive neuromuscular blockers (such as piperazine) prevent the binding of the neurotransmitter acetylcholine to its cognate receptors. In contrast, depolarizing neuromuscular blockers (levamisole, pyrantel, and morantel) bind to and activate the acetylcholine receptors, but the depolarizing effect on the muscle fiber is prolonged because the drugs are not degraded quickly. In that way, the muscle fiber becomes unresponsive to normal nerve signals. Cholinesterase inhibitors, such as dichlorvos and trichlorfon, achieve a similar effect by blocking the action of enzymes that degrade acetylcholine.

Inhibition of the neuronal system. Paralysis of the parasite can also be induced by activating G-protein-coupled receptors at the neuromuscular junction (with a drug such as emodepside), which stimulates the release of neuropeptides that impair muscle function. Macrocyclic lactones, such as avermectins and milbemycins, act on nerve cells by binding to gated chloride channels, thereby increasing cell permeability and hyperpolarization. These compounds paralyze the pharyngeal pumping mechanism of helminths and appear to prevent the secretion of proteins needed to evade the host immune system.

Inhibition of energy metabolism. Benzimidazoles (such as thiabendazole, mebendazole, and albendazole) act against helminths and some protozoa by binding to beta-tubulin; this prevents the formation of microtubules, which are needed for the cellular uptake of glucose. In addition, benzimidazoles appear to inhibit fumarate reductase (an enzyme important in anaerobic respiration) and to degrade the endoplasmic reticulum and mitochondria, which reduces the production of adenosine triphosphate needed for energy transfer.

The drugs clorsulon, sodium stibogluconate, and meglumine antimoniate inhibit glycolysis, and nitazoxanide inhibits electron transfer by blocking pyruvate-ferredoxin oxidoreductase, an enzyme unique to parasites. Atovaquone is a ubiquinone analog that appears to inhibit electron transport in mitochondria through an interaction with cytochrome B, and niclosamide targets the mitochondria by inhibiting oxidative phosphorylation. Primaquine also appears to disrupt mitochondrial function, although the precise mechanism of action is not clear.

Damaging membrane integrity. Damaging the cellular membrane of muscle cells results in calcium release from intracellular stores. Praziquantel and epsiprantel are two drugs that produce this effect in helminths, thereby causing paralysis and stimulating muscular contractions. The drugs also disrupt the parasite's surface membrane to expose antigens, which are then recognized by the host immune system.

Interfering with reproduction. Several drugs target the reproductive cycle of parasites. The inhibitory effect of benzimidazoles against microtubule formation is also responsible for their ovicidal and larvicidal effects. The drug fumagillin inhibits the proliferation of microsporidia, possibly by blocking the action of methionine aminopeptidase 2, an enzyme involved in protein translation. One of the actions of macrocyclic lactones, which bind to ion channels in nerve and muscle cells, is to paralyze the reproductive tract in adult female helminths.

IMPACT

Parasitic infections are a significant health burden for many of the world's poorest people. These diseases are on the rise because of the use of immunosuppressive drugs, because of immigration, and because of increased travel to affected regions. Many parasitic infections cannot be treated with the drugs that are now available, so further research and development is warranted, and necessary.

Kathleen LaPoint, M.S.

FURTHER READING

Crompton, D. W. T., et al., eds. *Controlling Disease Due to Helminth Infections.* Geneva: World Health Organization, 2003. Available at whqlibdoc.who.int/publications/2003/9241562390.pdf. A collection of articles on helminth infection around the world and strategies for disease control.

Moore, Thomas. "Agents Active Against Parasites and *Pneumocystis.*" In *Mandell, Douglas, and Bennett's Principles and Practice of Infectious Diseases*, edited by Gerald L. Mandell, John E. Bennett, and Raphael Dolin. 7th ed. New York: Churchill Livingstone/Elsevier, 2010. An alphabetical list of treatments for all major parasitic infections that includes each drug's mechanism of action, if known.

Pearson, Richard. "Antiparasitic Therapy." In *Cecil Medicine*, edited by Lee Goldman and Dennis Arthur Ausiello. 23d ed. Philadelphia: Saunders/Elsevier, 2008. Features treatments for parasitic infections organized by type of parasite: helminths, protozoa (further distinguished by ability to live under aerobic or anaerobic conditions), and kinetoplastids, which have specialized mitochondrial structures.

WEB SITES OF INTEREST

Centers for Disease Control and Prevention
http://www.cdc.gov/parasites

Microbiology and Immunology On-line: Parasitology
http://pathmicro.med.sc.edu/book/parasit-sta.htm

National Institute of Allergy and Infectious Diseases
http://www.niaid.nih.gov/topics/tropicaldiseases

National Institutes of Health
http://health.nih.gov/topic/parasiticdiseases

Partners for Parasite Control
http://www.who.int/wormcontrol

See also: Antiparasitic drugs: Types; Children and infectious disease; Developing countries and infectious disease; Diagnosis of parasitic diseases; Emerging and reemerging infectious diseases; Globalization and infectious disease; Immune response to parasitic diseases; Parasites: Classification and types; Parasitic diseases; Parasitology; Pathogens; Prevention of parasitic diseases; Treatment of parasitic diseases; Tropical medicine.

Antiparasitic drugs: Types

CATEGORY: Treatment

DEFINITION

Antiparasitic drugs are drugs used to treat infections by parasites, organisms that live at the expense of another organism, or host. Parasites include helminths (worms), protozoa, and ectoparasites.

ANTHELMINTICS

Helminths are parasites that are frequently found in the digestive tracts of humans and other mammals. Other sites of infestation include blood, liver, the lungs, and the skin, and can be dictated by the particular life cycle of the helminth. Helminths include the nematodes (roundworms), cestodes (flatworms), and trematodes (flukes).

The ultimate goal of an anthelmintic drug is to eliminate the worm infestation from the host. Broadly, anthelmintics can be classified as vermifuges, which stun the worm, and vermicides, which kill the worm. Once worms are killed or incapacitated, they are eliminated by the host's digestive and immune systems.

Anthelmintic drugs include piperazines, tetrahydropyrimidines, imidazothiozoles, benzimidazoles, salicylanilides, nitroaryls, tetrahydroquinolines, isoquinolines, and organometallics. The effectiveness of these drugs varies from parasite to parasite. Mebendazole, one of the benzimidazoles, inhibits the formation of worm microtubules and depletes the worm's glucose. Mechanisms of action vary from drug to drug.

Efforts have also been made to develop anthelmintic vaccines. These attempts have focused primarily on formulations of helminth antigens, which would sensitize the immune systems of humans and animals against the organism. Initial vaccine efforts have focused on the hookworm.

ANTIPROTOZOALS

Protozoa are unicellular eukaryotes. Of the six protozoan phyla, Sarcomastigophora and Apicomplexa include the most important species that cause human disease. Notable Apicomplexa parasites in humans include *Plasmodium falciparum*, which causes malaria, and *Toxoplasma gondii*, which causes toxoplasmosis. Other protozoan parasites include *Giardia intestinalis*, *Cryptosporidium* species, *Trypanosoma* species, and various amebas.

Antiprotozoal drugs include quinolines, nitroheterocycles, antifolates, bisamidines, haloacetamides, and organometallics. Quinine, an antimalarial drug, inhibits nucleic acid and protein syntheses, and glycolysis, but the exact mechanism of this inhibition is not completely understood. Metronidazole, an antiamebal, interacts with deoxyribonucleic acid (DNA), causing a loss of helical DNA structure and strand breakage.

ECTOPARASITICIDES AND ENDECTOCIDES

Ectoparasiticides, broadly defined, are substances that kill external parasites, the vectors that carry them, and the vectors that carry internal parasites to their hosts. Ectoparasiticides include scabicides, insecticides, and insect repellents, and comprise a more diverse collection of compounds because of their more varied modes of action. Common examples are lindane, which is used to treat lice and scabies infestations, and insect repellents such as NN-diethyl metatoluamide (DEET).

Endectocides are compounds that possess antiparasitic qualities against both interior (endoparasites) and exterior (ectoparasites) parasites. One example of an endectocide is ivermectin, one of the avermectin class, which can be used against intestinal threadworms and lice and scabies. Avermectins bind to glutamate-gated chloride ion channels in invertebrate nerve and muscle cells, which results in an increase in permeability of the cell membrane to chloride ions. This change in permeability leads to hyperpolarization of the cell, resulting in paralysis and death of the parasite. Other mechanisms of action may vary.

ANTIPARASITIC NATURAL PRODUCTS AND HISTORY

A limited number of studies have been conducted outside the scope of the pharmaceutical industry in the use of natural products to eradicate parasitic infestations. These products include kalanji, myrrh, onion, oregano, papaya, and wormwood.

One of the first natural products to be successfully used against a parasite was the bark of the cinchona tree, which contains quinine. Quinine has been used against *Plasmodium*, the parasite that causes malaria. It should be noted that these products often require a process to formulate them into the preparation given in these studies, and it should not be inferred that consuming the source product necessarily will give the same effect. Many of these products also require further testing to validate their use.

IMPACT

Parasitic infections are common in areas in which sanitation and water cleanliness standards do not achieve a level required to prevent their transmission. In these areas, antiparasitic drugs are often the best defense against infectious agents such as helminths and amebas. In addition to gaining entry to the human body through oral and oral-fecal routes, certain parasites, such as the hookworm, can gain entry through breaks in the skin. Often because of poverty, people do not wear shoes that would protect them against soil-transmitted parasites like the hookworm. Other parasites, such as the pinworm, can be contracted by inhaling aerosolized eggs.

In 2008, it was estimated that, worldwide, 2.5 billion persons were infected with helminths alone. The bulk of this burden falls on the developing countries, although parasites, such as *Trypanosoma* and *Plasmodium*, can be carried to industrialized areas from regions where parasitic infections are endemic. Immunocompromised persons should be monitored for infection more closely, as parasites have been found outside their usual target organs or in greater numbers when the immune system cannot mount its normal defense.

Resistance to antiparasitic drugs has increased. This resistance is now presenting its own challenges to the elimination of parasites.

Andrew J. Reinhart, M.S.

FURTHER READING

Abdi, Yakoub Aden, et al., eds. *Handbook of Drugs for Tropical Parasitic Infections*. 2d ed. Bristol, Pa.: Taylor & Francis, 2003. A practical reference for indicating the proper drug for a particular parasite. Also describes clinical trials and side effects of the drugs.

Cairncross, Sandy, Ralph Muller, and Nevio Zagaria. "Dracunculiasis (Guinea Worm Disease) and the Eradication Initiative." *Clinical Microbiology Reviews* 15, no. 2 (2002): 223-246. This scientific review details successful measures to eliminate the guinea worm, which is not sensitive to drug therapy.

Hotez, Peter J., et al. "Helminth Infections: The Great Neglected Tropical Diseases." *Journal of Clinical Investigation* 118, no. 4 (2008): 1311-1321. This scientific review contains information on helminth epidemiology, immunobiology, genomics, and control strategies.

Roberts, Larry S., and John Janovy, Jr. *Gerald D. Schmidt and Larry S. Roberts' Foundations of Parasitology*. 8th ed. Boston: McGraw-Hill, 2009. A classic work focusing on the parasites of humans and domestic animals.

Sharma, Satyavan. *Approaches to Design and Synthesis of Antiparasitic Drugs*. New York: Elsevier Science, 1997. A brief review of a variety of parasites and common methods of transmission, followed by a review of drugs used to treat them. Includes discussions of biochemistry and mode of action.

WEB SITES OF INTEREST

Centers for Disease Control and Prevention
http://www.cdc.gov/parasites

National Center for Biotechnology Information
http://pubchem.ncbi.nlm.nih.gov

See also: Antiparasitic drugs: Mechanisms of action; Developing countries and infectious disease; Diagnosis of parasitic diseases; Epidemiology; Fecal-oral route of transmission; Hosts; Microbiology; Parasites: Classification and types; Parasitic diseases; Parasitology; Tropical medicine; Vectors and vector control; Worm infections.

Antiviral drugs: Mechanisms of action

CATEGORY: Treatment

DEFINITION

Antiviral drugs are used to prevent the replication of viruses in the cells of the human body. Viruses, the smallest agents of infection, consist of either deoxyribonucleic acid (DNA) or ribonucleic acid (RNA) and typically are enclosed within a protein coat (capsid). Viruses lack their own metabolism, so to replicate, they must infect a living organism (host) and use that host's cellular machinery.

The viral life cycle is similar for most viruses. Attachment to the host cell is achieved through interaction between viral and host surface proteins. The virus crosses the host cell membrane (entry), the capsid proteins protecting the viral genome are shed (uncoating), and the genome is transcribed into mRNAs (messenger RNA), which are translated. After uncoating, retroviruses (which have the ability to replicate themselves in a host cell) require additional steps: converting the RNA genome to DNA (reverse transcription) and integration into the host genome (strand transfer). After genome replication, the virus self-assembles and is released from the cell by lysis or budding.

Therapies Against Viral Infection

Therapies for viral infections can be classified into agents (antivirals) that inhibit viral replication within the cell, agents (antibodies, virucides) that block viral infection of the host cell, and agents (immunomodulators) that modulate the host response to the viral infection. To selectively inhibit viral replication, drugs exploit the differences between viral and human proteins. Most antiviral drugs target viral nucleic acid synthesis.

Inhibition of Attachment, Entry, and Uncoating

The human immunodeficiency virus (HIV) drugs enfuvirtide and maraviroc are small molecules that inhibit the entry of a virus to its target cell by interacting with viral surface glycoproteins. Enfuvirtide is a peptide that is similar to the HIV glycoprotein gp41; it appears to block the conformational change in gp41 required for fusion and entry. Maraviroc binds to the HIV protein gp120, which prevents its interaction with the host chemokine receptor CCR5. The drug *n*-docosanol is a 22-carbon saturated fatty acid that appears to block entry of lipid-enveloped viruses into target cells.

Amantadine and rimantadine target the viral uncoating step by blocking matrix protein, which forms a transmembrane proton channel in the influenza A lipid envelope. After fusion with the host cell endosome, the passage of hydrogen ions through the proton channel into the virion acidifies the interior, which alters interactions among nucleocapsid proteins and initiates viral uncoating. Pleconaril is another drug that blocks viral uncoating; its high-affinity binding to a hydrophobic pocket of the main capsid protein increases capsid stability and inhibits release of the viral genome.

Inhibition of Genome Replication and Expression

Viral replication is most often targeted by drugs that inhibit the viral polymerase. Nucleoside and nucleotide analog drugs are used as substrates by the viral polymerase, the enzyme that links nucleotide monomers covalently into DNA or RNA. Nucleotides contain one or more phosphate groups, whereas nucleosides require intracellular phosphorylation before they can be incorporated into nucleic acid strand.

For example, acyclovir, an analog of the nucleoside guanosine, inhibits replication of herpes simplex virus (HSV) types 1 and 2 and varicella zoster virus (VZV). It lacks the 3 hydroxyl group needed to create a bond to the next nucleotide in the growing nucleic acid chain; therefore, it is a chain terminator of viral DNA elongation. Because it prevents binding of the normal substrate to the enzyme, it is a competitive inhibitor. Valacyclovir is a more bioavailable form of acyclovir; it is inactive until chemically converted within the cell (that is, as a prodrug of acyclovir). Other guanosine/guanine inhibitors include penciclovir (prodrug famciclovir); ganciclovir (prodrug valganciclovir), which is modified to increase activity against cytomegalovirus (CMV) infections; and ribavirin, which inhibits viral RNA polymerase activity and inhibits the 5 capping of viral mRNA. Ribavirin also appears to enhance the host T-cell-mediated immune response and to inhibit the host inosine monophosphate dehydrogenase, thereby decreasing the intracellular pool of guanosine triphosphate needed for viral replication and acting as a virus mutagen.

Penciclovir (prodrug famciclovir) is another guanine analog, but unlike acyclovir, it is sometimes incorporated into the DNA. It is active against VZV, HSV, and Epstein-Barr virus (EBV). Other nucleoside/nucleotide analogs include cidofovir, a cytosine analog that is active against HSV and poxviruses; vidarabine, an adenosine analog; and the thymidine analogs brivudine, idoxuridine, and trifluridine. Similarly, the reverse transcriptase of retroviruses can be inhibited by nucleotide/nucleoside inhibitors, including zidovudine (the first antiretroviral drug approved for HIV treatment), emtricitabine, abacavir, didanosine, and lamivudine. Retroviruses also require the enzyme integrase for stable integration of the viral DNA into the host genome. The drug raltegravir is the first integrase inhibitor approved for clinical use.

Viral replication can also be blocked by noncompetitive inhibition of the polymerase. Foscarnet is a pyrophosphate analog that binds the pyrophosphate-binding site of herpesvirus DNA polymerase and HIV reverse transcriptase. This binding blocks pyrophosphate cleavage from nucleotides, which prevents their incorporation into the DNA chain.

Fomivirsen is a 21-nucleotide antisense molecule complementary to the mRNA encoding intermediate-early region 2 of CMV, but it also appears to prevent attachment and viral DNA synthesis through unknown mechanisms. Antisense molecules bind to the target mRNA and block its translation. Fomivirsen is modified to block its degradation by nucleases. One of the oxygens in the phosphodiester backbone is replaced with a sulfur, making it a phosphorothioate.

INHIBITION OF VIRAL MATURATION AND RELEASE

For many viruses, the maturation of viral proteins by a protease is essential before the virions are released. A number of drugs have been developed that inhibit the HIV protease by binding to its active site; they include tipranavir, indinavir, saquinavir, nelfinavir, and fosamprenavir.

Viral release is targeted by zanamivir and oseltamivir, which are sialic acid analogs that are competitive reversible inhibitors of neuraminidase, an enzyme expressed on the surface of influenza A and B viruses. Viral neuraminidases cleave sialic acid residues on host receptors recognized by viral hemagglutinin; this releases new viruses from the infected cell, allowing them to spread and infect other cells. Neuraminidase inhibitors, therefore, limit the spread of the virus.

IMPACT

Considerable progress has been made in the development of effective therapies for viral infections.

Better understandings of the physiology of viral replication will reveal more drug targets and increase the therapeutic options for viral infections, especially for emerging viruses such as coronavirus and chronic viral diseases such as hepatitis B and C.

Kathleen LaPoint, M.S.

FURTHER READING

Driscoll, John S. *Antiviral Drugs.* Hoboken, N.J.: John Wiley & Sons, 2006. Presents the most commonly used antiviral drugs and discusses the mechanisms by which the drugs exert their therapeutic effects.

Mahy, Brian W. J., and Marc H. V. van Regenmortel, eds. *Desk Encyclopedia of Human and Medical Virology.* Boston: Academic Press/Elsevier, 2010. Describes common and rare viruses in detail, along with their treatments.

Neal, M. J. *Modern Pharmacology at a Glance.* 6th ed. Hoboken, N.J.: Wiley-Blackwell, 2009. An introduction to pharmacology that explains how drugs, including antiviral drugs, work.

Wagner, Edward K., and Martinez J. Hewlett. *Basic Virology.* 3d ed. Malden, Mass.: Blackwell Science, 2008. An undergraduate text covering issues of virology and viral disease, properties of viruses and virus-cell interaction, working with viruses, and replication patterns of specific viruses.

WEB SITES OF INTEREST

International Consortium on Anti-Virals
http://icav-citav.ca

Universal Virus Database
http://www.ictvdb.org

Viral Zone
http://www.expasy.org/viralzone

See also: AIDS; Antibodies; Antiviral drugs: Types; Autoimmune disorders; Blood-borne illness and disease; HIV; Immunodeficiency; Integrase inhibitors; Maturation inhibitors; Protease inhibitors; Retroviral infections; Retroviridae; Reverse transcriptase inhibitors; Treatment of viral infections; Viral infections; Viruses: Types.

Antiviral drugs: Types

Category: Treatment

Definition

Antiviral drugs are medications used to prevent the replication of viruses in the cells of the human body during infection.

HIV and AIDS Medications

Antivirals targeted at the human immunodeficiency virus (HIV) make up more than one-half of the available antivirals. These antivirals can be divided into six subclasses: nucleoside reverse transcriptase inhibitors (NRTIs), non-nucleoside reverse transcriptase inhibitors (NNRTIs), protease inhibitors (PIs), integrase strand transfer inhibitors (INSTIs), CCR5 antagonists, and fusion inhibitors. Each class targets a different HIV enzyme or receptor.

Nucleoside reverse transcriptase inhibitors. NRTIs are competitive substrate inhibitors that complete with naturally occurring deoxynucleotides. NRTIs inhibit the enzyme, reverse transcriptase, thereby blocking the transcription of viral ribonucleic acid (RNA) to host deoxyribonucleic acid (DNA), preventing HIV from replicating, and preventing incorporation into the host genome. Available NRTIs include zidovudine, didanosine, stavudine, lamivudine, abacavir, and emtricitabine.

Non-nucleoside reverse transcriptase inhibitors. NNRTIs prevent viral RNA from being converted into DNA through the inhibition of reverse transcriptase. Available NNRTIs include efavirenz, nevirapine, delavirdine, and etravirine.

Protease inhibitors. HIV protease is an enzyme that exerts its effect after HIV has successfully entered the host cell and been incorporated into the host genome. Protease is responsible for breaking large protein strands called polyproteins into smaller viral particles, which then mature and become infectious to the host. Protease inhibitors prevent this cleaving of polyproteins and, therefore, prevent HIV particles from maturing and replicating. Available protease inhibitors include atazanavir, darunavir, fosamprenavir, indinavir, lopinavir/ritonavir, nelfinavir mesylate, ritonavir, saquinavir, and tipranavir.

Integrase strand transfer inhibitors. Integrase is an enzyme that facilitates insertion of viral HIV DNA into the host cell DNA. By inhibiting incorporation of the viral DNA, there is no formation of the provirus and, therefore, no viral reproduction within the host. The only available ISTI is raltegravir.

CCR5 antagonists. CCR5, along with CXCR4, is an important coreceptor facilitating the entry of HIV into the host cells. CCR5 antagonists inhibit CCR5, changing the conformation of the coreceptor and, therefore, preventing fusion of the host cell membrane and HIV. The only available CCR5 antagonist is maraviroc.

Fusion inhibitors. Fusion inhibitors bind to the viral envelope glycoprotein and block the conformational change that, if carried out, would result in the fusion on the HIV viral and host cell membrane. The only available fusion inhibitor is enfurvirtide.

Influenza Medications

Four antiviral medications are available, either as treatment or prophylaxis, for influenza A or B. These drugs can be divided into M2 inhibitors and neuraminidase inhibitors. M2 inhibitors can be used prophylactically or for treatment of influenza A; however, the U.S. Food and Drug Administration has issued a statement that for the treatment of influenza A, M2 inhibitors are not recommended for current flu strains.

M2 inhibitors work by inhibiting the uncoating of the influenza A virus, thereby blocking entrance of the virus into the host. Available M2 inhibitors include amantadine and rimantadine.

Neuraminidase inhibitors are the drug of choice for current influenza strains and are active against both A and B strains. Both are approved for both prophylaxis and treatment. Neuraminidase enzyme is an enzyme that plays a role in preparing the glycoproteins to which the influenza virus can attach. Available neuraminidase inhibitors are zanamivir and oseltamivir.

Herpesvirus Medications

Another virus that can lead to a variety of symptoms and complications is the herpes simplex virus (HSV). HSV can be divided into two types, HSV-1 and HSV-2. Additional viruses within the herpes family include cytomegalovirus (CMV), Epstein-Barr virus (EBV), and varicella zoster virus (VZV). The herpesvirus can cause an array of infections affecting various body structures, including genital, orolabial, dermatologic, and ocular. Agents used to treat HSV-1 and HSV-2 include acyclovir, famiciclovir, and valacyclovir.

Acyclovir and related agents work by inhibiting DNA polymerase, stopping viral DNA synthesis.

HEPATITIS MEDICATIONS

Treatment for hepatitis C includes a regimen of pegylated interferon alpha-2a in combination with ribavirin, an antiviral. Ribavirin inhibits viral protein synthesis by preventing both replication of viral genome and elongation of RNA fragments.

IMPACT

The antivirals covered here represent some of the most common antivirals used. Viral diseases that respond to antiviral treatment include HIV and AIDS, influenza, HSV, and viral hepatitis. Mechanisms of action vary among agents, even those used to treat a specific virus. It is important that the differentiation between bacterial and viral pathology is made by clinicians to correctly treat ailments that may have similar presentations.

Allison C. Bennett, Pharm.D.

FURTHER READING

Aberg, Judith A., Jonathan E. Kaplan, and H. Libman. "Primary Care Guidelines for the Management of Persons Infected with Human Immunodeficiency Virus." *Clinical Infectious Diseases* 49, no. 5 (2009): 651-681. Comprehensive guidelines for the treatment of HIV, including treatment-naïve and treatment-experienced regimens. Includes first-line agent recommendations and drug information of the treatments covered.

Clerq, Eric De. "Antiviral Drugs in Current Clinical Use." *Journal of Clinical Virology* 30 (2004): 115-133. Thorough discussion of the mechanism of action of antivirals used for various disease states. Includes chemical compound structure and some pharmacokinetic and pharmacodynamic information.

Driscoll, John S. *Antiviral Drugs.* Hoboken, N.J.: John Wiley & Sons, 2006. Presents the most commonly used antiviral drugs and discusses the mechanisms by which the drugs exert their therapeutic effects.

Mahy, Brian W. J., and Marc H. V. van Regenmortel, eds. *Desk Encyclopedia of Human and Medical Virology.* Boston: Academic Press/Elsevier, 2010. Describes common and rare viruses in detail, along with their treatments.

Yost, Raymond, et al. "A Coreceptor CCR5 Antagonist for Management of HIV Infection." *American Journal of Health-System Pharmacy.* Covers the pharmacology of maraviroc, including mechanism of action, pharmacology, pharmacokinetics, and clinical efficacy. Also covers its place in therapy in the treatment of HIV/AIDS.

WEB SITES OF INTEREST

International Consortium on Anti-Virals
http://icav-citav.ca

Universal Virus Database
http://www.ictvdb.org

Viral Zone
http://www.expasy.org/viralzone

See also: AIDS; Antibodies; Antiviral drugs: Mechanisms of action; Herpesvirus infections; HIV; HIV vaccine; Immunodeficiency; Influenza; Influenza vaccine; Integrase inhibitors; Maturation inhibitors; Protease inhibitors; Reverse transcriptase inhibitors; Treatment of viral infections; Viral hepatitis; Viral infections; Viruses: Structure and life cycle; Viruses: Types.

Appendicitis

CATEGORY: Diseases and conditions
ANATOMY OR SYSTEM AFFECTED: Abdomen, appendix, digestive system, gastrointestinal system, intestines

DEFINITION

Appendicitis is inflammation of the appendix, a structure that arises from the wall of the cecum (a pouch at the beginning of the large intestine). Persons have a 7 percent lifetime risk of developing appendicitis, which is most frequently seen in the second and third decades of life. Acute appendicitis is one of the most frequent reasons for abdominal surgery.

CAUSES

Obstruction of the lumen of the appendix is the most common cause of appendicitis. The most frequent causes of obstruction include fecaliths (dry, compacted feces), calculi (stones), tumors, parasites, foreign bodies, and, rarely, barium (a radiologic dye used in imaging). Secondary bacterial invasion of the appendix also can lead to the development of appendicitis.

Risk Factors

The risk of developing appendicitis is related to the risk of developing an appendiceal obstruction. In young persons, infection is the most likely cause of obstruction. With a person's increasing age, his or her appendix can be obstructed by a tumor or by scar tissue. In endemic areas, parasites can cause obstruction in any age group.

Symptoms

Pain is commonly the first symptom of appendicitis. Initially, the pain is vague and located around or above the umbilicus. Nausea and vomiting normally ensue after the appearance of the initial pain. The pain reaches its peak in about four hours, by which time it migrates to the right lower quadrant of the abdomen. Fever and a lack of appetite can also be associated with appendicitis. The symptoms of appendicitis are not specific and, frequently, not all symptoms are present.

Screening and Diagnosis

Appendicitis is often a clinical diagnosis, in which a doctor takes a person's medical history and conducts a physical examination. Diagnostic tests include blood and urine samples and imaging. A computed tomography (CT) scan is the gold standard in establishing the diagnosis of appendicitis; however, in children and in women who might become pregnant, an ultrasound is performed to prevent exposure to radiation. Once the suspicion of appendicitis is confirmed, the doctor will refer the infected person to a general surgeon.

Treatment and Therapy

Appendicitis is managed both medically and surgically. Patients are normally given IV (intravenous) fluids and antibiotics before surgery. Most commonly, the surgery to remove the appendix, called an appendectomy, is performed through either laparoscopy or laparotomy. In a laparoscopy, small incisions are made in the abdomen, through which surgical instruments are placed and the appendix is removed under camera guidance. A laparotomy, in contrast, involves an open incision into the abdomen and direct visualization and removal of the appendix. This approach, as it is more invasive, is reserved for special circumstances, including for a ruptured appendix and for cases involving an obese patient.

In cases of a ruptured appendix, antibiotics also are given postoperatively. In persons who have an abscess (which is seen during diagnostic imaging), the abscess must be drained. If an inflammatory mass is present, one should avoid surgery and undergo conservative treatment instead.

Prevention and Outcomes

Prevention of appendicitis is not normally feasible; however, prompt recognition of symptoms and appropriate intervention can significantly reduce the morbidity associated with this disease.

Ravinder Pandher, M.D.

Further Reading

"Appendicitis." In *Sabiston Textbook of Surgery*, edited by Courtney M. Townsend et al. 18th ed. Philadelphia: Saunders/Elsevier, 2007.

Blaser, Martin, eds. *Infections of the Gastrointestinal Tract.* 2d ed. Philadelphia: Lippincott Williams & Wilkins, 2002.

Kirschner, Barbara S., and Dennis D. Black. "The Gastrointestinal Tract." In *Nelson Essentials of Pediatrics*, edited by Karen J. Marcdante et al. 6th ed. Philadelphia: Saunders/Elsevier, 2011.

Kumar, Vinay, et al. "Appendicitis." In *Robbins and Cotran Pathologic Basis of Disease*, edited by Vinay Kumar, Abul K. Abbas, and Nelson Fausto. 8th ed. Philadelphia: Saunders/Elsevier, 2010.

Silen, William. *Cope's Early Diagnosis of the Acute Abdomen.* 21st ed. New York: Oxford University Press, 2005.

Zinner, Michael J., et al., eds. *Maingot's Abdominal Operations.* 11th ed. New York: McGraw-Hill, 2007.

Web Sites of Interest

American College of Gastroenterology
http://www.acg.gi.org

American Gastroenterological Association
http://www.gastro.org

Canadian Association of Gastroenterology
http://www.cag-acg.org

See also: *Clostridium difficile* infection; Diverticulitis; Enterobiasis; Gastritis; Infection; Inflammation; Intestinal and stomach infections; Pancreatitis; Peptic ulcer; Peritonitis; *Yersinia pseudotuberculosis*.

Arenaviridae

CATEGORY: Pathogen
TRANSMISSION ROUTE: Direct contact, inhalation

DEFINITION

The arenaviridae family comprises highly infectious, virulent, zoonotic, viral pathogens that are transmitted to humans by rodents. Each arenavirus is associated with a specific host that is native to its geographical region.

Two branches classify arenaviruses: Old World and New World. These branches represent the geographical origin and its subsequent evolutionary pathway to its current locale. The pathway also represents a complicated coevolution between the host and its ribonucleic acid (RNA), with point mutations during genome replications allowing for a large diversity in the arenavirus family.

Taxonomic Classification for Arenaviridae

Order: Unassigned
Family: Arenaviridae
Genus: *Arenavirus*
Species:
Lassa virus
Lymphocyte choriomeningitis
Tacaribe virus

NATURAL HABITAT AND FEATURES

The arenavirus is a beaded nucleocapsid with two single-stranded RNA segments with negative polarity. The virus particles are spherical with an average diameter of 110 to 130 nanometers (nm) and are enveloped in a lipid membrane. The genome includes RNA only. The virus's replication strategy involves forming virions that are spheroid and 50 to 300 nm. They virions bead off from the host cells, giving off a grainy or sandlike appearance, hence the name "arena," meaning "sand" in Latin.

The Old World or Lassa virus derives from the rodent family Muridae, subfamily Muridnae, for which viruses including Lassa and lymphocyte choriomeningitis were derived.

The New World or Tacaribe virus comes from rats, bats, and mice of the family Muridae, subfamily Sigmodontinae. These viruses include Amapari, Guanarito, Junin, Latino, Machupo, Sabia, Tacaribe, and Whitewater Arroyo.

Most of the Old World viruses are found in sub-Saharan Africa, with the exception of lymphocyte choriomeningitis, which was first discovered in the United States (Missouri) and is now found throughout the world. Three of the New World viruses are found in the southwestern regions of the United States; Tacaribe is found in Trinidad. Most of the remaining viruses are found in South America. Specialists indicate that a new arenavirus is discovered every three years.

The habitats of the arenaviruses include any location with rodents and mice. Agricultural areas, barns, homes (especially poorly maintained ones), and dry savannas are especially vulnerable to epidemics. Other areas of possible infection are laboratories that use mice or rodents and homes with pet mice, rats, or hamsters. Secondary and nosocomial infections are especially problematic for Lassa and Machupo viruses.

PATHOGENICITY AND CLINICAL SIGNIFICANCE

Arenaviruses are considered highly infectious, virulent pathogens. There are nine arenaviruses associated with human disease. Five of these, Lassa, Junin, Machupo, Guanarito, and Sabia, are known to cause severe hemorrhagic syndromes and have led to regional epidemics. Lymphocytic choriomeningitis causes an acute central nervous system disease that can lead to congenital malformation. Other viruses are virulent to humans but have caused limited, nonlethal, and nonepidemic cases only or have been grown only in the laboratory.

Lassa fever was first seen in Nigeria in 1969. Since then, it has spread throughout West Africa and, because of widespread international travel, has appeared throughout the world. A reported 100,000 to 300,000 cases occur each year, with 5,000 deaths in West Africa alone. In addition to the expected transmission routes, persons in this area consume rodents, leading to infection caused by ingestion. Nosocomial rates are very high too. Pregnant women are especially at risk, and they risk miscarriage caused by infection at a rate of 75 percent.

The incubation time for Lassa fever is seven to eighteen days, after which the infected person has a fever, is weak, and has general malaise. Cough, severe headaches, sore throat, and gastrointestinal symptoms follow. The next stage of the illness involves vascular permeability, such as facial edema and pleural effusions; if a patient reaches this stage of the illness, the prognosis becomes poor. Rapid deterioration follows, with pulmonary edema, shock, seizures, and coma. Another significant feature of this illness is sensineural deafness in up to 15 percent of patients.

The South American hemorrhagic fevers (Argentine hemorrhagic fever, Guanarito, Machupo, Junin, and Sabia) are usually found in agricultural areas or in hot, dry landscapes, such as the Argentine pampas. Argentine hemorrhagic fever has a mortality rate of 15 to 30 percent. Incubation is one to two weeks, after which the patient experiences fever, malaise, mild neurological symptoms, and vascular damage.

Lymphocytic choriomeningitis usually affects young adults. One common cause in industrialized nations is a bite from a pet hamster. The illness manifests with fever, headache, leucopenia, and thrombocytopenia. After three to four days, the fever may dissipate, but it can return two to four days later with a severe headache and meningitis. Lymphocytic choriomeningitis can cause severe damage to the central nervous system, including hydrocephalus and chorioretinitis.

DRUG SUSCEPTIBILITY

No drug combats all of the arenaviruses. Some success has been found, however, with the use of ribavirin, a nucleoside analogue that has shown to help reduce morbidity and mortality in Lassa, Machupo, and Junin infections. Ribavirin must be given early in the course of the infection to target the viral life cycle. In general, patients with a lower viral load tend to have lower morbidity and mortality rates.

No vaccines are available for any of the arenaviruses. The U.S. Army Medical Research Institute of Infectious Diseases has taken a special interest in the South American hemorrhagic viruses as potential biological warfare agents. The institute is also assisting researchers in developing vaccines.

S. M. Willis, M.S., M.A.

FURTHER READING

De la Torre, Juan C. "Reverse Genetics Approaches to Combat Pathogenetic Arenaviruses." *Antiviral Research* 80 (2008): 239-250. Details new antiviral strategies and includes comprehensive explanations of the pathogenicity of the most virulent arenaviruses.

Gonzalez, J. P., et al. "Arenaviruses." *Current Topics in Microbiology and Immunology* 315 (2007): 253-288. An overview of the history of arenaviruses, including their coevolution with rodent species. Includes a description of the genetics and pathogenicity of arenaviruses.

Kunz, Stefan. "The Role of the Vascular Endothelium in Arenavirus Haemorrhagic Fevers." *Thrombosis and Haemostasis* 102 (2009): 1024-1029. A detailed look at arenaviruses and hemorrhagic fevers, highlighting the vascular damage they cause.

Norkin, Leonard. *Virology: Molecular Biology and Pathogenesis.* Washington, D.C.: ASM Press, 2010. Using the framework of the Baltimore classification scheme, the author provides a detailed account of virus structure and replication and of the basis for disease pathology.

WEB SITES OF INTEREST

Centers for Disease Control and Prevention, Special Pathogens Branch
http://www.cdc.gov/ncidod/dvrd/spb

Virus Pathogen Database and Analysis Resource
http://www.viprbrc.org/brc

See also: Adenoviridae; Hemorrhagic fever viral infections; Lassa fever; Rodents and infectious disease; Viral infections; Viral meningitis; Viruses: Structure and life cycle; Viruses: Types; Zoonotic diseases.

Arthropod-borne illness and disease

CATEGORY: Diseases and conditions
ANATOMY OR SYSTEM AFFECTED: All
ALSO KNOWN AS: Insect-borne illness and disease, vector-borne illness and disease

DEFINITION

Arthropod-borne illnesses are diseases that are spread by arthropods (insects) and are commonly seen in tropical and subtropical climates. The phylum Arthropoda, a term that comes from *arthro* (meaning "joint") and *poda* (meaning "foot"), is the largest phylum in the animal kingdom. This phylum consists of invertebrates (animals that lack a backbone) that manifest bilateral symmetry (in which both halves of the body are identical), an exoskeleton (an external skeleton), a segmented body (a body divided into sections), and jointed legs.

The most diverse category in the Arthropoda phylum is class Insecta, which includes some well-known disease carriers: mosquitoes, ticks, and flies. Other arthropods are mites, fleas, and lice.

According to the World Health Organization (WHO), one in every six persons has an arthropod-borne illness at any given time. Rarely are these diseases caused by the arthropod itself; rather, they are typically caused by pathogenic bacteria, viruses, and protozoa that are carried by a vector. Any arthropod that carries disease-causing microbes is called a vector or carrier.

CAUSES

Pathogenic microbes that move from an infected host to a healthy host through insect bites include bacteria, viruses, protozoa, and helminths. Examples of insect-borne illnesses that are caused by bacteria include Lyme disease, plague, and tularemia. Common insect-borne diseases that are of viral origin include West Nile encephalitis, Chikungunya, yellow fever, and dengue fever. These viruses typically belong to the arbovirus (arthropod-borne viruses) family. Parasitic protozoa cause diseases such as leishmaniasis, Chagas' disease, and malaria. Helminths cause diseases such as ascariasis and lymphatic filariasis.

A vector can be used by a pathogen in many different ways. Sometimes the vector simply offers a means of mechanical transfer from one point to another, such as when a housefly picks up a pathogen from a garbage bin and then deposits the pathogen on food that is consumed by humans. In other instances, such as in the case of malaria, the malarial parasite *Plasmodium* multiplies in the gut of the female *Anopheles* mosquito (a vector) before being transmitted to a healthy host by an insect bite (via the mosquito's saliva). Thus, in this case the vector serves as an intermediate host required to complete the life cycle of the pathogenic protozoan *Plasmodium*. The pathogen also can be deposited on the host's skin through the insect's feces, which then enters the host either through the bite site or through another open wound, as is the case in Chagas' disease.

RISK FACTORS

Persons who are not native to high-risk regions of the world, namely tropical regions, are considered most at risk because they have no common knowledge of these illnesses and have not become immune to secondary infections. Another risk factor is staying in the adobe houses used by locals; some vectors, such as the Triatomine bugs (also called kissing bugs) that transmit Chagas' disease, for example, live in the mud walls and thatched roofs of rural houses in tropical regions.

SYMPTOMS

Symptoms depend on the disease origin (bacterial, viral, protozoan, or helminthic).

Bacterial origin. Lyme disease is the most common tickborne disease in the United States and is caused by a corkscrew-shaped bacterium called *Borrelia burgdorferi.* Early symptoms of Lyme disease include one or more of the following: a characteristic skin rash called erythema migrans, tiredness, headache, chills, muscle and joint pain, and inflammation of the lymph glands. If the early symptoms are not pronounced or go untreated for any reason, later symptoms include arthritis (inflammation and pain in joints, which can become chronic), nervous system problems such as meningitis (marked by a fever, a stiff neck, and a severe headache), and Bell's palsy (paralysis of facial muscles).

Another bacteria-caused arthropod-borne disease is plague, one of the most ancient diseases known to affect humans (an epidemic of the fourteenth century wiped out about one-third of the human population). It is caused by the fleaborne bacteria *Yersinia pestis.*

There are two kinds of plague: bubonic and pneumonic plague. Bubonic plague produces symptoms such as high fever, headache, chills, and painful swollen lymph nodes (also known as buboes). Pneumonic plague symptoms include fever, headache, and pneumonia-like symptoms such as shortness of breath, cough, chest pain, and blood in the sputum.

Tularemia, another disease of bacterial origin, produces signs and symptoms based on the portal (path) of entry of the pathogen. The most common form of tularemia is spread by tick or deer fly bites and produces high fever accompanied by skin ulcers and inflammation (pain and swelling) of the lymph nodes. If left untreated, the infection can become more severe and cause pneumonia-like symptoms such as chest pain, cough, and difficulty in breathing.

Viral origin. West Nile encephalitis is caused by the West Nile encephalitis virus and is classified as a neuroinvasive disease because several forms of this disease affect the nervous system. About 80 percent of people who are exposed to this virus are asymptomatic. However, in persons without symptoms, the disease typically starts with fever, headache, and chills, which can lead to convulsions, neck stiffness, and even paralysis.

Yellow fever, another arthropod-borne illness of viral origin, is named for the yellowish skin coloration that is commonly associated with the better-known liver disease called jaundice. Most yellow fever infections are relatively mild and can remain undetected. However, about 15 percent of persons exposed to the yellow fever virus face a severe life-threatening condition characterized by fever, aches, nausea, abdominal pain, and vomiting that later progresses to melena (blood in the stool), hematemesis (vomiting blood), jaundice, and coma.

Chikungunya, another arthropod-borne illness, was first reported in the mid-twentieth century and was seen primarily in the developing world; hence, very little is known about this disease. The disease has reemerged in more temperate climates, such as Italy and France. Chikungunya resembles dengue fever, in that they both produce symptoms such as high fever, rash, and arthralgia (pain in the joints). Even though most of the symptoms of Chikungunya recede with time, the arthralgia often becomes chronic or relapses frequently after short breaks.

Protozoal origin. Leishmaniasis affects about two million people worldwide annually. It is caused by the protozoan *Leishmania* and is spread by bites of infected sandflies. Among the different types of leishmaniasis, the most common are cutaneous leishmaniasis (marked by skin sores) and visceral leishmaniasis, also known as kala azar, which is characterized by bouts of fever, splenomegaly (an enlarged spleen), weight loss, and anemia.

Chagas' disease has an acute phase and a chronic phase. In the acute phase, the symptoms, if any, are mild and may include fever, fatigue, rash, aches, swollen spleen, and lymph nodes. Chronic symptoms can include irregular heartbeat, cardiomyopathy (an enlarged heart), and congestive heart failure.

Malaria is a greater threat in the tropics, but every year, about fifteen hundred cases are reported in the United States. Malaria is characterized by symptoms such as fever with chills, anemia, nausea, headaches, vomiting, and a feeling of malaise. Usually, malaria is treatable, but a certain *Plasmodium* species, *P. falciparum*, can cause fatal cerebral malaria if left untreated.

Helminthic origin. Ascariasis, if mild, may not produce symptoms. However, moderate to heavy infestation may lead to vomiting, diarrhea, bloody stools, abdominal pain, and worm in the stool.

Lymphatic filariasis (elephantiasis), seen only in a small percentage of infected persons, will produce swelling in the limbs from lymphedema, an accumulation of lymph caused by lymphatic system dysfunction. Because the lymphatic system is part of the body's immune defense, affected people are more prone to bacterial infections in the skin and lymph. This leads to chronic hardening and thickening of the skin surface (in which skin texture resembles those of elephants) called elephantiasis.

SCREENING AND DIAGNOSIS

Persons who have an arthropod-borne disease are diagnosed based on clinical signs and symptoms. For some diseases, such as bubonic plague, characteristic signs help with a definitive diagnosis. Lyme disease is often diagnosed by the classic symptom of a circular skin rash called erythema nigrans. Because not all persons who have been exposed to arthropods such as ticks and who suspect they might develop Lyme disease will get a skin rash, doctors will often order laboratory tests such as ELISA (enzyme linked immunosorbent assay) to test for either an antigen (unique to the pathogen) or an antibody (made in the host to fight the antigen). Persons who test positive in the ELISA test are then recommended for the Western blot assay, which is much more specific.

In case of an arboviral infection, once the preliminary diagnosis has been made on the basis of clinical signs, cerebrospinal fluid or serum is tested to check levels of virus-specific IgM (immunoglobulin M) and other neutralizing antibodies. Occasionally, in severe cases, specialized tests such as immunohistochemistry and virus cultures with tissue samples isolated from the affected individual are used. Diagnostic procedures that involve PCR (polymerase chain reaction) are also widely used because they offer a simple and sensitive method for confirming the diagnosis.

For diagnosing protozoan arthropod-borne diseases such as malaria, health care specialists will use techniques that include a microscopic examination of the blood to check for the presence of the malarial parasite and an RDT (rapid diagnostic test) to look for the presence of antigens borne by a malarial parasite. The RDT is usually available in dipstick or cassette format and, therefore, results can be obtained within a few minutes.

For persons who have symptoms of arthropod-borne diseases of helminthic origin, diseases such as ascariasis, stool samples are tested for the presence of the illness-causing worm. In other diseases of the same family, such as filariasis, blood samples are collected at night and tested for the presence of microfilariae (larval forms of filaria). The blood sample has to be collected from the patient at night because the microfilariae are circulating in the patient's blood at that time.

TREATMENT AND THERAPY

Arthropod-borne illness and disease have become points of major concern because, for most of these diseases, no easy treatments or vaccinations exist. Indeed, the treatments for certain vector-borne diseases can be difficult and dangerous. Diseases of bacterial origin, such as Lyme disease, are treated with antibiotics such as doxicillin and amoxicillin. If started in the early stages of illness, these antibiotics can completely cure the patient.

Arthropod-borne diseases of viral origin have no specific treatment, and treatment for protozoan diseases, such as malaria, involves the use of antimalarial drugs such as quinine and chloroquine; leishmaniasis is treated with drugs such as liposomal amphotericin B. Helminthic origin diseases are treated with drugs such as albendazole, mebendazole, or a yearly dose of diethycarbamazine, which kills circulating microfilariae.

PREVENTION AND OUTCOMES

Because these diseases are spread by insect bites, the simplest measures to prevent illness are to block insects from accessing the host and to practice good sanitation and hygiene. Therefore, one should wear covered clothing such as long-sleeve shirts and pants when outdoors and should use insect repellants such as permethrin or those with NN-diethyl metatoluamide, or DEET (about 20 to 30 percent). Similarly, to minimize the chance of insect bites, one should avoid wooded areas in the late evening or nighttime hours and should routinely check clothes and accessories for ticks and fleas after returning indoors. In the case

of diseases such as malaria, additional preventive measures include using insecticide-sprayed sleeping nets (around the bed) and using chemoprophylaxis (taking malaria-prevention drugs over time). Finally, for diseases such as ascariasis, helpful prevention strategies include avoiding soil that is infested with the worm that causes the disease and washing and peeling all fruits and vegetables. A proper understanding of these preventive measures is especially important because many of these diseases are included on the World Health Organization's list of emerging infectious diseases.

Sibani Sengupta, Ph.D.

FURTHER READING

Ashford, R. W., and W. Crewe. *The Parasites of "Homo sapiens": An Annotated Checklist of the Protozoa, Helminths, and Arthropods for Which We Are Home.* 2d ed. New York: Taylor & Francis, 2003. An examination of the parasites that are familiar to the human body.

Atkinson, P. W., ed. *Vector Biology, Ecology, and Control.* New York: Springer Science, 2010. This book is a good source for the reader who needs a detailed study of vectors and latest methods for effective vector control.

Busvine, James R. *Disease Transmission by Insects: Its Discovery and Ninety Years of Effort to Prevent It.* New York: Springer, 1993. This book provides a historical perspective on the evolution of and progress in the study of arthropod-borne diseases.

Jong, Elaine C., and Russell McMullen, eds. *Travel and Tropical Medicine Manual.* 4th ed. Philadelphia: Saunders/Elsevier, 2008. A useful reference manual with advice on preventing, evaluating, and managing diseases that can be acquired in tropical environments and countries outside the United States.

Marquardt, William C., ed. *Biology of Disease Vectors.* 2d ed. New York: Academic Press/Elsevier, 2005. This textbook is geared to graduate students and researchers, but most of the information is accessible to general readers.

O'Hanlon, Leslie Harris. "Tinkering with Genes to Fight Insect-Borne Disease: Researchers Create Genetically Modified Bugs to Fight Malaria, Chagas', and Other Diseases." *The Lancet* 363 (April 17, 2004): 1288. Discusses genetic engineering techniques and their anticipated results.

Tortora, Gerard J., Berdell R. Funke, and Christine L. Case. *Microbiology: An Introduction.* 10th ed. San

Francisco: Benjamin Cummings, 2010. A great reference for exploring the microbial world. Provides readers with an appreciation of the pathogenicity and usefulness of microorganisms.

WEB SITES OF INTEREST

Emerging and Reemerging Infectious Diseases Resource Center
http://www.medscape.com/resource/infections

National Center for Emerging and Zoonotic Infectious Diseases
http://www.cdc.gov/ncezid

National Institute of Allergy and Infectious Diseases
http://www.niaid.nih.gov/topics/vector

See also: Ascariasis; Bacterial meningitis; *Borrelia*; Bubonic plague; Chagas' disease; Chikungunya; Dengue fever; Ehrlichiosis; Elephantiasis; Encephalitis; Filariasis; Fleas and infectious disease; Flies and infectious disease; Insect-borne illness and disease; Leishmaniasis; Lyme disease; Malaria; Mites and chiggers and infectious disease; Mosquitoes and infectious disease; Parasitic diseases; Parasitology; Pathogens; Plague; Protozoan diseases; Ticks and infectious disease; Tropical medicine; Tularemia; Vectors and vector control; Viral infections; West Nile virus; Yellow fever; *Yersinia.*

Artificial joint infections. *See* Prosthetic joint infections.

Ascariasis

CATEGORY: Diseases and conditions
ANATOMY OR SYSTEM AFFECTED: Gastrointestinal system, heart, intestines, lungs, respiratory system, stomach, throat
ALSO KNOWN AS: Roundworm

DEFINITION

Ascariasis is an intestinal worm infestation. It is present worldwide, though mostly in tropical climates. *Ascaris lumbricoides* is a nematode (roundworm) parasite that can reach up to 40 centimeters (16 inches) in length. Like most parasites, *Ascaris* has a complex life cycle that begins with a person ingesting its eggs. After the parasite hatches in the gut, immature forms of the parasite travel to the heart and lungs, causing a type of pneumonia. They then migrate into the throat, where they are swallowed, reenter the gut, and develop into adult worms. The eggs the adults lay (240,000 per worm per day) pass out with feces to begin their cycle again when contaminated food or water is ingested.

CAUSES

Ascariasis is caused by ingesting food or water contaminated by feces containing *Ascaris* eggs.

RISK FACTORS

Those persons who have an increased chance of developing ascariasis include preschool age or younger children, travelers to developing countries, persons living in the southern United States, persons who eat unsanitary food, and persons who drink unclean water.

SYMPTOMS

A person with any of the following symptoms should not assume the symptoms are caused by ascariasis. These symptoms may be caused by other health conditions. Persons who experience any one of these symptoms, and who have been exposed to risks, should consult a doctor. The symptoms include pneumonia (dry cough and fever); wheezing; abdominal cramps; vomiting; malnutrition, especially in children; and passing a worm by mouth, nose, or rectum. Symptoms also include those of the diseases caused by *Ascaris* worms: gallbladder disease, liver abscess, pancreatitis, appendicitis, and peritonitis.

SCREENING AND DIAGNOSIS

A doctor will ask about symptoms and travel and medical history, and will perform a physical exam. The patient may then be referred to a gastroenterologist or a specialist in tropical diseases. Tests may include blood and urine tests, stool specimens to search for worm eggs, intestinal X rays, or ultrasound imaging.

TREATMENT AND THERAPY

It is common to have more than one intestinal parasite, leading to treatment for several. Treatment options include drugs such as mebendazole, albendazole, and pyrantel pamoate, which are all effective

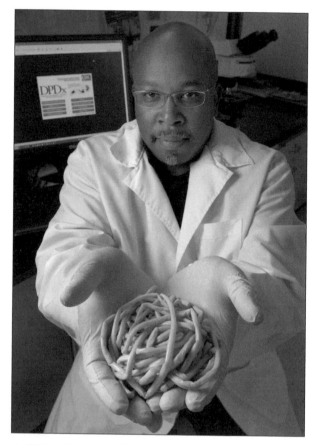

A CDC technician holds a mass of Ascaris lumbricoides *worms, which had been passed by a child in Kenya who was infected with ascariasis.* (CDC)

medications that kill *Ascaris* worms, and endoscopy or surgery, because an intestinal obstruction of many worms may require further intervention.

PREVENTION AND OUTCOMES

To help reduce the chance of getting ascariasis, one should avoid foods prepared without proper sanitary precautions (such as unwashed hands); avoid water and other drinks that might have come from contaminated sources; should peel, cook, or wash vegetables in an appropriate cleaning solution if there is a chance those vegetables came from soil fertilized with human excrement; and should wash hands when leaving a toilet area.

Ricker Polsdorfer, M.D.;
reviewed by David L. Horn, M.D., FACP

FURTHER READING

Berger, Stephen A., and John S. Marr. *Human Parasitic Diseases Sourcebook.* Sudbury, Mass.: Jones and Bartlett, 2006.

Despommier, Dickson D., et al. *Parasitic Diseases.* 5th ed. New York: Apple Tree, 2006.

EBSCO Publishing. *DynaMed: Ascariasis.* Available through http://www.ebscohost.com/dynamed.

Icon Health. *Roundworms: A Medical Dictionary, Bibliography, and Annotated Research Guide to Internet References.* San Diego, Calif.: Author, 2004.

Porter, Robert S., et al., eds. *The Merck Manual Home Health Handbook.* 3d ed. Whitehouse Station, N.J.: Merck Research Laboratories, 2009.

Roberts, Larry S., and John Janovy, Jr. *Gerald D. Schmidt and Larry S. Roberts' Foundations of Parasitology.* 8th ed. Boston: McGraw-Hill, 2009.

Weller, P. F., and T. B. Nutman. "Intestinal Nematodes." In *Harrison's Principles of Internal Medicine*, edited by Anthony Fauci et al. 17th ed. New York: McGraw-Hill, 2008.

WEB SITES OF INTEREST

American Society of Tropical Medicine and Hygiene
http://www.astmh.org

Centers for Disease Control and Prevention
http://www.cdc.gov/parasites

Nemours Foundation
http://kidshealth.org

World Health Organization
http://www.who.int

See also: Amebic dysentery; Capillariasis; Cryptosporidiosis; Developing countries and infectious disease; Diverticulitis; Fecal-oral route of transmission; Foodborne illness and disease; Giardiasis; Hookworms; Intestinal and stomach infections; Norovirus infection; Parasites: Classification and types; Parasitic diseases; Peritonitis; Pinworms; Roundworms; Strongyloidiasis; Travelers' diarrhea; Tropical medicine; Waterborne illness and disease; Whipworm infection; Worm infections.

Aseptic technique

CATEGORY: Prevention

DEFINITION

Aseptic technique involves applying preventive measures to minimize the chance of introducing into clinical settings the microorganisms, such as viruses and harmful bacteria (pathogens), that cause disease. In other words, its purpose is to maintain asepsis, or the absence of pathogens, in clinical settings. Aseptic technique is intended to protect the patient and the health care worker from pathogens and to prevent their spread.

Pathogens may introduce infection to a patient through contact with the environment, with personnel, or with medical equipment. The environment contains potential hazards that may disseminate pathogens through movement, touch, or proximity.

Aseptic technique involves a set of procedures designed to remove or kill microorganisms on hands and objects, reducing a patient's risk of exposure. It includes the use of sterile instruments and of barriers such as personal protective equipment, adequate handwashing, patient preparation, and maintenance of sterile fields and a safe environment in surgical and other areas for medical procedures.

MINIMIZING CONTAMINATION DURING SURGERY

Interventions such as minimizing surgical-room traffic, isolating a patient to reduce airborne contamination, and using low-particle-generating surgical attire contribute to reducing environmental hazards. Equipment or supplies can be sterilized through chemical treatment, radiation, gas, or heat.

The most prominent example of aseptic technique occurs in the operating room, in which clinicians work to prevent postoperative infection. Aseptic technique protocols include patient skin preparation, handwashing and surgical scrub, barrier protection for the patient (draping) and the surgical team (surgical attire), and maintenance of the sterile field.

Hand hygiene among medical personnel is the most important aspect of reducing contamination. Adequate handwashing involves removing jewelry, avoiding contact with the sink, and performing vigorous hand scrubbing. Thorough drying is critical because moist surfaces encourage pathogen growth. Bare hands are potential sources of infection, and glove use is important.

Sterile surgical clothing and protective devices such as gloves, face masks, goggles, and transparent eye and face shields serve as barriers against microorganisms. Surgical attire must be worn with deliberate care to prevent contact of sterile surfaces with nonsterile objects, including skin. Procedures for putting on surgical attire include covering facial hair, tucking hair out of sight, and removing jewelry or other dangling objects that may contain microorganisms. Personnel assist the surgeon in putting on gloves and the surgical gown and in arranging equipment to minimize the risk of contamination. Creating surgical fields with drapes, which are sterilized linens placed on the patient or around the field to define sterile areas, helps maintain asepsis in the operating room or during other invasive procedures.

Other principles applied to maintain asepsis include ensuring that all items in a sterile field are actually sterile. Also sterile packages should be opened as close as possible to time of use.

Moist areas are not considered sterile. Contaminated items must be removed immediately, and nonsterile items should not cross a sterile field. Edges of sterile fields are not considered sterile, and a margin of safety is maintained between sterile and nonsterile objects. Drapes or wrapped kits of equipment are opened in a manner to prevent contents from touching nonsterile surfaces. Others who work close to the sterile field, such as anesthesia personnel, also must follow aseptic technique. During a procedure, staff members are positioned so that those who have undergone surgical scrub and are wearing sterile attire are closest to the patient while unscrubbed staff members remain on the perimeter to obtain supplies, acquire assistance, and communicate with outside personnel.

NONSURGICAL CLINICAL SETTINGS

Aseptic technique is also used in a variety of settings outside the operating room. A primary difference between the operating room and other clinical environments is that areas outside the operating room generally do not allow for the same rigorous level of asepsis. Avoiding potential infection is still the goal, however. For example, changing a surgical dressing at the patient's bedside should still include thorough handwashing, use of gloves and other protective garb,

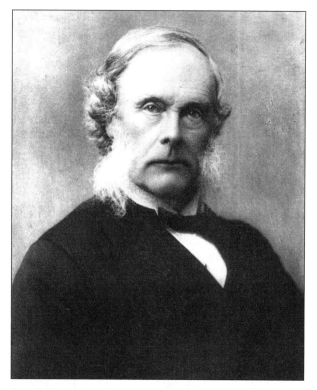

Joseph Lister is credited with helping to start the practice of sterilizing operating rooms. (Library of Congress)

creation of a sterile field, and avoidance of contact with nonsterile items.

Typical situations that require aseptic measures include insertion of intravenous lines, urinary catheters, and drains; changing of wound dressings; vaginal exams during labor; and respiratory suction. General habits such as prompt disposal of contaminated needles or blood-soaked bandages and dressings and the prevention of accumulation of drained bodily fluids through regular emptying of receptacles help preserve and maintain a clean medical environment and keep it as free of microorganisms as possible.

IMPACT

Practices that clean (remove dirt and other impurities), sanitize (reduce the number of microorganisms), or disinfect (remove most microorganisms) are not always adequate to prevent infection. The Centers for Disease Control and Prevention estimates that more than 27 million surgical procedures are performed in the United States each year. Surgical site infections are the third-most-common nosocomial, or hospital-acquired, type of infection and result in longer hospital stays and greater patient costs. Aseptic technique is vital in reducing the morbidity and mortality associated with surgical infections. Aseptic technique is especially important in cases involving patients who have compromised (weak) immune systems.

C. J. Walsh, Ph.D.

FURTHER READING

Clancy, Carolyn. "Simple Steps Can Reduce Health Care-Associated Infections: Navigating the Health Care System." Rockville, Md.: Agency for Healthcare Research and Quality, 2008. Available at http://www.ahrq.gov/consumer/cc/cc070108.htm. An advice column written by a general internist and researcher who is an expert in engaging consumers in their health care.

Farb, Daniel, and Gordon Bruch. *Infection Control in Healthcare Facilities Guidebook: A Concise Compliance Guide for Healthcare Staff and Management.* Los Angeles: UniversityOfHealthCare, 2006. A manual for clinical staff in health care facilities, including standards for infection control. Features detailed prevention procedures.

Kennamer, Mike. *Basic Infection Control for Health Care Providers.* 2d ed. Clifton, N.Y.: Thomas Delmar Learning, 2007. An instructional guide to preventing the spread of contagious and infectious diseases. Includes examinations of the disease process.

Peleg, Anton Y., and David C. Hooper. "Hospital-Acquired Infections Due to Gram-Negative Bacteria." *New England Journal of Medicine* 362, no. 19 (2010): 1804-1813. Explains how hospital-acquired infections are a major but often preventable challenge to patient safety, representing the sixth leading cause of death in the United States.

Perry, Christine. *Infection Prevention and Control.* Malden, Mass.: Blackwell, 2007. A concise text geared to nursing students and newly qualified nursing staff. Serves as an invaluable guide to essential principles of infection prevention and control.

Westin, Debbie. *Infection Prevention and Control: Theory and Practice for Healthcare Professionals.* Hoboken, N.J.: John Wiley & Sons, 2008. Includes background information to support the rationale behind basic principles of infection control and how to apply them using evidence-based recommendations on infection control management.

Workman, Barbara A., and Clare L. Bennett. *Key Nursing Skills*. London: Whurr, 2003. Each chapter focuses on a specific area of care and related skills. Includes a chapter on aseptic technique.

WEB SITES OF INTEREST

Association for Professionals in Infection Control and Epidemiology
http://www.knowledgeisinfectious.org

Association of Perioperative Registered Nurses
http://www.aorn.org

Clean Hands Coalition
http://www.cleanhandscoalition.org

Healthcare Infection Control Practices Advisory Committee
http://www.cdc.gov/hicpac

See also: Bacterial infections; Bloodstream infections; Chemical germicides; Contagious diseases; Decontamination; Disinfectants and sanitizers; Epidemiology; Hospitals and infectious disease; Hygiene; Iatrogenic transmission; Infection; Prevention of bacterial infections; Prevention of viral infections; Public health; Superbacteria; Transmission routes; Viral infections; Wound infections.

Aspergillosis

CATEGORY: Diseases and conditions
ANATOMY OR SYSTEM AFFECTED: Lungs, respiratory system

DEFINITION

Aspergillosis is an infection caused by the common fungus *Aspergillus*, which is found around the world. The infection can cause severe problems in the lung.

This type of infection is rare, and it is more common in people with chronic lung disease, human immunodeficiency virus (HIV) infection, and acquired immunodeficiency syndrome (AIDS), and in people undergoing prolonged chemotherapy and those using steroids. Most of these conditions weaken the immune system. The body is less able to fight infections.

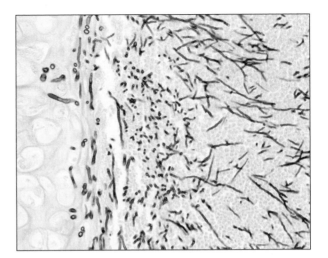

A microscopic image of pulmonary invasive aspergillosis. (CDC)

In these cases, the fungus can spread to other organs. This can include the eye, sinuses, and brain. Aspergillosis is a serious condition that requires treatment. Another form of aspergillosis—allergic bronchopulmonary aspergillosis, a type of allergic reaction to environmental agents—affects people with asthma.

CAUSES

Inhaling fungus spores is often the first step in the development of aspergillosis.

RISK FACTORS

The factors that increase the chance of developing aspergillosis include a compromised immune system; AIDS; drugs that accompany an organ transplant; certain cancer treatments; long-term, high-dose cortisone-like drugs; poorly functioning or too few white blood cells (neutropenia); chronic lung disease; bronchiectasis; tuberculosis; sarcoidosis; histoplasmosis; and asthma.

SYMPTOMS

Symptoms of aspergillosis include a chronic productive (mucus-producing) cough, coughing up blood, fever, shortness of breath, and wheezing.

SCREENING AND DIAGNOSIS

A doctor will ask about symptoms and medical history and will do a physical exam. The patient may be referred to a specialist in lung diseases or infectious diseases. One such specialist, a pulmonologist, focuses on the lungs. Tests for aspergillosis include blood and urine sampling, sputum sampling, a chest X ray, a magnetic resonance imaging (MRI) scan, a computed tomography (CT) scan, and bronchoscopy (in which a special thin scope is used to look into the lungs).

TREATMENT AND THERAPY

Treatment includes medications such as intravenous amphotericin B, which is given for a prolonged time and might damage the kidneys. Another medication is voriconazole, which is found to be highly effective for invasive aspergillosis and is a preferred treatment option for many persons. Still another medication is itraconazole, which is effective in some cases.

Surgery also is a treatment option. Part of the lung may need to be removed if it contains a large mass of fungus.

PREVENTION AND OUTCOMES

Aspergillus is everywhere in the environment, which makes it impossible to avoid. To avoid the fungi, one should avoid the conditions that are associated with it.

Ricker Polsdorfer, M.D.;
reviewed by David L. Horn, M.D., FACP

FURTHER READING

Barnes, Penelope D., and Kieren A. Marr. "Aspergillosis: Spectrum of Disease, Diagnosis, and Treatment." *Infectious Disease Clinics of North America* 20 (2006): 545-561.

Bennett, J. E. "Aspergillosis." In *Harrison's Principles of Internal Medicine*, edited by Anthony Fauci et al. 17th ed. New York: McGraw-Hill, 2008.

DynaMed: Aspergillosis. Available through http://www.esbcohost.com/dynamed.

Ferri, Fred F., ed. *Ferri's Clinical Advisor 2011: Instant Diagnosis and Treatment.* Philadelphia: Mosby/Elsevier, 2011.

Patterson, Thomas F. "*Aspergillus* Species." In *Mandell, Douglas, and Bennett's Principles and Practice of Infectious Diseases*, edited by Gerald L. Mandell, John F. Bennett, and Raphael Dolin. 7th ed. New York: Churchill Livingstone/Elsevier, 2010.

Richardson, Malcolm D., and Elizabeth M. Johnson. *Pocket Guide to Fungal Infection.* 2d ed. Malden, Mass.: Blackwell, 2006.

WEB SITES OF INTEREST

American Lung Association
http://www.lungusa.org

Canadian Lung Association
http://www.lung.ca

Centers for Disease Control and Prevention
http://www.cdc.gov

See also: Allergic bronchopulmonary aspergillosis; *Aspergillus*; Atypical pneumonia; *Bordetella*; Bronchiolitis; Bronchitis; Cryptococcosis; Diagnosis of fungal infections; Fungal infections; Fungi: Classification and types; Histoplasmosis; Legionnaires' disease; Nocardiosis; Pneumonia; Respiratory route of transmission; Soilborne illness and disease; Tuberculosis (TB); Waterborne illness and disease; Whooping cough.

Aspergillus

CATEGORY: Pathogen
TRANSMISSION ROUTE: Blood, direct contact, inhalation

DEFINITION

Aspergillus is a common fungus (mold) that frequently causes life-threatening infections in immunocompromised persons. *Aspergillus* species also produce many mycotoxins and allergens that can cause cancer, can damage the immune and nervous systems, and can increase the risk for developing asthma and sinus problems.

NATURAL HABITAT AND FEATURES

Aspergillus is a ubiquitous aerobic mold that is found on vegetation, decomposing matter, soil, food, water, and feces, and in outdoor and indoor air. The asexual spores (conidia) are small (2 to 5 microns) and are borne in chains formed on spherical or oblong vesicles. *Aspergillus* is often fast growing and can sporulate in a few days after germination.

Aspergillus is present mainly in the anamorphic or asexual phase. Some *Aspergillus* species also have a telemorphic phase and produce ascospores. Some of the more common *Aspergillus* ascospore forms include *Eurotium amstelodami*, which is the teleomorph of *A. vitis*,

Taxonomic Classification
for *Aspergillus*

Kingdom: Fungi
Phylum: Ascomycota
Class: Eurotiomycetes
Order: Eurotiales
Family: Trichocomaceae
Genus: *Aspergillus*
Species:
A. candidus
A. clavatus
A. flavus
A. fumigatus
A. niger
A. ochraceus
A. oryzae
A. paristicus
A. tamari
A. terreus
A. ustus
A. versicolor

and *E. herbariorum*, which is the teleomorph of *A. glaucus*.

Aspergillus is often a part of plant and food spoilage and plays an important role in the decomposition of leaves and other organic matter. It also is involved in the production of certain enzymes, pharmaceuticals, and organic acids.

PATHOGENICITY AND CLINICAL SIGNIFICANCE

Aspergillus can adversely affect humans by three mechanisms that include infection and the production of mycotoxins (fungal toxins) and allergens. Both superficial and disseminated invasive *Aspergillus* infections are common. Invasive *Aspergillus* infections cause a minimum of five thousand deaths annually in the United States. The most common species that causes infection is *fumigatus*, with *flavus*, *niger*, and *terreus* also causing many infections. Even with hospitalization and antifungal drugs, invasive *Aspergillus* infections have a 32 to 99 percent fatality rate.

Aspergillus infections are especially common in people with compromised immune systems, including persons with human immunodeficiency virus infection, lymphoma, or leukemia; malnourished persons; and persons on immunosuppressive drugs following bone or organ transplantation. *Aspergillus* infections are also more common in hospitalized persons who are recovering in rooms that are close to water damage or building construction. As many as 2 to 15 percent of persons with bone-marrow transplants, 6 to 13 percent of persons with a lung transplant, and up to 8 percent of persons with leukemia or lymphoma develop *Aspergillus* infections. Disseminated *Aspergillus* infections usually begin in the respiratory tract and can cause breathing troubles, coughing, hemoptypsis, high fever, growth of lung fungal balls, and death. *Aspergillus* can also produce localized infections, especially in the lungs and nasal sinuses. Exposure to *Aspergillus* during heart surgery can produce serious heart valve infections.

Aspergillus also produces dozens of mycotoxins. The strongly carcinogenic aflatoxin mycotoxins are produced by *flavus* and *parasiticus*. *Aspergillus* frequently produces aflatoxins on damp or otherwise poorly stored crops, especially peanuts and corn (maize). Eating aflatoxin-contaminated food has been associated with significantly higher levels of liver cancer. Other common mycotoxins produced by *Aspergillus* include ochratoxin, patulin, gliotoxin, verrucologen, fumitremorgin, and strerigmatocystin.

Aspergillus produces dozens of allergens that can worsen asthma, sinusitis, and allergies. A number of studies have reported that exposure to high airborne levels of *Aspergillus* and other fungi are associated with higher levels of asthma and sinus problems. Exposure to airborne *Aspergillus* can also produce a serious hypersensitivity condition called allergic bronchopulmonary aspergillosis.

The best way to prevent *Aspergillus* infection is to limit exposure in persons with compromised immune systems. Many studies have reported that housing bone and organ transplant patients in rooms with air filtration significantly reduces the incidence of *Aspergillus* infections and mortality from these infections. Using positive-pressure hospital rooms, adequately cleaning the patient's room, having walls covered in antifungal paint, promptly cleaning up water damage, and avoiding construction areas can also significantly reduce *Aspergillus* infection rates.

Invasive *Aspergillus* infections are often hard to diagnose in the early stages, as persons may not exhibit obvious symptoms until the infection is advanced and life-threatening. High resolution computed tomography (CT) scans are often useful in detecting invasive fungal infections. The CT scan usually will show a halo sign in images of early-stage infection (infections beginning less than five days before scan) and an air crescent sign in images of late-stage infection.

Serological tests are often used to detect the presence of invasive *Aspergillus* infections, with the most common test being the galactomannan assay. A meta-analysis of twenty-five galactomannan studies reported that the overall sensitivity and specificity were found to be 71 and 89 percent, respectively. Polymerase chain reaction (PCR) assays can also be used to detect deoxyribonucleic acid (DNA) from various *Aspergillus* species.

DRUG SUSCEPTIBILITY

Traditionally, the drugs used most often for *Aspergillus* infections include amphotericin B and azole drugs, such as fluconazole and itraconazole. These drugs have only modest success in persons with invasive *Aspergillus* infections. Systemic amphotericin B also has many serious side effects, including fever, vomiting, and headache, and damage to the kidneys, liver, and heart. These side effects often force the discontinuation of amphotericin B.

A newer class of drugs, echinocandins, has been developed. This class blocks cell-wall synthesis in *Candida* and *Aspergillus*. Echinocandin drugs include anidulafungin, caspofungin, and micafungin. Studies have reported that the echinocandin drugs are about as effective in treating invasive *Aspergillus* infections as amphotericin B but have a much lower risk of side effects.

Luke Curtis, M.D.

FURTHER READING

Chandrasekar, Pranatharthi. "Diagnostic Challenges and Recent Advances in the Early Management of Invasive Fungal Infections." *European Journal of Haematology* 84 (2009): 281-290. This article discusses the challenges of getting an early diagnosis for invasive *Aspergillus* and other fungal infections.

Gullo, Antonio. "Invasive Fungal Infections." *Drugs* 69 (2009): 65-73. This paper reports on twenty-first century advances in the development of antifungal drugs.

Marr, Kieren, Thomas Patterson, and David Denning. "Aspergillosis: Pathogenesis, Clinical Manifestations, and Therapy." *Infectious Disease Clinics of North America* 16 (2002): 875-894. This article provides a good overview of *Aspergillus* infections, lung-imaging studies, early diagnosis, and treatments.

Patridge-Hinckley, Kimberly, et al. "Infection Control Measures to Prevent Invasive Mould Diseases in Hematopoietic Stem Cell Transplant Recipients." *Mycopathologica* 168 (2009): 329-337. This article discusses the use of air filters and other environmental controls to reduce the risk of *Aspergillus* infections in immunocompromised persons.

Patterson, Thomas F. "*Aspergillus* Species." In *Mandell, Douglas, and Bennett's Principles and Practice of Infectious Diseases,* edited by Gerald L. Mandell, John F. Bennett, and Raphael Dolin. 7th ed. New York: Churchill Livingstone/Elsevier, 2010. A thorough review of *Aspergillus* species in a respected text on infectious diseases.

Samson, Robert, Ellen Hoesktra, and Jens Frisvad. *Introduction to Food and Airborne Fungi.* 7th ed. Utrecht, the Netherlands: Central Bureau for Fungal Cultures, 2004. This guide has much useful information about *Aspergillus*, common indoor fungi, and their identification. Includes useful photos and diagrams.

WEB SITES OF INTEREST

American Lung Association
http://www.lungusa.org

Canadian Lung Association
http://www.lung.ca

See also: Airborne illness and disease; Allergic bronchopulmonary aspergillosis; Antifungal drugs: Types; Aspergillosis; Diagnosis of fungal infections; Echinocandin antifungals; Food-borne illness and disease; Fungal infections; Fungi: Classification and types; *Fusarium;* Hospitals and infectious disease; Immune response to fungal infections; Mycetoma; Soilborne illness and disease; *Stachybotrys;* Waterborne illness and disease.

Asplenia

CATEGORY: Diseases and conditions
ANATOMY OR SYSTEM AFFECTED: Abdomen, immune system, spleen

DEFINITION

Asplenia is the absence of a working spleen. The

spleen is located in the upper left side of the abdomen and is roughly the size of a person's fist. Asplenia can be anatomical, in which the spleen is actually missing, or functional, in which the spleen is present but not functioning.

Although originally considered a nonessential organ, the spleen is now recognized as a vital part of the immune system. It is also part of the body's system that manages waste material. The spleen has two different tissue types: white pulp and red pulp. White pulp makes white blood cells that, in turn, produce antibodies (infection-fighting proteins). Red pulp filters foreign or abnormal materials from the blood. It also destroys old or abnormal red blood cells.

Causes

Some persons are born without a spleen. This can be part of a genetic condition that also causes problems with other organs (usually the heart). Sometimes only the spleen is missing and other organs are functioning properly. This can happen if, for example, the artery leading to the spleen does not develop normally in the fetus.

Sometimes the spleen has to be removed, as when it is damaged. Because the spleen stores blood cells, any injury to the spleen can cause severe, uncontrolled bleeding. Doctors commonly used to remove the spleen after such injuries, but this practice changed once the importance of the spleen to the immune system became clear.

The spleen also can stop working as a result of a disease that damages it. Sickle cell anemia, for instance, causes red blood cells to have an abnormal shape. This abnormal shape blocks the blood flow to the spleen and can cause irreparable damage.

Infection Risks

Because the spleen plays an important role in immunity, the absence of a spleen makes a person vulnerable to infections such as bacterial pneumonia and bacterial meningitis. Younger persons are more at risk for overwhelming, fatal infection in the absence of a spleen.

The heightened risk of infections can be somewhat alleviated by making sure persons without a functioning spleen receive several important vaccines: pneumococcal vaccine (which protects against several types of bacterial pneumonia), meningitis vaccine,

hepatitis A and B vaccines, influenza vaccine, and *Haemophilus influenzae* type B (Hib) vaccine. (Hib does not cause the flu, despite its name. It is a bacterium that causes several types of dangerous infections throughout the body.)

Impact

The absence of a spleen is manageable, but caution and education are required to prevent potential life-threatening complications. Persons without a spleen are often treated with preventive antibiotics for long periods of time, and they require specific vaccinations. Adults who lose their spleen do better than children born without one, but in either case, patients or their caregivers should be taught to watch for early signs of illness and should seek any needed medical attention sooner rather than later, so that infections do not flare out of control.

Adi R. Ferrara, B.S., ELS

Further Reading

DeFranco, Anthony, Richard Locksley, and Miranda Robertson. *Immunity: The Immune Response in Infectious and Inflammatory Disease.* Sunderland, Mass.: Sinauer, 2007.

Geha, Raif, and Fred Rosen. "Congenital Asplenia." In *Case Studies in Immunology.* Hoboken, N.J.: Taylor & Francis, 2010.

Lichtman, Marshall A., et al., eds. *Williams Hematology.* 7th ed. New York: McGraw-Hill, 2006.

National Library of Medicine. "Immune System and Disorders." Available at http://www.nlm.nih.gov/medlineplus/immunesystemanddisorders.html.

Web Sites of Interest

National Heart, Lung, and Blood Institute
http://www.nhlbi.nih.gov

National Institute of Diabetes and Digestive and Kidney Diseases
http://www2.niddk.nih.gov

See also: Antibodies; Babesiosis; Brucellosis; Idiopathic thrombocytopenic purpura; Immunity; Mononucleosis; Neutropenia; Pneumococcal infections; Pneumococcal vaccine; Vaccines: Types.

Athlete's foot

CATEGORY: Diseases and conditions
ANATOMY OR SYSTEM AFFECTED: Feet, skin
ALSO KNOWN AS: Tinea pedis

DEFINITION

Athlete's foot is a fungal infection that typically occurs on the feet. Because the infection is common among people who exercise or play sports, it was named athlete's foot. However, anyone can experience athlete's foot.

CAUSES

Fungi thrive in warm, dark, and moist places, such as inside a shoe, in locker rooms and showers, and around swimming pools. When a person walks through an area contaminated with fungi, his or her bare feet come in contact with the fungus. If the feet or the area between the toes stays moist, the fungus will grow.

RISK FACTORS

Risk factors for athlete's foot include prior athlete's foot infection, walking barefoot in locker rooms or public places, not keeping feet clean and dry, wearing airtight or poorly ventilated shoes or boots, sweaty feet, hot and humid weather, and disorders of the immune system.

SYMPTOMS

Athlete's foot symptoms usually start between the toes. As the infection progresses, it may spread to the soles or arches of the feet or to the toenails.

Symptoms often occur in combination and may include dry skin; itching, which worsens as the infection spreads; scaling; cracking; redness; a white, wet surface; and blisters, which may open and become painful.

SCREENING AND DIAGNOSIS

A doctor will ask about symptoms and medical history, and will perform a physical exam. The doctor will then likely scrape a small sample from the infected skin and look at it under the microscope. Infections caused by bacteria, rather than a fungus, may cause similar symptoms. Other conditions may also mimic athlete's foot. Getting an accurate diagnosis is important for successful treatment.

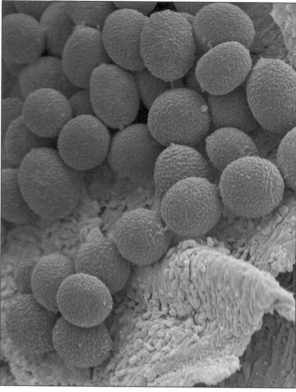

A micrograph of the fungal spores that cause athlete's foot, seen here (as spherical shapes) on human skin.

TREATMENT AND THERAPY

Treatment aims to rid the body of the infection. Therapy may include good foot hygiene or medication; many over-the-counter antifungal medications are available. However, if the infection persists for two weeks or more, one should seek medical care.

Other treatments are to wash feet often (daily) with soap and water and completely dry all areas, including between the toes; put a dusting of antifungal foot powder on feet or in shoes to absorb moisture, and change shoes and socks frequently; and avoid swimming or using public locker rooms if one already has athlete's foot. This will help prevent spreading the infection to others.

Over-the-counter (OTC) topical antifungals may be helpful, but if there is no improvement within two weeks of trying the OTCs, one should consult a doctor. Prescription topical or oral medications may be more effective, and the doctor may prescribe an antifungal medication to be taken by mouth or applied to the feet. Topical medications include miconazole, haloprogin, clotrimazole, ciclopirox, terbinafine, butenafine, tolnaftate, econazole, ketoconazole, naftifine, oxiconazole, sulconazole, and griseofulvin (a prescription oral medication). Other oral drugs may also be prescribed. One should wash his or her hands after applying topical medications.

Medication should not be stopped without a doctor's approval, even if the infected areas look better. Treatment generally lasts four to eight weeks. Shortening the treatment plan often results in another infection.

PREVENTION AND OUTCOMES

Preventing athlete's foot can be difficult, but keeping feet clean and dry will help. Suggestions for preventing athlete's foot include the following: Wash feet daily using soap and water, dry carefully between the toes, wear shoes that are comfortable and that allow feet to breathe, wear sandals in the summer, change shoes often, wear cotton socks that wick moisture from skin, change socks when they become damp, apply an antifungal foot powder to feet or shoes, take off shoes and socks and walk barefoot at home when possible, do not walk barefoot in damp places, wear shower shoes or sandals in public locker rooms, and do not wear other people's shoes.

Debra Wood, R.N.;
reviewed by David L. Horn, M.D., FACP

FURTHER READING

Alexander, Ivy L., ed. *Podiatry Sourcebook.* 2d rev. ed. Detroit, Mich.: Omnigraphics, 2007.

American Academy of Family Physicians. "Tinea Infections: Athlete's Foot, Jock Itch, and Ringworm." Available at http://www.aafp.org/afp/980700ap/980700b.html.

Donowitz, Leigh G., ed. *Infection Control in the Child Care Center and Preschool.* 5th ed. Philadelphia: Lippincott Williams & Wilkins, 2001.

Mandell, Gerald L., John E. Bennett, and Raphael Dolin, eds. *Mandell, Douglas, and Bennett's Principles and Practice of Infectious Diseases.* 7th ed. New York: Churchill Livingstone/Elsevier, 2010.

Pleacher, M. D., and W. W. Dexter. "Cutaneous Fungal and Viral Infections in Athletes." *Clinics in Sports Medicine* 26, no. 3 (2007).

Richardson, Malcolm D., and Elizabeth M. Johnson. *The Pocket Guide to Fungal Infection.* 2d ed. Malden, Mass.: Blackwell, 2006.

Tanaka, K., et al. "Preventive Effects of Various Types of Footwear and Cleaning Methods on Dermatophyte Adhesion." *Journal of Dermatology* 33, no. 8 (2006): 528-536.

Weedon, David. *Skin Pathology.* 3d ed. New York: Churchill Livingstone/Elsevier, 2010.

Woodfolk, J. A. "Allergy and Dermatophytes." *Clinical Microbiology Reviews* 18 (2005): 30-43.

WEB SITES OF INTEREST

American Academy of Dermatology
http://www.aad.org

American Podiatric Medical Association
http://www.apma.org

College of Family Physicians of Canada
http://www.cfpc.ca

See also: Antifungal drugs: Types; Chromoblastomycosis; Dermatomycosis; Fungal infections; Fungi: Classification and types; Jock itch; Onychomycosis; Plantar warts; Prevention of fungal infections; Ringworm; Skin infections; Tinea capitis; Tinea corporis; Tinea versicolor; *Trichophyton.*

Atypical pneumonia

CATEGORY: Diseases and conditions
ANATOMY OR SYSTEM AFFECTED: Lungs, respiratory system
ALSO KNOWN AS: *Mycoplasma* pneumonia, viral pneumonia, walking pneumonia

DEFINITION

Atypical pneumonia is a lung infection. It tends to be a mild illness in comparison with typical pneumonia, which is a severe illness. Typical pneumonia is usually caused by bacteria such as *Streptococcus pneumoniae, Haemophilus influenzae,* or *Klebsiella pneumoniae,* and it tends to strike older persons, especially those with heart or lung conditions.

In contrast, atypical pneumonia is caused by a different assortment of bacteria or viruses, and it usually strikes healthy young people. All types of pneumonia are potentially serious conditions that require care from a doctor.

Causes

Atypical pneumonia is usually caused by bacteria such as *Mycoplasma pneumoniae*, *Chlamydia*, *Coxiella burnetii*, and *Legionella*, and by viruses.

Risk Factors

The following factors increase the chance of developing atypical pneumonia: being a child, adolescent, or young adult; living in closed communities, such as dormitories in boarding schools or colleges and in military barracks; cigarette smoking; lung disease; and a weakened immune system.

Symptoms

The following symptoms are not necessarily caused by pneumonia and might be caused by other, less serious health conditions: fever (mild); enlarged lymph nodes; red eyes; chills; cough, often dry; sore throat; phlegm (sputum) production; muscle aches and pains; decreased appetite; headache; chest pain; shortness of breath; fast breathing; intense fatigue; weakness; vomiting; diarrhea; and skin rash.

Screening and Diagnosis

A doctor will ask about the infected person's symptoms and medical history and will perform a physical exam. Tests may include a chest X ray; blood tests (testing white blood cells, which can determine if the person has a bacterial or viral infection); other blood tests, which might identify the presence of certain bacteria or viruses; blood cultures (in which bacteria or viruses may be grown from blood samples); and a sputum test. If the person is coughing up sputum, he or she may be asked to collect some of that sputum in a sterile container for testing; this test can reveal what type of bacterium is causing the illness.

Treatment and Therapy

If diagnosed with pneumonia, one should follow instructions from the doctor. Usually, atypical pneumonia caused by bacteria can be treated with oral antibiotics at home. However, more severe pneumonia may require intravenous antibiotics in a hospital. Some of the antibiotics used to treat atypical pneumonia include erythromycin, azithromycin, and clarithromycin.

Viral pneumonia will not respond to antibiotic treatment. If the person is severely ill from pneumonia, he or she may need extra oxygen.

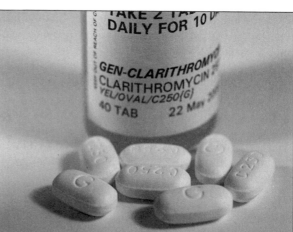

Atypical pneumonia is often treated with the macrolide antibiotic clarithromycin.

Prevention and Outcomes

To help reduce the chances of getting pneumonia, one should use good handwashing technique, should avoid contact with other ill people, and should be treated for any chronic conditions.

Rosalyn Carson-DeWitt, M.D.;
reviewed by Christine Colpitts, M.A., CRT

Further Reading

Blasi, F., et al. "*Chlamydia pneumoniae* and *Mycoplasma pneumoniae*." *Seminars in Respiratory and Critical Care Medicine* 26 (2005): 617-624.

Cunha, B. A. "The Atypical Pneumonias: Clinical Diagnosis and Importance." *Clinical Microbiology and Infection* 12, suppl. 3 (2006): 12-24.

_____. "Atypical Pneumonias: Current Clinical Concepts Focusing on Legionnaires' Disease." *Current Opinion in Pulmonary Medicine* 14 (2008): 183-194.

Goetz, M. B. "Pyogenic Bacterial Pneumonia, Lung Abscess, and Emphysema." In *Murray and Nadel's Textbook of Respiratory Medicine*, edited by Robert J. Mason et al. 5th ed. Philadelphia: Saunders/Elsevier, 2010.

Mandell, Gerald L., John E. Bennett, and Raphael Dolin, eds. *Mandell, Douglas, and Bennett's Principles and Practice of Infectious Diseases.* 7th ed. New York: Churchill Livingstone/Elsevier, 2010.

Rosenow, E. "Walking Pneumonia: What Does It Mean?" Mayo Clinic. Available at http://www.mayoclinic.com.

Schlossberg, D. "Mycoplasmal Infection." In *Andreoli*

and Carpenter's Cecil Essentials of Medicine, edited by Thomas E. Andreoli et al. 8th ed. Philadelphia: Saunders/Elsevier, 2010.

Thibodeau, K. P., and A. J. Viera. "Atypical Pathogens and Challenges in Community-Acquired Pneumonia." *American Family Physician* 69 (2004): 1699-1706.

West, John B. *Pulmonary Pathophysiology: The Essentials.* 7th ed. Philadelphia: Wolters Kluwer/Lippincott Williams & Wilkins, 2008.

WEB SITES OF INTEREST

American Lung Association
http://www.lungusa.org

Canadian Lung Association
http://www.lung.ca

National Institute of Allergy and Infectious Diseases
http://www.niaid.nih.gov

Public Health Agency of Canada
http://www.phac-aspc.gc.ca

See also: Adenovirus infections; Bacterial infections; *Chlamydia*; *Chlamydophila pneumoniae* infection; Histoplasmosis; Influenza; *Legionella*; Legionnaires' disease; *Mycoplasma*; *Mycoplasma* pneumonia; Nocardiosis; *Pneumocystis*; Pneumocystis pneumonia; Pneumonia; Q fever; Viral infections; Viral upper respiratory infections.

Autoimmune disorders

CATEGORY: Diseases and conditions
ANATOMY OR SYSTEM AFFECTED: All
ALSO KNOWN AS: Autoimmune diseases

DEFINITION

Normally, the immune system protects the body from infection and disease and does not trigger an immune response. If a person's immune system goes awry, that person is said to have an autoimmune disorder (AD). ADs are characterized by the loss of what is known as immunological tolerance (the ability of the body to ignore "self" while reacting to "nonself") and by the presence of self-reactive T cells, autoanti-bodies, and inflammation. In other words, a person's immune system malfunctions by failing to differentiate between self (the body) and nonself (foreign substances, such as invading microorganisms). The immune system produces autoantibodies that mistakenly attack the body's own healthy tissues and cells, while impaired T cells fail to protect them.

This misdirected immune response puts people at risk for infection. Additionally, many of the medications given to control the autoimmune response are powerful drugs with side effects that tend to lower the body's ability to fight disease. This makes affected persons highly susceptible to infectious diseases.

There are more than 80 known types of ADs and more than 150 different autoimmune-related diseases, classified as either organ-specific or systemic. In organ-specific disorders, the autoimmune response is localized and directed to antigens of a single organ or tissue; the body part affected depends on what autoimmune disease a person has. Other organ systems may become affected too, because the damage these disorders cause tends to extend beyond the targeted site. In a systemic AD, the autoimmune response is widespread throughout the body, affecting multiple organs. This can be followed by complications and life-threatening events.

CAUSES

To understand how autoimmunity and ADs evolve requires some knowledge of how the body's immune system works. The immune system is a complex network of specialized cells and organs that serves as the body's defense system against attacks by antigens, those invading microorganisms or foreign substances that trigger an immune response. The components of the immune system include white blood cells (called T and B lymphocytes, or T and B cells) and chemicals and proteins in the blood, such as antibodies, complement proteins, and interferon. T cells attack antigens directly and release chemicals, known as cytokines, which control the entire immune response. B cells produce the antibody proteins that attach to a specific antigen and help immune cells destroy the antigen.

There are two types of immunity: innate and acquired (sometimes called adaptive). Innate immunity is the defense system humans have at birth. Examples of innate immunity are the cough reflex, tear and skin oil enzymes, mucus, stomach acid, and skin. The innate immune system consists of circulating white blood cells called leukocytes, two types of which are called granulocytes and monocytes. Once released from the bloodstream, they act as phagocytes to engulf and digest microorganisms, foreign substances, and cellular debris, preventing harmful substances from entering the body.

Acquired immunity develops as a person matures. The development of the components of acquired immunity takes time. As lymphocytes start to mature, they learn to tell the difference between body tissues and foreign substances. Being able to recognize a threat versus a nonthreat is the basis of immunological tolerance. Once the T and B cells are formed, the immune system utilizes the attack mechanism of the T cells and the antibodies produced by the B cells to fight invading antigens. Exposure to these various antigens enables the immune system to build a defense that is specific to each antigen.

The innate and adaptive immune systems are designed to work together in protecting the body from disease. If the innate immune system malfunctions, a person is susceptible to what are called autoinflammatory disorders. When the acquired immune system malfunctions and attacks its own tissues by mistake, the diseases that develop are called autoimmune disorders.

Autoimmunity itself is an etiology, meaning it causes disease. Exactly how or why the immune system stops recognizing the difference between healthy body tissues and antigens is unknown. It has been speculated that antibodies or T cells may attack normal cells if part of their structure resembles part of the structure of the antigen or if B cells have malfunctioned and made the wrong kind of antibody.

Despite these conjectures, ADs generally do not have a single cause; a combination of heredity and environmental factors are strongly implicated. ADs tend to run in families, and there are several genes known to put people at higher risk for developing them. However, what is inherited is a susceptibility to these disorders, not the disorder itself. Thus, ADS are hereditary, not genetic, diseases. Examples of environmental triggers that can cause a disorder to surface are viral or bacterial infections and tissue damage from exposure to sunlight or certain solvents or drugs.

RISK FACTORS

Approximately fifty million Americans (or about 16 percent of the population of the United States)

have one or more ADs. ADs usually develop in the adult years, and women are much more likely than men to be affected. This statistic would place young women at particular risk. It also has raised speculation that hormones may be involved in the autoimmune process.

People with a family history of ADs or those who have inherited certain genes are more susceptible to developing these disorders. It is not uncommon for multiple ADs to occur in one family. ADs can erupt from exposure to certain environmental triggers or from an injury to body tissue. Some ADs are more prevalent in people of certain races or ethnic backgrounds. For example, type 1 diabetes occurs more often in Caucasians, and lupus is more prevalent among African Americans and Hispanics.

ADs themselves put people at higher risk for infection because the immune system does not function normally. Tuberculosis is an especially common threat to persons who are immunocompromised, and persons with ADs are routinely screened for the disease. Most prescribed AD drugs have immunosuppressant properties, which compounds the risk of infection. Immunosuppressants have serious adverse effects that can cause bone marrow suppression, can increase the risk of infection, and can remain in the body long after the treatment has ended.

SYMPTOMS

Rather than characterized as progressive, most ADs are characterized by flare-ups and relapses, in which triggers provoke the sudden and severe onset of symptoms, followed by a period of remission. Multiple sclerosis is a prime example. Each AD has its own set of symptoms, but there are certain symptoms that are universal, such as fatigue, dizziness, and low-grade fever. Other common symptoms include weight gain or loss, swelling, and menstrual irregularities.

Over time, the misdirected immune responses can destroy single types of cells or tissue, can cause an organ to increase in size, or can interfere with its function, resulting in damage to one or more parts of the body. The organs and tissues most frequently affected by ADs include the endocrine glands (thyroid, pancreas, and adrenal glands), components of the blood (usually red blood cells), connective tissue, the skin, muscles, and joints. Persisting symptoms that may signify damage to any of these body parts may indicate an AD and include the following: heat and cold sensitivity; changes in blood pressure or pulse; changes in mood or thinking; hair loss or excessive growth; changes in hair texture; skin rashes, ulcers, bruising, thinning, thickening, and sun sensitivity; blurred or double vision; eye pain, inflammation, or dry eyes; dry mouth, mouth sores, excessive thirst, difficulty swallowing, changes in voice quality, choking sensation, or feeling of a lump in throat; muscle, bone, and joint pain; all-over body pain and tenderness; muscle weakness and joint stiffness; deformed joints; backache; nausea or vomiting; diarrhea; constipation; bloody or foul-smelling stools; abdominal bloating and pain; gas; frequent urination; lack of coordination or balance; numbness or tingling; and tremors.

Screening and Diagnosis

The sheer number and complexity of ADs present challenges for diagnosis and generally require multiple laboratory tests to pinpoint a specific disease. Such a diagnostic battery includes basic tests, such as a complete blood count, basic and comprehensive metabolic panels, and the erythrocyte sedimentation rate, in addition to many more specialized tests specific to the diagnosis of individual ADs. Antibody blood tests include the following:

Antineutrophil cytoplasmic antibodies (ANCA). Performed when autoimmune vasculitis (Wegener's granulomatosis) is suspected; uses indirect immunofluorescence microscopy.

Rheumatoid factor (RF). Performed when rheumatoid arthritis or Sjögren's syndrome is suspected; detects and measures whether high levels of RF are present in the blood; test is used to diagnose rheumatoid arthritis in conjunction with X rays showing evidence of swollen joint capsules and loss of cartilage and bone.

Cyclic citrullinated peptide antibody test (CCPA). An assay used to detect the presence of citrulline antibodies in the blood. CCPA is a new test that helps to diagnose early rheumatoid arthritis when the RF test is negative.

Antinuclear antibody test(ANA). Performed to screen for ADs and when systemic lupus erythematosus (SLE) is suspected; uses enzyme-linked immunosorbent assay (ELISA) or indirect immunofluorescence microscopy.

Smooth muscle antibody. Ordered with ANA to help diagnose autoimmune hepatitis or to rule out liver damage caused by viral infection.

Extractable nuclear antigen antibodies (ENA panel). Or-

dered when a person has symptoms of an AD and has had a positive ANA test. The four-test ENA is used to help diagnose mixed connective tissue disease, SLE, and Sjögren's syndrome. A six-test ENA helps in diagnosing scleroderma and polymyositis.

Thyroid peroxidase antibody (TPOAb), triiodothyronine (T3), thyroxine (T4), thyroid-stimulating hormone receptor antibody (TSH). TPOAb is measured when Hashimoto's thyroiditis is suspected; T3 is used to diagnose Graves' disease; T4 helps in evaluating thyroid gland function and helps diagnose hypothyroidism and hyperthyroidism; TSH is used to monitor the effects of Graves' disease therapy.

Islet cell cytoplasmic autoantibodies (ICCA). Measures a group of islet cell autoantibodies targeted against several kinds of islet cell proteins. ICCA are diabetes autoantibodies and are used to distinguish type 1 diabetes from diabetes from other causes; this test is not routinely used because it is labor-intensive and requires skill to interpret results.

Antimitochondrial antibody. High levels help in diagnosing primary biliary cirrhosis; lower levels may be present in other ADs, such as autoimmune hepatitis or SLE.

Other tests include the following:

C-reactive protein. Detects the presence of inflammation and is performed when infection or certain ADs are suspected.

Complement levels (C3 and C4). Used to help diagnose the cause of recurrent microbial infections and to monitor the activity of acute or chronic autoimmune diseases.

Human leukocyte antigen B27 (HLA-B27). The presence of HLA-B27 is genetic; this test is preformed to support suspected diagnosis of ankylosing spondylitis (AS), reactive arthritis, or juvenile rheumatoid arthritis; nondiagnostic on its own.

It should be noted that most laboratory tests for autoimmune diseases are not entirely sensitive or specific and must be interpreted with care. Different techniques and assays may give different results for the same antibody test. Diagnosing can be difficult because titers of autoantibodies can be low in healthy persons and in those who are symptomatic.

Treatment and Therapy

Similar to diagnosing an AD, treatment of an AD requires multiple drugs and therapies. Also, treatment poses numerous risks. Once a diagnosis is made, the next step is to reduce the immune system response. One of the challenges in doing this is to find a balance of medications that controls the disease and maintains the body's ability to fight disease and infection. Serious adverse reactions, some of which are life-threatening, can occur with virtually all of the drugs used to treat ADs. Increased risk of infection also can occur. The action of these drugs can damage rapidly dividing tissues, such as bone marrow, requiring that persons be monitored carefully to avoid infection. Skin reactions and rashes are also common in all AD drug therapies and in many of the ADs.

Corticosteroids have been the mainstay in the treatment of ADs, especially the systemic disorders. Corticosteroids are a group of natural and synthetic analogs of the hormones secreted by the pituitary gland and include the glucocorticoids, which are anti-inflammatory agents. Another group, called nonsteroidal anti-inflammatory drugs (NSAIDs), has been used in less severe forms of these disorders and in other ADs to relieve symptoms.

A group of antimetabolite/cytotoxic agents called disease-modifying antirheumatic drugs (DMARDs) have begun to replace the corticosteroids and NSAIDs as primary therapies for many of the systemic ADs. These powerful immunosuppressants are more steroid-sparing, yet they still induce or maintain remission. By the 1990's, biologic DMARDs became available. Since then, they have revolutionized the treatment of many systemic ADs.

Major classes of AD drugs include the following:

Corticosteroids. Prednisone and methylprednisolone are glucocorticoid analogs that suppress inflammatory mediator production and immune effector cells and promote T lymphocyte apoptosis (death). They are used during acute periods of disease. Complications arise with high doses and prolonged therapy. Major adverse affects are bone marrow suppression, gastrointestinal complications, cataracts, and glaucoma.

DMARDs. Azathioprine (AZA) is a purine analog (6-mercaptopurine) that inhibits synthesis of deoxyribonucleic acid (DNA), ribonucleic acid (RNA), and proteins and interferes with purine metabolism and mitosis, suppressing delayed hypersensitivity responses and cell-mediated cytotoxicity. Common adverse effects include leukopenia, pancreatitis, hepatitis, bone marrow suppression, potential malignancies, and pulmonary disease.

Cyclophosphamide is a nitrogen-derived alkylating agent/cytotoxic immunosuppressant that cross-links DNA and RNA strands, inhibiting cell functions and protein synthesis. It has a dose-dependent effect on the immune system, and at high doses, it can induce an aberrant anti-inflammatory immune effect on lymphocyte activity, can affect regulatory T cells, and can cause a state of serious immunosuppression that includes major bone-marrow suppression, leukopenia, anemia, and thrombocytopenia. There also can be adverse effects on the gastrointestinal or renal-genitourinary tracts and the cardiovascular system, and there can be increased risk of malignancy and pulmonary toxicity.

Methotrexate (MTX). A dihydrofolate reductase inhibitor and antimetabolite approved for treatment of rheumatoid arthritis and psoriasis. Despite its efficacy, MTX has major toxic effects with prolonged use, including liver damage, cytopenias, and several pulmonary diseases, the most frequently reported of which is hypersensitivity pneumonitis.

Hydroxychloroquine. An antimalarial agent with immunosuppressant properties. The drug has cardiovascular effects that can cause toxic myopathy, cardiomyopathy, and peripheral neuropathy.

Biological DMARDs. Adalimumab is a monoclonal antibody and tumor necrosis factor (TNF) inhibitor that binds TNF-alpha and blocks its interaction with cell surface receptors. Adverse events include renal-genitourinary effects and dyslipidemia.

Infliximab is a chimeric (part human/part synthetic) monoclonal antibody and anti-TNF agent that binds TNF-alpha and blocks its interaction with cell surface receptors. A twofold risk of infection is the most common adverse event, and the risk of developing tuberculosis may be greater than with other anti-TNF agents. Skin and subcutaneous tissue infections and apoptosis-inducing activity (cell death) can occur.

Etanercept is a TNF receptor antagonist that inhibits binding of TNF-alpha and TNF-beta to cell surface receptors, preventing its interaction with TNF receptors and rendering it biologically inactive. Its use can cause infections of the respiratory tract, skin, or subcutaneous tissue. All three biological DMARDs are approved for the treatment of rheumatoid arthritis, psoriasis, ankylosing spondylitis, ulcerative colitis, and Crohn's disease.

PREVENTION AND OUTCOMES

ADs are lifelong, chronic diseases that cannot be prevented or cured, but they can be managed. Being compliant with therapy, knowing the triggers, living a healthy lifestyle, and reducing stress can help to alleviate symptoms and reduce the damaging effects of these complicated diseases.

Barbara Woldin, B.S.

FURTHER READING

Firestein, Gary S. "The Inflammatory Response." In *Cecil Medicine*, edited by Lee Goldman and Dennis Ausiello. 23d ed. Philadelphia: Saunders/Elsevier, 2008. Explains the immune response and how the immune system protects the body from foreign substances and from infection by bacteria and viruses. Describes antigens and antibodies and how they function.

Goronzy, J. J., and C. M. Weyand. "The Innate and Adaptive Immune Systems." In *Cecil Medicine*, edited by Lee Goldman and Dennis Ausiello. 23d ed. Philadelphia: Saunders/Elsevier, 2008. Explains the two types of immunity, describes the components of both types, and shows how they work together.

Shlomchik, Mark J. "Immunologic Basis of Hematology: Tolerance and Autoimmunity." In *Hematology: Basic Principles and Practice*, edited by Ronald Hoffman et al. 5th ed. Philadelphia: Churchill Livingstone/Elsevier, 2009. Explains self-reactive lymphocytes and the origin, control, and breakdown of self-tolerance in autoimmune diseases. Also discusses implications and therapy.

WEB SITES OF INTEREST

American Autoimmune Related Disease Association
http://www.aarda.org

Immune Deficiency Foundation
http://www.primaryimmune.org

National Institute of Arthritis and Musculoskeletal and Skin Diseases
http://www.niams.nih.gov

See also: Agammaglobulinemia; AIDS; Antibodies; Creutzfeldt-Jakob disease; Gerstmann-Sträussler-Scheinker syndrome; Guillain-Barré syndrome; HIV; Idiopathic thrombocytopenic purpura; Immunity; Immunoassay; Immunodeficiency; Incubation period; Inflammation; Neutropenia; Opportunistic infections; Progressive multifocal leukoencephalopathy; Reinfection; Reiter's syndrome; Retroviral infections; Seroconversion; T lymphocytes; Virulence.

Avian influenza

CATEGORY: Diseases and conditions
ANATOMY OR SYSTEM AFFECTED: All
ALSO KNOWN AS: Bird flu, H5N1 infection

DEFINITION

Avian influenza, often called bird flu, is a strain of influenza that mainly infects birds, with some cases of avian influenza in humans in Asia. Health experts are concerned that the virus could become more efficient at infecting humans, which could lead to a pandemic (a worldwide outbreak).

CAUSES

Viruses belonging to the A type of influenza viruses cause avian influenza. Sometimes a virus can mutate. These mutations can allow a bird virus to infect pigs or humans. Humans who have close contact with infected birds or pigs can then contract the virus. There is also concern that the virus can mutate to allow it to pass between humans.

The virus is not contracted through eating poultry, eggs, or pork products. It is passed through contact with an infected animal's saliva, nasal secretions, and droppings.

RISK FACTORS

The following factors increase the chance of developing avian influenza: close contact with infected animals, such as ducks, geese, chickens, turkeys, and pigs; and travel to an area known to have cases of avian influenza, such as Thailand, Hong Kong, China, Vietnam, Cambodia, Malaysia, Indonesia, South Korea, Laos, and the Netherlands.

SYMPTOMS

The following symptoms do not necessarily point to avian flu. These symptoms may be caused by other conditions: flu symptoms, such as fever, chills, cough, sore throat, general aches, diarrhea, vomiting, and abdominal and chest pain. In more severe cases, the symptoms include pneumonia (with worsening fever and cough with shortness of breath), problems with blood clotting, and organ failure (involving kidney, liver, lungs, and heart).

SCREENING AND DIAGNOSIS

A doctor will ask about the patient's symptoms and medical history and will perform a physical exam. The virus can be identified through a blood test. Samples are also usually sent to the Centers for Disease Control and Prevention (CDC), which identifies the specific strain of the virus.

TREATMENT AND THERAPY

One should consult a doctor about the best treatment plan. Research is underway to find an antiviral agent that works against the virus. Some current agents are ineffective against the virus. Antiviral agents that appear effective against the avian flu include zanamivir (Relenza), which may worsen asthma or chronic obstructive pulmonary disease (COPD), and oseltamivir, or Tamiflu (and perhaps zanamivir), which is the preferred medication to treat avian flu,

but which may increase the risk of self-injury and confusion shortly after taking, especially in children. Children should be closely monitored for signs of unusual behavior.

These medications do not cure the flu, but they may help relieve symptoms and decrease the duration of the illness. One should take the drugs within forty-eight hours of the first symptoms.

PREVENTION AND OUTCOMES

To help reduce the chance of getting avian influenza, one should avoid traveling to areas with avian influenza outbreaks. Updated travel restrictions are available from the CDC (http://www.cdc.gov/travel). One should also avoid contact with potentially infected poultry or swine, avoid farms or open-air markets, and avoid eating raw eggs, as egg shells may be contaminated with bird droppings. Raw poultry could be contaminated with bird droppings, saliva, or mucus. Also, one should cook poultry thoroughly, carefully clean hands after handling the poultry, and clean all cooking surfaces, utensils, and cutting boards. Cooked poultry will not transmit the avian influenza virus. Also, a person should wash his or her hands thoroughly when in an area in which exposure to the avian influenza virus is possible, and should use a hand sanitizer if clean water is not available for washing.

In 2007, the U.S. Food and Drug Administration approved the first vaccine in the United States to protect against the avian influenza virus in adults ages eighteen through sixty-four years. The U.S. government has stored this vaccine in its Strategic National Stockpile in case of a national emergency.

Rosalyn Carson-DeWitt, M.D.;
reviewed by David L. Horn, M.D., FACP

FURTHER READING

Beigel, John, and Mike Bray. "Current and Future Antiviral Therapy of Severe Seasonal and Avian Influenza." *Antiviral Research* 78 (2008): 91-102.
Clark, Larry, and Jeffrey Hall. "Avian Influenza in Wild Birds: Status as Reservoirs and Risks to Humans and Agriculture." In *Current Topics in Avian*

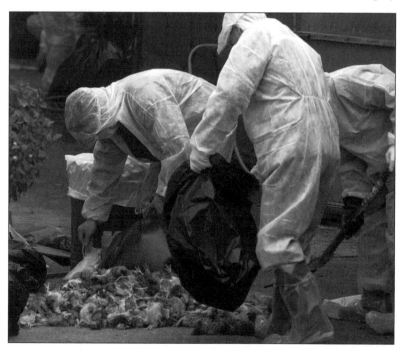

Health workers in Hong Kong collect chickens killed by avian influenza in 2002. (AP/Wide World Photos)

Disease Research: Understanding Endemic and Invasive Diseases, edited by Rosemary K. Barraclough. Washington, D.C.: American Ornithologists' Union, 2006.

Cohen, Jonathan, William G. Powderly, and Steven E. Opal. *Infectious Diseases*. 3d ed. St. Louis, Mo.: Mosby/Elsevier, 2010.

EBSCO Publishing. *DynaMed: Avian Influenza*. Available through http://www.ebscohost.com/dynamed.

_____. *Health Library: The Avian Flu Vaccine*. Available through http://www.ebscohost.com.

Sfakianos, Jeffrey N. *Avian Flu*. New York: Chelsea House, 2006.

Wehrwein, Peter, ed. "Bird Flu: Don't Fly into a Panic." *Harvard Health Letter* 31, no. 8 (June, 2006): 1-3.

Weir, E., T. Wong, and T. Gemmill. "Avian Influenza Outbreak: Update." *Canadian Medical Association Journal* 170 (2004): 785-786.

WEB SITES OF INTEREST

Centers for Disease Control and Prevention
http://www.cdc.gov/flu

Flu.gov
http://www.flu.gov

Public Health Agency of Canada
http://www.phac-aspc.gc.ca

World Health Organization
http://www.who.int

See also: Birds and infectious disease; Ebola hemorrhagic fever; Epidemics and pandemics: Causes and management; Fecal-oral route of transmission; Foodborne illness and disease; H1N1 influenza; Histoplasmosis; Influenza; Influenza vaccine; Pigs and infectious disease; Psittacosis; Tropical medicine; Viral infections; Zoonotic diseases.

B

Babesiosis

CATEGORY: Diseases and conditions
ANATOMY OR SYSTEM AFFECTED: All

DEFINITION

Babesiosis in humans is a rare and potentially fatal intraerythrocytic parasitic infection caused by the *Babesia* protozoan. It is transmitted through the bite of an infected *Ixodes* tick, which also is responsible for the transmission of Lyme disease. Some cases of transfusion and transplacental transmission have been documented as well.

CAUSES

The first case of human babesiosis was reported in 1957 in an Eastern European farmer with asplenia (abnormal spleen function); several hundred cases have been reported since. In the United States (northeastern and midwestern states), babesiosis is caused primarily by *B. microti.* In Europe, the disease is typically caused by *B. divergens* and occurs mostly in Ireland, the United Kingdom, and northern France. Episodic cases have been reported in Japan, Korea, China, Mexico, South Africa, and Egypt. The parasite is typically spread by the young nymph stage of the tick.

RISK FACTORS

Babesiosis is most frequently seen in elderly people, persons who are asplenic, and persons with compromised immune systems. Coinfection with Lyme disease occurs in approximately 20 percent of cases.

SYMPTOMS

It may take from one to eight weeks or longer for symptoms to appear, although the infection can also be asymptomatic. In the majority of cases, babesiosis is a mild-to-moderate disease with nonspecific flulike symptoms such as fever, chills, sweats, headache, musculoskeletal pain, loss of appetite, nausea, and generalized weakness. Hemolytic anemia, jaundice, and dark urine that persists from several days to several months are frequent. Babesiosis can have a severe and fulminant course (with severe hemolysis, thrombocytopenia, disseminated intravascular coagulation, renal failure, pulmonary edema, hepatosplenomegaly, spontaneous splenic rupture, and shock). If left untreated, the disease may be fatal. Among infected persons who have symptoms, the mortality rate is 10 percent in the United States and 50 percent in Europe.

SCREENING AND DIAGNOSIS

Diagnosis is based on medical history, a physical examination, and laboratory identification of the parasite in red blood cells. An immunofluorescence antibody test may be necessary to confirm the diagnosis.

TREATMENT AND THERAPY

Treatment in asymptomatic cases is usually started if parasitemia (condition in which parasites are in the blood) persists for more than three months. Symptomatic persons are treated with a combination of quinine plus clindamycin (a first-line treatment for persons with severe symptoms) or with atovaquone plus azithromycin (a first-line treatment for mild and moderate disease). To reduce the level of parasitemia in symptomatic persons, one should begin therapy immediately after diagnosis. Persons with severe babesiosis (having high parasitemia, significant hemolysis, or renal, hepatic, or pulmonary dysfunction) may need supportive care that includes antipyretics, vasopressors, blood or exchange transfusions (or both), mechanical lung ventilation, and dialysis.

PREVENTION AND OUTCOMES

The use of prevention measures is especially important for persons at increased risk (such as asplenic persons) for severe babesiosis. *Ixodes* ticks are most frequently found in wooded, brushy, and grassy areas during warm months. Simple preventive measures include avoidance or minimization of exposure to tick-infested areas, application of tick repellents (products containing 10 to 35 percent NN-diethyl metatoluamide, or DEET) on skin and clothes before entering a tick-infested area, wearing light-colored clothing (which allows for simple tick discovery), tucking pants into socks and shirt into pants, and the careful examination of skin after exposure. Early removal of ticks is recommended because the tick must remain attached for at least twenty-four hours to transmit the parasite. One can also insist on public health measures that reduce the density of the tick population (such as the use of acaricides in conjunction with other methods).

Katia Marazova, M.D., Ph.D.

FURTHER READING

Gelfand, Jeffrey A., and Edouard Vannier. "Babesiosis." In *Harrison's Principles of Internal Medicine*, edited by Joan Butterton. 17th ed. New York: McGraw-Hill, 2008.

Goddard, Jerome. *Physician's Guide to Arthropods of Medical Importance*. 4th ed. Boca Raton, Fla.: CRC Press, 2003.

Hunfeld, K.-P., A. Hildebrandt, and J. S. Gray. "Babesiosis: Recent Insights into an Ancient Disease." *International Journal for Parasitology* 38 (2008): 1219-1237.

Mylonakis, Eleftherios. "When to Suspect and How to Monitor Babesiosis." *American Family Physician* 63 (May, 2001): 1969-1974, 1976.

Sheorey, Harsha, John Walker, and Beverley-Ann Biggs. *Clinical Parasitology*. Melbourne, Vic.: University of Melbourne Press, 2003.

Wormser, Gary P., et al. "The Clinical Assessment, Treatment, and Prevention of Lyme Disease, Human Granulocytic Anaplasmosis, and Babesiosis: Clinical Practice Guidelines by the Infectious Diseases Society of America." *Clinical Infectious Diseases* 43, no. 9 (2006): 1089-1134.

WEB SITES OF INTEREST

American Lyme Disease Foundation
http://www.aldf.com

Centers for Disease Control and Prevention
http://www.cdc.gov/babesiosis

See also: Acariasis; Arthropod-borne illness and disease; Asplenia; Colorado tick fever; Lyme disease; Mediterranean spotted fever; Mites and chiggers and infectious disease; Parasitic diseases; Protozoan diseases; Rocky Mountain spotted fever; Ticks and infectious disease; Vectors and vector control.

Bacteria: Classification and types

CATEGORY: Pathogen
TRANSMISSION ROUTE: Direct contact, ingestion, inhalation

DEFINITION

Bacteria are small, primarily microscopic, single-celled organisms defined as members of the group prokaryotes, which lack internal membrane-enclosed organelles such as a nucleus.

Microbial classification has its roots, like those of more evolved organisms (such as plants and animals), in the system originally developed by Swedish botanist Carolus Linnaeus in the mid-eighteenth century; such systems reflect the evolutionary relationships among these organisms as largely confirmed in DNA (deoxyribonucleic acid) studies during the latter half of the twentieth century. Members of the same genus are considered closely related and may even interbreed. Members within the same order or family are not as closely related, yet they still reflect a common ancestry. An example is that of the class Mammalia, which includes both humans and whales. The lowest levels of the taxonomic hierarchy are the genus and species, with their Latinized binomial nomenclature considered the scientific name.

The system is applied to bacteria in an attempt to bring a sense of order in defining genetic relationships: Members of the same genus are considered closely related, while members of different genera are considered relatively unrelated. Variants within the same species are designated as subspecies or serovars, representing variations in surface molecules.

However, naming and classification of bacteria have often drawn on historical aspects of the organisms, such as the person who first isolated or characterized the bacterium (Theodor Escherich) or the disease (cholera). Members of different genera may actually be variants of the same species; the pathogens *Shigella*, the etiological agent of bacterial dysentery, and *Escherichia*, which is associated with a variety of gastrointestinal or urinary tract infections, are really variations of the same species. Among the reasons for the confusion in taxonomy is the instability of genetic material.

Bacteria have the ability to carry out horizontal transfer of genetic material: Large segments of DNA readily pass or are exchanged not only among different

Taxonomic Classification for Bacteria

Domain: Bacteria
Phylum: Firmicutes
Class: Bacilli
Order: Bacillales
Family: Bacillaceae
Genus: *Bacillus*
Species: *B. anthracis*
Family: Staphylococcaceae
Genus: *Staphylococcus*
Species: *S. aureus*
Order: Lactobacillales
Family: Streptococcaceae
Genus: *Streptococcus*
Species: *S. pyogenes*
Class: Clostridia
Order: Clostridiales
Family: Clostridiaceae
Genus: *Clostridium*
Species:
C. botulinum
C. tetani
C. perfringens
Phylum: Proteobacteria
Class: {agr}-Proteobacteria

Order: Rickettsiales
Family: Rickettsiaceae
Genus: *Rickettsia*
Species:
R. prowazekii
R. rickettsia
Class: {bgr}-Proteobacteria
Order: Neisseriales
Family: Neisseriaceae
Genus: *Neisseria*
Species:
N. gonorrhoeae
N. meningitidis
Class: {ggr}-Proteobacteria
Order: Enterobacteriales
Family: Enterobacteriaceae
Genera: *Escherichia, Salmonella,*
Shigella, Yersinia, Klebsiella
Species:
E. coli
Salmonella species
Shigella dysenteriae
Y. pestis
K. pneumoniae

Order: Legionellales
Family: Legionellaceae
Genus: *Legionella*
Species: *L. pneumophila*
Order: Pasteurellales
Family: Pasteurellaceae
Genus: *Haemophilus*
Species: *H. influenzae*
Order: Pseudomonadales
Family: Pseudomonadaceae
Genus: *Pseudomonas*
Species: *P. aeruginosa*
Order: Vibrionales
Family: Vibrionaceae
Genus: *Vibrio*
Species: *V. cholerae*
Class: {egr}-Proteobacteria
Order: Campylobacterales
Family: Campylobacteraceae
Genus: *Campylobacter*
Species: *C. jejuni*
Family: Helicobacteraceae
Genus: *Helicobacter*
Species: *H. pylori*

genera but also among different orders. In this manner, not only do the genetic characteristics of bacteria change, but harmless organisms may acquire the ability to cause disease. Despite these shortcomings of bacterial taxonomy, modern genetic analysis has resulted in more accurate classification that reflects the relationships among bacteria. Also, new names for genera as the underlying molecular biology of microorganisms becomes better understood.

Bacteria are classified into two general categories, depending upon their cell-wall structure: gram-positives, which have a wall predominately composed of peptidoglycan (polysaccharide and protein), and gram-negatives, which have a cell wall composed primarily of lipopolysaccharide (lipids and polysaccharides). Gram-positives include members of the phylum Firmicutes, while gram-negatives represent most of the rest. The gram "characteristic" is named for Hans Christian Gram, a nineteenth and twentieth century German scientist.

NATURAL HABITAT AND FEATURES

Organisms that are etiological agents of disease generally associate with the host in two ways: as members of the normal flora, or microbiota, or as pathogens that must enter the body through "openings" such as respiratory passages (the nose or mouth), the gastrointestinal tract, or the genitourinary tract.

Resident pathogenic bacteria survive in the host primarily within niches that allow their survival. For example, the skin provides both a natural barrier to sterile regions within the body and a surface environment inhibitory to many types of microorganisms. The secretion of fatty acids in sebum creates an environment of low pH (acidity), and the secretion of NaCl (sodium chloride, or salt) in body sweat creates an environment of high salt. Organisms that become part of the microbiota on the skin, primarily members of the staphylococci and certain streptococci, must be able to survive under these conditions.

The microbiota of the colon consists of large num-

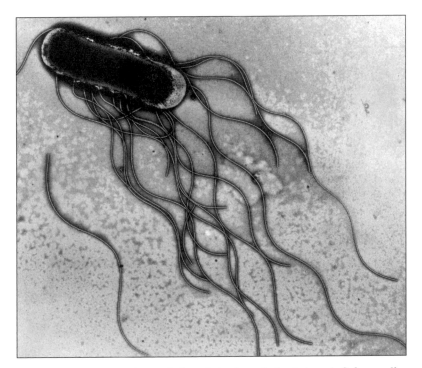

A common gram-negative, rod-shaped, pathogenic bacterium is Salmonella, *which causes food-borne illness and disease.*

bers of primarily anaerobic, nonpathogenic bacteria, with an estimate of about one thousand bacteria in one gram of feces. Competition from the resident flora is generally sufficient to prevent transient pathogens from becoming established. In turn, anything that disrupts the resident flora can allow pathogens to become established. For example, the use of broad-spectrum antibiotics may remove the normal bacteria in the colon. *Clostridium difficile*, commonly present in a dormant spore state in the colon, can establish itself under these conditions and produce toxins that result in severe ulcerative colitis.

To carry out infection, pathogenic bacteria must exhibit characteristics that not only allow transmission between hosts but also allow them to survive and colonize within the new host. Such features are referred to as virulence factors, and they represent whatever means bacteria use to resist the host defenses and to produce the symptoms of disease. The most obvious examples are those of toxins, which are placed in two general categories: endotoxins, pharmacologically active chemicals that compose a portion of the lipid component of the cell-wall structure of gram-negative bacteria, and exotoxins, which are secreted by some, primarily gram-positive, bacteria. Other virulence factors include a polysaccharide or protein capsule that surrounds some bacteria and prevents destruction by white blood cells (phagocytes) of the host's immune system, and fimbriae, hairlike structures on the cell surface that allow attachment and colonization in the host.

PATHOGENICITY AND CLINICAL SIGNIFICANCE

The transmission of bacteria varies significantly and depends upon the environmental niche of the organism in the host. Respiratory infections such as whooping cough or tuberculosis are transmitted through respiratory secretions, such as droplets resulting from sneezes or coughs, which are inhaled by the recipient. Sexually transmitted diseases such as gonorrhea or syphilis are passed through sexual contact. Some illnesses, such as staphylococcal infections, may be transmitted by direct contact or by ingestion of contaminated foods.

Staphylococci. Members of the family Staphylococcaceae, a group of gram-positive cocci, include some of the most common pathogenic organisms that also can produce some of the most deadly infections. There are more than forty species of *Staphylococcus*, most of which are harmless. The two species of clinical importance are *S. epidermidis*, a member of the skin microbiota, and *S. aureus*, commonly found on the skin and nasal passages.

The staphylococci are differentiated from the streptococci, which they physically resemble, by their ability to produce catalase, an enzyme that, when mixed with peroxide, produces bubbles of oxygen. *S. aureus* in particular has the ability to be a significant pathogen because of the large variety of toxins various strains may produce. Most strains of *S. aureus* produce several forms of coagulase, an enzyme that causes serum to clot and that may play a role in the formation of boils. In addition, various strains may produce enzymes that lyse red blood cells (β-hemolysins), may produce white blood cells (leukocidins), and may induce severe shock (toxic shock syndrome toxin). The experience with which most persons encounter the staphylococci is in the form of what is commonly known as food poisoning, the result of exposure to a heat-stable staphylococcal enterotoxin.

Streptococci. The streptococci are gram-positive cocci that physically resemble the staphylococci, but are genetically different and are differentiated from the latter by their lack of production of catalase. The streptococci is a large and diverse collection of species that were originally classified into groups by Rebecca Craighill Lancefield in the 1930's on the basis of surface carbohydrates; the Lancefield classification scheme is still used.

Group *A, which includes Streptococcus pyogenes* ("pus-creator"), is the most important of the streptococci. Most commonly associated with strep throat, infection with *S. pyogenes* can potentially lead to rheumatic fever or glomerulonephritis. *S. pyogenes* can produce a variety of toxins, any of which may contribute to virulence. Such toxins include enzymes that can lyse red blood cells (streptolysins) and can cause impetigo, erythrogenic toxins (scarlet fever), and severe shock (toxic shock syndrome toxin). Other species of streptococci may contribute to the formation of dental carries (*S. mutans*) and to meningitis in infants (group B *S. agalactiae*). *S. pneumoniae* is a common cause of bacterial pneumonia, and before the discovery of antibiotics, it was associated with a high proportion of deaths in the elderly.

Enteric bacteria. The family Enterobacteriaceae, more commonly called the enteric bacteria, is a diverse group of gram-negative bacteria that are part of the microbiota of the intestinal tract in both warm-blooded and cold-blooded organisms. Not all are pathogens, however. Most provide a benefit to the host by suppressing the colonization of pathogens while at the same time producing B and K vitamins for that host.

The species perhaps best known to the general public is *Escherichia coli*. Most types of *E. coli* are harmless. However, some types or strains have acquired the ability to invade host intestinal cells or to produce a variety of enterotoxins associated with food poisoning.

E. coli infections are routinely classified on the basis of the type of disease and are placed in the following five categories: enterotoxigenic, which causes the illness commonly referred to as travelers' diarrhea, the result of two forms of toxins produced by this strain, one of which is nearly identical to that associated with cholera; shiga-toxin-producing, which produces a toxin that likely originated with *Shigella*, the cause of bacterial dysentery (the most noted strain is *E. coli* O157:H7, which produces a potentially life-threatening hemolytic anemia); enteropathogenic, which is a cause of severe diarrhea in infants; enteroinvasive, which is capable of invading intestinal cells; and enteroaggregative, which is associated with chronic diarrhea in persons in developing countries.

Salmonella and *Shigella* are the two other major pathogens among the enterics. *Salmonella* is a common contaminant of cold-blooded animals, birds, and ruminants such as cattle and sheep. The most common result of infection in humans is severe enterocolitis, usually the result of fecal contamination of food or water. Historically *S. typhi* was the etiological agent of typhoid fever, a significant cause of mortality in cities in which sewage was untreated. *Shigella* is the cause of bacterial dysentery, a disease also transmitted through contaminated food or water.

Another enteric, *Yersinia pestis*, is the agent of bubonic plague, a major killer between the fourteenth and nineteenth centuries. Plague is endemic to many rodents and is transmitted to humans through the bite of a flea.

Clostridia. The clostridia are gram-positive rods that form spores, allowing them to survive in the soil or as part of the intestinal microbiota. While most are nonpathogenic, helping to degrade organic material, several are important pathogens because of the toxins they encode. The diseases they cause are in part the result of their being strictly anaerobic (oxygen free).

C. tetani spores are ubiquitous. If they enter a cut or wound, or any anaerobic environment, the spores may germinate, producing a toxin associated with tetanus. If the infected person has not been immunized against the toxin, the disease produces a loss of control of motor neurons, resulting in a spastic paralysis (lockjaw). Botulinum toxin, produced by *C. botulinum*, is among the most potent toxins known. While rare, botulism poisoning usually results from canned vegetables that have not been properly sterilized.

Campylobacter and *Helicobacter*, members of the ε-Proteobacteria, are among the most recently discovered pathogens. *Campylobacter* is an important cause of infant diarrhea, particularly in developing countries. *Helicobacter* infections of the stomach were found to be associated with the development of stomach ulcers. As a result of this connection, the treatment of ulcers with antibiotics rather than with palliative methods (antacids) was found to be more effective in preventing ulcer recurrence.

DRUG SUSCEPTIBILITY

Toxic substances such as mercury, which could be used to treat diseases such as syphilis, have been known since the seventeenth century. However, the concept of a "magic bullet," a safe antimicrobial agent that would kill germs and cure disease, dates to the 1880's, when the germ theory of disease was evolving. The first success in this area of research was the arsenic compound salvarsan, developed by German physician Paul Ehrlich, who was able to successfully treat syphilis with the compound. However, this also was too toxic for general use. Arguably, the primary impetus in researching antimicrobial drugs grew from the enormous number of casualties of World War I, in which infection was as likely to result in death as was the wound itself.

The first success in antimicrobial therapy was the discovery of sulfa drugs by German physician Gerhard Domagk. Working closely with the dye industry in the 1920's and 1930's, Domagk discovered that sulfur derivatives, the sulfonamides, could kill streptococci, among the deadliest of bacteria. German dictator Adolf Hitler and the Nazi Party limited research to finding ways to improve the effectiveness of the drugs, and it was not until after World War II that the full potential of sulfa drugs was seen. Meanwhile, penicillin, discovered by British scientist Alexander Fleming in 1928, became the first broad-spectrum antibiotic effective against most major bacteria.

Antimicrobials fall into four general categories: analogs such as the sulfa drugs, which block DNA replication; inhibitors of cell-wall synthesis, such as the penicillins, cephalosporins, and vancomycin; inhibitors of cell-membrane function, such as polymyxin; and inhibitors of bacterial protein synthesis, such as tetracycline, chloramphenicol, streptomycin, and erythromycin.

Bacteria have evolved a variety of means to resist antibiotic functions. In some cases, resistance is a natural function of bacterial structure. For example, the penicillins inhibit cross-linking of the cell-wall peptidoglycan in gram-positive cells such as the staphylococci and streptococci. Because most gram-negative bacteria such as *E. coli* and *Salmonella* have cell-wall struc-

tures containing limited amounts of peptidoglycan, historically they were more resistant. Some bacteria have acquired genetic information to produce enzymes that destroy or inactivate antibiotics. In particular, most staphylococci have developed a penicillinase that inactivates penicillin, rendering the drug useless. Other bacteria have acquired genetic information to enzymatically modify other antibiotics. Bacteria may also become resistant by changing the target of the drug; altered ribosome structures confer resistance to erythromycin or streptomycin. Likewise, bacteria may acquire mechanisms to pump the antibiotic out of the cell.

Richard Adler, Ph.D.

FURTHER READING

Brooks, George, et al. *Jawetz, Melnick, and Adelberg's Medical Microbiology.* 25th ed. New York: McGraw-Hill, 2010. A medical text that summarizes the major groups of pathogens, with concise descriptions of virulence factors associated with disease.

Hager, Thomas. *The Demon Under the Microscope.* New York: Harmony Books, 2006. Story behind the first "miracle drug," the sulfa drugs that were effective in treating streptococcal infections. Largely a biography of Gerhard Domagk, their discoverer, the story also delves into antibiotic research and the politics and economics behind the work.

Koch, Arthur L. *The Bacteria: Their Origin, Structure, Function, and Antibiosis.* Bloomington, Ind.: Springer, 2006. Evolutionary history of bacteria. Focuses on how the evolution of the cell-wall structure led to the diversification of bacterial species.

Murray, Patrick, et al., eds. *Manual of Clinical Microbiology.* 9th ed. Washington, D.C.: ASM Press, 2007. Provides extensive coverage of pathogenic bacteria and mechanisms of disease. The detailed discussions are not for the casual science reader, but the book does serve as an excellent resource for the subject.

Singleton, Paul. *Bacteria in Biology, Biotechnology, and Medicine.* 6th ed. New York: John Wiley & Sons, 2004. A concise description of bacteria and their roles in nature. Included are chapters on bacterial structure, staining, and methods of classification and identification.

Willey, Joanne, et al. *Prescott's Microbiology.* 8th ed. New York: McGraw-Hill, 2011. Outstanding textbook of microbiology. Specific chapters detail the most important organisms, including pathogens. The authors summarize pathogenic mechanisms in a manner that will not overwhelm readers.

WEB SITES OF INTEREST

American Society for Microbiology
http://www.microbeworld.org

Todar's Online Textbook of Bacteriology
http://www.textbookofbacteriology.net

Virtual Museum of Bacteriology
http://www.bacteriamuseum.org

See also: Antibiotic resistance; Antibiotics: Types; Bacteria: Structure and growth; Bacterial infections; Bacteriology; Diagnosis of bacterial infections; Immune response to bacterial infections; Infection; Microbiology; Mutation of pathogens; Pathogenicity; Pathogens; Prevention of bacterial infections; Superbacteria; Treatment of bacterial infections; Virulence.

Bacteria: Structure and growth

CATEGORY: Pathogen

DEFINITION

Bacteria are single-celled organisms that reside in every habitat, including the human body. Bacteria are a necessary part of the normal flora of the human body; very few species actually cause illness, and many are beneficial. Bacteria are the smallest known organisms that can reproduce independently.

GENERAL STRUCTURE

Bacteria are the most common life-form on Earth. These single-celled organisms come in a variety of shapes and sizes. The millions of known species of bacteria live in a wide range of environments, from vents deep in the ocean floor to the recesses of the human digestive tract. The vast majority of bacteria are harmless to humans; some are actually helpful and necessary for human health, while a small fraction are pathogenic. Despite these diverse features, all types of bacteria have fundamental characteristics in common.

Bacteria have a simpler structure than plant and animal cells, which are higher life-forms called eukary-

otes. Eukaryotes have cells that are divided into smaller compartments by membranes. Each compartment, or organelle, carries out specialized functions. Bacteria are prokaryotes, which have no organelles. They consist of just one compartment that is separated from the outside world by a cell membrane and a cell wall. The interior of the cell, called cytoplasm, contains a solution of sugars, salts, vitamins, enzymes, and other substances dissolved in water. Suspended in the cytoplasm are large numbers of ribosomes and a nucleoid made of DNA (deoxyribonucleic acid).

The cell membrane is a semipermeable barrier that separates the inside of the cell from the outside. This thin structure is vital to the survival of the cell. The membrane is created by the assembly of phospholipids and proteins into a bilayer. The inner and outer surfaces of the bilayer are charged and, thus, are attracted to the water molecules inside and outside the cell. The center layer of this structure is composed of fatty acids, which repel water. These chemical properties of the cell membrane ensure that the watery contents of the cell cannot leak through.

The structure of cell membranes also allows for the selective passage of certain molecules. This important feature ensures that necessary nutrients are allowed to enter the cell and that waste products are allowed to exit. While some substances cross the membrane through passive diffusion, most are transported actively by processes that require energy. The active transport of molecules across the membrane is mediated by proteins that are embedded in the cell membrane.

The cell membrane also serves as a site for the attachment of proteins involved in essential biochemical reactions. One example is the electron transport system, which generates adenosine triphosphate (ATP), the cell's energy currency. In bacteria, ATP is generated by a chain of proteins bound to the inner side of the cell membrane. In eukaryotes, this process occurs on the inner membranes of mitochondria. The bacterial cell membrane thus provides some of the functions carried out by organelles in eukaryotes.

The cell wall is a tough network of fibers that encloses and protects the bacterial cell. The substance that makes up the cell wall is a unique polymer called peptidoglycan, which is not found in eukaryotes. Peptidoglycan is made of long sugar molecules that are connected to each other by short peptides. Bacteria can be divided into two major groups based on the structure of their cell walls. Gram-positive bacteria have a thicker peptidoglycan cell wall that will turn purple when treated with a Gram's stain. The cell walls of gram-negative bacteria are surrounded by an outer membrane, which prevents the adhesion of a Gram's stain. The extra protection provided by the more complex cell wall of gram-negative bacteria makes them less sensitive to some antibiotics, which can penetrate the cell walls of only the gram-positive bacteria.

Several classes of antibiotics target the cell walls of bacteria. Penicillins, cephalosporins, and vancomycin interfere with cell-wall construction, causing the bacteria to rupture and die. The goal in treating bacterial infections with antibiotics is to kill the intended organisms without damaging the cells of the host. Because human and animal cells lack cell walls, they are not affected by such drugs.

The internal components of bacteria use nutrients in the environment to allow the organisms to grow and reproduce. The bacterial cytoplasm is rich with ribosomes. As in eukaryotic cells, bacterial ribosomes carry out protein synthesis and are made of ribonucleic acid (RNA). Slight differences in the structure of eukaryotic and prokaryotic ribosomes make the ribosome a target for antibiotic action. Multiple classes of antibiotics, including streptomycin (and its relatives), tetracycline, and erythromycin, disrupt protein synthesis in bacteria but not in the cells of the host.

Bacterial DNA is organized into one large ring-shaped chromosome. In contrast to eukaryotes, the bacterial chromosome is not encased in a nucleus. The bacterial chromosome contains all the information needed to provide for the basic functions of the organism. Bacteria may also contain circular DNA structures called plasmids. The genes on plasmids are not usually necessary for survival, but they may become so in certain environments; plasmids can carry genes for antibiotic resistance, allowing the host bacteria to survive in the presence of a drug that is normally deadly to its species.

SPECIALIZED FEATURES

The variety of specialized features found in bacteria reflects their adaptation to the broadest range of environments of any organism on Earth. Bacteria are diverse in their size and morphology. Although the average size of a bacterial cell is 1 to 5 micrometers (μm) in diameter, they range in size from 0.1 to 750 μm in diameter. One of the most distinguishing features of bacterial cells is their shapes, which can be used diagnostically. The most common shapes are spheres (cocci), rods (bacilli), comma shapes (vibrios), and spirals (spirochetes and spirillum).

Many bacteria have developed specialized structures that allow them to move in their environment. Some have flagella, which are long filaments that protrude from the cell wall and are used to produce a swimming motion. The arrangement of flagella on the bacterial cell depends on the species. A cell can have a single flagellum or multiple flagella, either clumped at one end of the cell or spread over the entire surface. Some bacteria exhibit a gliding motion, which is created by structures known as pili. These cell surface projections can extend and retract, causing the bacteria to move. Bacteria also use pili to attach to surfaces and to each other. Some aquatic bacteria use gas vesicles to adjust their position in their environment. Gas vesicles are hollow structures made of protein. When present, they increase the buoyancy of the organism, making it rise to the water surface. Gas vesicles disintegrate and reassemble according to the concentration of nutrients in the cell.

Capsules are specialized structures that add an extra layer of protection to the exterior of some bacterial cells. The capsule is made of a polysaccharide-containing material that forms rigid layers on the cell wall's exterior. Species that have capsules are extremely resistant to the action of phagocytes, cells of the host immune system that engulf and kill bacteria. Capsule-bearing strains of *Streptococcus pneumoniae*, for example, cause a particularly invasive and dangerous form of pneumonia.

Some species of bacteria can survive harsh conditions by forming endospores, which allow the bacteria to become dormant. Endospores, small cells that develop within bacterial cells, contain DNA and a portion of the cytoplasm. A strong wall surrounds and protects the endospore. Once the bacteria die, the endospores are released into the environment, where they can survive indefinitely. These tough structures are resistant to heat, radiation, chemicals, and desiccation. When environmental conditions improve, the endospore rapidly germinates and develops into a bacterial cell. Endospore-forming bacteria include *Bacillus anthracis*, which causes anthrax, and *Clostridium botulinum*, responsible for a serious form of food poisoning called botulism.

BACTERIAL GROWTH

Bacteria possess all the machinery necessary to grow and reproduce independently of other cells. They are the smallest creatures on Earth that have this capacity. While they may use a host organism as a habitat, nearly all bacteria can reproduce without invading host cells. This feature sets them apart from viruses, which carry their own genetic material but require host-cell components for reproduction. The small size and relatively simple structure of bacteria allow them to grow and reproduce much faster than eukaryotic cells.

Bacteria reproduce asexually by dividing in half, in a process called binary fission. Individual bacterial cells grow continuously, making copies of their components and duplicating their DNA. The two copies of the chromosome move toward opposite ends of the cell, ensuring that each "daughter" cell will receive this essential DNA. When enough new material is present to sustain two cells, the cell membrane begins to pinch inward at the center. A cell wall grows to form a partition that divides the cell into two daughter cells. Because bacterial reproduction is asexual, each daughter will be identical to the parent cell.

Populations of bacteria grow at a rate determined by the time it takes individual cells to grow and divide, creating the next generation. The population doubles in size with each generation. The time required for a population of cells to double is known as the doubling time. Bacterial doubling times vary with the species, ranging from a few minutes to several hours. The nearly explosive growth rate of bacteria is about one hundred times faster than that of eukaryotic cells. Rapid binary fission allows bacteria to become extremely numerous in a short amount of time. If one bacterium with a doubling time of twenty minutes were allowed to grow for forty-four hours, the resulting mass of bacteria produced would equal the mass of the earth.

FACTORS AFFECTING BACTERIAL GROWTH RATES

The actual occurrence of exponential bacterial growth is greatly limited by environmental factors, both in natural habitats and in laboratories. Long before a bacterial population could grow to match the earth's mass, the supply of nutrients in the environment for the bacteria would be depleted. Bacterial growth rates are highly dependent on many factors, including temperature, the availability of nutrients, pH (acidity), and oxygen concentrations. Measures that reduce the rate of bacterial growth can be used to prevent illnesses caused by bacteria; most pathogenic bacteria must be present in large numbers to cause illness.

The optimal temperature for bacterial growth depends upon the species. Bacteria that live inside humans, including those of medical significance, thrive at an optimal temperature of about 98.6° Fahrenheit (37° Celsius). They can survive at temperatures generally ranging from 50° to 118.4° F (10° to 48° C), but their growth rates will be significantly reduced at lower temperatures. Their ability to survive below the optimal temperature may allow them to live outside a host for short periods until they enter a new host. This temperature tolerance facilitates the spread of bacteria from one host to another.

Bacterial growth rates can be reduced by controlling the temperature of the environment. Refrigeration of food slows the growth of bacteria, keeping their numbers low enough to prevent illness. Aqueous solutions heated to boiling 212° F (100° C) for thirty minutes will kill all bacteria in the solution. Medical instruments and solutions can be sterilized in an autoclave by heating above 248° F (120° C), which kills bacteria and heat-tolerant endospores.

Bacteria take in nutrients from their environment. Specific nutrients will vary depending on the habitat of a given species. General nutritional requirements of most bacteria include a carbon-source for energy, such as sugar; a nitrogen source, such as ammonia or nitrate; a variety of minerals and salts; vitamins; and other growth factors.

Bacteria are sensitive to the pH of their environment and can live only within a relatively narrow pH range. Most species of bacteria grow optimally in neutral environments, with a pH level between 6 and 8. Some species are specially adapted to live in extremely acidic or basic environments. The optimal pH of a given species will determine where it thrives, even within the human body. The stomach, with a pH of 2, is home to low numbers of acid-tolerant species of lactobacilli and streptococci. The large intestine, with a neutral pH of 7, is a much more popular residence; enormous numbers of bacteria from a minimum of ten different species live in the large intestine. The sensitivity of most bacteria to low pH can be used to inhibit bacterial growth, as occurs when foods are pickled in vinegar.

The presence of oxygen in the environment is another factor that affects bacterial growth. Most species, the aerobes, require oxygen for growth. For these species, low oxygen will cause a decrease in growth rate; if oxygen levels fall too low, they will not survive. For other species, the anaerobes, oxygen is not necessary for growth. Oxygen is toxic to some species; these obligate anaerobes cannot survive in environments where oxygen is present. Oxygen tolerance is an attribute used to identify bacterial species.

Impact

Bacteria are ubiquitous, and they will remain so. They have developed diverse traits that allow them to thrive in an amazing variety of habitats, including unimaginably harsh conditions. Their demonstrated adaptability should give pause and guide future scientific and medical strategies for preventing and treating bacterial illnesses.

Kathryn Pierno, M.S.

Further Reading

Braude, Abraham I., Charles E. Davis, and Joshua Fierer. *Infectious Diseases and Medical Microbiology.* 2d ed. Philadelphia: W. B. Saunders, 1986. Microbiology from a medical perspective, designed for medical students. Provides a systematic approach, with highly detailed information about pathogens.

Brooker, Robert J., et al. *Biology.* New York: McGraw-Hill Higher Education, 2008. A standard biology textbook for undergraduate college students. Bacterial structure and reproduction covered in a concise manner, with excellent photographs.

Koch, Arthur L. *The Bacteria: Their Origin, Structure, Function, and Antibiosis.* Bloomington, Ind.: Springer, 2006. Evolutionary history of bacterial structures. Focuses on how the evolution of the cell-wall structure led to diversification of bacterial species. Covers the mechanism of action of cell-wall antibiotics and presents an evolutionary perspective on antibiotic resistance.

Madigan, Michael T., and John M. Martinko. *Brock Biology of Microorganisms.* 12th ed. Upper Saddle River, N.J.: Pearson/Prentice Hall, 2010. A standard microbiology textbook for undergraduate students, with detailed descriptions of cell structures and clear illustrations. Includes evolutionary perspectives and covers pathogenesis.

Web Sites of Interest

American Society for Microbiology
http://www.microbeworld.org

Todar's Online Textbook of Bacteriology
http://www.textbookofbacteriology.net

Virtual Museum of Bacteriology
http://www.bacteriamuseum.org

See also: Antibiotic resistance; Antibiotics: Types; Bacteria: Classification and types; Bacterial infections; Bacteriology; Contagious diseases; Diagnosis of bacterial infections; Immune response to bacterial infections; Infection; Inflammation; Microbiology; Mutation of pathogens; Opportunistic infections; Pathogenicity; Pathogens; Prevention of bacterial infections; Superbacteria; Treatment of bacterial infections; Virulence.

Bacterial endocarditis

CATEGORY: Diseases and conditions
ANATOMY OR SYSTEM AFFECTED: Blood, cardiovascular system, heart, tissue
ALSO KNOWN AS: Infective endocarditis

Definition

The endocardium is a thin membrane that covers the inner surface of the heart. Bacterial endocarditis is an infection of this membrane. Infection occurs when bacteria attach to the membrane and grow.

The infection is most common when the heart or heart valves have already been damaged. It can be life-threatening, and it can permanently impair the heart valves. This can lead to serious health problems, such as congestive heart failure.

The infection can also cause growths on the valves or other areas of the heart. Pieces of these growths can break off and travel to other parts of the body. This can cause serious complications.

Causes

Bacteria can travel to the heart through the blood. They can enter the blood from an infection elsewhere in the body. They can also enter through breaks in the skin or mucous membranes caused by dental work, surgery, or IV (intravenous) drug use. Only certain bacteria cause this infection, the most common of which are streptococci, staphylococci, and enterococci.

The bacteria may then be able to attach to the endocardium. Some heart conditions can increase the chance of infections. These conditions may cause blood flow to be obstructed or to pool, providing a place for the bacteria to build up.

Risk Factors

The following conditions place a person at greater risk for bacterial endocarditis during certain procedures: heart valve scarring from rheumatic fever or other conditions; artificial heart valve; congenital heart defect; cardiomyopathy; prior episode of endocarditis; and mitral valve prolapse, with significant regurgitation (abnormal backflow of blood).

The foregoing conditions increase the risk of the infection with certain activities, including IV drug use (risk is extremely high when needles are shared); any dental procedure, even cleanings; removal of tonsils or adenoids, and other procedures involving the ears, nose, and throat; bronchoscopy (viewing the airways though a thin, lighted tube); and surgery on the gastrointestinal or urinary tracks, including the gallbladder and prostate.

Symptoms

Symptoms of bacterial endocarditis vary from mild to severe, depending on the bacteria causing the infection, the amount of bacteria in the bloodstream, the extent of structural heart defects, the body's ability to fight infection, and overall health. The symptoms, which can begin within two weeks of the bacteria entering the bloodstream, include fever, chills, fatigue, weakness, malaise, unexplained weight loss, poor appetite, muscle aches, joint pain, coughing, shortness of breath, bumps on the fingers and toes, and little red dots on the skin, inside the mouth, or under the nails. The first symptom may be caused by a piece of the infected heart growth breaking off.

Screening and Diagnosis

A doctor will ask about symptoms and medical history and will perform a physical exam, which includes listening to the patient's heart for a murmur. Tests may include blood cultures to check for the presence of bacteria; blood tests to look for signs of infections

and complications related to endocarditis; a computed tomography (CT) scan (a detailed X-ray picture that identifies abnormalities of fine tissue structure); an electrocardiogram (ECG or EKG), which is a test that records the heart's activity by measuring electrical currents through the heart muscle; an echocardiogram, which is a test that uses high-frequency sound waves (ultrasound) to examine the size, shape, and motion of the heart; and a transesophageal echocardiogram, in which ultrasound is passed through the patient's mouth and then into the esophagus to better visualize the heart valves.

Treatment and Therapy

Treatment, including medications and possible surgery, focuses on getting rid of the infection from the blood and heart. Antibiotics are given through an IV into a vein. The patient must be admitted to the hospital for this treatment, which could take four to six weeks to complete. If the antibiotics fail to remove the bacteria, or if the infection returns, surgery may be needed. Surgery may also be necessary if the infection has damaged the heart or valves.

Prevention and Outcomes

The best way to prevent endocarditis is to avoid the use of illegal IV drugs. Certain heart conditions may increase the risk too. To find out if the patient is at increased risk for this condition, the doctor should be consulted.

The American Heart Association (AHA) recommends that people with high and moderate risk should take antibiotics before and after certain dental and nondental medical procedures. In addition, the AHA recommends taking an antibiotic just before and after any procedure that may put a person at risk.

The patient should tell his or her dentist and other health professionals about the heart condition. Other preventive measures include maintaining good oral hygiene, brushing teeth twice daily, flossing daily, visiting a dentist for a cleaning at least every six months, and seeing a dentist if dentures cause discomfort. Finally, people should seek medical care immediately for symptoms of an infection.

Debra Wood, R.N.; reviewed by David N. Smith, M.D.

Further Reading

Bonow, R. O., et al. "ACC/AHA 2006 Guidelines for the Management of Patients with Valvular Heart

Disease." *Journal of the American College of Cardiology* 48 (2006).

Durack, David T., and Michael H. Crawford, eds. *Infective Endocarditis*. Philadelphia: W. B. Saunders, 2003.

Fauci, Anthony, et al., eds. *Harrison's Principles of Internal Medicine*. 17th ed. New York: McGraw-Hill, 2008.

Giessel, Barton E., Clint J. Koenig, and Robert L. Blake, Jr. "Information from Your Family Doctor: Bacterial Endocarditis, a Heart at Risk." *American Family Physician* 61, no. 6 (March 15, 2000): 1705.

Hoen, B. "Epidemiology and Antibiotic Treatment of Infective Endocarditis: An Update." *Heart* 92 (2006): 1694-1700.

Rakel, Robert E., Edward T. Bope, and Rick D. Kellerman, eds. *Conn's Current Therapy 2011*. Philadelphia: Saunders/Elsevier, 2010.

Zipes, Douglas P., et al., eds. *Braunwald's Heart Disease: A Textbook of Cardiovascular Medicine*. 8th ed. Philadelphia: Saunders/Elsevier, 2008.

WEB SITES OF INTEREST

American Dental Association
http://www.ada.org

American Heart Association
http://www.heart.org

Canadian Dental Association
http://www.cda-adc.ca

Heart and Stroke Foundation of Canada
http://www.heartandstroke.com

See also: Bacterial infections; Behçet's syndrome; Bloodstream infections; Endocarditis; *Enterococcus*; Iatrogenic infections; Myocarditis; Pericarditis; Rheumatic fever; Septic arthritis; *Staphylococcus*; *Streptococcus*; Vancomycin-resistant enterococci infection.

Bacterial infections

CATEGORY: Diseases and conditions
ANATOMY OR SYSTEM AFFECTED: All

DEFINITION

Bacteria are microscopic, single-celled organisms that are present everywhere on Earth. They have adapted to every conceivable environment, including fresh water and salt water, soil, and the atmosphere; they also live in a wide range of temperatures. Bacteria are present in the skin, gastrointestinal tract, and lungs of all humans.

Bacteria that are normally present in an area of the body are known as that body's normal flora. Some bacteria are beneficial to human health; for example, lactobacilli in the intestinal tract aid in the digestion of food. Many bacteria are harmless, and others can cause severe illness and death.

In addition to their scientific name of genus and species, bacteria are classified by their shape, their appearance after a Gram's stain is applied, and their need for oxygen. Bacterial shapes include bacilli (rods), cocci (spheres), and spirochetes (helixes or spirals). Bacteria are designated as either gram-positive (those that stain blue) or gram-negative (those that stain red). Aerobic bacteria require oxygen to survive; anaerobic bacteria do not require oxygen. Some bacteria are known as facultative bacteria and can survive with or without oxygen. An example of a bacterial classification is *Streptococcus* (genus) *pneumonia* (species), which is a gram-positive aerobic coccus that causes pneumonia.

CAUSES

Only a small percentage of bacteria can cause disease. These bacteria, known as pathogens, cause disease by producing toxins, which damage surrounding cells; some pathogens invade or destroy tissues and other pathogens do both. Bacteria can enter and multiply in the bloodstream and can then develop into a condition referred to as bacteremia. Common areas of bacterial infections are the throat, ears, sinuses, gastrointestinal tract, lungs, and urinary tract.

Certain types of bacteria are present at different locations in the body (for example, the mouth, throat, stomach, and colon) and are the normal bacterial flora for that region of the body. These bacteria can become harmful if they invade another area of the body. For example, a tear in the intestinal lining can release bacteria into the abdominal cavity. In other cases, bacteria can become harmful if they multiply, disproportionately. For example, an antibiotic may kill off harmless (commensal) bacteria and allow harmful (pathogenic) bacteria to increase.

Representative types of bacteria that cause human disease include *Vibrio cholerae*, *Clostridium*, *Neisseria*

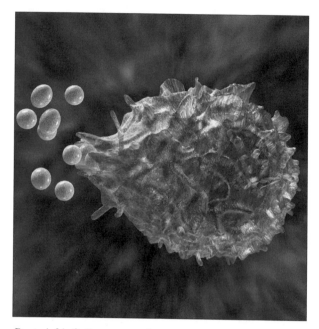

Bacterial infections, most often, are met with a fierce response by the immune system. A macrophage, right, engulfs pathogenic bacteria to try to stop the infection.

gonorrhoeae, *Staphylococcus*, *Streptococcus*, and *Treponema pallidum*.

V. cholera. The bacterium *V. cholera* causes cholera, an acute diarrheal infection with an incubation period ranging from two hours to five days; the infection can cause death within hours. It is contracted by ingesting food or water contaminated with the bacteria. An estimated 3 to 5 million cases occur annually, resulting in 100,000 to 120,000 deaths. Epidemics can occur because of cholera's rapid incubation.

Clostridium. The anaerobic bacterium *Clostridium* is found in the intestinal tract of 4 to 8 percent of healthy adults. Clostridia are also present in nonhuman animals, in decaying vegetation, and in soil. The bacteria cause disease by producing a toxin either before or after entering a body. In some cases, the bacteria invade the bloodstream and produce widespread bacteremia and then sepsis, which quickly can be fatal. Botulism can occur if a person eats raw or undercooked food contaminated by *C. botulinum* toxin. Gas gangrene is caused by *C. perfringens*, *C. novyi*, and other clostridia species. The bacteria can enter a muscle through a wound, can multiply in necrotic (dead) tissue, and can produce powerful toxins. These toxins destroy surrounding healthy tissue and generate gas.

Tetanus is caused by a toxin produced by the bacterium *C. tetani*. Spores of this bacterium, which are present in soil, dust, saliva, and manure, enter the body through a cut and develop into bacteria, which multiply and produce a toxin. The toxin causes a spasm of skeletal muscles, which leads to death in more than 50 percent of cases. The incubation period ranges from eight days to several months.

C. perfringens also causes food poisoning, which occurs when a person eats food (usually beef) contaminated with the bacterial spores. These spores develop into bacteria in the food and then multiply; further multiplication occurs in the intestinal tract. The bacteria produce a toxin that leads to abdominal cramping and watery diarrhea. These infections are usually mild; however, they can be fatal, particularly in persons with a weakened state of health.

C. difficile produces toxins that damage the intestinal wall, resulting in watery diarrhea. This bacterium might be part of the intestinal flora or contracted from the environment, another person, or a pet. If a person takes a course of antibiotics, competing organisms are destroyed and *C. difficile* multiplies. Clostridial toxic shock syndrome (TSS) is a rare but serious infection of the female reproductive organs caused by *C. sordellii*.

N. gonorrhoeae. Gonorrhea is a sexually transmitted disease caused by the *N. gonorrhoeae* bacterium. Often, infected persons have no symptoms; however, the disease can be transmitted through sexual contact (vaginal, oral, or anal). In women, the disease can damage the Fallopian tubes, resulting in infertility. It also can spread into the abdominal cavity, resulting in pelvic inflammatory disease (PID). In men, it can cause urethritis (inflammation of the urinary outlet), which can progress to narrowing or obstruction of the urethra. It sometimes spreads to other parts of the body and can cause arthritis and can damage the heart valves.

Staphylococcus. Staphylococci are gram-positive aerobic bacteria that cause a wide variety of diseases, ranging from mild to life-threatening. These organisms, commonly known as staph, are part of the normal flora of the nose and skin. Most infections are caused by *S. aureus*. A break in the skin can result in a localized staph infection (an abscess, furuncle, or boil), which can progress to cellulitis (inflammation of connective tissue beneath the skin). Staph infections can invade the bloodstream and cause bacteremia. Staphylococcal sepsis is a major cause of shock and circulatory collapse. The organism can cause pneumonia, particularly in people in poor health or with underlying lung disease. It can spread to the bones and cause osteomyelitis (bone-muscle infection). *S. aureus* can produce toxins, which can result in TSS, staphylococcal food poisoning (SFP), and staphylococcal scalded-skin syndrome (SSSS). As with other bacteria, staph has evolved to resist antibiotics. One strain that is a global health concern is methicillin-resistant *S. aureus* (MRSA). MRSA is resistant to a number of antibiotics, including penicillin, methicillin, and cephalosporins.

Streptococcus. Like staphylococci, streptococci are gram-positive aerobic bacteria, which cause a wide variety of diseases ranging from mild to life-threatening. They are a common cause of sore throats (strep throat), scarlet fever, and rheumatic fever. The bacteria can also cause two rapidly progressive, severe infections: necrotizing fasciitis, which attacks fascia (sheathes around the muscles), and TSS.

T. pallidum. Syphilis is a sexually transmitted disease caused by a spirochete, *T. pallidum*. It is initially characterized by a chancre (nonpainful ulcer). Over time it can produce severe damage to the heart, joints, and central nervous system.

Risk Factors

Poor health, crowded living conditions, and poor sanitation increase the risk of infection. Hospital workers are at increased risk through direct patient contact and indirectly through contact with needles, syringes, and bodily fluids. For example, MRSA infections commonly occur in hospitals and other health care facilities, such as nursing homes. MRSA acquired in a hospital is known as hospital-acquired-MRSA. The risk of cholera increases if drinking water is not treated through boiling, chlorination, or other measures. The risk of botulism increases if a person ingests improperly home-canned food. The risk of tetanus is increased if one has not been vaccinated against tetanus or does not receive a booster after experiencing a deep puncture wound. Improper cleansing of a deep wound also increases the risk of tetanus and gas gangrene. The risk of *C. difficile* increases after taking a course of antibiotics, particularly those that are more potent. The risk of food poisoning from clostridia or staph increases if food is left sitting in the sun for prolonged periods after preparation. The risk of gonorrhea and syphilis increases with unprotected sex (no condom) unless the partner is known to be disease-free.

Symptoms

Cholera is characterized by the sudden onset of severe, watery diarrhea and vomiting. Early symptoms of botulism may be a dry mouth and throat or nausea and vomiting (or all of these). However, botulism usually begins with weakness of the muscles supplied by the twelve cranial nerves; these nerves control eye movements, facial muscles, and the muscles involved in chewing and swallowing. Weakness spreads to the arms, then the legs. Respiratory muscles can be affected too, causing difficulty breathing and respiratory failure. Gas gangrene is characterized by rapidly progressive necrosis of muscle tissue accompanied by swelling from the produced gas. Tetanus produces spasm of the skeletal muscles. It usually begins with spasm of the jaw muscles; thus, its common name of lockjaw. *C. perfringens* food poisoning and *C. difficile* infections are characterized by watery diarrhea.

Gonorrhea infections may be asymptomatic. Common symptoms for males are a discharge from the penis and dysuria (painful urination). Females may also experience dysuria. The infection may flare during the menstrual period when the bacteria feed on blood products and progress into the uterus and Fallopian tubes. As the disease progresses, pelvic pain occurs.

The symptoms of staphylococci infection depend on the affected organ. Skin infections appear as abscesses, furuncles, boils, or, in more advanced cases, cellulitis. Infections of the respiratory system can range from sinus congestion to pneumonia. Staphylococcal food poisoning is characterized by nausea, vomiting, and diarrhea. TSS is characterized by fever, low blood pressure, and generalized rash, which resembles a sunburn. It can progress rapidly to shock, cardiorespiratory failure, and death. SSSS is characterized by blistering of the skin, which spreads to generalized, painful reddening of the skin.

Like staphylococci, streptococci-infection symptoms depend on the affected organ. Scarlet fever causes a red rash, facial reddening, fever, and a very sore throat. Lymph nodes in the neck are swollen and the person has difficulty swallowing. Rheumatic fever causes abdominal pain, fever, joint pain and swelling, nosebleeds, and skin nodules. The bacteria can damage the heart valves, resulting in rheumatic heart disease. Necrotizing fasciitis, also known as flesh-eating disease, sometimes begins as redness and swelling of the skin. The skin later turns violet with blisters. Subsequently, necrosis of deeper tissues occurs. Often, TSS begins with two to three days of a low-grade fever, muscle aches, and chills. Subsequently, the infected person spikes a high fever. A red, sunburn-like rash then appears across most of the body. Muscle aches and headache are also common. The disease can affect most organs in the body (skin, lungs, liver, and kidneys). Cardiorespiratory failure and death are then likely

With a syphilis infection, a chancre (nonpainful ulcer) forms at the point of sexual contact; this is known as primary syphilis. Secondary syphilis manifests as a rash on the palms and soles of the feet. Tertiary syphilis appears one to ten years after the initial infection and can produce damage to the heart, joints, and central nervous system.

SCREENING AND DIAGNOSIS

Diagnosis involves taking a sample from the site of infection (such as from skin abscesses, sputum, blood, skin, or urine). The sample can undergo Gram staining and can then by viewed under a microscope. The stained specimen may yield a diagnosis; however, to make a definitive diagnosis, it is necessary to culture the sample. Specific culture media are required for the type of bacteria suspected. For example, *N. gonorrhoeae* requires a chocolate agar medium, and gram-negative bacteria can be cultured on MacConkey agar. The coagulase test is used to differentiate *S. aureus* from other types of staphylococci. *S. aureus* is coagulase positive and causes blood serum to clot.

TREATMENT AND THERAPY

Death from cholera can be prevented by prompt administration of fluids and electrolytes (body salts). In severe cases, the fluid replacement can be given intravenously. With fluid and electrolyte replacement, recovery is most common.

In any clostridial infection, antibiotics such as penicillin are given to eradicate the bacteria. If botulism is diagnosed early, it can be treated with an antitoxin that blocks the action of the neurotoxin in the bloodstream. Supportive care is essential to increase the chance of recovery. Gas gangrene requires debridement (excision of infected, dead tissue) and wound irrigation with antiseptics. Amputation is sometimes

necessary. Prompt intramuscular injection of immunoglobulin can treat nonimmunized persons suspected of exposure to tetanus bacteria. Bed rest, quiet conditions, and sedation are helpful. Paralysis of the muscles with muscle relaxing agents and mechanical ventilation with a respirator may be administered to control muscle spasms. The treatment for *C. perfringens* food poisoning is primarily supportive therapy. *C. difficile* also requires supportive therapy. The antibiotic metronidazole is effective for eradicating the bacteria.

Gonorrhea is susceptible to many antibiotics, including penicillin, cephalosporins, and tetracycline. Resistant strains have developed, particularly to penicillin.

Staph and strep infections are treated with antibiotics such as penicillin, cephalosporins, and tetracycline. These bacteria commonly mutate to resistant strains. One noteworthy example is MRSA. The antibiotic vancomycin is the drug of choice for these infections. However, strains resistant to vancomycin have developed. Finally, syphilis is commonly cured with penicillin.

PREVENTION AND OUTCOMES

Cholera can be prevented by boiling or otherwise sterilizing water and by avoiding eating any food that might be contaminated. Protective clothing and masks should be worn by persons caring for people with cholera.

Botulism can be prevented by using proper home-canning techniques and by avoiding canned goods that might be contaminated (a bloated can or one with evidence of puncture). Thorough cooking destroys the toxin. Gas gangrene can be prevented by thorough cleansing of a wound and by seeking prompt medical attention if redness, swelling, or pain occurs. Tetanus can be prevented by immunization and receiving a booster shot every ten years or after sustaining a deep puncture wound. *C. perfringens* food poisoning can be prevented by eating food promptly after cooking. *C. difficile* infections can be reduced by prescribing antibiotics only when appropriate.

Gonorrhea and syphilis can be prevented by safer sex practices, such as wearing a condom and by avoiding sexual relations with persons who might be infected.

Complete prevention of staph and strep infection is impossible; however, the risk of infection can be reduced by thorough cleansing of wounds and by the avoidance of contact with a person who is or might be infected. Bacterial infection can be avoided by washing one's hands before eating and by disinfecting objects such as telephone mouthpieces (which can harbor bacteria).

Robin Wulffson, M.D., FACOG

FURTHER READING

Brogden, K., et al. *Virulence Mechanisms of Bacterial Pathogens.* 4th ed. Washington, D.C.: ASM Press, 2007. An overview of the latest knowledge regarding the mechanisms used by bacterial pathogens to cause disease. Includes proven strategies for overcoming these mechanisms.

Gillespie, S. *Management of Multiple Drug-Resistant Infections.* Totowa, N.J.: Humana Press, 2004. Multidrug-resistant and, therefore, difficult to treat, infections continue to occur and are clearly increasing in some areas. This book covers the management of these challenging infections.

Hart, T. *Microterrors: The Complete Guide to Bacterial, Viral, and Fungal Infections That Threaten Our Health.* Buffalo, N.Y.: Firefly Books, 2004. Covers the hidden dangers surrounding the human environment, namely, the threat of deadly, unseen organisms such as resistant strains of bacteria, which can survive the strongest antibiotics, and deadly new biological weapons, which are being cultured in laboratories worldwide

Robbins, J. *Bacterial Vaccines.* New York: Praeger, 1987. Covers advances in vaccine research and illustrates the need for continuing research.

Rotbat, H. *Germ Proof Your Kids: The Complete Guide to Protecting (Without Overprotecting) Your Family from Infections.* Washington, D.C.: ASM Press, 2007. An easy-to-read guide for parents who wish to reduce the risk of infections in their children.

World Health Organization. *WHO Model Prescribing Information: Drugs Used in Bacterial Infections.* Geneva: Author, 2001. Provides prescribing information for essential drugs used in the treatment of bacterial infections. It also covers prophylaxis against rheumatic fever, meningitis, and bacterial infection during surgery.

WEB SITES OF INTEREST

Centers for Disease Control and Prevention
http://www.cdc.gov

Clean Hands Coalition
http://www.cleanhandscoalition.org

Todar's Online Textbook of Bacteriology
http://www.textbookofbacteriology.net

See also: Antibiotic resistance; Antibiotics: Types; Bacteria: Classification and types; Bacteria: Structure and growth; Bacteriology; Bloodstream infections; Contagious diseases; Diagnosis of bacterial infections; Epidemiology; Immune response to bacterial infections; Infection; Inflammation; Microbiology; Mutation of pathogens; Opportunistic infections; Pathogenicity; Pathogens; Prevention of bacterial infections; Superbacteria; Treatment of bacterial infections; Virulence.

Bacterial meningitis

CATEGORY: Diseases and conditions
ANATOMY OR SYSTEM AFFECTED: Brain, central nervous system, respiratory system, spinal cord, tissue
ALSO KNOWN AS: Spinal meningitis

DEFINITION

The brain and spinal cord are encased by layers of tissue. These layers are called the meninges. Certain bacteria can cause an infection in these layers called bacterial meningitis, a serious infection that can cause death within hours. A quick diagnosis and treatment are vital.

CAUSES

Many times, the bacteria first cause an upper respiratory tract infection. Then the bacteria travel through the bloodstream to the brain. Worldwide, three types of bacteria cause the majority of cases of acute bacterial meningitis: *Streptococcus pneumoniae* (the bacterium that causes pneumonia); *Neisseria meningitidis*; and *Haemophilus influenzae* type B (Hib). In the United States, widespread immunization has almost eliminated meningitis caused by Hib. Other forms of bacterial meningitis include *Listeria monocytogenes* meningitis, *Escherichia coli* meningitis, *Mycobacterium tuberculosis* meningitis, and group B *Streptococcus* meningitis.

Newborn babies and the elderly are more prone to get sick. Some forms are spread by direct contact with

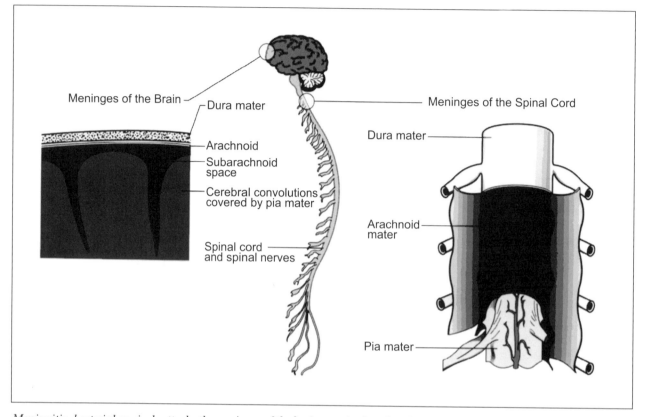

Meningitis, bacterial or viral, attacks the meninges of the brain or spinal cord, or both.

fluid from the mouth or throat of an infected person. This can happen during a kiss or by sharing eating utensils. In general, meningitis is not spread by casual contact.

RISK FACTORS

Risk factors for bacterial meningitis are close and prolonged contact with persons with meningitis caused by Hib or *N. meningitidis*; a weakened immune system caused by human immunodeficiency virus (HIV) infection or other conditions; alcoholism; smoking (for meningitis caused by *N. meningitidis*); and living in proximity to others, such as in dormitories and military barracks (for meningitis caused by *N. meningitidis*). At higher risk are infants, young children, and persons older than age sixty years.

SYMPTOMS

Classic symptoms can develop over several hours or may take one to two days. These symptoms are a high fever, headache, and a stiff, sore neck. Other symptoms may include red or purple skin rash, cyanosis (bluish skin), nausea, vomiting, photophobia (sensitivity to bright lights), sleepiness, and mental confusion.

In newborns and infants, symptoms are hard to see. As a result, infants younger than three months of age with a fever are often checked for meningitis. Symptoms in newborns and infants may include inactivity; unexplained high fever or any form of temperature instability, including a low body temperature; irritability; vomiting; jaundice (yellow color to the skin); feeding poorly or refusing to eat; tautness or bulging of soft spots between skull bones; and difficulty awakening. As the illness progresses, seizures or hearing loss, or both, can occur. This can happen to patients of all ages.

SCREENING AND DIAGNOSIS

A doctor will ask about symptoms and medical history and will conduct a physical exam. Tests may include a spinal tap (removal of a small amount of cerebrospinal fluid to check for bacteria); other cultures (testing of samples of blood, urine, mucus, and pus from skin infections); magnetic resonance imaging (a scan that uses radio waves and a powerful magnet to produce detailed computer images) to be sure the inflammation is not from some other cause, such as a tumor; and a computed tomography scan (a detailed X-ray picture that identifies abnormalities of fine tissue structure).

TREATMENT AND THERAPY

More than 90 percent of all people with this infection survive when they receive immediate care that includes antibiotics and corticosteroids, which are often given together, and fluids. Options include antibiotics, which are given intravenously (IV). This is started as soon as the infection is suspected. The antibiotics may be changed once tests name the exact bacterial cause. The patient usually stays in the hospital until his or her fever has fallen. The fluid around the spine and the brain must also be clear of infection.

Another treatment option is corticosteroids. These are usually given by IV early in treatment. They control brain pressure and swelling and reduce the body's production of inflammatory substances. This treatment can prevent further damage. Also, fluids can be lost because of fever, sweating, or vomiting. They may be replaced through an IV, but replaced carefully to avoid complications of fluid overloading. The doctor might prescribe pain medications and sedatives, and also anticonvulsants to prevent seizures.

PREVENTION AND OUTCOMES

To help reduce the chances of infection with bacterial meningitis, one should consider getting the recommended vaccines (for oneself and one's child). The vaccines include Hib vaccine (for babies), pneumococcal vaccine (for children younger than two years of age, for adults older than age sixty-five years, and for others with certain medical conditions), and meningococcal vaccine (for children age eleven to twelve years and for others at high risk; people in the high-risk group may need to be vaccinated every five years).

Persons such as health care workers, who have close contact with someone who is infected, should take preventive antibiotics. Another preventive measure is to use only pasteurized milk and milk products, which can prevent meningitis caused by *L. monocytogenes*. Women and girls who are pregnant will be monitored by a doctor to ensure the infection is not passed to the fetus.

Krisha McCoy, M.S.; reviewed by David L. Horn, M.D., FACP

FURTHER READING

American Academy of Family Physicians. "Diagnosis of Acute Meningitis in Adult Patients." Available at http://www.aafp.org/afp/20000115/tips/9.html.

Centers for Disease Control and Prevention. "An Updated Recommendation from the Advisory Committee on Immunization Practices (ACIP) for Revaccination of Persons at Prolonged Increased Risk for Meningococcal Disease." *Morbidity and Mortality Weekly Report* 58, no. 37 (2009): 1042-1043.

EBSCO Publishing. *Health Library: Meningococcal Vaccine.* Available through http://www.ebscohost.com.

Ferreiros, C. *Emerging Strategies in the Fight Against Meningitis.* New York: Garland Science, 2002.

National Institute of Neurological Disorders and Stroke. "Meningitis and Encephalitis Fact Sheet." Available at http://www.ninds.nih.gov.

Shmaefsky, Brian. *Meningitis.* Rev. ed. Philadelphia: Chelsea House, 2010.

Tunkel, Allan R. *Bacterial Meningitis.* Philadelphia: Lippincott Williams & Wilkins, 2001.

WEB SITES OF INTEREST

Centers for Disease Control and Prevention
http://www.cdc.gov

Meningitis Foundation of America
http://www.musa.org

Meningitis Research Foundation of Canada
http://www.meningitis.ca

National Institute of Neurological Disorders and Stroke
http://www.ninds.nih.gov

See also: Acanthamoeba infection; Bacterial infections; Children and infectious disease; Encephalitis; *Escherichia coli* infection; Guillain-Barré syndrome; *Haemophilus; Haemophilus influenzae* infection; *Listeria*; Listeriosis; Meningococcal meningitis; Meningococcal vaccine; Mosquito-borne viral encephalitis; *Neisseria*;

Oxazolidinone antibiotics; Pneumococcal infections; Pneumococcal vaccine; Pneumonia; Poliomyelitis; Saliva and infectious disease; *Streptococcus*; Viral meningitis.

Bacterial vaginosis

CATEGORY: Diseases and conditions
ANATOMY OR SYSTEM AFFECTED: Genitalia, reproductive system, skin, vagina

DEFINITION

Bacterial vaginosis is a mild infection of the vagina. Although it is usually treated easily, it may be a sign of another, more serious condition. It can also lead to complications during pregnancy, such as low birth weight and premature delivery, and a higher risk of pelvic inflammatory disease if the bacteria infect the uterus and Fallopian tubes.

There is an association between bacterial vaginosis and a higher risk of being infected with the human immunodeficiency virus (HIV) or other sexually transmitted diseases. If a woman has HIV and also bacterial vaginosis, she risks transmitting HIV to her partner during unprotected sex.

CAUSES

Bacterial vaginosis is caused when the normal balance of bacteria in the vagina is disrupted. Normally, the vagina has helpful or commensal bacteria (lactobacilli) and harmful bacteria (anaerobes), bacteria that do not need oxygen to live. Sometimes the harmful bacteria overgrow, reducing the amount of helpful bacteria in the vagina. The cause of this overgrowth is not understood. In some cases, it may be related to sexual activity through transfer of harmful bacteria from a sexual partner.

RISK FACTORS

The factors that increase the chance of developing bacterial vaginosis include smoking, using douches or feminine sprays, having unprotected sex (sex without a condom), having a new sexual partner or multiple partners, and using an intrauterine device (IUD) for birth control.

SYMPTOMS

Some women with bacterial vaginosis do not have any symptoms. Others experience abnormal, white or gray vaginal discharge with a thin consistency and a fishy odor, especially after sex. Other symptoms include a burning feeling while urinating, itching around the vagina, vaginal irritation, and pain during sex.

If any of these symptoms appear, one should not assume they are caused by bacterial vaginosis. These symptoms may be caused by other conditions. However, one should contact a health care provider if these symptoms appear.

SCREENING AND DIAGNOSIS

A doctor will ask about symptoms and medical history and will perform a physical exam. Tests may include a pelvic exam to look for signs of bacterial vaginosis and obtaining a sample of fluid from the vagina to test for signs of infection.

TREATMENT AND THERAPY

Bacterial vaginosis should be treated as soon as the patient experiences symptoms, or, if the patient is pregnant, treatment should begin even without symptoms. Bacterial vaginosis is easily treated with antibiotics, in the form of pills or vaginal creams prescribed by a doctor.

PREVENTION AND OUTCOMES

To help reduce the chance of getting bacterial vaginosis, one should abstain from sex or remain monogamous, use condoms during sex, avoid using douches or feminine sprays, and visit a doctor for regular pelvic exams. To avoid a recurrence of bacterial vaginosis, patients should finish all prescribed medication, even if the symptoms go away. One should also wash diaphragms and other reusable birth control devices thoroughly after use, avoid wearing panty hose and clothing that traps moisture in the vagina, and, after bowel movements, wipe oneself from front to back (away from the vagina).

Nicky Lowney, M.A.;
reviewed by Adrienne Carmack, M.D.

FURTHER READING

Centers for Disease Control and Prevention. "Bacterial Vaginosis." Available at http://www.cdc.gov/std/bv/stdfact-bacterial-vaginosis.htm.
EBSCO Publishing. *DynaMed: Bacterial Vaginosis.*

Available through http://www.ebscohost.com/dynamed.

Martin, H. L., et al. "Hormonal Contraception, Sexually Transmitted Diseases, and Risk of Heterosexual Transmission of Human Immunodeficiency Virus Type 1." *Journal of Infectious Diseases* 178 (1998): 1053-1059.

_____. "Vaginal Lactobacilli, Microbial Flora, and Risk of Human Immunodeficiency Virus Type 1 and Sexually Transmitted Disease Acquisition." *Journal of Infectious Diseases* 180 (1999): 1863-1868.

Myer, L., et al. "Bacterial Vaginosis and Susceptibility to HIV Infection in South African Women: A Nested Case-Control Study." *Journal of Infectious Diseases* 192 (2005): 1372-1380.

_____. "Intravaginal Practices, Bacterial Vaginosis, and Women's Susceptibility to HIV Infection: Epidemiological Evidence and Biological Mechanisms." *Lancet Infectious Diseases* 5 (2005): 786-794.

Taha, T. E., et al. "Bacterial Vaginosis and Disturbances of Vaginal Flora: Association with Increased Acquisition of HIV." *AIDS* 12 (1998): 1699-1706.

Van de Wijgert, J. H., et al. "Bacterial Vaginosis and Vaginal Yeast, but Not Vaginal Cleansing, Increase HIV-1 Acquisition in African Women." *JAIDS: Journal of Acquired Immune Deficiency Syndromes* 48 (2008): 203-210.

WEB SITES OF INTEREST

Centers for Disease Control and Prevention
http://www.cdc.gov/std

EngenderHealth
http://www.engenderhealth.org

National Women's Health Information Center
http://www.womenshealth.gov

Women's Health Matters
http://www.womenshealthmatters.ca

See also: AIDS; Cervical cancer; Endometritis; HIV; Pelvic inflammatory disease; Pregnancy and infectious disease; Sexually transmitted diseases (STDs); Urinary tract infections; Vaginal yeast infection; Women and infectious disease.

Bacteriology

CATEGORY: Epidemiology

DEFINITION

Medical bacteriology is the study of the physiologic relationship of bacteria to human health and disease. Once focused solely on bacterial pathogenicity, the field of medical bacteriology has evolved to encompass the study of the broader roles of bacteria, including beneficial symbiosis and factors that contribute to opportunism.

HISTORY

The concept of passing disease from person to person through unseen entities had been postulated centuries before the development of the technological capacity to culture and visualize bacteria. In the seventeenth century, Antoni van Leeuwenhoek's and Robert Hooke's inventions of the single-lens and compound microscopes, respectively, ushered in the field of bacteriology. Through the work of Joseph Lister, Louis Pasteur, Robert Koch, and their contemporaries in the nineteenth century, the causative relationship of specific bacteria to known infectious diseases was established, opening the door to targeted prevention and control with antimicrobials.

CLINICAL SIGNIFICANCE

Bacterial diseases have been a significant cause of morbidity and mortality through human history. Despite marked successes, facilitated by advances in public hygiene, by mass immunization, and by antimicrobial therapy, bacterial infectious disease remains a serious threat. Bacterial pneumonia and sepsis remain among the leading causes of death in the United States.

Sexually transmitted bacterial diseases, including chlamydia, gonorrhea, and, to a lesser extent, syphilis, continue to circulate among populations globally, with a high incidence of annual new infections. Respiratory infections, including whooping cough (pertussis), pneumococcal pneumonia, and tuberculosis, remain as lethal infectious diseases. Outbreaks of food-borne and waterborne bacterial illnesses caused by *Salmonella*, Shiga toxin-producing *Escherichia coli*, *Campylobacter*, *Listeria*, *Shigella*, *Staphylococcus aureus*, and *Vibrio cholerae* occur in both impoverished and developed nations. Vector-borne bacterial infections,

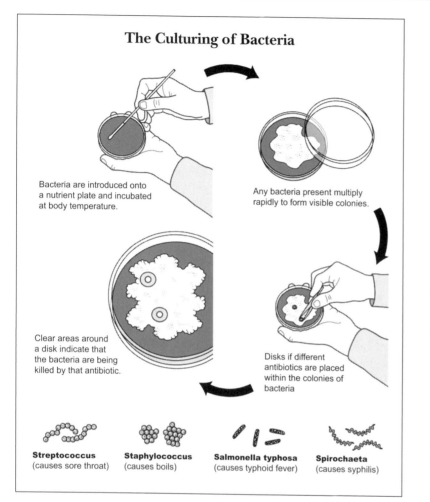

The Culturing of Bacteria

Bacteria are introduced onto a nutrient plate and incubated at body temperature.

Any bacteria present multiply rapidly to form visible colonies.

Clear areas around a disk indicate that the bacteria are being killed by that antibiotic.

Disks if different antibiotics are placed within the colonies of bacteria

Streptococcus
(causes sore throat)

Staphylococcus
(causes boils)

Salmonella typhosa
(causes typhoid fever)

Spirochaeta
(causes syphilis)

Bacteriology involves the use of cultures to identify types of bacteria and to develop and test antibiotics. Pathogenic bacteria include Streptococcus, Staphylococcus, Salmonella, *and the spirochetes.*

including Lyme disease and rickettsial fevers, persist despite vector-control efforts.

EMERGING RESISTANCE

The discovery of penicillin by Alexander Fleming in 1928 launched a new era in medical bacteriology, wherein previously untreatable infections could be cured with short-term antibiotic therapy. Beginning in the late 1940's, the mass production of antibiotics fueled the burgeoning use of these pharmaceuticals in medicine and agriculture. Predictably, a few years following the introduction of antibiotics into the human bacteriological milieu, acquired drug resistance emerged in several bacterial species.

Driven by natural selection in an environment rife with broad-spectrum antibiotics, antimicrobial resistance among many species of pathogenic bacteria has grown alarmingly prevalent, with many organisms exhibiting resistance to multiple antibiotics. Bacteria develop antimicrobial resistance through spontaneous mutation and natural selection (vertical evolution) or through acquisition of deoxyribonucleic acid (DNA) from other bacteria that encodes for specific resistance (horizontal evolution).

Many common bacterial pathogens exhibit significant levels of antibiotic resistance. These pathogens include *S. aureus* (methicillin-resistant and vancomycin-resistant), group B *Streptococcus, S. pneumoniae, Neisseria meningitidis, N. gonorrhea, Klebsiella pneumoniae, E. coli, Shigella, Acinetobacter, Enterococcus* (vancomycin-resistant), and *Mycobacterium tuberculosis.* Once found primarily in health care settings, antibiotic-resistant strains of common bacterial pathogens are increasingly common in community-acquired infections.

THERAPEUTIC BACTERIA

The normal bacterial flora of the human gastrointestinal tract perform beneficial functions, including breaking down plant-derived carbohydrates and synthesizing vitamin K and certain B-complex vitamins. Additionally, normal gut flora compete with potentially pathogenic bacteria, including *S. aureus* and *L. monocytogenes.* Building on observations of the beneficial functions of normal intestinal flora, bacteriologists and health care professionals are exploring the potential uses of probiotics for a variety of gastrointestinal and other medical disorders. Probiotics, according to the Food and Agriculture Organization of the United Nations and the World Health Organization, are live microorganisms that, when administrated in adequate amounts, confer a health benefit on the host.

The National Center for Complementary and Alternative Medicine of the National Institutes of Health reports that bacterial probiotics may prove useful for treating rotavirus-induced diarrhea, irritable bowel syndrome, female genitourinary tract infections, *Clostridium difficile* enterocolitis, and atopic dermatitis. Large-scale, controlled clinical trials of various probiotic formulations for specific indications and ongoing bacteriologic research help clarify the potential role of bacteria as therapeutic agents.

IMPACT

The relationship between bacteria and human health remains dynamic, as bacterial species evolve and biomedical discoveries open new possibilities for interrupting pathogenicity and utilizing these ubiquitous organisms to promote health. Bacteriology is the interface between these opposing aspects of humanity's relationship with the ever-changing bacterial world.

Tina M. St. John, M.D.

FURTHER READING

Beekman, Susan E., and David K. Henderson. "Infections Caused by Percutaneous Intravascular Devices." In *Mandell, Douglas, and Bennett's Principles and Practice of Infectious Diseases*, edited by Gerald L. Mandell, John F. Bennett, and Raphael Dolin. 7th ed. New York: Churchill Livingstone/Elsevier, 2010. Infectious disease text with referenced discussion of the epidemiology, pathogenesis, microbiology, and antimicrobial resistance of nosocomial (hospital acquired) infections associated with intravascular devices.

Blaser, Martin J. "Introduction to Bacteria and Bacterial Diseases." In *Mandell, Douglas, and Bennett's Principles and Practice of Infectious Diseases*, edited by Gerald L. Mandell, John F. Bennett, and Raphael Dolin. 7th ed. New York: Churchill Livingstone/ Elsevier, 2010. Infectious disease text with referenced information on bacterial classification, virulence factors, pathogenicity, and evolution.

Craven, Donald E., and Alexandra Chroneou. "Nosocomial Pneumonia." In *Mandell, Douglas, and Bennett's Principles and Practice of Infectious Diseases*, edited by Gerald L. Mandell, John F. Bennett, and Raphael Dolin. 7th ed. New York: Churchill Livingstone/Elsevier, 2010. Infectious disease text with referenced discussion of the epidemiology, patho-genesis, microbiology, and antimicrobial resistance of health-care-acquired pneumonia.

Klevens, R. Monina, et al. "Invasive Methicillin-Resistant *Staphylococcus aureus* Infections in the United States." *Journal of the American Medical Association* 298 (2007): 1763-1771. Epidemiology of invasive MRSA infections in the United States from July, 2004, through December, 2005, based on data from the Active Bacterial Core Surveillance/ Emerging Infections Program network.

Petrof, Elaine O. "Probiotics and Gastrointestinal Disease: Clinical Evidence and Basic Science." *Anti-inflammatory and Anti-allergy Agents in Medicinal Chemistry* 8 (2009): 260-269. Review of the uses, mechanisms of action, and clinical evidence of three therapeutic, probiotic formulations.

Sleator, Roy D. "Probiotics: A Viable Therapeutic Alternative for Enteric Infections Especially in the Developing World." *Discovery Medicine* 10 (2010): 119-124. Review of clinical research data supporting the use of probiotics for the prevention and management of infectious diarrhea and possible applications of genetically engineered probiotics.

Tenover, Fred C. "Mechanisms of Antimicrobial Resistance in Bacteria." *American Journal of Medicine* 119 (2006): S3-S10. Case-history-based essay on the selective pressures and emergence of antimicrobial resistance among three common bacterial pathogens.

WEB SITES OF INTEREST

Centers for Disease Control and Prevention, Emerging Infections Program
http://www.cdc.gov/ncpdcid/deiss/eip

National Institute of Allergy and Infectious Diseases, Emerging and Reemerging Infectious Diseases
http://www.niaid.nih.gov/topics/emerging

Todar's Online Textbook of Bacteriology
http://www.textbookofbacteriology.net

See also: Antibiotic resistance; Antibiotics: Experimental; Antibiotics: Types; Bacteria: Classification and types; Bacteria: Structure and growth; Bacterial infections; Biosurveillance; Centers for Disease Control and Prevention (CDC); Contagious diseases;

Emerging and reemerging infectious diseases; Epidemiology; Infectious disease specialists; Microbiology; National Institute of Allergy and Infectious Diseases; National Institutes of Health; Opportunistic infections; Outbreaks; Pathogens; Primary infection; Public health; Secondary infection.

Balantidiasis

CATEGORY: Diseases and conditions
ANATOMY OR SYSTEM AFFECTED: Gastrointestinal system, intestines, stomach
ALSO KNOWN AS: Balantidiosis

DEFINITION

Balantidiasis is an infectious gastrointestinal illness caused by the protozoan parasite *Balantidium coli*, a single-celled microbial organism that also infects pigs, rodents, horses, sheep, and goats.

CAUSES

Balantidiasis is caused by ingestion of *B. coli*, which reside in animal and human intestines and are excreted in feces in cyst (dormant) form. Humans ingest the cysts by eating contaminated food or water. Inside the colon, intestinal enzymes dissolve the cysts' protective covering, releasing the active (trophozoite) form of the organism. The organism secretes a substance that breaks down the intestinal mucosa, causing ulceration and various other gastrointestinal symptoms.

RISK FACTORS

Balantidiasis occurs throughout the world but is most prevalent in locations where exposure to animal excrement is common, such as facilities where pigs or other infected animals are raised, slaughtered, or prepared as food. Living or working in such environments and poor sanitary conditions increase the risk of infection.

SYMPTOMS

Not everyone infected with *B. coli* develops balantidiasis. Persons with impaired immunity or who are generally unwell because of malnutrition, cancer, or alcoholism are more likely than healthy persons to manifest symptoms. Balantidiasis can cause gastrointestinal disease ranging from mild fever and stomach pain to severe diarrhea, vomiting, weight loss, and dehydration. Rarely, patients with balantidiasis develop a tear (perforation) in the lining of the intestines or develop pneumonia or inflammation of the lymph nodes.

SCREENING AND DIAGNOSIS

The patient's recent history will typically reveal exposure to infected animals or contact with someone who has had gastrointestinal symptoms. *B. coli* cysts and trophozoites can be identified by stool culture or by colonoscopy, a procedure during which a flexible scope is used to examine and biopsy the intestines. If the patient's symptoms indicate a need, an X ray or a computed tomography (CT) scan may be ordered to examine the lungs or lymph nodes.

TREATMENT AND THERAPY

Balantidiasis is treated with the antibiotic medications tetracycline and metronidazole, together with intravenous fluids for patients who are dehydrated. Most patients experience a complete recovery with antibiotic therapy.

PREVENTION AND OUTCOMES

Balantidiasis can be prevented by practicing good hygiene, especially when preparing food, and by avoiding environments where potentially infectious animals are handled.

Carita Caple, M.S.H.S., R.N.

FURTHER READING

Escobedo, Angel A., et al. "Treatment of Intestinal Protozoan Infections in Children." *Archives of Disease in Childhood* 94 (2009): 478-482.

Feldman, Mark, Lawrence S. Friedman, and Lawrence J. Brandt, eds. *Sleisenger and Fordtran's Gastrointestinal and Liver Disease: Pathophysiology, Diagnosis, Management*. New ed. 2 vols. Philadelphia: Saunders/Elsevier, 2010.

Kapadia, Cyrus R., James M. Crawford, and Caroline Taylor. *An Atlas of Gastroenterology: A Guide to Diagnosis and Differential Diagnosis*. Boca Raton, Fla.: Pantheon, 2003.

Nilles-Bije, Lourdes, and Windell L. Rivera. "Ultrastructural and Molecular Characterization of *Balantidium coli* Isolated in the Philippines." *Parasitology Research* 2 (2010): 932-113.

Schuster, Frederick, L., and Lynn Ramirez-Avila. "Current World Status of *Balantidium coli.*" *Clinical Microbiology Reviews* 12 (2008): 626-638.

Weller, Peter F. "Protozoal Intestinal Infections and Trichomoniasis." In *Harrison's Principles of Internal Medicine*, edited by Joan Butterton. 17th ed. New York: McGraw-Hill, 2008.

WEB SITES OF INTEREST

American College of Gastroenterology
http://www.acg.gi.org

Centers for Disease Control and Prevention
http://www.cdc.gov

National Center for Emerging and Zoonotic Infectious Diseases
http://www.cdc.gov/ncezid

See also: Amebic dysentery; Antibiotic-associated colitis; Ascariasis; Bacterial infections; *Campylobacter*; Campylobacteriosis; Cholera; Cryptosporidiosis; Fecal-oral route of transmission; Food-borne illness and disease; Giardiasis; Intestinal and stomach infections; Protozoan diseases; *Salmonella*; *Shigella*; Travelers' diarrhea; Trichinosis; Waterborne illness and disease; Worm infections; Zoonotic diseases.

Bartonella infections

CATEGORY: Diseases and conditions
ANATOMY OR SYSTEM AFFECTED: All
ALSO KNOWN AS: Bacillary angiomatosis, bacteremia, bartonellosis, cat scratch fever, endocarditis, Oroya fever, trench fever, urban trench fever

DEFINITION

The bacterium *Bartonella* is a member of the family Bartonellaceae. An infection by these bacteria is called bartonellosis. *Bartonella* is named for Alberto Leonardo Barton Thompson, who discovered *B. bacilliformis* in 1905 as the cause of Oroya fever, also known as Carrion's disease.

Twenty-four species of *Bartonella* have been identified, ten of which cause infectious diseases in humans. *Bartonella* infections include Oroya fever, cat scratch fever, trench fever, endocarditis, bacteremia, and bacillary angiomatosis.

CAUSES

Bartonella infection is caused by *Bartonella* bacteria entering the body of humans and other mammals by the bites of fleas, sandflies, and ticks or by animal bites or scratches. The bacteria travel through the bloodstream and cause infections that can be mild or life-threatening, involve different body systems and organs, and present in different ways.

RISK FACTORS

During World War I, factors such as malnutrition, poor hygiene, alcohol abuse, compromised immunity, and flea, fly, and tick infestations led to an infection from *B. quintana* that came to be called trench fever. Epidemic fever led to widespread morbidity of troops and prisoners. Today, some of these same factors occur in homeless populations, leading to the reemergence of infection. This "new" infection is referred to as urban trench fever. Also, researchers have determined that veterinary and animal shelter staff and animal groomers and trainers are at an increased risk for *Bartonella* infection because of daily exposure to animals, animal feces, and parasites.

SYMPTOMS

Symptoms of *Bartonella* infection depend on the bacteria involved and on the degree of infection. One of the most common infections, Oroya fever, has initial symptoms of fever, jaundice, and anemia. Once Oroya fever has progressed from the acute to chronic phase, infected persons develop verruga peruana (Peruvian warts), which are blood-filled warts. Trench fever may present with symptoms of high fever, severe headache, eye pain, and muscle pain in the back and shins. Cat scratch fever, caused by *B. henselae*, may present as swollen lymph nodes but then progresses to much more severe symptoms and conditions, such as encephalopathy, convulsions, and hepatitis.

SCREENING AND DIAGNOSIS

Screening and diagnosis of *Bartonella* infection relies on epidemiologic data for an affected population and confirmation by laboratory evaluation. Because of the wide range of presenting symptoms and organ involvement, diagnosis is most commonly made using polymerase chain reaction testing and serology to detect antibodies. The Centers for Disease Control and Prevention recommends an immunofluorescent antibody assay.

TREATMENT AND THERAPY

Persons with otherwise healthy immune systems often do not receive treatment for mild or moderate *Bartonella* infection, but severely infected persons or those with compromised immune systems may be treated with a course of oral or intravenous antibiotic drugs such as erythromycin, doxycycline, and azithromycin.

PREVENTION AND OUTCOMES

Animals and household pets represent a large reservoir for many types of *Bartonella* bacteria that may infect humans. Immunocompromised persons should limit animal or pet exposure.

April Ingram, B.S.

FURTHER READING

Lamps, L. W., and M. A. Scott. "Cat-Scratch Disease: Historic, Clinical, and Pathologic Perspectives." *American Journal of Clinical Pathology* 121, suppl. (2004): S71-80.

Maguiña, Ciro, Guerra, Humberto, and Palmira Ventosilla. "Bartonellosis." *Clinics in Dermatology* 27 (2009): 271-280.

Marquardt, William C., ed. *Biology of Disease Vectors.* 2d ed. New York: Academic Press/Elsevier, 2005.

Minnick, Michael F., and James M. Battisti. "Pestilence, Persistence, and Pathogenicity: Infection Strategies of *Bartonella*." *Future Microbiology* 4 (2009): 743-758.

Schaller, James L. *The Diagnosis, Treatment, and Prevention of "Bartonella": Atypical "Bartonella" Treatment Failures and Forty Hypothetical Physical Exam Findings.* Tampa, Fla.: Hope Academic Press, 2008.

WEB SITES OF INTEREST

Centers for Disease Control and Prevention: Healthy Pets Healthy People
http://www.cdc.gov/healthypets/diseases/catscratch.htm

National Center for Emerging and Zoonotic Infectious Diseases
http://www.cdc.gov/ncezid

See also: Bacterial infections; Brucellosis; Bubonic plague; Cat scratch fever; Cats and infectious disease; Colorado tick fever; Dogs and infectious disease; Fleas and infectious disease; Lyme disease; Lymphadenitis; Mosquitoes and infectious disease; Pasteurellosis; Plague; Rocky Mountain spotted fever; Tularemia; Vectors and vector control; Wound infections; Zoonotic diseases.

Bats and infectious disease

CATEGORY: Transmission

DEFINITION

Bats are flying mammals belonging to the order Chiroptera (meaning "hand-wing"). With 925 described species, bats make up one-fifth of all mammals. The order is one of the most widespread on Earth, inhabiting all continents except Antarctica. Bat wingspans range in size from 150 millimeters to 2 meters. The first bats evolved about 52 million years ago, making the order ancient. The genome of many species is highly conserved, meaning the species has not changed significantly over time.

In addition to being the only mammal that flies, bats also have a highly specialized sensory specialization of echolocation. Echolocation requires considerable energy and neuronal capacity. Bats are relatively small, but because they fly, they can inhabit large ranges; some migrate hundreds of miles. They also tend to spend a great deal of time living in large, multispecies colonies at densities as high as three hundred bats per square foot.

ZOONOTIC DISEASE

Historically, bats have been associated with disease and danger to humans, perhaps in part because some bats are hematophagous (blood-eating). Bats do transmit rabies to both humans and domestic animals (even more so if they are hematophagous), but their contribution to the transmission of rabies is relatively small worldwide.

Bats have become a concern because they are increasingly associated with the emergence of previously unknown viruses. The severe acute respiratory syndrome (SARS) epidemic, caused by a newly recognized coronavirus, was traced to bats. Also, newly rec-

Bat Facts

TAXONOMIC CLASSIFICATION

Kingdom: Animalia
Subkingdom: Metazoa
Phylum: Chordata
Subphylum: Verbetrata
Class: Mammalia
Subclass: Theria
Order: Chiroptera (bats)
Suborders: Megachiroptera (flying foxes),
   Microchiroptera (bats)
Families:
Pteropopidae (flying foxes)
Rhinopomatidae (mouse-tailed bats)
Emballonuridae (sheath-tailed bats)
Craseonycteridae (hog-nosed bats)
Nycteridae (slit-faced bats)
Megadermatidae (false vampire bats)
Rhinolophidae (horseshoe bats)
Hipposideridae (leaf-nosed bats)
Mormoopidae (leaf-chinned bats)
Noctilionidae (bulldog bats)
Mystacinidae (short-tailed bats)
Phyllostomidae (spear-nosed bats)
Desmodontinae (vampire bats)
Natalidae (funnel-eared bats)
Furipteridae (thumbless bats)
Thyropteridae (disk-winged bats)
Myzopodidae (sucker-footed bats)
Vespertilonidae (common or vesper bats)
Molossidae (free-tailed bats)

Geographical location: Every continent except
   Antarctica
Habitat: Mostly forests and deserts; some grasslands
Gestational period: Three to ten months, with
   delayed implantation
Life span: Generally three to five years; up to thirty
   years in captivity
Special anatomy: Head, body, tail, two wings, each
   supported by upper arm, forearm, hand; knee
   joints bend backward, enabling the bat to hang
   upside down and remain ready to take flight easily

ognized strains of lyssavirus and new paramyxoviruses arose from virus reservoirs in bats. In addition, bats are potential sources of bacterial and fungal pathogens such as histoplasmosis. Research continues to isolate previously unknown viruses from bats, although most are not dangerous to humans.

NATURAL HISTORY AND RISK FACTORS

Knowledge of the natural history of bats helps explain their fitness as reservoirs for potential pathogens for other species. Bat species are ancient; their genome contains conserved information likely to be shared by many mammalian species. Thus, cellular receptors recognized by bat viruses may be homologous and identical to receptors conserved in many other mammalian species.

Bat behavior promotes the long-term harboring of pathogens. Bats often spend much of their lives in a state of torpor or hibernation. In this state of lowered metabolism, pathogens may remain latent and depressed immune systems may fail to clear them from their systems. As bats are flying mammals, their range is large, increasing the probability of transmission of pathogens over a large area. Some bats migrate, some as far as eight hundred miles, increasing the range for dispersal of pathogens significantly.

Bats often rest en masse in caves, in colonies that often run in the millions, often including more than one species. Direct contact can increase transmission rates for pathogens. In addition, bats use echolocation and make high-pitched sounds that are emitted with great pressure, resulting in aerosolization of droplets from their respiratory tracts. The droplets could carry pathogens and be easily passed among bats.

Bats have remarkably long lives for such small mammals. Life expectancy for some species is commonly twenty-five years. A bat with a latent infection could continue in a carrier state and transmit pathogens for decades. This may contribute to the apparent capability of bats to carry pathogens in a subclinical state for long periods.

BAT-ASSOCIATED DISEASES

Rabies. Bats transmit rabies, a type of viral encephalitis that is nearly 100 percent fatal once signs have set in. A number of different bat species propagate their own rabies variant, and genetic sequencing identifies specific strains. Globally, the number of rabies cases caused by exposure to bats is negligible in comparison with those transmitted by dogs and terrestrial wildlife. Nonetheless, in developed nations where dog rabies has been eradicated, bat rabies make up an

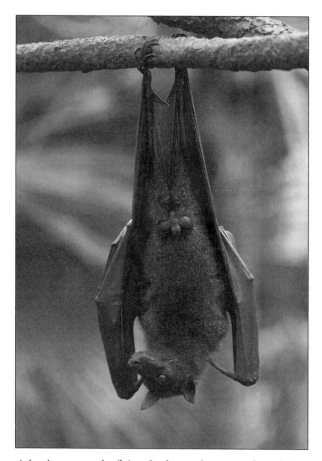

A bat known as the flying fox hangs from a tree branch in a rainforest. (©Dreamstime.com)

increasing proportion of cases. In addition, many rabies infections occur in persons who have no known history of exposure. In South America, vampire bats transmit rabies to humans and domestic animals during their normal feeding behavior.

Lyssavirus. A genus of the family Rhadoviridae, which includes rabies, lyssavirus also causes severe forms of encephalitis that are indistinguishable from rabies. Between 1996 and 1998, a novel lyssavirus was isolated from a flying fox in New South Wales, Australia; two women died of the virus after exposure to sick bats.

SARS and coronavirus. In late 2002, a new disease emerged from the wildlife meat markets of China. In nine months, SARS had spread from southern China to cause a near pandemic around the world, infecting eight thousand people in thirty-seven countries and killing nearly eight hundred persons. The disease was caused by a coronavirus that was isolated from masked palm civets and raccoon dogs, but, ultimately, the origin of the virus was believed to be in Chinese horseshoe bats.

Henipavirus. Flying foxes were implicated as sources for another novel pathogen, the paramyxoviruses known as hendra virus and nipah virus (a family of viruses that includes measles, rinderpest, and canine distemper viruses), which emerged to cause outbreaks of acute respiratory syndromes respectively in horses and humans in Hendra, Australia, and in pigs and humans in Malaysia from 1994 to 2004. The diseases were often fatal, killing 105 of 265 people in Malaysia and resulting in the culling (slaughter) of more than one million pigs. Nipah virus also has been found in flying foxes in Bangladesh, India, and Cambodia. It is unlikely that people can contract these viruses from bats directly.

Ebola virus. The Ebola virus causes hemorrhagic disease that is fatal in 80 percent of cases. The disease has occurred as localized outbreaks in Africa and has been exported to Europe and North America with nonhuman primates. The natural reservoir has not yet been discovered, but Ebola virus RNA has been detected in bat tissues.

Histoplasmosis. Humans exposed to dust from large bat colonies may contract the pulmonary infection known as fungal histoplasmosis. The disease is generally mild, flulike, and self-limiting, but it can be severe if exposure is significant or is suffered by immunocompromised persons.

IMPACT

While bats constitute a unique threat as reservoirs for emerging viruses, the magnitude of the threat may be exaggerated, particularly if weighed against the positive contributions of bats to the world's ecosystems. As effective insectivores, bats save millions of dollars in damage to crops and probably prevent more vector-borne diseases in humans than they cause.

Cynthia L. Mills, D.V.M.

FURTHER READING

Calisher, Charles H., et al. "Bats: Important Reservoir Hosts of Emerging Viruses." *Clinical Microbiology Reviews* 39 (2006): 531-545. A comprehensive review of bat natural history and a survey of emerging viral pathogens associated with bats.

Brown, Corrie. "Emerging Zoonoses and Pathogens of Public Health Significance: An Overview." *World Organization for Animal Health: Scientific and Technical Review* 23 (2004): 435-442. An introduction and general look at emerging diseases and human factors increasing exposures to potential pathogens.

McCall, Bradley J., et al. "Potential Exposure to Australian Bat Lyssavirus, Queensland, 1996-1999." *Emerging Infectious Disease* 6 (2000): 259-264. A report of the emergence of a novel lyssavirus and related outbreaks from 1996 through 1999.

Philbey, Adrian W., et al. "An Apparently New Virus (Family Paramyxoviridae) Infectious for Pigs, Humans, and Fruit Bats." *Emerging Infectious Disease* 4 (1998): 268-271. A report of the emergence of Nipah virus.

Poon, L. L. M., et al. "Identification of a Novel Coronavirus in Bats." *Journal of Virology* 79 (2005): 2001-2009. A report of the identification of the virus that causes SARS.

WEB SITE OF INTEREST

National Center for Emerging and Zoonotic Infectious Diseases
http://www.cdc.gov/ncezid

See also: Birds and infectious disease; Ebola hemorrhagic fever; Histoplasmosis; Rabies; SARS; Transmission routes; Zoonotic diseases.

BCG vaccine. *See* Bacillus Calmette-Guérin vaccine.

Behçet's syndrome

CATEGORY: Diseases and conditions
ANATOMY OR SYSTEM AFFECTED: Blood vessels, circulatory system
ALSO KNOWN AS: Adamantiades-Behçet's disease, Behçet's disease

DEFINITION

Behçet's syndrome is an uncommon form of vasculitis, or inflammation of the blood vessels, that can affect multiple body systems. The syndrome is more prevalent in nations of the Mediterranean and the East, and it first appears in persons who are between twenty and forty years of age.

CAUSES

The exact cause of Behçet's syndrome has not been determined. Multiple causes have been proposed, however, including viral and bacterial infection, autoimmune response, and genetic predisposition. Behçet's appears to be more common among people with a certain variation of the HLA-B5 gene. Some experts believe that genetic susceptibility in combination with an environmental trigger is necessary for Behçet's to develop.

RISK FACTORS

Risk is difficult to determine because the cause of Behçet's is unknown. People in countries of the Mediterranean and the East are affected at higher rates; Turkey reports most cases of Behçet's syndrome, followed by Japan. Men are affected twice as frequently as women and often have more severe symptoms. Behçet's is rare in the United States.

SYMPTOMS

Behçet's is a chronic syndrome with symptoms that wax and wane. Primary symptoms include recurrent ulcers on the skin, genitals, and in the mouth. Other manifestations include inflammation of the tissues of the eye (uveitis, glaucoma), hearing loss, arthritis, neurological impairment, increased allergic response (pathergy), and the formation of blood clots (thrombosis). Serious complications such as total vision loss, aneurysm, and stroke may occur. Younger age at onset of Behçet's is associated with a more serious course of illness.

SCREENING AND DIAGNOSIS

Behçet's syndrome is diagnosed by the appearance of symptoms and by laboratory and diagnostic tests that reveal widespread inflammation. A pathergy test may be conducted, which involves pricking the skin with a sterile needle; patients with Behçet's will experience an exaggerated inflammatory response (swelling) at the site. Imaging tests may be conducted on patients with Behçet's to identify areas of vascular inflammation and neurological injury; these tests include magnetic resonance imaging and a computed tomography scan.

TREATMENT AND THERAPY

Behçet's is treated with immunosuppressive and anti-inflammatory drugs. Corticosteroids, which are used to treat many symptoms, may be applied topically to areas of skin and mouth ulceration, administered as eye drops, injected into the joints for arthritis symptoms, and administered intravenously or in pill form for the treatment of systemic (widespread) inflammation.

PREVENTION AND OUTCOMES

There is no known method of prevention for Behçet's syndrome.

Carita Caple, M.S.H.S., R.N.

FURTHER READING

Davatchi, F., et al. "HLA-B51 in Behçet's Disease." *Acta Medica Iranica* 46 (2008): 507-510.

Hirohata, Shunsei, and Hirotoshi Kikuchi. "Behçet's Disease." *Arthritis Research and Therapy* 5 (2003): 181-184.

Lee, Sungnack, et al., eds. *Behçet's Disease: A Guide to Its Clinical Understanding.* New York: Springer, 2001.

Moutsopoulous, Haralampos M. "Behçet's Syndrome." In *Harrison's Principles of Internal Medicine*, edited by Joan Butterton. 17th ed. New York: McGraw-Hill, 2008.

Parker, James N., and Philip M. Parker, eds. *The Official Patient's Sourcebook on Behçet's Disease.* San Diego, Calif.: Icon Health, 2002.

Zeis, Joanne. *Essential Guide to Behçet's Disease.* Uxbridge, Mass.: Central Vision Press, 2002.

WEB SITES OF INTEREST

Genetic and Rare Diseases Information Center
http://rarediseases.info.nih.gov/gard

National Heart, Lung, and Blood Institute
http://www.nhlbi.nih.gov

See also: Bacterial endocarditis; Bloodstream infections; Disseminated intravascular coagulation; Endocarditis; Myocarditis; Pericarditis; Rheumatic fever; Rocky Mountain spotted fever.

Bell's palsy

CATEGORY: Diseases and conditions
ANATOMY OR SYSTEM AFFECTED: Central nervous system, head, mouth, muscles
ALSO KNOWN AS: Facial palsy, idiopathic peripheral facial palsy

DEFINITION

Bell's palsy occurs when the seventh cranial nerve that controls muscles in the face swells or becomes inflamed. One side of the face may droop, causing a crooked smile. The eye on the affected side may not close, and normal facial movements are difficult. Tears, taste, and saliva may also be affected, as may a bone in the middle ear. Bell's palsy is temporary and usually goes away in three to six months. In some people, prolonged facial drooping may occur or a second episode may develop.

CAUSES

Viral infections are the primary cause of Bell's palsy. The herpes simplex virus associated with genital herpes and cold sores is the primary cause, but other viruses can also lead to problems. These viruses include herpes zoster, which causes chickenpox and shingles; Epstein-Barr virus, which causes mononucleosis; and cytomegalovirus.

RISK FACTORS

Bell's palsy is seen in the latter stages of pregnancy or soon after birth in women, in people with respiratory infections or influenza, and in people with diabetes. There may be a genetic tendency for Bell's palsy, and episodes may be seen among family members.

SYMPTOMS

A sudden onset of drooping on one side of the face is the most common symptom of Bell's palsy, but in rare cases drooping may occur on both sides of the face. Jaw pain and ear pain on the affected side often occurs. Headache and sensitivity to noise, changes in the taste of food or drink, and noticeable changes in saliva and tears may also be seen.

SCREENING AND DIAGNOSIS

There is no screening test for Bell's palsy. Diagnosis is made by evaluating symptoms and taking a careful history to determine if there has been a recent viral infection. Because the symptoms of Bell's palsy may resemble stroke, tumors, Lyme disease, and other infections, a doctor may order a computed tomography scan, magnetic resonance imaging, or electromyography, which measures nerve impulses to the muscle.

TREATMENT AND THERAPY

There are some treatments for Bell's palsy that may cause symptoms to subside more rapidly, but recovery usually occurs with or without treatment. Antiviral medicines such as acyclovir or valcyclovir may be used if the cause is linked to a viral infection. Steroids may be used alone, or in combination with an antiviral drug, to decrease inflammation of the nerve. In rare cases, surgery may be used to widen the bony corridor where the nerve passes through to the face. Physical therapy may be ordered by the doctor to keep the facial muscles in shape during the disease. The patient is taught how to exercise and massage the facial area.

Because the affected eye may not close completely, lubricating drops or ointments and eye protection may be used. Moist wet heat applied to the face may ease discomfort. Medications for pain may be prescribed.

PREVENTION AND OUTCOMES

There is no single known cause for Bell's palsy, so the best prevention is to avoid infection. Helpful preventive measures are careful handwashing, avoiding contact with sick people, and practicing safer sex.

Patricia Stanfill Edens, R.N., Ph.D., FACHE

FURTHER READING

Bradley, Walter G., et al., eds. *Neurology in Clinical Practice.* 5th ed. Philadelphia: Butterworth Heinemann/Elsevier, 2007.

Hazin, R., B. Azizzadeh, and M. T. Bhatti. "Medical and Surgical Management of Facial Nerve Palsy." *Current Opinion in Ophthalmology* 20, no. 6 (November, 2009): 440-450.

Parker, James N., and Philip M. Parker, eds. *The Official Patient's Sourcebook on Bell's Palsy.* San Diego, Calif.: Icon Health, 2002.

Woodson, Gayle E. *Ear, Nose, and Throat Disorders in Primary Care.* Philadelphia: W. B. Saunders, 2001.

WEB SITES OF INTEREST

All Bell's Palsy
http://allbellspalsy.info

National Institute of Neurological Disorders and Stroke
http://www.ninds.nih.gov

See also: Acute cerebellar ataxia; Autoimmune disorders; Bacterial endocarditis; Creutzfeldt-Jakob disease; Endocarditis; Gerstmann-Sträussler-Scheinker syndrome; Guillain-Barré syndrome; Herpes simplex infection; Inflammation; Meningococcal meningitis; Myocarditis; Pericarditis; Pregnancy and infectious disease; Rheumatic fever; Tetanus; Viral infections.

Biochemical tests

CATEGORY: Diagnosis

DEFINITION

Biochemical tests play an essential role in infectious disease diagnosis, screening, prognosis, and treatment. Screening may be advisable for at-risk groups and for checking disease prevalence in a given population.

A physician begins a diagnosis by examining a person's symptoms. Samples of blood, urine, feces, and tissues may be collected. The samples are sent to various departments in a medical laboratory for examination. These lab departments include bacteriology (culturing), immunology, and pathology.

Biochemistry departments aid in identifying pathogenic species or in distinguishing organisms from other species. Biochemical tests detect distinctive differences in metabolism of a species. These metabolic differences result in the formation of acid, gas, or other chemical products that can be detected by color changes or other means.

Many tests are named according to the enzyme active in the test; the enzyme names end with the letters *ase*. An evaluation of test results, together with a person's clinical history, can lead to a prognosis, or a prediction of the course or outcome of the disease. Biochemical tests can also be important during the treatment phase to monitor changes in body metabolism or function.

Bacteria can be divided into two physiological groups depending on whether they retain a Gram's stain or not. These bacteria are either gram-positive or gram-negative. Bacteria can assume various shapes, such as spherical (cocci) or rodlike (bacilli). Biochemical tests can be classified into three categories

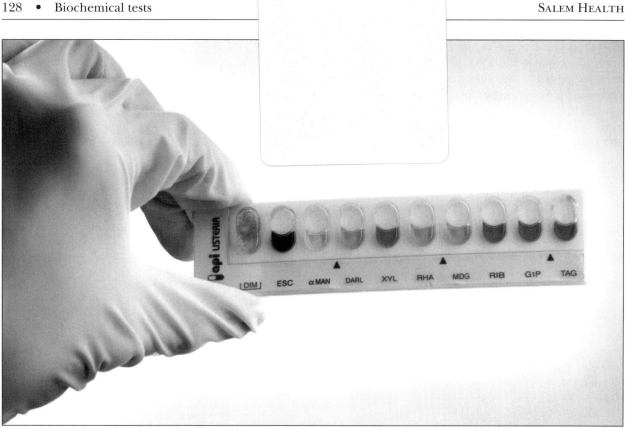

A microbiologist holds a test panel containing chemicals and bacteria.

according to the characteristics of the bacteria being tested: gram-negative bacilli, gram-positive cocci, and gram-negative cocci.

ENTEROBACTERIACEAE

The Enterobacteriaceae is a large family of gram-negative rods that inhabits the intestinal tract. Most Enterobacteriaceae are harmless normal flora of the intestines, but some can become pathogenic. Important genera in this family include *Escherichia, Salmonella, Shigella, Klebsiella, Citrobacter,* and *Proteus.* Many biochemical tests are involved in the identification and differentiation of members of this family.

A series of four tests known collectively by the acronym IMViC is used to differentiate between *Escherichia, Enterobacter,* and other genera. The indole test is positive for organisms that have tryptophanase. The methyl red and Voges-Proskauer tests examine differences in glucose fermentation among species. The citrate test is positive for species that are able to use citrate as a sole source of carbon.

Other tests are available to differentiate Enterobacteriaceae. The urease, phenylalanine deaminase, and decarboxylase tests detect differences in enzyme activities among species. The Kliger's iron agar test differentiates Enterobacteriaceae based on how the species ferment lactose and glucose. Hippurate hydrolysis is a positive test for *Campylobacter.*

Haemophilus influenzae is another gram-negative rod. The X and V factors test can differentiate this species (which requires the factors) from other *Haemophilus* species.

STAPHYLOCOCCI AND STREPTOCOCCI

Staphylococci and streptococci are gram-positive cocci usually grouped in clusters and chains. The catalase test is valuable for distinguishing between the genera; *Staphylococcus* is positive and *Streptococcus* is negative. The coagulase test is positive for *Staphylococcus aureus.* Lysostaphin is an enzyme that specifically breaks down *Staphylococcus* strains. The bile solubility and optochin disk tests are positive for *Streptococcus pneumonia* but negative for other beta hemolytic streptococci. The litmus milk test differentiates among streptococci based on lactose fermentation. Finally, the CAMP factor test is positive for group B *Streptococcus*.

NEISSERIA SPECIES

The *Neisseria* genus is a gram-negative diplococci with a characteristic doughnut shape. *Neisseria* can cause gonorrhea and meningitis, so several tests have been developed to differentiate the species. The nitrate reduction test is negative for *N. gonorrhea* but positive for closely related species. The DNase test is also negative for *N. gonorrhea*. The acid detection test detects *Neisseria* species that metabolize carbohydrates by oxidative pathway rather than by the more common fermentative pathway. The oxidase test is positive for *Neisseria* and *Moraxella* and can also help to differentiate among many related species in conjunction with other tests. The carbohydrate utilization test distinguishes between *N. gonorrhea* that ferments glucose only and *N. meningitis* that ferments both glucose and maltose.

IMPACT

Clinical biochemistry laboratories are responsible for most of the tests performed on samples sent to diagnostic laboratories by clinicians. The results of biochemical tests are used by medical staff for diagnosis in approximately 70 percent of all cases. Compared with other medical tests, biochemical tests are generally easier to perform but are relatively expensive. They can help prevent misdiagnosis by distinguishing between closely related species.

David A. Olle, M.S.

FURTHER READING

Forbes, Betty A., Daniel F. Sahm, and Alice S. Weissfeld. *Bailey and Scott's Diagnostic Microbiology.* 12th ed. St. Louis, Mo.: Mosby/Elsevier, 2007.

MacFadden, Jean F. *Biochemical Tests for Identification of Medical Bacteria.* 3d ed. Philadelphia: Lippincott Williams & Wilkins, 2000.

Mandell, Gerald L., John E. Bennett, and Raphael Dolin, eds. *Mandell, Douglas, and Bennett's Principles and Practice of Infectious Diseases.* 7th ed. New York: Churchill Livingstone/Elsevier, 2010.

Murray, Patrick R., Ken S. Rosenthal, and Michael A. Pfaller. *Medical Microbiology.* 6th ed. Philadelphia: Mosby/Elsevier, 2009.

Murray, Robert K., et al. *Harper's Illustrated Biochemistry.* 27th ed. Stamford, Conn.: Appleton & Lange, 2006.

Pagana, Kathleen Deska, and Timothy J. Pagana. *Mosby's Diagnostic and Laboratory Test Reference.* 9th ed. St. Louis, Mo.: Mosby/Elsevier, 2009.

Truant, Allan L. *Manual of Commercial Methods in Clinical Microbiology.* Washington, D.C.: ASM Press, 2002.

Volk, Wesley A., et al. *Essentials of Medical Microbiology.* Philadelphia: Lippincott Williams & Wilkins, 1995.

Winn, Washington C., Jr., et al. *Koneman's Color Atlas and Textbook of Diagnostic Microbiology.* 6th ed. Philadelphia: Lippincott Williams & Wilkins, 2006.

WEB SITES OF INTEREST

Biochemical Society
http://www.biochemistry.org

Protocolpedia
http://www.protocolpedia.com

Virtual Library of Biochemistry, Molecular Biology, and Cell Biology
http://www.biochemweb.org

See also: Acid-fastness; Bacterial infections; Bacteriology; Biostatistics; Diagnosis of bacterial infections; *Enterobacter*; Gram staining; Immunoassay; Microbiology; Microscopy; Pathogens; Polymerase chain reaction (PCR) method; Pulsed-field gel electrophoresis; Serology; Viral infections; Virology.

Biological weapons

CATEGORY: Transmission

DEFINITION

Biological weapons, comprising infectious biological agents, most often bacteria or viruses, are used to harm human, animal, and plant life.

EARLY USE

With increased scientific understanding of the agents of disease, called pathogens, comes an increase in the use of these biological agents as weapons. In the past, the use of biological weapons was based on an intuitive understanding that introducing a biological agent into an environment, such as by poisoning a water source or by using a natural poison, could cause harm. How a biological agent harmed was not always understood; that it did harm was all that mattered.

The ancient world also appears to have used biological weapons, mostly involving simple activities, such as poisoning a well, dumping rotting animal carcasses into water courses or near human habitation, using poisoned arrows or spear points, or destroying crops. Some researchers believe that disease agents, such as plague, had been used as weapons during this time, but this claim has been difficult to document.

For example, historians have claimed that Roman troops sowed the soil of Carthage with salt to destroy agricultural productivity after the Third Punic War in the second century B.C.E. It is sometimes said that the Mongols spread plague to the inhabitants of the city of Caffa in 1346 by catapulting plague-infected human bodies over the city walls, leading to the pandemic known as the Black Death. A more likely scenario is a "natural" one: that rats with plague-carrying fleas found entrance into the city and infected its inhabitants.

One often discredited example of the use of a biological agent reportedly occurred in 1763. In response to the uprising known as Pontiac's Rebellion in 1763, British troops allegedly gave to indigenous American Indians blankets that were infected with the smallpox virus. Although difficult to document, this episode is plausible because the British knew from firsthand experience that clothing or blankets used by persons with smallpox could be lethal for the next user. In addition, the American Indian population had no immunity to the disease, as had been seen in earlier smallpox epidemics that decimated Indian villages.

Much later, participants in World War I resorted to the use of poison gas, but they made no use of biological weapons. It is impossible to say whether this failure to use biological weapons stemmed from a lack of understanding or from a revulsion at their use. Even though they did not use biological weapons during World War I, several countries began to experiment with their development in the postwar years.

In partial response to the horrors of the war, most of the major powers agreed, in 1925, to the Geneva Protocol, which banned the use of chemical and biological weapons. Some countries signed with reserva-

tions, and the United States did not sign the agreement until 1975. The Geneva Protocol had no enforcement power, so some nations continued to engage in weaponizing biological agents. Most of the industrialized nations, including the United States, the United Kingdom, and Germany, experimented with biological weapons through the end of World War II.

Japan went even further in developing and using biological weapons, more so than any other country before 1945. Starting in 1932, Japan had developed several biological-war research facilities in China, especially at Pin Fan in Manchuria. The Japanese biological warfare research units investigated a variety of human diseases but concentrated on anthrax and plague (they also tried to spread cholera in Burma, now Myanmar). Research facilities such as that of unit 731 at Pin Fan engaged in extensive experimentation on humans, usually Chinese persons, in barbaric circumstances. These experiments included vivisection to gain experimental data. The Japanese also investigated the different means of dispersal of the biological agents, including trying to develop plague bombs that would deliver plague carrying fleas. At the end of World War II, the United States acquired the data from the Japanese biological warfare research units in return for not prosecuting for war crimes General Shiro Ishii, the head of Japanese biological weapons research, and others involved in Japanese biological-weapons research.

THE HEIGHT OF BIOLOGICAL WARFARE

During the Cold War, several nations experimented with biological agents and developed the means for delivering them. This experimentation was partially defensive in nature, but it was also geared to weapons development. The United States, the United Kingdom, and the Soviet Union were leaders in the process of weaponizing biological agents, often building on research carried out by the Japanese or the Germans during World War II.

The British started researching biological weapons in the late 1930's at the Porton Down facility in Wiltshire. Porton Down remained the center of British bio-war research throughout the Cold War. During World War II, the British had placed most of their emphasis on developing anthrax as a weapon (with some laboratory tests of plague), conducting tests with anthrax bombs on Gruinard Island off the coast of

Biological Warfare Agents and Associated Diseases, by Emergency Priority (A-C = Highest-Lowest)

Category	Biological agents and associated disease
A	• *Bacillus anthracis* (anthrax) • *Clostridium botulinum* toxin (botulism) • Filoviruses/arenaviruses (hemorrhagic fevers) • *Variola major* virus (smallpox) • *Francisella tularensis* (tularemia) • *Yersinia pestis* (plague)
B	• Alphaviruses (encephalitis) • *Brucella* species (brucellosis) • *Burkholderia mallei* (glanders) • *Burkholderia pseudomallei* (melioidosis) • *Chlamydia psittaci* (psittacosis) • *Clostridium perfringens* (epsilon toxin) • *Coxiella burnetii* (Q fever) • *Ricinus communis* (ricin toxin) • *Rickettsia prowazekii* (typhus fever) • *Salmonella* species, *Escherichia coli* O157:H7, *Shigella* (food-borne illnesses) • Staphylococcal enterotoxin B • *Vibrio cholerae, Cryptosporidium parvum* (water-borne illnesses)
C	• Emerging infectious diseases such as Nipah virus and hantavirus

Source: Centers for Disease Control and Prevention

Scotland. The tests concluded prematurely in August, 1943, when the bodies of sheep killed in the tests washed ashore on the mainland. Gruinard Island remained contaminated and quarantined for forty-eight years. The United States also began to conduct experiments with biological weapons at Camp (later Fort) Detrick, Maryland, concentrating on developing bombs that could deliver biological agents. After 1945, U.S. research remained centered at Fort Detrick, with some research carried out at the Plum Island facility off the coast of Long Island and in Pine Bluff, Arkansas. Field testing was conducted at the Dugway Proving Ground in Utah. U.S. researchers worked with both human pathogens and crop-destroying and defoliating agents during the war.

The U.S. acquisition of Japanese bio-war research in return for some Japanese immunity helped push U.S. biological weapons research forward in the postwar years, yet it also had profound implications for future policy. The secrecy of the agreement meant that no open discussion of biological weapons would be held, so the program expanded, and decision-making rested solely with military authorities.

The Soviet Union began research into the development and use of biological weapons long before World War II. Its Revolutionary Military Council ordered research into turning typhus into a battlefield weapon in 1928. The Soviets obtained some captured Japanese documents at the end of World War II, which spurred further research. New research facilities were established, one at Sverdlovsk in the Ural Mountains and several others in locations around the country. To camouflage the nature of the work, some of these research facilities were located in urban centers. These facilities included the Institute of Ultra-Pure Biopreparations in Leningrad and the new "research city" of Obolensk, just south of Moscow. By the 1970's, Soviet researchers were conducting extensive aerosol testing with harmless biological agents in Asiatic Russia and tests in the Moscow subway system.

The Soviets experimented with a variety of biological agents, including plague, anthrax, tularemia, smallpox, and, ultimately, Ebola hemorrhagic fever. In some cases the Soviets experimented with combining two pathogens into a new "superbug." The Soviet research was often carried out in haste and with little concern for safety. In April, 1979, for example, a major accident occurred at the Sverdlovsk facility and led to the release of anthrax in the surrounding area.

Although the British gradually phased out their bio-war research, the research of the United States increased during the 1950's. Because the United States was not a signatory to the Geneva Protocol that banned chemical and biological weapons, its bio-war research, like that of the Soviet Union, was considered an offensive move militarily. The Chinese and

North Korean governments accused the United States of using biological weapons during the Korean War, but this was denied by the United States.

During the 1960's, the United States stepped up its experimental work and conducted numerous field tests with bio-war agents at Dugway Proving Ground and with harmless biological agents in places such as National Airport (now Ronald Reagan Washington National Airport) in Washington, D.C., and the New York subway system in 1966. In addition to working with anthrax and plague, U.S. researchers also considered pathogens that acted as incapacitating agents; these pathogens included the viruses that cause Q fever, Venezuelan equine encephalitis, and Rift Valley fever.

The United States and the Soviet Union were not the only countries that experimented with biological weapons in the years after 1945. The Canadian and French governments also engaged in biological weapons research. The South African government phased out its biological weapons research program in the 1990's, although there is suspicion that some of that country's research results may have reached other countries. During the 1990's, the government of Iraq engaged in biological weapons research too, although its efforts were not as well-developed as first thought.

FUTURE OF BIOLOGICAL WARFARE

Opposition to U.S. development of biological weapons had been growing during the 1960's, but it was U.S. president Richard Nixon who took the step to ban biological weapons. On November 25, 1969, he announced a ban on U.S. biological weapons and placed restrictions on the development of chemical weapons. He then sent the 1925 Geneva Protocol to the U.S. Senate, which ratified it in 1975. Nixon also supported a draft British treaty to ban the development, production, possession, and stockpiling of all biological weapons. Initially opposed by the Soviet Union, the Convention on the Prohibition of the Development, Production, and Stockpiling of Bacteriological (Biological) and Toxic Weapons and on Their Destruction (commonly known as the Biological Warfare Convention, or BWC) came to be supported by most nations of the world. Nixon signed the convention on behalf of the United States on April 10, 1972, and it came into force in 1975. It seems that Nixon intended that biological weapons research be transformed into research on epidemic disease worldwide.

Soon, he refocused Fort Detrick toward disease eradication and renamed it the U.S. Army Medical Research Institute of Infectious Diseases.

The BWC lacked strong compliance provisions, so the Soviet Union, which had signed the treaty, intensified its bio-weapons research and its development efforts in the 1970's. Much of the Soviet effort remains secret, but the defection of the deputy director of Biopreparat, Ken Alibek, and the subsequent publication of his book, *Biohazard*, in 1999, revealed some of the work of the Soviets. Biopreparat reportedly continued with bio-weapons research and continued building related facilities, such as that at Stepnogorsk in Kazakhstan, which produced large amounts of pathogens, including the smallpox virus. It is not known, however, if the Soviet military developed plans for the use of the biological weapons.

By 1988, the United States and the Soviet Union were reaching accord on nuclear arms control and the Cold War was coming to an end. Nonetheless, several Soviet biological research facilities remained closed to Western observers for another ten years. One of these facilities, at Sergiev Posad, was alleged to be experimenting with smallpox and an Ebola-smallpox cocktail during the 1990's. Most Soviet bio-war facilities were closed with the collapse of the Soviet Union, and others, such as Obolensk, turned to disease-prevention research. However, the disposition of the weapons stocks and research material in the post-Soviet era remains troubling, as some observers indicate that this material may be finding its way to other nations or even to terrorist groups.

IMPACT

Although several nations have engaged in biological weapons research in the twentieth century, most have been unwilling to make use of these weapons. Still, research continues in several countries in hopes of curtailing the effect of infectious biological agents. The greatest threat today is the possible use of biological weapons by terrorist groups.

Anthrax and smallpox are likely the most feared agents for biological weapons of terror. Anthrax is easily and anonymously transmitted. Smallpox, once it becomes an epidemic, can be transmitted readily from one person to another. Also, few people have any immunity to the disease. Other pathogens that continue to be a threat as bio-war agents are those that cause plague, tularemia, cholera, SARS, and influenza, and the pathogens *Salmonella*, Ebola virus, hantavirus, and botulinum toxin.

In some cases, such as for influenza or smallpox, vaccines exist; in other cases, such as plague, vaccines are being developed. In other cases, such as cholera, the disease, in industrialized nations, can be readily treated and prevented. In a few other cases, such as for Ebola, no vaccine or treatment exists.

Weaponizing some of these disease agents continues to be a challenge. Especially difficult is developing genetically modified agents; also difficult is finding a suitable delivery system. Access to virus and bacteria cultures of most bio-war agents has become a challenge for unauthorized persons, yet is not impossible for a clever and determined group to obtain these cultures.

John M. Theilmann, Ph.D.

FURTHER READING

Alibek, Ken. *Biohazard.* New York: Delta, 1999. Account of Soviet bio-weapons research by the former deputy director of Biopreparat.

Clark, William R. *Bracing for Armageddon? The Science and Politics of Bioterrorism in America.* New York: Oxford University Press, 2008. Examines the possible use of biological weapons by terrorist groups.

Clunan, Anne L., Peter R. Lavoy, and Susan B. Martin, eds. *Terrorism, War, or Disease? Unraveling the Use of Biological Weapons.* Stanford, Calif.: Stanford University Press, 2008. Essays examine the legal and political questions concerning bio-war and the possibility of bio-war events.

Fong, I. W., and Kenneth Alibek, eds. *Bioterrorism and Infectious Agents: A New Dilemma for the Twenty-first Century.* New York: Springer, 2009. Updated discussion of biological agents and treatments.

Guillemin, Jeanne. *Biological Weapons: From the Invention of State-Sponsored Programs to Contemporary Bioterrorism.* New York: Columbia University Press, 2005. Comprehensive coverage of the development of biological weapons since the early twentieth century. Excellent starting point for further research.

Harris, Sheldon H. *Factories of Death: Japanese Biological Warfare, 1932-1945, and American Cover-up.* Rev. ed. New York: Routledge, 2002. An account of Japanese biological warfare efforts, and U.S. knowledge of these efforts, through World War II.

Mayor, Adrienne. *Greek Fire, Poison Arrows, and Scorpion Bombs: Biological and Chemical Warfare in the Ancient World.* Woodstock, N.Y.: Overlook Duckworth, 2003. Interesting although not always convincing account of the use of biological and chemical weapons in the ancient world.

Spiers, Edward M. *A History of Chemical and Biological Weapons.* London: Reaktion Books, 2010. An examination of the threat posed by the accessibility of chemical and biological weapons since 2001.

Wheelis, Mark, Lajos Rózsa, and Malcolm Dando, eds. *Deadly Cultures: Biological Weapons Since 1945.* Cambridge, Mass.: Harvard University Press, 2006. Essays deal with various national and potential terrorist bio-war programs.

Zubay, Geoffrey L., et al. *Agents of Bioterrorism: Pathogens and their Weaponization.* New York: Columbia University Press, 2005. Essays explore various pathogens, how they have been turned into weapons, and antipathogen methods.

WEB SITES OF INTEREST

Center for Biosecurity
http://www.upmc-biosecurity.org

Centers for Disease Control and Prevention
http://www.bt.cdc.gov/bioterrorism

Disaster Information Management Research Center
http://sis.nlm.nih.gov/enviro/biologicalwarfare.html

U.S. Army Medical Research Institute of Infectious Diseases
http://www.usamriid.army.mil

See also: Airborne illness and disease; Anthrax; Bacterial infections; Bioterrorism; Botulinum toxin infection; Disease eradication campaigns; Infectious disease specialists; Plague; Public health; SARS; Smallpox; Transmission routes; U.S. Army Medical Research Institute of Infectious Diseases.

Biostatistics

CATEGORY: Epidemiology

DEFINITION

Biostatistical analyses are essential to epidemiological studies. The analyses are used to summarize the data obtained in research on disease outbreaks and in disease surveillance. The statistics can describe risks of the disease, compare risk among community groups, and develop hypotheses about the causes of disease. Determining the causes of differences in risk among groups leads to better prevention and control measures.

ANALYZING DATA

Two basic definitions are important in biostatistics, also called biometrics or biometry. "Incidence" is the rate at which new cases occur in a population during a specified period, whereas "prevalence" is the proportion of a population that is a case at a point in time.

The data collected in a study are notable for their variability. The types of variability can be classified as either categorical or continuous. Categorical variables can be either nominal (with no natural order), such as the variables race or gender, or ordinal (with an order), such as the variable of symptom severity. Continuous data can have any value within an interval, such as age or weight. Mortality data are special cases of continuous data, because some people are still alive at the end of the study. The survivors are known as censored data, so calculations, such as median survival time, are measured from a Kaplan-Meier curve.

Biostatistics seeks to determine if the differences between groups of data, in this case the differences in morbidity or mortality between exposed and unexposed groups, could be caused by chance. The mean or statistical measurement of central tendency is calculated on mortality or other criteria of interest in groups. The type of statistical analysis performed is dependent on the way the data is distributed.

Parametric tests assume the data are normally distributed, while nonparametric tests are used if the data are not normally distributed. It is important to realize that if the analysis shows that the differences are statistically significant, the analysis does not prove that there is a difference. For example, a significant level of p .05 simply means that there is less than a 5 percent chance that there is no difference. The calculation of confidence intervals around the means provides a range of values that is believed to encompass the actual population value.

STUDY DESIGNS

Biostatistical analyses are performed on three types of epidemiological studies: prospective, retrospective, and cross-sectional. These types of studies are known as observational, which involves observing people and comparing groups without influencing their treatment or care. These studies are in contrast to randomized controlled studies, such as clinical trials, which involve active intervention in the selection, treatment, and care of subjects. Randomized studies are usually not feasible for epidemiology because of ethical and practical considerations.

Observational studies vary according to the time of the study. Case-control or retrospective studies collect cases of a disease and identify control subjects free of the disease that are otherwise as similar as possible to the case subjects. Through medical records and subject interviews, the researcher goes back in time to identify exposure to a factor or factors that could be the cause or causes of the disease. Case-control studies are particularly useful in studying rare diseases. Prospective (cohort) studies involve selecting well-defined subsets of the population, persons known as cohorts, who are exposed or unexposed to the risk factor. The cohorts are then followed over time to examine subsequent incidence of mortality or morbidity.

Both case-control and prospective studies are longitudinal because they study changes over time. Cross-sectional studies examine a sample of the population at a point in time, so they study disease prevalence and attempt to relate the disease to a risk factor. Frequently, cross-sectional studies are descriptive in nature rather than analytical.

MEASURES OF RISK

A risk is the probability of an event occurring. Absolute risk measures the probability of an event or outcome occurring in the group of people under study. Attributable risk is the portion of the incidence of the disease in the exposed population that is caused by exposure. Relative risk is the risk of the exposed group contracting the disease compared with that of people who are unexposed. Relative risk cannot be calculated in case-control studies because of the way participants are selected. The appropriate statistical measure of association for case-control studies is the odds ratio, which is the odds that a subject with the condition was exposed to the risk factor divided by the odds that a control was exposed.

SOURCES OF ERROR IN STATISTICS

The conclusions drawn from observational studies are inherently more error prone than from randomized trials, although with well-designed trials, statistical analyses can partially correct these errors. Because observational studies include participants from a broader spectrum of the population than do randomized trials, the results of the study may have more general applications.

Bias occurs when systematic factors in a trial design or implementation influence the outcome of a trial in an erroneous way. Selection bias occurs when study participants are not representative of the larger population at risk for the disease. Information bias results in incorrect data being obtained because of different measurements of exposure or different detections of outcomes between exposed and unexposed participants. Recall bias is particularly important for case-control studies because subjects with the disease are more likely to recall exposure to the risk factor than are subjects without the disease. Confounding occurs when a factor is associated with both exposure and outcome, which could lead to the erroneous conclusion that an unrelated factor caused the outcome.

IMPACT

Biostatistics is integral to interpreting the results of epidemiological studies. To draw valid conclusions, the studies must be well-designed and executed and the limitations of statistical analyses must be clearly understood.

David A. Olle, M.S.

FURTHER READING

Armitage, Peter, and Theodore Colton, eds. *Encyclopedia of Biostatistics.* 2d ed. Hoboken, N.J.: Wiley Interscience, 2005.

Bowers, David. *Medical Statistics from Scratch.* 2d ed. Hoboken, N.J.: Wiley, 2007.

Brase, Charles Henry, and Corrinne Pellillo Brase. *Understandable Statistics.* 9th ed. Boston: Brooks/Cole, 2009.

Daniel, Wayne W. *Biostatistics: A Foundation for Analysis in the Health Sciences.* 9th ed. Hoboken, N.J.: John Wiley & Sons, 2009.

Phillips, John L. *How to Think About Statistics.* 6th ed. New York: Henry Holt, 2002.

Porta, Miquel, ed. *A Dictionary of Epidemiology.* 5th ed. New York: Oxford University Press, 2008.

Sahai, Hardeo, and Anwer Khurshid. *Statistics in Epidemiology: Methods, Techniques, and Applications.* Boca Raton, Fla.: CRC Press, 1996.

Wassertheil-Smoller, Sylvia. *Biostatistics and Epidemiology: A Primer for Health and Biomedical Professionals.* 3d ed. New York: Springer, 2004.

WEB SITES OF INTEREST

Collection of Biostatistics Research Archive
http://biostats.bepress.com/repository

International Biometric Society
http://www.tibs.org

See also: Biosurveillance; Centers for Disease Control and Prevention (CDC); Disease eradication campaigns; Emerging and reemerging infectious diseases; Emerging Infections Network; Epidemics and pandemics: Causes and management; Epidemic Intelligence Service; Epidemiology; Infectious disease specialists; Koch's postulates; Mathematical modeling; Outbreaks; Public health.

Biosurveillance

CATEGORY: Epidemiology
ALSO KNOWN AS: Biological surveillance, biomonitoring

DEFINITION

Biosurveillance is a systematic process of surveying the environment for viruses, bacteria, fungi, and other pathogens to detect disease in humans, animals, and plants. The process also characterizes outbreaks of such disease.

OVERVIEW

Biosurveillance combines disease surveillance with public health surveillance, both of which depend upon data collection and analysis with the goal of early disease detection to thwart a potential outbreak. Diseases may be defined by incubation and infectious periods, source, and transmission route, while outbreak characterization uses general analytic techniques, such as spatiotemporal distribution, incidence, mortality, and cohort or case-control studies. Biosurveillance proceeds from continuous data collection to confirmation of cases with a feedback loop back to data aggregation. Environmental investigations include food chains, vectors, weather, geography, the number of people who became ill, and those at risk.

In the United States, the major use of biosurveillance is to track emerging and reemerging infectious diseases such as H1N1 influenza, food-borne diseases caused by resistant strains of *Escherichia coli* and *Salmonella*, sexually transmitted diseases (STDs), and human immunodeficiency virus infection, which may also be transmitted by contaminated blood products or through maternal transmission.

In the United States, government agencies conduct biosurveillance at the levels of state and local health departments, which then report to federal agencies such as the Centers for Disease Control and Prevention (CDC), a division of the Department of Health and Human Services (HHS). The CDC is responsible for collecting, analyzing, and distributing national disease occurrence and mortality rates to state and local health authorities and to the public. Other federal agencies conducting biosurveillance include the Department of Defense (DoD), the Department of Homeland Security (DHS), and, globally, U.S. collaborative partners such as the World Health Organization (WHO), the Pan American Health Organization (PAHO), and the South East Asia Regional Office (SEARO).

Before 2000, biosurveillance systems included the National Electronic Telecommunications System for Surveillance (NTESS) and PulseNet, the national subtyping network comprising state and local public health laboratories and federal food regulatory laboratories that perform molecular surveillance of food-borne infections. Systems in place after 2000 include BioSense and other early warning systems, such as the Real-time Outbreak and Disease Surveillance System (RODS).

Numerous decision-making tools, such as Bayesian inference, may be applied to the detection of an outbreak of infectious disease. The importance of the decision-making process cannot be overestimated when providing alerts to the public. The costs versus benefits of false alerts must be weighed against the goal of protecting the population at risk.

INFLUENZA SURVEILLANCE

The CDC maintains a comprehensive surveillance system for influenza viruses, which mutate from year to year, requiring the collection and characterization of varying types of pathogens. Flu vaccines have to be annually updated in accordance with surveillance data to include relevant strains. Treatment for influenza is determined by laboratory surveillance for antiviral resistance. The impact of influenza on hospitalizations and mortality must also be assessed.

The epidemiology and prevention branch of the influenza division at the CDC collects and analyzes information on influenza activity throughout the year in the United States. This surveillance results in "FluView," a weekly report, which is issued from October through mid-May of each year. The influenza surveillance system is a collaborative effort between the CDC and its many partners in state, local, and territorial health departments; public health and clinical laboratories; health care providers; clinics; and emergency departments.

The CDC employs five categories of influenza surveillance: viral, outpatient influenza-like illness (ILI), mortality, hospitalization, and Flu-SurvNET. ILI is defined as a fever (100° Fahrenheit or 37.8° Celsius or greater) and a cough or sore throat (or both) in the absence of a known cause other than influenza. Flu-SurvNET provides population-based, laboratory-confirmed estimates of influenza-related hospitalizations. Each week, approximately eighteen hundred outpatient care sites around the United States provide data to the CDC. This data includes the total number of patients with ILI, according to age group. The data by age had confirmed, for example, that young people were more adversely affected by H1N1 influenza in 2009, relative to those age sixty-five years and older (when compared with seasonal flu).

Also included in national data are human infections with novel influenza A viruses, pneumonia, influenza mortality from the 122 Cities Mortality System, influenza-associated pediatric deaths, and Aggregate Hospitalizations and Death Reporting Activity. The Emerging Infections Program (EIP) is a population-based network of the CDC and state health departments that assesses the public health impact of emerging infections and examines ways to prevent and control these infections.

VIRAL SURVEILLANCE

Approximately eighty U.S. and WHO collaborating laboratories and sixty labs from the National Respiratory and Enteric Virus Surveillance System (NREVSS) participate in influenza surveillance. The U.S.-WHO and NREVSS collaborating labs report to the CDC the total number of respiratory specimens tested and the number of positives for influenza types A and B each week. Reports from both U.S.-WHO and NREVSS are combined and presented in "FluView."

Routine seasonal surveillance does not count individual flu cases, hospitalizations, or deaths (except for pediatric influenza deaths); rather, it monitors flu activity levels, trends, and viral characteristics through a nationwide surveillance system. The reporting of hospitalizations and deaths by state health departments was initiated at the start of the pandemic H1N1 outbreak in 2009. To avoid the underestimation of cases, the CDC altered this system and asked states to report both laboratory confirmed hospitalizations and deaths and presumed influenza or pneumonia deaths on cases coded as ICD-9 (International Classification of Diseases). The CDC also created a Web-based data application for states to submit their numbers each week. This data is compiled for publication in the CDC's *Morbidity and Mortality Weekly Report* (MMWR) and in "FluView."

HIV AND AIDS SURVEILLANCE

The annual *HIV Surveillance Report* provides an overview of the most up-to-date epidemiology data on HIV infection in the United States and five U.S. territories. The CDC funds state and territorial health departments so they can collect data on persons with HIV infection; all personal identifiers are removed before data is transmitted to the CDC through a secure data network. Data are analyzed by the CDC and then displayed by age, race and ethnicity, gender, and transmission category, a significant change in the operation of the surveillance system. Moreover, the *HIV Surveillance Report* for 2012 (to be issued in 2014) marks the first time that data is included from each of the fifty states.

In 2008, changes were made to the case definition of HIV infection. To accurately track the epidemic, emphasis is now be placed on HIV surveillance rather than on acquired immunodeficiency disease syndrome (AIDS) surveillance. HIV testing and linkage to care are essential for identifying persons early.

Approximately 1.1 million persons in the United States are HIV-positive. The CDC used 2001 to 2009 data from the National Health Interview Survey to estimate percentages of persons age eighteen through sixty-four years who reported being tested (at any time) for HIV in the United States. Data from the national HIV surveillance system were employed to estimate cases and rates of HIV infection, AIDS diagnoses, and late diagnoses of HIV infection. In turn, these data were used to determine the populations and regions most affected by HIV and AIDS and to determine the trends in HIV testing and late diagnoses.

FOOD-BORNE DISEASE OUTBREAK SURVEILLANCE

Food-borne pathogens cause an estimated seventy-six million illnesses annually in the United States. Data from outbreak surveillance provides insights into the etiology of these illnesses, the foods in question, and their settings. State, local, and territorial health departments use a standard, Web-based form to report food-borne outbreaks to the Foodborne Disease Outbreak Surveillance System.

As reported to the CDC, 1,097 food-borne outbreaks occurred in 2007, which resulted in 21,244 cases of illness and 18 deaths; of the single, laboratory confirmed agents of outbreak-associated illnesses, 12,767 were caused by norovirus (47 percent) and *Salmonella* (27 percent). In July, 2010, the CDC collaborated with public health officials in several states and with the HHS, FDA, and the Department of Agriculture (USDA) Food Safety and Inspection Service to investigate a nationwide rise in *S. enteritidis* (SE) infections. Investigators used deoxyribonucleic acid (DNA) analysis of SE bacteria obtained through diagnostic testing to identify cases of illness. They also identified restaurant and event clusters that may have been associated with this outbreak. Investigators determined that eggs contaminated by *Salmonella* were responsible for the outbreak. In late November, 2010, following a recall and ban, the FDA issued permits to some of the affected farms, allowing the resumption of egg sales.

IMPACT ON GLOBAL PUBLIC HEALTH

The age of public health globalization has arrived. Global health and global health surveillance have come to the fore, in part because of newly emerging and reemerging infectious diseases. In addition, climate change, poor hygiene and sanitation, lack of economic and food security, political unrest, war, and accelerating threats of bioterrorism have greatly increased global morbidity and mortality from infectious diseases, especially in developing countries.

To counter these challenges, global health surveillance procedures have been updated. Changes were made to the new International Health Regulations (IHR), new global networks were developed, and specific guidelines to monitor emerging diseases and acts of bioterrorism were developed. Global surveillance now provides real-time information about potential outbreaks and epidemics.

Global response to the 2009 H1N1 influenza pandemic demonstrated the benefits of the new global monitoring systems and the importance of WHO in coordinating the global public-health community. As a result, valuable models were developed on how to respond to novel strains of influenza and other pathogenic entities, such as the severe acute respiratory syndrome (SARS) virus. As the number of cases H1N1 influenza cases increased and rapidly spread, it was apparent that significant resources, intervention, and biosurveillance at the international level would be necessary.

Cynthia F. Racer, M.P.H., M.A.

FURTHER READING

Burkle, F. M., Jr, and P. G. Greenough. "Impact of Public Health Emergencies on Modern Disaster Taxonomy, Planning, and Response." *Disaster Medicine and Public Health Preparedness* 2 (2008): 192-199. Examines disaster taxonomy and how it defines variability, unique characteristics, and classification of disasters. Also looks at how compromised public health infrastructure and systems may impact public health consequences, especially those that are "widespread, population dense, and prolonged."

DeFraites, Robert F., and William C. Chambers. "Gaining Experience with Military Medical Situational Awareness and Geographic Information Systems in a Simulated Influenza Epidemic." *Military Medicine* 172 (2007): 1071-1076. Examines the practice of medical situational awareness in integrating relevant medical and operational information to bolster decision making.

Giles-Vernick, Tamara, and Susan Craddock, eds. *Influenza and Public Health: Learning from Past Pandemics.* London: Earthscan, 2010. Discusses from a historical perspective the lessons learned from past flu pandemics about transmission patterns and successful (and not so successful) interventions.

Lazarus, R., et al. "Using Automated Medical Records for Rapid Identification of Illness Syndromes (Syn-dromic Surveillance): The Example of Lower Respiratory Infection." *BMC Public Health* 1 (2001): 9. Discusses how information gleaned from automated medical records complements current surveillance programs by evaluating most episodes of illness for which no etiologic agent is defined.

Lober, W. B., L. Trigg, and B. Karras. "Information System Architectures for Syndromic Surveillance." *Morbidity and Mortality Weekly Report* 5, suppl. (2004): 203-208. Describes the information-architecture components of a particular surveillance data system. Discusses existing and potential approaches to data integration.

O'Neil, Eileen A., and Elena N. Naumova. "Defining Outbreak: Breaking Out of Confusion." *Journal of Public Health Policy* 28 (2007): 442-455. Illustrates the complexity of defining terms used to describe emerging and reemerging infectious diseases that have resulted in the use of emotionally charged terms such as "outbreak." Argues that public health may benefit from strengthening the definitions of key terms.

WEB SITES OF INTEREST

Centers for Disease Control and Prevention, OutbreakNet Team
http://www.cdc.gov/outbreaknet

Emerging and Reemerging Infectious Diseases Resource Center
http://www.medscape.com/resource/infections

Global Health Council
http://www.globalhealth.org

World Health Organization
http://www.who.int

See also: Biostatistics; Centers for Disease Control and Prevention (CDC); Disease eradication campaigns; Emerging and reemerging infectious diseases; Epidemics and pandemics: Causes and management; Epidemiology; Globalization and infectious disease; Infectious disease specialists; Infectious Diseases Society of America; Outbreaks; Pathogenicity; Public health; Social effects of infectious disease; Virulence; World Health Organization (WHO).

Bioterrorism

Category: Epidemiology

Definition

Bioterrorism, or biological terrorism, is the intentional release of bacteria or viruses into a civilian population to harm that population and, thereby, achieve a political or social end.

Biological Agents

Found in nature, biological agents threaten human populations when terrorists engineer these agents for release. The agents are cultivated to make them more resistant to medicines and vaccines and more easily transmitted in a population. The Centers for Disease Control and Prevention (CDC) in the United States classifies biological terror agents by their likelihood for use by terrorist groups and by their risk to a population. The CDC groups bioterrorism agents into categories A, B, and C.

Category A Agents

Cited as highest priority are category A agents, which are rare in the United States. These agents are easily transmitted and would cause a high death rate and would demand a proactive public health preparedness strategy. A agents include anthrax (*Bacillus anthracis*), botulism (*Clostridium botulinum* toxin), plague (*Yersinia pestis*), smallpox (*Variola major*), tularemia (*Francisella tularensis*), and viral hemorrhagic fever filoviruses, such as Ebola and Marburg, and arenaviruses, such as Lassa and Machupo.

Anthrax. An anthrax infection is triggered by *B. anthracis*, a bacterium that forms spores, or dormant cells that reawaken under certain conditions. There are three types of anthrax infection: those that involve the skin (cutaneous), the lungs (inhalation), and the digestive tract (gastrointestinal). Anthrax does not spread from person to person. People normally contract an anthrax infection by handling or ingesting infected animal products. Symptoms can appear within seven days. For cutaneous anthrax infection, symptoms include the appearance of nonpainful skin blisters with a black area in the center. For gastrointestinal anthrax, symptoms are nausea, loss of appetite, bloody diarrhea, fever, and stomach pain. For inhalation anthrax, symptoms are similar to those of a common cold: significant chest congestion and shortness of breath.

Botulism. Spread by the bacterium *C. botulinum*, botulism is a muscle-paralyzing disease. It is not spread from person to person. People normally contract botulism from infected food or from an infected wound. Infants can contract the disease from the presence of the bacterium in their digestive tract. The food-borne form of botulism has a potential for becoming a public health emergency, as the toxin can contaminate large amounts of food. After ingesting the toxin, symptoms of double vision, dry mouth, slurred speech, and muscle weakness appear. Gradually, paralysis spreads throughout the body. Though most treated persons recover within weeks, untreated persons can die from paralysis of the breathing muscles.

Plague. Caused by the *Y. pestis* bacterium, plague originates with rodents and their fleas. Though bubonic plague is transmitted through a rodent or flea bite, pneumonic plague can be transmitted through the air from person to person or through a deliberate aerosol release. Once exposed, a person experiences symptoms within one to six days that include cough, shortness of breath, chest pain, nausea, and abdominal pain. Plague is diagnosed through blood, sputum, or lymph-node aspirate sampling and is treated with antibiotics. Untreated, plague results in respiratory failure.

Smallpox. The two forms of smallpox are *V. major*, which is severe and most common, and the less common and less deadly *V. minor*. The four types of *V. major* smallpox are ordinary, modified, flat, and hemorrhagic. Ordinary *V. major*, causing 90 percent of known cases, has a fatality rate of 30 percent, according to the CDC. The flat and hemorrhagic types are rare and usually fatal. Humans are the only known carriers of smallpox, and they spread the disease to others through close personal contact. Following an incubation period of seven to seventeen days, an infected person becomes contagious and experiences fever, head and body aches, and a rash of small red spots (first in the mouth and throat, then over the entire body). The last known case of smallpox in the United States was in 1949, and the last known case worldwide was in Somalia in 1977. The *Variola* virus exists only in science laboratories.

Tularemia. Tularemia is caused by the bacterium *F. tularensis*, which is found in rodents and rabbits. A human contracts the disease upon being bitten by an infected tick or fly, by handling an infected carcass, by ingesting contaminated food or water, or by inhaling

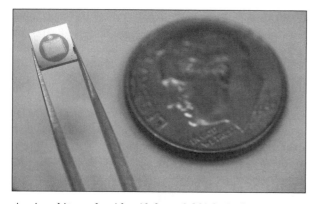

A microchip used to identify harmful biological agents, especially those used in an act of bioterrorism. (AP/Wide World Photos)

the airborne bacteria. Appearing within three to five days after exposure, symptoms include spiked fever, chills, headache, diarrhea, muscle aches, joint pain, dry cough, and weakness. Tularemia is treated with antibiotics.

Viral hemorrhagic fevers. Filovirus viral hemorrhagic fevers (VHFs), such as Ebola and Marburg, and arenavirus VHFs, such as Lassa and Machupo, are known by the CDC as severe multisystem syndrome diseases. VHFs attack multiple systems of the body, an attack accompanied by bleeding. Persons experience symptoms of fever, achiness, and fatigue before seeing bleeding under the skin and from the mouth, eyes, and ears. VHF may progress to nervous system damage or kidney failure. Initially transmitted from contact with rodents and their bodily excretions or by mosquito or tick bites, some VHFs (as Ebola, Marburg, and Lassa) can spread through human-to-human contact. Though there is no direct treatment for VHFs, the antiviral drug ribavirin is sometimes administered to persons with a VHF disease.

CATEGORY B AGENTS

Ranked by the CDC as second highest priority, category B agents are moderately easy to transmit and result in lower mortality rates. B agents include brucellosis (*Brucella* species); epsilon toxin of *Clostridium perfringens*; food safety threats (*Salmonella, Escherichia coli*, and *Shigella*); glanders (*Burkholderia mallei*); melioidosis (*B. pseudomallei*); psittacosis (*Chlamydophila psittaci*); Q fever (*Coxiella burnetii*); ricin toxin from *Ricinus communis* (castor beans); staphylococcal enterotoxin B; typhus fever (*Rickettsia prowazekii*); viral

encephalitis Alphaviruses, such as Venezuelan equine encephalitis, eastern equine encephalitis, and western equine encephalitis; and water-safety threats, such as *Vibrio cholerae* and *Cryptosporidium parvum*.

CATEGORY C AGENTS

The agents with the third highest priority are those in category C; they include emerging pathogens. Newly discovered diseases such as nipah virus and hantavirus infections are in category C and are rated according to availability, ease of production, and potential for causing death.

HISTORY OF BIOLOGICAL WEAPONS

At the end of the nineteenth century, scientists discovered a link between microorganisms and the outbreak of illness. They began to understand how diseases are spread through air, food and water supplies, person-to-person contact, and insect bites. Upon uncovering these facts, scientists rapidly found ways to protect people against the outbreak of several diseases.

By the early twentieth century, some Western governments began to explore the harvesting and use of biological agents for use as weapons. In World War I, Germany undertook the first-known state-sponsored biological weapons program, deliberately infecting the horses and mules of enemy forces. In the 1920's, the French conducted research in biological weapon aerosols, increasing research in the mid-1930's.

In 1942, American biologists Theodor Rosebury and Elvin A. Kabot noted that *B. anthracis*, in its dormant-spore state, can easily be used as a biological weapon. The spores can withstand disbursement in hot or cold environments. Viewing this pathogen as a potential threat, Rosebury and Kabot recommended the development of an anthrax vaccine. They also described how plague bacillus, if freeze-dried, could also be weaponized in an aerosol. As a result of Rosebury and Kabot's findings on the potential for use of biological weapons, Allied soldiers were administered antibiotics and vaccines during World War II.

The September 11, 2001, terrorist attacks in the United States prompted a surge in support and funding for defense against bioterror threats. This support and funding led to the development of technologies for detecting airborne threats and for treatment of disease caused by bioterror attacks. In *Biological Weapons* (2005), Jeanne Guillemin writes that the establishment of the U.S. Department of Homeland

Security (DHS) in 2003 "far outweighed the diffuse, decentralized domestic preparedness project of the previous decade."

THREATS

The Homeland Security Act of November 25, 2003, incorporated the Federal Emergency Management Agency (FEMA), which immediately dedicated resources to investigate the threat of biological terrorism. FEMA concluded that three groups of biological agents could be used as weapons: bacteria, viruses, and toxins. Though terrorists may choose biological warfare over other tactics, most known agents are difficult to cultivate and are quickly destroyed once exposed to dry air and sunlight. For example, though the airborne spread of plague is possible, *Y. pestis* bacteria survive up to one hour only once released. Some agents, like the smallpox virus, are spread only through human contact, while others, like anthrax, infect only those exposed to a primary source of the germs. However, terrorists could choose to release germs that infect animals bred for human consumption or could choose to contaminate water supplies.

In December, 2008, a bipartisan panel commissioned by the U.S. Congress to analyze the threat of unconventional weapons warned that, unless the international community commits to preventive measures and additional security, "it is more likely than not that a weapon of mass destruction will be used in a terrorist attack somewhere in the world by the end of 2013." The panel called for the strengthening of international organizations dedicated to preventing unconventional warfare, to improving rapid-response and bioforensic capabilities, to heightening security at research institutions housing biological pathogens, and to forming an international conference on biosecurity. Notably, the report concluded that weaponizing biological agents is extremely difficult and likely outside the range of capabilities for a rogue, non-state-supported group. Before leaving office in January, 2009, U.S. president George W. Bush signed an executive order on laboratory biosecurity that established an interagency body dedicated to regulating and overseeing research programs and laboratories.

The warning about the potential for breaching the security of state-sponsored programs relates to lessons learned following events in 2001, when anthrax was spread through an infected powder sent with letters through the U.S. postal system. The anthrax-laced let-

ters were targeted to persons in media and politics, resulting in twenty-two documented cases of anthrax infection. Analysis of the infected letters pointed to the Ames strain, the form grown and studied in the U.S. program. A federal investigation later identified the anthrax source as the laboratory of Bruce Ivins of the U.S. Army research facility at Fort Detrick, Maryland.

Federal agencies and politicians continue to incorporate the threat of biological terrorism into national security regulations and policies. The next-generation threat to U.S. security is lax security at labs researching diseases that could be cultivated for biological weapons. In mid-October, 2010, Jacek Bylica, head of the Weapons of Mass Destruction Centre of the North Atlantic Treaty Organization, said that the spread of weapons of mass destruction, their delivery, and the chance that terrorists will acquire them are major, significant threats. In November, bioterrorism security concerns were again raised when U.S. senator Richard G. Lugar and Pentagon officials visited Uganda's ministry of agriculture, animals, industry, and fisheries. Discovered there were research specimens of anthrax and the Ebola and Marburg viruses, stored in an unlocked refrigerator in an unsecured building.

RESPONSE

In response to the threat of bioterrorism, the DHS seeks works to determine the agents that are easiest to grow and deliberately release and seeks to develop methods for identifying the natural outbreak of a disease from a bioterrorism attack. In 2004, the DHS established the Knowledge Center, which provides a collaborative forum for experts in biological pathogens and political terrorism to share information and assess bioterror threats.

The CDC and the American Red Cross prepare populations for a bioterrorism attack through multimedia educational programs that urge families to store supplies, that show how to detect signs and symptoms of biological terror agents, and that show how to deal with exposure to suspected biological agents, among other topics. According to FEMA, optimal prevention against a bioterrorism attack includes installing a high-efficiency particulate-air filter in furnaces and ensuring that recommended immunizations are updated for all persons.

In preparation for a possible aerosol attack of the pneumonic plague agent or the tularemia agent, national and state health centers have stockpiled antibiotics. The CDC also maintains an antitoxin to treat botulism. Though there have been no known cases of smallpox since 1977, and routine vaccination against the disease has been discontinued, the United States now secures research and treatment stockpiles of the *Variola* virus. No plague vaccine is available in the United States, but research for such a vaccine continues.

PREVENTION

A June, 2010, report from the Center for Biosecurity at the University of Pittsburgh Medical Center stated that from 2008 through 2010, government spending to support biodefense programs increased. Bioterrorism prevention and intervention are top priorities, according to Department of Health and Human Services secretary Kathleen Sebelius, who, in early 2010, announced a new national health security strategy of focusing resources on first-responder teams and front-line health care. On October 7, the National Institute of Allergy and Infectious Diseases announced its investment of $68 million in research projects for the development of vaccines to protect against biological terror. These projects include those looking into a needle-free dengue vaccine, an orally administered anthrax vaccine, and an anthrax vaccine administered with an adjuvant to stimulate the immune system. On November 5, the Biomedical Advanced Research and Development Authority of the HHS awarded Northrop Grumman a one-year contract to develop a biodefense system to allow first-responders to rapidly screen and triage persons exposed to a biological agent.

IMPACT

Because there have been few incidents of bioterrorism, there is little historical data on its impact. However, scientific predictions about likely effects on populations have led to response strategies and to investment in prevention and detection technologies.

Melissa Walsh

FURTHER READING

Guillemin, Jeanne. *Biological Weapons.* New York: Columbia University Press, 2005. Covers the history of terrorist- and state-sponsored development of biological weapons.

Isikoff, Michael. "The Case Still Isn't Closed." *Newsweek*, August 18, 2008, p. 152.

Kron, Josh. "Uganda Seen as a Front Line in the Bioterrorism Fight." *The New York Times*, November 11, 2010, A8.

Miller, Judith, et al. *Germs: Biological Weapons and America's Secret War.* New York: Simon & Schuster, 2002. An investigation into state-sponsored biological weapons programs.

Rosebury, Theodor. *Peace or Pestilence: Biological Warfare and How to Avoid It.* New York: McGraw-Hill, 1949. A frequently referenced early work about the weaponization of biological agents.

Spiers, Edward M. *A History of Chemical and Biological Weapons.* London: Reaktion Books, 2010. An examination of the threat posed by the accessibility of chemical and biological weapons since 2001.

WEB SITES OF INTEREST

American Red Cross
http://www.redcross.org/preparedness

Centers for Disease Control and Prevention
http://www.bt.cdc.gov/bioterrorism

U.S. Department of Homeland Security
http://www.ready.gov

U.S. Food and Drug Administration
http://www.fda.gov/oc/opacom/hottopics/bioterrorism

See also: Airborne illness and disease; Bacterial infections; Biological weapons; Botulinum toxin infection; Centers for Disease Control and Prevention (CDC); Decontamination; Disease eradication campaigns; Infectious disease specialists; Public health; Transmission routes; U.S. Army Medical Research Institute of Infectious Diseases.

Bird flu. *See* Avian influenza.

Birds and infectious disease

CATEGORY: Transmission

DEFINITION

Wild and domestic birds are at risk for infections with pathogens that may lead to disease in other birds and in humans. Each type of bird may carry infections that lead to different clinical diseases. Wild birds have adapted to urban environmental settings, increasing the risk of domestic infections.

Even though infections may be spread from birds to humans, a resulting human illness is rare. Newborns, young children, and immunocompromised persons are at greatest risk for disease transmission.

AVIAN FLU

Avian flu, or bird flu, is typically found in asymptomatic wild birds. However, domestic birds such as farm chickens and ducks may become sick and spread the disease through saliva or droppings. The avian flu does not pass easily from bird to human or from human to human. Typically, the avian flu is spread to pigs and other animals that can contract both bird and human flu strains. The bird and human flu strains combine to form a new mutant strain to which humans are susceptible. The avian flu is caused by strain H5N1.

Mild symptoms resemble the seasonal flu: fever, sore throat, and muscle aches. More severe symptoms include eye infection and pneumonia and other respiratory difficulties. The risk for mortality is high because humans have no immunity to the avian flu strains. More than one-half of all persons who have been diagnosed with the avian flu have died.

Certain antiviral medications are effective, but the seasonal influenza vaccine cannot protect against avian flu. Newer vaccine combinations appear promising.

WEST NILE VIRUS

West Nile virus is a flavivirus that is spread by a mosquito that first bites an infected bird and then, newly infected, bites a human. West Nile virus was first documented in the United States in 1999, and it spread rapidly. Urban communities have a higher risk than rural populations. Symptoms may be mild, with a rash, muscle weakness, and flulike symptoms, or they may be more severe, with meningitis, encephalitis, or a lack of cognitive clarity.

In 2004, 2,200 human cases were reported; 73 of these cases ended in death. Although the virus is not as prevalent in the human population now as it was during the original outbreak, West Nile virus remains a subject of medical research. Scientists continue to work on identifying the types of birds that carry the disease and on what mechanism causes the disease to

infect both humans and birds. Antibiotics are not effective, and antiviral medication trials are ongoing.

BACTERIAL INFECTIONS

Psittacosis. Parrots and parakeets often carry the bacterium *Chlamydophila psittaci.* The disease is rare in humans; only a few hundred cases are reported each year in the United States. Veterinarians, pet-store employees, and bird owners between the age of thirty and sixty years are at greatest risk; the disease is rarely reported in children. Symptoms are usually flulike, with a cough, and are treated with antibiotics. Rarely, the presentation is more severe and includes pneumonia, infection of the heart, hepatitis, and death.

Salmonellosis. Baby chicks and ducklings often have the bacterium *Salmonella* in their intestines, hence they shed it in their droppings. *Salmonella* is also found on the feathers and beaks of birds. Chicks will not typically display signs of infection. Humans may develop salmonellosis either by holding the bird or by touching a contaminated object. Children are at greatest risk because of their improper handwashing technique and because of their tendency to put their fingers in their mouths after petting birds. Persons who are immunocompromised, elderly, or pregnant should avoid touching birds, especially chicks and ducklings. Salmonellosis results in diarrhea, fever, stomach pain, and other flulike symptoms within a few days of exposure. The symptoms typically resolve within one week.

FUNGAL DISEASES

Cryptococcosis. Cryptococcosis is a disease transmitted to humans from pigeons and chickens. The fungi *Cryptococcus neoformans,* which causes the disease, is found in soil droppings or in roosts, such as in attics and on ledges. Inhaling the spores causes the disease. Infections are usually asymptomatic or mild and include flulike symptoms, a cough, and a skin rash. In more severe forms, infection in the lungs may spread to the central nervous system and cause brain damage or become fatal. Cryptococcosis is treated with antifungal medication.

Histoplasmosis. Histoplasmosis, a disease transmitted to humans commonly from pigeons, starlings, blackbirds, and bats, is caused by the fungus *Histoplasma capsulatum.* Humans may contract the disease by inhaling air near affected soil, near roosts that have been maintained for several years, or near droppings

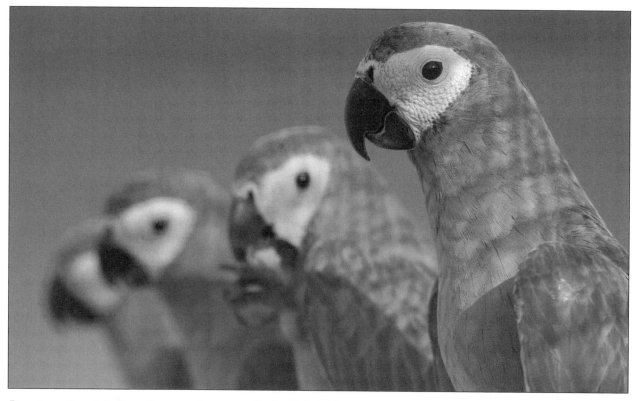

Parrots can pass infectious diseases to humans and other birds. (©Dreamstime.com)

(from bats). The spores may be airborne too and can travel great distances. Construction workers, gardeners, and those in other outdoor occupations are at highest risk because of the disruption of soil at work sites. Infections are typically mild with flulike symptoms. Rarely, the infection may lead to fever, blindness, and death. Young children, the elderly, and persons with lung disease are at greatest risk for these more significant symptoms.

IMPACT

Perhaps the greatest impact to global public health and the world economy can be found in the experiences of the bird flu pandemic of 1997. For example, government officials in Hong Kong who feared outbreaks and a significant number of deaths had ordered the slaughter of all poultry in that region (about 1.5 million birds) within three days. This slaughter led to economic problems in Hong Kong and elsewhere. The virus spread rapidly to other Asian countries, and with bird migration, the disease spread to Europe.

Continuing research into vaccines and proper edu-

cation about bird handling and care are vital to reducing the amount of human infections and preventing avian-disease-related pandemics. However, a balance should exist between preserving the wild and domestic bird populations and protecting humans.

Janet Ober Berman, M.S., CGC

FURTHER READING

Clark, Larry, and Jeffrey Hall. "Avian Influenza in Wild Birds: Status as Reservoirs and Risks to Humans and Agriculture." In *Current Topics in Avian Disease Research: Understanding Endemic and Invasive Diseases*, edited by Rosemary K. Barraclough. Washington, D.C.: American Ornithologists' Union, 2006. A good outline of the problem. Also considers human health, agricultural concerns, and the potential effect on wild bird populations.

Krauss, Hartmut, et al. *Zoonoses: Infectious Diseases Transmissible from Animals to Humans.* 3d ed. Washington, D.C.: ASM Press, 2003. Explores the myriad infections introduced by human-animal contact.

Ligon, B. "Avian Influenza Virus H5N1: A Review of

Its History and Information Regarding Its Potential to Cause the Next Pandemic." *Seminars in Pediatric Infectious Diseases* 16 (2005): 326-335. Examines the history of the bird flu and its possible future effects on global health.

Marquardt, William C., ed. *Biology of Disease Vectors.* 2d ed. New York: Academic Press/Elsevier, 2005. A biology text examining disease vectors, including bats and wild and domestic birds. Written for graduate students and researchers, but accessible to general readers.

National Association of State Public Health Veterinarians. "Compendium of Measures to Control *Chlamydophila psittaci* Infection Among Humans (Psittacosis) and Pet Birds (Avian Chlamydiosis)." 2010. Available at http://www.nasphv.org/documents/psittacosis.pdf.

Thomas, Nancy J., D. Bruce Hunter, and Carter T. Atkinson, eds. *Infectious Diseases of Wild Birds.* Ames, Iowa: Blackwell, 2007. A detailed description of the health risks to birds, other animals, and humans from avian-related infectious diseases.

WEB SITES OF INTEREST

American Veterinary Medicine Association
http://www.avma.org

Centers for Disease Control and Prevention: Healthy Pets Healthy People
http://www.cdc.gov/healthypets

National Center for Emerging and Zoonotic Infectious Diseases
http://www.cdc.gov/ncezid

See also: Airborne illness and disease; Avian influenza; Bats and infectious disease; Chlamydia; *Chlamydophila*; Coccidiosis; Cryptococcosis; Fecal-oral route of transmission; Fungi: Classification and types; *Histoplasma*; Histoplasmosis; Psittacosis; *Salmonella*; Soilborne illness and disease; Transmission routes; Vectors and vector control; West Nile virus; Zoonotic diseases.

Birth disorders. *See* Childbirth and infectious disease; Children and infectious disease; Pregnancy and infectious disease.

BK virus infection

CATEGORY: Diseases and conditions
ANATOMY OR SYSTEM AFFECTED: Kidneys, lungs, respiratory system, urinary system

DEFINITION

BK virus infection, a rare infection most commonly of the respiratory tract, is caused by the BK virus, a member of the Polyomavirus family. The BK virus was first isolated in 1971 from a kidney transplant patient with the initials "B. K."

CAUSES

It is not known exactly how the BK virus is transmitted. It is known, however, that the virus is spread from person to person (not from an animal source), possibly through saliva, air, cough, blood, needles, blood transfusions, sexual contact, pregnancy, or organ transplant.

RISK FACTORS

Elderly people are generally at higher risk of having BK infection. Males are also at higher risk. Injuries to the kidney may also cause the BK virus to become active.

Most people have unknowingly been infected with the BK virus at some point in their lives. It is likely they had the infection but had symptoms that were flulike (leading many, possibly, to believe they had the flu). The virus typically remains in a latent form and does not cause disease. It is thought that nearly 80 percent of the population contains a latent form of the BK virus. However, the virus can be reactivated if the immune system is compromised (weakened). A long-term illness, such as diabetes or acquired immunodeficiency syndrome, may weaken the immune system. Anti-rejection medications taken by organ transplant patients may also weaken the immune system.

SYMPTOMS

If symptoms do appear, they are generally mild (respiratory infection or fever). However, in immunocompromised persons, symptoms can be severe and include interstitial nephritis and narrowed ureters following kidney transplant; hemorrhagic cystitis following bone marrow transplant; increased risk of bladder cancer; encephalitis (swelling of the brain); retinitis (swelling of the retina); and pneumonitis (swelling of the lungs). Signs of BK virus infection also include stomach problems; blurry vision; brown or reddish-colored urine; burning pain or trouble when passing urine, or passing more urine than usual; cough, colds, or trouble breathing; muscle pain or weakness; and seizures.

SCREENING AND DIAGNOSIS

Diagnosis is made by blood and urine testing or biopsy. Polymerase chain reaction techniques are often used to identify the virus.

TREATMENT AND THERAPY

A mild BK infection may go away without treatment. In the severe cases seen in immunocompromised persons, decreasing immunosuppression therapy is the principle treatment. Leflunomide is frequently used because it has both immunosuppressive and antiviral properties. Quinolone antibiotics (such as ciprofloxacin) and intravenous immunoglobulin are also used. Additional treatments, such as pain medication, bladder irrigation, or hyperhydration, may be necessary.

PREVENTION AND OUTCOMES

Screening persons at high risk for BK virus infection (such as kidney transplant recipients) allows for early detection and prevention of symptomatic BK infection.

Anita P. Kuan, Ph.D.

FURTHER READING

Blanckaert, K., and A. S. De Vriese. "Current Recommendations for Diagnosis and Management of Polyoma BK Virus Nephropathy in Renal Transplant Recipients." *Nephrology Dialysis Transplant* 21 (2006): 3364-3367.

Egli, A., et al. "Prevalence of Polyomavirus BK and JC Infection and Replication in Four Hundred Healthy Blood Donors." *Journal of Infectious Diseases* 199 (2009): 837-846.

Grady, D. *Deadly Invaders: Virus Outbreaks Around the World, from Marburg Fever to Avian Flu*. Boston: Kingfisher, 2006.

WEB SITES OF INTEREST

National Kidney Foundation
http://www.kidney.org

National Organization for Rare Disorders
http://www.rarediseases.org

See also: Infection; Kidney infection; Opportunistic infections; Respiratory route of transmission; Respiratory syncytial virus infections; Viral infections; Viruses: Types.

Bladder infections. *See* Urinary tract infections.

Blastomyces

CATEGORY: Pathogen
TRANSMISSION ROUTE: Inhalation

DEFINITION

Blastomyces is a pathogenic, dimorphic, endemic soil fungus that causes a respiratory infection known as blastomycosis.

**Taxonomic Classification
for *Blastomyces***

Kingdom: Fungi
Phylum: Ascomycota
Order: Onygenales
Genus: *Blastomyces (Ajellomyces)*
Species: *B. dermatitidis*

NATURAL HABITAT AND FEATURES

Blastomyces is a soil fungus. Like other fungi, it can reproduce both sexually and asexually. The size, shape, and arrangement of cells are often very different between the sexual and asexual morphological forms of the same fungus. The sexual form of any fungus is called the teleomorph, in contrast to the asexual morphological form, called the anamorph. Technically, *Blastomyces* refers to the anamorph stage of the fungus only. *Ajellomyces dermatitidis* is the teleomorph stage and is the official name of the fungus. *Blastomyces* is one of only a few dimorphic fungi that can cause serious disease in humans. Infection by *Blastomyces* is called blastomycosis and has been recognized since the nineteenth century.

While most fungi are always either molds or yeast-like cells, dimorphic fungi can grow as either yeastlike cells or as filamentous forms (molds). Molds grow by branching and longitudinal extension (adding cells to the end of filament), while yeasts grow by budding or binary cell division. In soil or the environment, *Blastomyces* grow as filamentous molds. These molds produce conidia (asexual spores), which can become airborne and cause infection through inhalation. The conidia, after inhalation, lodge in the lungs, where infection begins. *Blastomyces* is thermally dimorphic, that is, the increased temperature of the host's body causes it to convert to yeastlike cells after infection.

Most dimorphic fungi (such as *Blastomyces, Coccidioides, Paracoccidioides,* and *Histoplasma*) are also considered endemic fungi because each of them is found primarily in a particular region of the world. For *Blastomyces,* the vast majority of cases are seen in certain regions of North America and Africa, although cases are seen worldwide. In the United States, areas endemic for *Blastomyces* are the central and southeast states, especially along the Mississippi and Ohio rivers and the upper Great Lakes region. In highly endemic areas, mean annual incidence rates can be as high as 40 per 100,000 persons. The exact ecological niche of *Blastomyces* is still unknown. Studies using molecular techniques to detect *Blastomyces* in endemic areas have generally failed to find it.

Blastomycosis is a common infection among dogs in endemic areas. Infection in dogs may serve as a warning of potential human outbreaks. Blastomycosis is also reported in other animals.

Blastomyces is infectious only in the filamentous mold form that grows in soil. Therefore, transmission occurs only through environmental sources; human-to-human or animal-to-human cases have not been reported.

PATHOGENICITY AND CLINICAL SIGNIFICANCE

Blastomycosis begins as a lung infection after inhalation of the *Blastomyces* conidia. After lodging in the lungs, the conidia germinate into the yeast form of the fungus. This change provides *Blastomyces* a distinct advantage for infection, as yeastlike cells are much more resistant to phagocytosis than are filamentous mold forms. Virulence factors are also produced in the yeast but not mold form of *Blastomyces.* The infection can then disseminate through the blood and lymphatics to other organs. The inflammatory immune response results in macrophage recruitment and, ultimately, granuloma formation.

In most immunocompetent people, the innate immune system (especially the action of alveolar macrophages) provides a natural resistance to infection with *Blastomyces.* Studies of epidemic exposures indicates that about 50 percent of people exposed to *Blastomyces* develop no symptoms (are asymptomatic).

Symptoms of blastomycosis are usually mild or nonexistent. If symptoms do appear, they include a dry cough, chest pain, hoarseness, and a low-grade fever. The symptoms may take several months to appear after the initial inhalation of the conidia. Because blastomycosis symptoms are similar to those of many other diseases, such as tuberculosis, acute pneumonia, histoplasmosis, and even influenza, diagnosis is often delayed or missed. Pneumonia is the most frequent symptom of blastomycosis, and, except in rare cases of skin infection, the lungs are the site of first infection. Infection of skin, bone, prostate, and the central nervous system are also seen in blastomycosis.

If the primary pulmonary infection does not resolve, severe progressive (chronic) blastomycosis can result. Chronic illness may resemble tuberculosis or lung cancer, with symptoms of low-grade fever, a productive cough, night sweats, and weight loss. It can sometimes be fatal. Blastomycosis can disseminate and spread infection to the skin, bones, urogenital tract, prostate, and the central nervous system. Dissemination outside the respiratory tract occurs more often in those who are immunocompromised and in persons with chronic pulmonary illness.

Reactivation of blastomycosis may occur after a pulmonary infection. In these cases, although the initial infection is resolved, live *Blastomyces* remains inside the host and are capable of causing secondary infection. Reactivation at extrapulmonary sites is very rare.

Immunocompromised persons are at much higher risk for developing severe *Blastomyces* infections. Prognosis is also much worse for immunocompromised persons with blastomycosis. Among people with human immunodeficiency virus infection or with acquired immunodeficiency syndrome, mortality rates for blastomycosis of 30 to 40 percent have been reported.

There are no known practical measures for the prevention of blastomycosis. Minimizing morbidity and mortality from blastomycosis depends primarily on early recognition and appropriate treatment of the disease.

DRUG SUSCEPTIBILITY

The in vitro drug susceptibility of *Blastomyces*, like many fungi, correlates poorly with treatment efficacy. That is, antifungal agents that may work well in the laboratory do not always work well in clinical cases. The primary antifungal drugs for treating *Blastomyces* infection are amphotericin B, itraconazole, flucanazole, ketoconazole. Amphotericin B has historically been the most effective antifungal for severe blastomycosis (especially in children). However, while effective, amphotericin B has many deleterious side effects and must be administered intravenously. Liposomal formulations of amphotericin B have with significantly less toxicity, and anecdotal reports suggest they may be effective against *Blastomyces*.

The azole class of antifungals is an equally effective and less toxic alternative to amphotericin B for treating mild-to-moderate blastomycosis. Azoles used to treat blastomycosis include itraconazole, flucanazole, and ketoconazole. While these oral drugs are less toxic than amphotericin B, they are often less effective at treating blastomycosis with central nerve system involvement. Because they most often resolve spontaneously, many cases of mild blastomycosis are treated by close supervision, rather than by antifungal therapy.

David M. Faguy, Ph.D.

FURTHER READING

Anaissie, Elias J., Michael R. McGinnis, and Michael A. Pfaller, eds. *Clinical Mycology*. 2d ed. New York: Churchill Livingstone, 2009. An advanced medical mycology textbook with chapters written by experts in their field.

Bradsher, R. W. "A Clinician's View of Blastomycosis." *Current Topics in Medical Mycology* 5 (1993): 181-200. Although somewhat dated, especially in regard to therapy for blastomycosis, this article is a well-written general review of the clinical features of *Blastomyces* infection.

Kauffman, C. A. "Endemic Mycoses: Blastomycosis, Histoplasmosis, and Sporotrichosis." *Infectious Disease Clinics of North America* 20 (2006): 645-662. A good review comparing these endemic fungal pathogens.

Saccente, Michael, and Gail L. Woods. "Clinical and Laboratory Update on Blastomycosis." *Clinical Microbiology Review* 23 (2010): 367-381. Detailed review of *Blastomyces* and blastomycosis, especially of laboratory identification methods.

WEB SITES OF INTEREST

American Lung Association
http://www.lungusa.org

Centers for Disease Control and Prevention, Division of Foodborne, Bacterial, and Mycotic Diseases
http://www.cdc.gov/nczved/divisions/dfbmd

Microbiology and Immunology On-line: Mycology
http://pathmicro.med.sc.edu/book/mycol-sta.htm

Systematic Mycology and Microbiology Laboratory
http://www.ars.usda.gov

See also: Allergic bronchopulmonary aspergillosis; Antifungal drugs: Types; Aspergillosis; *Aspergillus*; Blastomycosis; *Coccidioides*; Coccidiosis; Fungi: Classification and types; *Fusarium*; Histoplasmosis; Mold infections; Mycoses; *Paracoccidioides*; Paracoccidioidomycosis; Respiratory route of transmission; *Rhizopus*; Soilborne illness and disease; Sporotrichosis.

Blastomycosis

CATEGORY: Diseases and conditions
ANATOMY OR SYSTEM AFFECTED: Lungs, respiratory system
ALSO KNOWN AS: Gilchrist's disease

DEFINITION

Blastomycosis is an infection caused by *Blastomyces dermatitidis*, a fungus typically found in soil. It is endemic to the central and southeastern United States, Canada, and parts of Africa. This type of infection primarily affects the lungs but may spread to other parts of the body.

CAUSES

B. dermatitidis is a dimorphic fungus that exists as either a mold or a yeast, depending on the environment where it is found. The fungus is in mold form in wooded areas and waterways. Inhalation of fungal spores into the lungs causes a respiratory infection known as pulmonary blastomycosis. Once inside the body, the spores transform into a phagocytosis-resistant yeast form that creates cavities and then disperses. The most common extrapulmonary site of infection is the skin, followed by the bones, the prostate and other genitourinary organs, and the brain.

RISK FACTORS

All ages may be affected by the disease; however, the majority of reported cases involve healthy males with an outdoor occupation or hobby. Persons with diabetes mellitus or those with weakened immune systems, including organ transplant recipients and those on immunosuppressants, are more likely to have a severe form of the disease. Atypical for fungal infections, blastomycosis is not more likely to appear in persons with acquired immunodeficiency syndrome (AIDS).

SYMPTOMS

Some persons with pulmonary blastomycosis are asymptomatic, while others may have flulike symptoms that include fever, chills, myalgia, headache, cough, chest pain, weight loss, and fatigue. Extrapulmonary blastomycosis of the skin is indicated by ulcerated lesions on the face, neck, and extremities and is a significant indication of the disease. As the disease progresses, pain and lesions may occur on the bones, genitalia, parts of the central nervous system, and organs. Persons with severe disease may show symptoms simulating bacterial pneumonia, tuberculosis, lung cancer, or adult respiratory distress syndrome.

SCREENING AND DIAGNOSIS

Blastomycosis is a rare systemic infection. Primary care physicians often consult with an infectious disease specialist for diagnosis and treatment. Diagnostic tests include blood and urine analyses, tissue biopsy, sputum culture, chest X ray, and bronchoscopy. Definitive diagnosis of blastomycosis requires culture and analysis of infected tissue under a microscope.

TREATMENT AND THERAPY

Persons with blastomycosis should be treated based on the extent and severity of the disease. Amphotericin B and intraconazole are the drugs of choice. Oral intraconazole is recommended for persons with pulmonary blastomycosis. Intravenous amphotericin B is recommended for persons with severe disease. A blastomycosis infection has the potential to be fatal if untreated.

PREVENTION AND OUTCOMES

B. dermatitidis is a microscopic airborne fungus. The best form of prevention is to avoid endemic areas where the fungus is prevalent.

Rose Ciulla-Bohling, Ph.D.

FURTHER READING

Bradsher, Robert W. "Blastomycosis." In *Clinical Mycology*, edited by William E. Dismukes, Peter G. Pappas, and Jack D. Sobel. New York: Oxford University Press, 2003.

Bradsher, Robert W., and Anupama Menon. "Blastomycosis." In *Conn's Current Therapy 2011*, edited by Robert E. Rakel, Edward T. Bope, and Rick D. Kellerman. Philadelphia: Saunders/Elsevier, 2010.

Chapman, Stanley W., and Donna C. Sullivan. "Blastomycosis." In *Harrison's Principles of Internal Medicine*, edited by Joan Butterton. 17th ed. New York: McGraw-Hill, 2008.

Levitzky, Michael G. *Pulmonary Physiology.* 7th ed. New York: McGraw-Hill Medical, 2007.

McKinnell, James A., and Peter G. Pappas. "Blastomycosis: New Insights into Diagnosis, Prevention, and Treatment." In *Fungal Diseases*, edited by Kenneth S. Knox and George A. Sarosi. Philadelphia: Saunders/Elsevier, 2009.

Steele, Russell W., and Avinash Shetty. "Blastomycosis." Available at http://emedicine.medscape.com/article/961731-overview.

Webster, John, and Roland Weber. *Introduction to Fungi.* New York: Cambridge University Press, 2007.

WEB SITES OF INTEREST

American Lung Association
http://www.lungusa.org

British Mycological Society
http://fungionline.org.uk

Canadian Lung Association
http://www.lung.ca

See also: Airborne illness and disease; Allergic bronchopulmonary aspergillosis; Antifungal drugs: Types;

Aspergillosis; Chromoblastomycosis; Coccidiosis; Diagnosis of fungal infections; Fungal infections; Fungi: Classification and types; *Fusarium*; Histoplasmosis; Melioidosis; Mucormycosis; Mycetoma; Mycoses; Nocardiosis; Paracoccidioidomycosis; Respiratory route of transmission; *Rhizopus*; Soilborne illness and disease; *Stachybotrys*.

Blood-borne illness and disease

CATEGORY: Transmission

DEFINITION

Blood-borne illnesses and diseases are caused by pathogens that are transmitted through contact with contaminated blood. The most common blood-borne diseases are human immunodeficiency virus HIV), hepatitis B virus (HBV), and hepatitis C virus (HCV). HBV and HCV are both diseases of the liver. HIV is a virus that destroys immune cells, leaving the body unable to fight infection. HIV can eventually progress to acquired immune deficiency syndrome (AIDS).

EXPOSURE

Blood-borne illnesses and diseases are spread by direct contact with contaminated blood or other body fluids, such as semen. They also can be transmitted during childbirth from a woman to her fetus. Common methods of transmission include the following: having sex with a person who is infected with a blood-borne illness or disease; needle sharing during drug use; needle pricks or other puncture wounds made by sharp objects that are contaminated with infected blood or other body fluids; being splashed in the face with infected blood or body fluids (contact with eyes, nose, or mouth); sharing personal items, such as razors or toothbrushes, that have come in contact with the blood or body fluids of an infected person; getting contaminated blood or body fluid in an open sore or wound; contact with open sores on someone who has a blood-borne illness or disease; and blood transfusions.

Blood-borne illnesses and diseases cannot be transmitted through casual contact, such as hand-holding, kissing, hugging, shaking hands, or eating food prepared by someone who is infected. Also, these diseases are not transmitted through saliva unless the saliva is contaminated with blood.

There are some occupations that may put a person at risk of contacting potentially contaminated blood or body fluids. These include health care workers, sanitation workers, public safety personnel (such as police officers, emergency medical technicians, and firefighters), housekeepers, teachers, blood bank staff, dentists and dental hygienists, funeral home staff, and first aid workers.

Others who may be at increased risk of exposure to blood-borne illness and disease include men with same-sex partners, heterosexuals with multiple partners, people whose sex partners are infected, persons on hemodialysis, persons who have another sexually transmitted disease, men who are not circumcised, and injection-drug users.

Once someone has been exposed to a blood-borne pathogen, several variables may determine whether or not that person actually contracts a blood-borne illness or disease. These variables include the type of pathogen to which the person has been exposed, how the person was exposed to the pathogen, how much blood or body fluid the person came in contact with during the exposure, and the amount of virus in the infected person's blood at the time of the exposure.

PREVENTION

Some blood-borne illnesses and diseases (such as HBV) can be prevented through vaccination. The World Health Organization (WHO) and the Centers for Disease Control and Prevention (CDC) recommend that all infants be given the hepatitis B vaccine as part of their routine immunization schedule. WHO also recommends that all children under the age of eighteen years who were not vaccinated at birth be given the vaccine. It is also recommended that people in the following groups, who are considered at increased risk for exposure, should be vaccinated: people with multiple sex partners, men with same-sex partners, partners of people who are infected with HBV, injection drug users, people who frequently require blood or blood products, organ donation recipients, health care workers and other workers who are at increased risk of occupational exposure, and people traveling to countries with high rates of HBV.

There are also some high-risk settings in which many people may be at risk for HBV. The CDC recommends that all adults who receive care in the following high-risk settings be given the HBV vaccine: testing and treatment facilities for sexually transmitted dis-

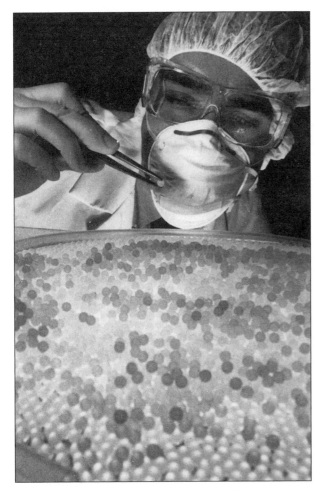

A technician inspects batches of biochemically treated beads used in a test to screen blood for evidence of early-stage HIV infection. (AP/Wide World Photos)

eases, drug abuse rehabilitation facilities, correctional facilities, hemodialysis facilities, and facilities for the developmentally disabled.

There is no vaccination for the prevention of HIV or HCV. The best way to prevent HIV, HCV, and other blood-borne illnesses and diseases for which there is no vaccination is to take the following precautions to avoid exposure to blood or body fluids of people who are or who may be infected: Wash hands before and after eating, after using the toilet, and after contact with another person's blood or body fluids; wear disposable gloves when touching anything that may have come in contact with blood or body fluids, including wound dressings; avoid sharing personal items, such as razors or toothbrushes; avoid sharing needles for injection-drug use; and use latex condoms during sex.

Health care should be using universal precautions when there is a possibility of being exposed to blood or body fluid. The CDC defines "universal precautions" as a set of precautions designed to prevent the transmission of HIV, HBV, and other blood-borne pathogens when providing first aid or health care. Universal precautions should be used when there is a potential for contact with blood, semen, vaginal secretions, or other types of body fluid, including cerebrospinal, synovial, pleural, peritoneal, pericardial, and amniotic fluids.

Universal precautions include the use of personal protective equipment (PPE), such as gloves, gowns, masks, and protective eye wear. Gloves should be worn when there is a potential for the hands to come in contact with blood or body fluids. Gloves should be changed between each patient, and hands should be washed after gloves are removed.

PPE should be worn during any procedure in which there is a potential that the health care worker may be splashed by blood or body fluids. The purpose of PPE is to keep the blood or body fluid from coming in contact with the worker's clothes, skin, eyes, mouth, or nose.

All health care workers should take precautions to prevent needle sticks by using safe practices, such as not recapping needles and disposing of needles in appropriate puncture-resistant containers. Also, a number of safety devices on the market are designed to prevent needle sticks. These devices should be used, when available.

Persons exposed to blood or to a potentially infectious body fluid can help prevent blood-borne illness or disease by taking the following measures: Areas stuck by a needle or other sharp object should immediately be washed with soap and water. Eyes splashed with blood or body fluid should be rinsed with clean water or saline. A nose or mouth splashed with blood or body fluids should be flushed with water.

A blood test may be needed following an exposure to see if the person involved has contracted a blood-borne disease or illness. Postexposure treatment may also be recommended, so immediate medical attention is critical. For example, a person who has been exposed to blood or body fluid and has not had the HBV vaccine should, according to the CDC, get the vaccine as a precautionary measure, even if the person whose blood he or she came in contact with has not been diagnosed with HBV. For persons exposed to HIV, the U.S. Public Health Service recommends a four-week course of antiretroviral drugs. There is no known postexposure treatment to prevent HCV infection.

SYMPTOMS

About 50 percent of people who are infected with HBV have no symptoms. Others may have any of the following symptoms: Fatigue, nausea and vomiting, loss of appetite, itching of the skin, pain in the upper right abdomen, dark urine, light-colored stools, or a yellowing of the skin and the whites of the eyes (jaundice).

Chronic HBV may eventually progress to cirrhosis of the liver, a scarring of the liver that prevents it from functioning properly. People who develop cirrhosis may have some or all of the symptoms associated with HBV, plus the following: bruising of the skin; swelling of the ankles and legs (edema); abdominal swelling; vomiting of blood; black, tarry stools; dizziness or fainting; confusion; and memory loss.

The severity of symptoms will depend on the progression of the disease. Cirrhosis can also increase a person's risk of developing liver cancer.

Around 80 percent of people with HCV do not have any symptoms, or only have mild symptoms, until the disease has progressed to a late stage. Symptoms of HCV are similar to those of HBV and may also include fatigue, nausea and vomiting, diarrhea, loss of appetite, pain in the upper right abdomen, dark urine, light-colored stools, and yellowing of the skin and the whites of the eyes (jaundice). Some people may live with HCV for many years without developing any major liver damage. Others will develop cirrhosis, liver cancer, or liver failure.

Symptoms of HIV vary depending on the stage of the illness. When HIV is first contracted, there may be no symptoms at all, or there may be a brief period of flulike symptoms, such as headache, fever, sore throat, and swollen lymph glands. These symptoms may also be accompanied by a skin rash. As immune cells begin to deteriorate over a period of years, the infected person may experience diarrhea, weight loss, fever, swollen lymph nodes, shortness of breath, and cough. When the disease progresses to AIDS, symptoms may include night sweats, fever, chills, diarrhea, mouth sores, cough, shortness of breath, fatigue, weight loss, skin rash, headache, and blurred vision.

TREATMENT

There is no cure for HBV, HCV, or HIV infection. Acute HBV usually resolves on its own, although medications are sometimes given to relieve symptoms. Chronic HBV is generally treated with antiviral medications that are intended to slow or stop the progression of the disease. HCV is also treated with antiviral medications and liver transplant, in extreme cases.

Liver transplant is often the only treatment option for HBV or HCV, when damage to the liver becomes severe enough to be life-threatening. If it is determined that the liver has sustained severe damage, a liver transplant may be required. Some people, however, may not be eligible for a liver transplant. These people include those who are actively abusing alcohol or drugs, those with cancer whose cancer has spread outside the liver, those who have other conditions that may make the transplant unlikely to be successful (such as advanced heart or lung disease or severe infection), those with major liver failure with associated brain injury, and those who are HIV-positive.

A liver transplant will not cure HBV or HCV, so treatment with antivirals will still be necessary following transplant surgery. Liver transplant patients will likely sustain damage to the new liver over time.

HIV is usually treated with a combination of anti-HIV drugs that are intended to control the virus. There are five different classes of drugs, and each class works in a different way to slow the spread of the virus. HIV drug classes include the following:

Non-nucleoside reverse transcriptase inhibitors (NNRTIs). NNRTIs keep the HIV virus from multiplying by interfering with a protein called reverse transcriptase.

Nucleoside/nucleotide reverse transcriptase inhibitors (NRTIs). Like NNRTIs, NRTIs keep HIV from multiplying by interfering with reverse transcriptase. The difference between the two drug classes is their method of interference.

Protease inhibitors (PIs). PIs keep HIV from multiplying by interfering with a protein called protease.

Entry inhibitors, including fusion inhibitors. Entry inhibitors and fusion inhibitors keep HIV from entering human immune cells.

Integrase inhibitors (IHs). IHs keep HIV from inserting its genetic material into human cells by interfering with the integrase enzyme.

Most persons with HIV infection are given drugs from more than one class, in case the HIV virus becomes resistant to a specific class of drugs.

IMPACT

According to WHO, approximately 2 billion people worldwide have been infected with HBV, and about 350 million people live with HBV at any given time. It is estimated that about 600,000 people die each year from complications of HBV.

WHO statistics show that HBV is endemic to China and other Asian countries, and that 8 to 10 percent of the adult population in that region is living with chronic HBV. Those same statistics show that in the Middle East, approximately 2 to 5 percent of the general population is living with chronic HBV. In Europe and North America, less than 1 percent of the population is chronically infected with HBV.

WHO estimates that about 3 percent of the world's population has been infected with HCV and that more than 170 million people are living with chronic HCV. According to WHO, in the United States, between 2 and 4 million people may be chronically infected with HCV. In Europe, between 5 and 10 million may be living with chronic HCV. In India, about 12 million people are estimated to have chronic HCV infection. Most do not know they are infected. WHO statistics also show that there are approximately 150,000 new cases of HCV in the United States and in Western Europe each year.

WHO estimates that there are 33.3 million people worldwide who are living with HIV. In 2009, there were 2.6 million people newly infected with the virus and 1.8 million people died from AIDS.

According to WHO, in sub-Saharan Africa, 22.5 million adults and children are living with HIV. There are 4.1 million people infected with the HIV virus in South Asia and Southeast Asia, 1.4 million in Central America and South America, 1.4 million in Eastern Europe and Central Asia, and 1.5 million in North America.

Julie Henry, R.N., M.P.A.

FURTHER READING

American College of Emergency Physicians. *Bloodborne Pathogens.* 5th ed. Sudbury, Mass.: Jones and Bartlett, 2008. A comprehensive manual on blood-borne illness and disease for health care workers.

Boyer, Thomas D., Teresa L. Wright, and Michael P. Manns, eds. *Zakim and Boyer's Hepatology: A Textbook of Liver Disease.* 5th ed. Philadelphia: Saunders/Elsevier, 2006.

Everson, Gregory T., and Hedy Weinberg. *Living with Hepatitis B: A Survivor's Guide.* Hobart, N.Y.: Hatherleigh, 2002. Explains hepatitis B and how it is spread, diagnosed, and treated; also examines liver transplants and living with liver disease.

_____. *Living with Hepatitis C: A Survivor's Guide.* 5th ed. New York: Hatherleigh Press, 2009. Explains hepatitis B and how it is spread, diagnosed, and treated; discusses associated emotional challenges and financial considerations; and covers liver transplants and living with liver disease.

Feldman, Mark, Lawrence S. Friedman, and Lawrence J. Brandt, eds. *Sleisenger and Fordtran's Gastrointestinal and Liver Disease: Pathophysiology, Diagnosis, Management.* New ed. 2 vols. Philadelphia: Saunders/Elsevier, 2010.

WEB SITES OF INTEREST

AIDS.gov
http://www.aids.gov

Centers for Disease Control and Prevention, National Center for HIV/AIDS, Viral Hepatitis, STD, and TB Prevention
http://www.cdc.gov/nchhstp

Hepatitis B Foundation
http://www.hepb.org

Hepatitis C Association
http://www.hepcassoc.org

See also: AIDS; Antiviral drugs: Mechanisms of action; Antiviral drugs: Types; Bacterial infections; Bloodstream infections; Cancer and infectious disease; Carriers; Childbirth and infectious disease; Contagious diseases; Epidemiology; Hepatitis B; Hepatitis C; Hepatitis vaccines; HIV; Infection; Liver cancer; Pathogens; Retroviral infections; Sexually transmitted diseases (STDs); Viral hepatitis; Viral infections.

Blood poisoning. *See* Bloodstream infections; Sepsis.

Bloodstream infections

CATEGORY: Diseases and conditions

ANATOMY OR SYSTEM AFFECTED: Blood, cardiovascular system

ALSO KNOWN AS: Bacteremia, blood poisoning, hematogenous infection, sepsis, septicemia

DEFINITION

A bloodstream infection involves the presence of large numbers of infectious microorganisms in circulating blood. The causative infectious agents are most often bacteria (leading to bacteremia) but may also be viruses, fungi, or parasites. Bacteria and other microorganisms multiplying in the bloodstream release harmful toxins, creating conditions sometimes referred to as blood poisoning. Infectious organisms in circulating blood may spread infection throughout the body (leading to sepsis), but not all bacteremia develops into widespread infection.

Initially, blood flow near an existing infected area may carry infective organisms into the bloodstream. Capillaries, the smallest blood vessels in the vascular system, may then transport microorganisms into organ tissue, sometimes affecting the function of body organs such as the heart, lungs, and kidneys (leading to systemic infection). Other biological factors can accelerate this process, including immune mediators, special infection-activated white blood cells, pro-inflammatory mediators, and coagulation factors.

Rapidly spreading bloodstream infection may overwhelm the body's immune system, resulting in a systemic inflammatory response (sepsis) with abnormal blood coagulation and interruption of oxygen delivery to body tissues. Sepsis is a serious complication of bloodstream infection that can progress to organ failure, severe hypotension (septic shock), and death. The seriousness and progression of bloodstream infection depends on a person's underlying health status and immune response.

CAUSES

Bloodstream infection may begin with bacteria migrating from an existing infection site, such as an open wound, a puncture wound, a burn, an ulcer, an infected prosthetic device, or a urinary tract infection. Other causes of bloodstream infection include infection of the skin (such as soft tissue infection or cellulitis), heart (endocarditis), lungs (such as pneu-monia or a lung abscess), or kidneys (such as pyelonephritis). Even a tooth abscess or dental work may cause oral infection that enters the bloodstream.

Common external sources of infection are indwelling intravascular and urinary catheters that are used frequently in persons in acute and long-term care. Central venous catheters are the most frequent cause of hospital-acquired (nosocomial) bloodstream infection; hemodialysis catheters are also causes.

Causative bacteria that have been identified in bloodstream infection include *Pseudomonas aeruginosa*, *Staphylococcus aureus*, pneumococcal and streptococcal organisms, and *Acinetobacter*, *Klebsiella*, and *Bacteroides* species. A definite source of infection is found in only 30 to 50 percent of all cases.

RISK FACTORS

Surgery, injury, and placement of indwelling catheters present high risk for bloodstream infection. Risk is increased in persons with existing acute or chronic infection, chronic disease (such as diabetes), or chronic alcoholism, and with persons who use IV (intravenous) drugs. People with compromised immune response, including the elderly, young children, persons with human immunodeficiency virus (HIV) infection or other immune disorders, and those being treated with chemotherapy, corticosteroids, or immunosuppressive drugs following transplantation, are at greater risk for bloodstream infection.

SYMPTOMS

Alternating chills and fever with prostration are early symptoms of bloodstream infection. Other symptoms vary depending on the primary infection site and overall health status. Progressive symptoms include mental confusion, changes in breathing and heart rate, and reduced urine output. Increased heart rate or low blood pressure may develop if the condition progresses rapidly toward sepsis.

SCREENING AND DIAGNOSIS

Early confirmation of bloodstream infection is crucial, and finding the infection source is important to treatment. A physical examination and the person's symptoms and history may help to locate existing infections. Infection derived from an intravenous catheter is suspected in hospitalized patients when no open wounds, urinary tract infection, or other obvious sources exist, especially if the intravenous line has

Blood Banks and Screening

Blood banks in the early twenty-first century faced growing challenges as new diseases threatened the purity of their blood supplies. In response to such threats, researchers attempted to design improved methods for blood banks to screen donors and blood for protection against contamination.

West Nile virus infection, a mosquito-borne disease, was first identified in the United States in 1999. In the fall of 2002, health officials discovered that organ transplant recipients had become infected with the virus through blood transfusions. The majority of persons with West Nile virus infection displayed no visible symptoms and had unintentionally donated contaminated blood. In November, the U.S. Food and Drug Administration (FDA) called for the development of a test before the outbreak of the 2003 mosquito season. Although some experts doubted that a screening method could be produced so quickly, two tests that detected minute fragments of the West Nile virus genes were in use by July 1, 2004. The tests also revealed the presence of viruses responsible for Japanese, St. Louis, and Murray encephalitis, permitting blood banks to reject blood contaminated with these diseases as well.

Although no conclusive evidence proved that either Creutzfeldt-Jakob disease (the human form of mad cow disease) or severe acute respiratory syndrome (SARS) were transmissible through blood transfusions, blood banks used verbal screening of potential donors to defend against these disease outbreaks. FDA guidelines mandated rejection or deferral of blood donations from people who might have had or might have been exposed to persons with either disease.

In 2002, the FDA approved nucleic acid amplification tests (NATs) for the hepatitis C virus (HCV) and the human immunodeficiency virus 1 (HIV1). Unlike existing tests for the presence of antibodies, which do not develop in the earliest stages of a disease, NAT reacts to small fragments of virus DNA (deoxyribonucleic acid) and can detect infections before the appearance of symptoms. The West Nile virus tests use similar methods.

Ongoing research into improved techniques for detecting bacteria and other blood pathogens, and into ways of using physical or chemical methods to destroy these organisms, may further improve blood supply safety.

Milton Berman, Ph.D.

---

been in place for one week or more. A history of kidney infection, kidney stones, or prostate disease suggests urinary tract infection, as does decreased mental function or confusion in the elderly.

Blood culture is the primary diagnostic measure in confirming bacteremia. The presence of any type of infection, fever of unknown origin, recent surgery, or placement of indwelling catheters, calls for a blood culture. The doctor will order a complete blood count with white-cell differential and will likely order an elevated white-blood-cell count. If routine urinalysis points to urinary tract infection, the doctor will order a urine culture and a urine Gram's stain.

Chest X rays may be taken to exclude lung tumor, pneumonia, or other lung infection. Diagnostic imaging such as ultrasound, computed tomography (CT), and magnetic resonance imaging (MRI) may help to identify or exclude an infection source, especially intra-abdominal infection. Hospitalized persons who have abnormal vital signs and respiratory or cardiac symptoms will need to be evaluated for evidence of sepsis.

TREATMENT AND THERAPY

An aggressive approach is crucial when bloodstream infection is suspected or confirmed. The core treatment for infection is intravenous broad-spectrum antibiotics, administered to eliminate the causative organism and prevent progression to sepsis. Ideally, antibiotic therapy is begun within two hours of a physical examination. Culture results may suggest a change in the type of antibiotics used in treatment.

Removing an infected catheter can be a critical step. Intravenous fluids, including blood transfusion, may be given dependent on urinary output. A respirator or oxygen may be needed to assist with breathing difficulty. Surgery is sometimes needed to drain an abscess or other localized infection. Oral antibiotics will be given for some time after the infection has diminished. Rarely, if kidney infection results in subsequent kidney failure, hemodialysis may be required.

PREVENTION AND OUTCOMES

Bloodstream infection cannot always be avoided, but seeking treatment early is important if fever or other signs of infection develop, particularly after injury or surgery, or in IV drug users. Hospital infection-control measures help prevent catheter-related bloodstream infection. These measures include the aseptic catheter insertion technique, the use of antibiotic-coated catheters, the use of chlorhexidine in central venous catheter protocols, and a reduction in the number of days catheters remain in place.

L. Lee Culvert, B.S., CLS

FURTHER READING

Barie, Philip S., and Steven M. Opal. "Infectious Complications Following Surgery and Trauma: Bloodstream Infection." In *Cohen and Powderly Infectious Diseases*, edited by Jonathan Cohen, Steven M. Opal, and William G. Powderly. 3d ed. Philadelphia: Mosby/Elsevier, 2010. Addresses the risk of opportunistic infection, especially bloodstream infection, following surgery or injury.

Centers for Disease Control and Prevention. "Prevention and Control of Intravascular Catheter-Related Bloodstream Infections." Available at http://www.cdc.gov/ncidod/dhap/dpac_iv.html. An online article on preventing bloodstream infections caused by misuse or poor use of intravascular catheters in health care settings.

Girard, T. D., and E. Wesley Ely. "Bacteremia and Sepsis in Older Adults." *Clinical Geriatric Medicine* 23, no. 3 (2007): 633-647. Examines the causes, diagnosis, and treatment of bacteremia and the outlook for elderly persons.

Goede, Matthew R., and Craig M. Coopersmith. "Catheter-Related Bloodstream Infection." *Surgical Clinics of North America* 89, no. 2 (2009): 463-474. A comprehensive look at catheter-related bloodstream infection and its treatment and prevention.

Que, Yok-Ai, and Philippe Moreillon. "Bloodstream Infections." In *Mandell, Douglas, and Bennett's Principles and Practice of Infectious Diseases*, edited by Gerald L. Mandell, John F. Bennett, and Raphael Dolin. 7th ed. New York: Churchill Livingstone/Elsevier, 2010. A discussion of bloodstream infection caused by staphylococcal organisms and of treatment to prevent sepsis as a consequence of bloodstream infection.

Strand, Calvin L., and Jonas A. Shulman. *Bloodstream Infections: Laboratory Detection and Clinical Considerations*. Chicago: American Society of Clinical Pathologists, 1988. A technical monograph reviewing the concepts and factors important in the selection and development of optimal blood culture systems for the detection of blood infection.

Zucker-Franklin, D., et al. *Atlas of Blood Cells: Function and Pathology*. 3d ed. Philadelphia: Lea & Febiger, 2003. An excellent pictorial presentation of blood components in different stages of function and disease.

WEB SITE OF INTEREST

National Heart, Lung, and Blood Institute
http://www.nhlbi.nih.gov

See also: AIDS; Bacterial endocarditis; Bacterial infections; Behçet's syndrome; Blood-borne illness and disease; Cellulitis; Disseminated intravascular coagulation; Endocarditis; HIV; Hospitals and infectious disease; Iatrogenic infections; Infection; Myocarditis; Neonatal sepsis; Neutropenia; Opportunistic infections; Pericarditis; Prosthetic joint infections; Sepsis; Septic arthritis; T lymphocytes; Wound infections.

Body lice

CATEGORY: Diseases and conditions
ANATOMY OR SYSTEM AFFECTED: Blood, skin
ALSO KNOWN AS: Pediculosis, *Pediculus humanus corporis*

DEFINITION

Body lice (*Pediculus humanus corporis*) are tiny parasites, up to one-eighth inch in length, that feed on human blood. They live and lay eggs (nits) in clothing folds and seams, then move to the skin to feed. An infestation or large number of body lice on one person is known as pediculosis, which is more of an embarrassment than a serious disorder.

Once off their host, lice usually die within five to seven days at room temperature, although the lice have been known to live up to thirty days. Body lice are larger and less common than their relatives, the pin-sized head or pubic lice.

CAUSES

Body lice infestations most often occur in overcrowded areas with poor hygiene. The parasites spread by direct contact. Lice do not jump or fly. Instead, they readily move from infested to noninfested persons, clothing, and linens.

RISK FACTORS

Risk factors for acquiring body lice include direct contact with infected people, clothing, or linens; not bathing regularly; wearing infected clothing; and using infected linens. Other risk factors include sleeping on reused mattresses and linens and on communal beds. Infestations are common among transients and have been known to occur during natural disasters or war.

SYMPTOMS

Body lice cause severe itching, especially at night, and red skin bumps. The lice most often accumulate under waist bands or in armpits. If present for any significant time, the infestation may cause skin sores around the waist and groin.

Long-term infestations can lead to a general tiredness and an increased chance of other diseases, such as relapsing or trench fever and louse-borne epidemic typhus. Louse-borne typhus is caused by a bacteria (*Rickettsia prowazèki*) that is found in louse droppings. Symptoms include a high fever, body ache, chills, cough, and a severe headache.

SCREENING AND DIAGNOSIS

Diagnosis is readily made by observation of the skin and clothing. It is not uncommon to self-diagnose a case of body lice. Adult body lice are light-colored (whitish-grey) and have six legs. Persons with body lice may also have head and pubic lice.

TREATMENT AND THERAPY

Treatment usually involves bathing and disposing of infected clothing and linens (such as towels and sheets). The clothes and linens can also be washed in very hot water (130° Fahrenheit) and machine dried on high heat for a minimum of twenty minutes. If lice or skin irritation continue, a physician may advise an over-the-counter (OTC) or prescription treatment. Calamine lotion, OTC steroids, or antihistamines may reduce the itching.

With careful treatment, regular bathing, and the use of clean clothing and linens (linens changed once or more per week), it is possible to completely eradicate all body lice.

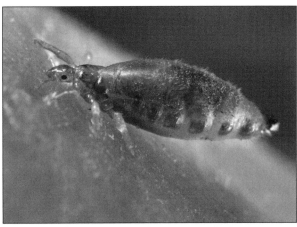

A female body louse, Pediculus humanus corporis, *getting a blood meal from a human host.* (CDC.)

PREVENTION AND OUTCOMES

To prevent lice from spreading, it is important to maintain careful hygiene and avoid contact with infected people, clothing, or linens. During a major lice outbreak, an insecticide may be used to prevent the spread of typhus.

Renée Euchner, R.N.

FURTHER READING

Ashford, R. W., and W. Crewe. *The Parasites of "Homo sapiens": An Annotated Checklist of the Protozoa, Helminths, and Arthropods for Which We Are Home.* 2d ed. New York: Taylor & Francis, 2003.

Despommier, Dickson D., et al. *Parasitic Diseases.* 5th ed. New York: Apple Tree, 2006.

Diaz, J. H. "Lice (Pediculosis)." In *Mandell, Douglas, and Bennett's Principles and Practice of Infectious Diseases*, edited by Gerald L. Mandell, John E. Bennett, and Raphael Dolin. 7th ed. New York: Churchill Livingstone/Elsevier, 2010.

"Ectoparasites." In *Textbook of Family Medicine*, edited by R. E. Rakel et al. 7th ed. Philadelphia: Saunders/Elsevier, 2007.

WEB SITES OF INTEREST

Centers for Disease Control and Prevention
http://www.cdc.gov/parasites

National Pediculosis Association
http://www.headlice.org

See also: Arthropod-borne illness and disease; Crab lice; Fleas and infectious disease; Flies and infectious disease; Head lice; Impetigo; Insecticides and topical repellants; Mites and chiggers and infectious disease; Parasitic diseases; Scabies; Skin infections.

Boils

CATEGORY: Diseases and conditions
ANATOMY OR SYSTEM AFFECTED: Skin
ALSO KNOWN AS: Carbuncle, cutaneous abscess, furuncle, skin abscess

DEFINITION

A boil is a swollen and painful red bump under the skin that is caused by an infection. Boils often start in an infected hair follicle. Bacteria then form an abscess, or a pocket of pus. Eventually, the pus may "come to a head" and drain out through the skin. Boils can occur anywhere, but common sites include the face, neck, armpits, buttocks, groin, and thighs.

There are several types of boils: a furuncle or carbuncle, an abscess caused by the bacteria *Staphylococcus aureus* or *Streptococcus pyogenes*, sometimes occurs as several boils in a group; a pilonidal cyst, an abscess that occurs in the crease of the buttocks and almost always requires medical intervention; cystic acne, an abscess that occurs when oil ducts become clogged and infected, more common among teenagers; and hidradenitis suppurativa, an uncommon disorder in which multiple abscesses occur in the armpit and the groin area.

CAUSES

Causes of boils may include bacteria, an ingrown hair, a splinter or foreign objected lodged in the skin, and a plugged sweat gland or oil duct.

RISK FACTORS

Factors that increase the chance of developing a boil include diabetes, poor nutrition, poor hygiene, a weakened immune system, and exposure to harsh chemicals.

SYMPTOMS

Symptoms include a skin lump or bump that is red, swollen, and tender. The lump becomes larger, more painful, and softer over time, and a pocket of pus may form on the boil (come to a head).

SCREENING AND DIAGNOSIS

A doctor will ask about symptoms and medical history, will perform a physical exam, and may take a bacterial culture of the boil. Some boils do not need medical attention and may drain on their own.

More serious symptoms associated with boils may require medical attention. These serious symptoms include the following: the boil worsens, persists, or becomes large or severe; patient has a fever; the skin around the boil turns red or red streaks appear; the boil does not drain; an additional boil or boils appear; the boil limits the patient's normal activities; the boil is on the face, near the spine, or in the anal area; the patient has diabetes; and many boils develop over several months.

TREATMENT AND THERAPY

A health care provider can drain the boil if necessary and treat the infection with antibiotics. Home treatment may include warm compresses (applying warm compresses to the boil for twenty minutes, three to four times a day). Depending on the area of the body affected, the boil can be soaked in warm water. These measures can ease the pain and help bring the pus to the surface. Once the boil comes to a head, repeated soakings will help the boil begin to drain.

Another treatment option is to have a doctor lance the boil, especially if the boil does not drain on its own or is unusually large. (The patient should not pop or lance the boil. Doing so can spread the infection and make it worse.) Whether the boil drains on its own or is lanced by a doctor, it must be kept clean. One should wash it with antibacterial soap and apply medicated ointment and a bandage. The affected area should be cleaned two to three times a day until the wound heals completely.

PREVENTION AND OUTCOMES

To help prevent boils, one should practice good hygiene, wash boil-prone areas with soap and water or an antibacterial soap, dry thoroughly, clean and treat any minor skin wounds, and avoid wearing clothes that are too tight.

Mary Calvagna, M.S.;
reviewed by Ross Zeltser, M.D., FAAD

Further Reading

Beers, Mark H., et al., eds. *The Merck Manual of Diagnosis and Therapy*. 18th ed. Whitehouse Station, N.J.: Merck Research Laboratories, 2006.

Crossley, Kent B., Kimberly K. Jefferson, and Gordon L. Archer, eds. *Staphylococci in Human Disease*. Hoboken, N.J.: John Wiley & Sons, 2009.

Turkington, Carol, and Jeffrey S. Dover. *The Encyclopedia of Skin and Skin Disorders*. 3d ed. New York: Facts On File, 2007.

Weedon, David. *Skin Pathology*. 3d ed. New York: Churchill Livingstone/Elsevier, 2010.

Web Sites of Interest

American Academy of Dermatology
http://www.aad.org

American Academy of Family Physicians
http://familydoctor.org

See also: Abscesses; Acne; Anal abscess; Bacterial infections; Methicillin-resistant staph infection; Pilonidal cyst; Skin infections; Staphylococcal infections; *Staphylococcus*; Streptococcal infections; *Streptococcus*.

Bordetella

Category: Pathogen
Transmission route: Inhalation

Definition

Most *Bordetella* species are obligate respiratory pathogens of animals and humans. *B. pertussis* causes a severe and potentially life-threatening disease (whooping cough, or pertussis) of infants and young children, characterized by repeated and violent coughing spells and the characteristic whooping sound that comes from breathing difficulties.

Natural Habitat and Features

The *Bordetella* species (except for *B. petrii*) are obligate respiratory pathogens of animals and humans. *B. pertussis* and *B. parapertussis* cause disease only in humans. The rest, except *B. petrii*, are found naturally in diseased animals, including birds. All have been

---

**Taxonomic Classification
for *Bordetella***

Kingdom: Monera
Phylum: Proteobacteria
Class: Betaproteobacteria
Order: Burkholderiales
Family: Alcaligenaceae
Genus: *Bordetella*
Species:
B. pertussis
B. parapertussis
B. bronchiseptica
B. avium
B. holmesii
B. hinzii
B. trematum
B. petrii

---

found, in rare cases, to cause disease in immunocompromised humans.

All *Bordetella* species are gram-negative coccobacilli that are nonfermentative and are strict aerobes. *B. pertussis* requires enriched media containing charcoal or blood (or both) to grow in the laboratory because of their sensitivity to unsaturated fatty acids and sulfur compounds in regular agar media. On Bordet-Gengou agar, *B. pertussis* forms small (less than 1 millimeter) smooth, transparent, shiny colonies with a circular edge in about five to seven days of incubation at 98.6° Fahrenheit (37° Celsius). *B. parapertussis* forms similar but larger, duller brownish colonies after two days, and *B. bronchiseptica* forms larger, rougher, and pitted colonies in one to two days on this medium. Other species can be grown successfully on less stringent media.

Bordetella species can be differentiated by growth, biochemical, and antigenic characteristics. Molecular methods, including fluorescent antibody and other immunological (serological), polymerase chain reaction (PCR), and 16S rRNA (ribosomal ribonucleic acid) gene sequencing, have been employed to identify and study properties of various species.

It has been shown through 16S rRNA (ribosomal ribonucleic acid) gene sequencing that *B. holmesii* is closely related to *B. pertussis*, *B. parapertussis*, and *B. bronchiseptica*, whereas *B. avium*, *B. hinzii*, *B. petrii*, and *B. trematum* have diverged through time.

PATHOGENICITY AND CLINICAL SIGNIFICANCE

All *Bordetella* species are pathogens. *B. pertussis* and *B. parapertussis* affect only humans and cause whooping cough. Whooping cough is most severe in infants less than one year of age, with significant morbidity and mortality rates. Roughly 85 to 90 percent of those exposed get the disease, with the majority being hospitalized. Patients with *B. parapertussis* normally have a less severe form of the disease, indistinguishable from a mild upper-respiratory-tract infection.

Older children, adolescents, and adults can also contract whooping cough. Cases are normally milder because of increased immunity; however, immunocompromised persons can experience severe disease. Research suggests that adolescents and adults can infect susceptible infants, and vice versa. Therefore, health authorities recommend giving adolescent siblings, parents, and health care workers an additional pertussis booster immunization.

B. pertussis has been studied most extensively, so its pathogenesis and the disease-causing roles of its many virulence factors are well understood. The incubation period lasts five to twenty-one days after exposure. During this time, the organism employs adhesins, including filamentous hemagglutinin, pertussis toxin, pertactin, and fimbriae proteins.

Recognizable symptoms occur during the catarrhal stage, when the pathogen multiplies rapidly. Because these symptoms resemble a common cold, the organism can be transmitted before patients realize they have a serious disease. This stage normally lasts one to two weeks, with persons exhibiting rhinorrhea, mild fever, coryza, and mild cough (although even at this stage, infants can exhibit apnea and respiratory distress).

The paroxysmal stage occurs when numerous toxins, including pertussis toxin, adenylate cyclase, dermonecrotic toxin, and tracheal cytotoxin, cause biochemical abnormalities and tissue destruction that advance the disease process and battle the host's immune defenses. During this stage, which lasts two to six weeks, characteristic multiple spasms of dry cough occur, often with projectile vomiting and exhaustion. In infants, the characteristic whoop occurs when he or she struggles to breathe.

During the convalescent stage (which last two to four weeks), patients have decreasing bouts of coughing and vomiting; however, secondary complications can occur, normally by other pathogens that can now colonize the host because of the biochemical and physical damage that occurred during *B. pertussis* pathogenesis. These complications include pneumonia, seizures, encephalopathy, and death. During this stage, recovery occurs when the host's defenses revive and when tissue, especially the ciliated epithelium, regenerates.

Most *Bordetella* species can infect animals (including birds) and immunocompromised humans. *B. bronchiseptica* can establish asymptomatic infections or serious respiratory infections in various mammals: kennel cough in dogs, atrophic rhinitis in pigs, snuffles in rabbits, and guinea pig bronchopneumonia. *B. avium* causes a potentially fatal respiratory disease of birds, including chickens and turkeys, which can result in significant economic loss. *B. hinzii* is found naturally as a commensal organism in the respiratory tracts of poultry. The least understood species, *B. trematum*, has been found associated with wounds and ear infections. *B. avium*, *B. hinzii*, and *B. petrii* have all been found in the lungs of persons with cystic fibrosis. Any disease-causing role is unclear.

DRUG SUSCEPTIBILITY

Treatment for whooping cough is primarily supportive; however, early antibiotic therapy can influence the severity and duration of the disease. It is critical to interfere with transmission to susceptible persons.

Traditionally, erythromycin has been used, but some infants experienced infantile hypertrophic pyloric stenosus. Another macrolide antibiotic, clarithromycin, has not been shown to be safe for infants. Azithromycin is effective and is preferred for infants younger than one month of age.

Azithromycin or clarithromycin are better for persons older than one month because they cause fewer side effects and less gastrointestinal upset. Persons older than two months of age who cannot tolerate a macrolide antibiotic can take trimethoprim-sulfamethoxazole for fourteen days. For persons exposed to clinically diagnosed pertussis cases, prophylaxis for five days with azithromycin or clarithromycin is recommended.

Although the efficacy of the pertussis portion of the diphtheria tetanus acellular pertussis (DTaP) vaccine is not 100 percent, immunization of infants, children, adolescents, and adults is the most effective way to combat the spread of pertussis.

Steven A. Kuhl, Ph.D.

FURTHER READING

EBSCO Publishing. *DynaMed: Pertussis.* Available through http://www.ebscohost.com/dynamed.

Levitzky, Michael G. *Pulmonary Physiology.* 7th ed. New York: McGraw-Hill Medical, 2007. A clinical text that describes and discusses the structure and function of the respiratory system.

Long, S. S. "Pertussis." In *Nelson Textbook of Pediatrics*, edited by Richard E. Behrman, Robert M. Kliegman, and Hal B. Jenson. 18th ed. Philadelphia: Saunders/Elsevier, 2007. A thorough chapter examining pertussis in children.

Mason, Robert J., et al., eds. *Murray and Nadel's Textbook of Respiratory Medicine.* 5th ed. Philadelphia: Saunders/Elsevier, 2010. Details basic anatomy, physiology, pharmacology, pathology, and immunology of the lungs.

Mattoo, Seema, and James D. Cherry. "Molecular Pathogenesis, Epidemiology, and Clinical Manifestations of Respiratory Infections Due to *Bordetella pertussis* and Other *Bordetella* Subspecies." *Clinical Microbiology Reviews* 18 (2005): 326-382. Details all aspects of *Bordetella*, including phylogeny, molecular and biological aspects of pathogenesis, and treatment options.

Sandora, Thomas J., Courtney A. Gidengil, and Grace M. Lee. "Pertussis Vaccination for Health Care Workers." *Clinical Microbiology Reviews* 21 (2008): 426-434. Examines the clinical aspects of pertussis epidemiology, treatment, and prevention and their affect on health care workers.

Weiss, Alison. "The Genus *Bordetella*." In *The Prokaryotes: A Handbook on the Biology of Bacteria*, edited by Martin Dworkin et al. Vol. 5. New York: Springer, 2006. Discusses aspects of the biology of *Bordetella*, including genus phylogeny and pathogenesis.

WEB SITES OF INTEREST

American Lung Association
http://www.lungusa.org

Canadian Lung Association
http://www.lung.ca

Centers for Disease Control and Prevention
http://www.cdc.gov

WhoopingCough.net
http://www.whoopingcough.net

See also: Airborne illness and disease; Allergic bronchopulmonary aspergillosis; Aspergillosis; *Aspergillus*; Bacterial infections; Bronchiolitis; Bronchitis; Children and infectious disease; *Chlamydophila pneumoniae* infection; DTaP vaccine; Immunization; Respiratory route of transmission; Tuberculosis (TB); Vaccines: Types; Whooping cough.

Borrelia

CATEGORY: Pathogen
TRANSMISSION ROUTE: Blood

DEFINITION

Borrelia are small, obligately parasitic spirochetes with linear DNA (deoxyribonucleic acid). They have very small genomes that lack information for many biosynthetic pathways and thus require nutrients from their hosts. They are the only spirochetes that require a blood-feeding arthropod as a vector.

Taxonomic Classification for *Borrelia*

Kingdom: Bacteria
Phylum: Spirochaetes
Class: Spirochaetes
Order: Spirochaetales
Family: Spirochaetaceae
Genus: *Borrelia*
Species:
  B. afzelii
  B. burgdorferi
  B. garinii
  B. hermsii
  B. parkeri
  B. recurrentis
  B. valaisiana

NATURAL HABITAT AND FEATURES

Borrelia spp., like all spirochetes, have a double envelope with a peptidoglycan-based wall between the plasma membrane and the outer envelope. The outer envelope contains lipopolysaccharides similar to those of gram-negative organisms and, on staining, these bacteria appear somewhat gram-negative. However, their cell walls do not contain the same lipopolysaccharides found in gram-negative bacteria, and the arrangement of the cell wall components is different. Because of this, they are not usually classified as either gram-negative or gram-positive.

Their genomes are very small, only about 900,000 base pairs compared with 4,600,000 for *Escherichia coli*, and are incomplete, lacking genes for most biosynthetic enzymes, including those for production of amino acids, nucleotides, and cofactors. They do possess numerous genes coding for production of the wide array of lipopolysaccharides and proteins found in their outer envelopes. They also possess the enzymes for glycolysis, but they lack enzymes for the Krebs cycle and aerobic respiration. Thus, they obtain most of their energy by fermentation of simple sugars.

As extracellular parasites, *Borrelia* spp. obtain their missing nutrients from their hosts. Culturing *Borrelia* spp. is difficult, but the bacteria can be grown on a complex artificial medium supplemented with rabbit serum. They grow best under microaerobic conditions at 89.6° Fahrenheit (32° Celsius) and grow slowly with generation times as long as twenty-four hours.

An unusual feature is that *Borrelia*, unlike most other bacteria, has a linear chromosome. In addition to a linear genome, the bacterium has as many as twenty or more linear and circular plasmids, many of which are thought to be involved in virulence and host specificity. The total number of plasmid base pairs can be one-third or more of the entire number of base pairs in the organism. For example, one well-studied *burgdorferi* strain contains nine circular and twelve linear plasmids that total more than 600,000 base pairs, compared with the 910,000 base pairs in its linear chromosome.

PATHOGENICITY AND CLINICAL SIGNIFICANCE

Borrelia is unique among the spirochetes in that it can be transmitted only by blood-feeding arthropods. Transmission of most *Borrelia* spp. is through various species of ticks. Ticks, small mammals, and birds serve as the main reservoirs. Humans and other large mammals usually become accidental hosts of the bacteria when they come in contact with infected ticks.

In the tick, *Borrelia* usually inhabits the gut and migrates to the salivary glands and finally the mouthparts during a blood meal. In hard ticks, the usual vector of Lyme disease, this migration is prolonged, and infection rarely occurs unless the tick has remained attached to its host for more than twenty-four

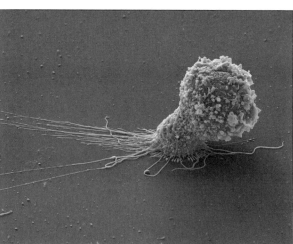

Borrelia *bacteria being engulfed by a macrophage, a type of white blood cell that eliminates microbial intruders from the human body.*

hours. Soft ticks, the usual vector of tick-borne relapsing fever, can transmit the bacteria in less than one hour.

Recurrentis, the cause of louse-borne relapsing fever, is transmitted by the human body louse; thus, humans serve as its only reservoir. In the United States, *burgdorferi* has been isolated from the gut fleas and other *Borrelia* spp. have been isolated in the guts of mosquitoes in the Czech Republic and China. Thus, fleas and mosquitoes may also be able to transmit these bacteria. None of these bacteria secrete toxins; instead, they induce severe inflammatory responses that cause most of the symptoms of borreliosis.

The major diseases of humans caused by *Borrelia* spp. are Lyme disease and relapsing fever. Lyme disease is the most common arthropod-transmitted disease in the United States and is common throughout the entire Northern Hemisphere. Usually starting with a characteristic bulls-eye rash, it can progress, if untreated, to arthritis, neuropathy, meningitis, and even permanent paraplegia. Relapsing fever is characterized by intermittent febrile episodes with relatively long afebrile periods between. Louse-borne relapsing fever shows the more severe symptoms and can become epidemic.

Borrelia spp. are often able to evade the immune system because, by turning on and off genes, they can readily change their surface proteins and lipopolysaccharides. This change in surface antigens is also the cause of the recurring fever episodes in both tick-borne and louse-borne relapsing fever.

DRUG SUSCEPTIBILITY

In all borrelioses, early treatment is the most effective. For early Lyme disease in children, two- to four-week treatments of amoxicillin are preferred. The same treatment regimen with doxycycline is used for adults. Cefuroxime and ceftriaxone are also effective. There is less agreement on the proper treatment for later chronic Lyme disease. One suggestion is two weeks of intravenous ceftriaxone followed by three months of oral amoxicillin or doxycycline. Louse-borne relapsing fever usually responds to a single dose of tetracycline, doxycycline, or erythromycin. The same antibiotics are used for tick-borne relapsing fever for five to ten days.

Richard W. Cheney, Jr., Ph.D.

FURTHER READING

Gray, Jeremy. *Lyme Borreliosis.* Wallingford, England: CABI, 2002. This book gives a good introduction to *Borrelia* infections, especially Lyme disease.

Krieg, Noel R., et al., eds. *Bergey's Manual of Systematic Bacteriology.* 2d ed. New York: Springer, 2010. Volume 4 of this multivolume work describes the Spirochaetes in detail.

Madigan, Michael T., and John M. Martinko. *Brock Biology of Microorganisms.* 12th ed. Upper Saddle River, N.J.: Pearson/Prentice Hall, 2010. This text outlines many common bacteria and describes their natural history, pathogenicity, and other characteristics.

Samuels, D. Scott, and Justin D. Radolf, eds. *Borrelia: Molecular Biology, Host Interaction, and Pathogenesis.* Norwich, England: Caister Academic Press, 2010. A comprehensive source of information about the genus *Borrelia* and its species.

WEB SITES OF INTEREST

Todar's Online Textbook of Bacteriology
http://www.textbookofbacteriology.net

Virtual Museum of Bacteriology
http://www.bacteriamuseum.org

See also: Arthropod-borne illness and disease; Bacteria: Classification and types; Blood-borne illness and disease; Body lice; Lyme disease; Microbiology; Parasites: Classification and types; Parasitic diseases; Ticks and infectious disease; Transmission routes; Vectors and vector control.

Botulinum toxin infection

CATEGORY: Diseases and conditions
ANATOMY OR SYSTEM AFFECTED: All

DEFINITION

Botulinum toxin is the most poisonous substance known to humans. Even a small amount is lethal. It is produced by bacteria in the *Clostridium* genus. The U.S. State Department reports that a number of countries that support terrorism are developing or have the toxin as a biological weapon. Some terrorists have attempted attacks using botulinum toxin that was produced from bacterial spores found in dirt. As a weapon, the toxin might be released in the air or placed in the food supply.

The toxin causes the disease botulism. In tiny doses, however, the toxin is injected as a treatment for eyelid muscle spasms, migraine headaches, and other conditions.

CAUSES

Botulinum toxin poses a great health threat. It is easy to produce and transport. Only one gram of the toxin evenly released and inhaled could lead to the deaths of one million people. However, the toxin is difficult to keep stable for release in the air. Some experts believe it would not work in stopping a military enemy. U.S. troops receive a botulinum toxoid vaccine, but release of the toxin in a civilian population would present serious results. Botulinum toxin is colorless and odorless. The toxin cannot be passed from one person to another.

RISK FACTORS

The number-one risk factor for botulinum toxin poisoning is being exposed to the toxin after its release in a biological terrorism attack. Rarely, one can be exposed to the toxin from food contamination, especially if the contaminated food was not packaged properly or was served undercooked (heat, however, destroys the toxin).

SYMPTOMS

Experts predict that symptoms from airborne bioterrorism would begin twelve to seventy-two hours after exposure. Symptoms from a food attack could start within two hours or as long as eight days after eating food with the toxin. The severity and speed of onset might vary depending on the amount of toxin absorbed. Symptoms include double or blurred vision; trouble swallowing; difficulty speaking; weakness in clenching the jaw; droopy eyelids; loss of head control; weakness, on both sides, starting at the head and working down the body; constipation; and paralysis.

SCREENING AND DIAGNOSIS

A doctor will ask about symptoms, medical history, and possible source of exposure, and will perform a physical exam. Blood, stool, and stomach contents will be tested for the toxin. Samples of questionable food may also be tested. The existence of other cases of botulism in the area may alert health care workers to the possibility of a bioterrorism attack. Special tests to confirm a diagnosis take days to complete. Tests to rule out other medical conditions include a magnetic resonance imaging scan (a scan that uses radio waves and a powerful magnet to produce detailed computer images), spinal fluid analysis, an electromyogram, and a nerve conduction test.

TREATMENT AND THERAPY

Early therapy with an antitoxin is essential to decrease resulting nerve damage. Treatment should start without waiting for confirming diagnostic test results.

If started early, an antitoxin can stop the paralysis from progressing and may shorten the duration of symptoms. It does not reverse the disease process. The most serious complication is respiratory failure. Treatment aims to maintain adequate oxygen supply. Patients may require a ventilator and close monitoring in an intensive care unit. Feeding through a tube also may be needed. Recovery occurs after the body produces new nerve fibers, a process that may take weeks or months.

Methods to eliminate the toxin include enemas, suctioning of stomach contents, and medication to stimulate vomiting. One should wash contaminated clothing and surfaces with a bleach solution, or the surfaces and clothing should be left untouched for days. Medical staff have been instructed to report all cases to public health officials.

PREVENTION AND OUTCOMES

Antitoxin could be given after a known release of the toxin, but there are limited supplies of antitoxin. In the event of a terrorism attack, the antitoxin likely would be given at the first signs of illness.

Laboratory workers and military personnel can receive a toxoid vaccine to prevent the disease by building immunity. The botulinum antitoxin is available from the Centers for Disease Control and Prevention through state and local health departments.

No warning systems exist to alert authorities that the toxin has been released. The success of an attack would depend on its secrecy, the size of the toxin particle, and weather conditions at the time of release. Persons who are aware of an attack should prepare to cover their mouth and nose with clothing or a handkerchief. Experts predict that some of the released toxin could live in dry, cool air for up to two days.

Botulinum toxin in food or drink can be inactivated by heating the food to 185° Fahrenheit (85° Celsius) for a minimum of five minutes. The toxin is also degraded under general environmental conditions. Exposed objects can be decontaminated by washing them with a 0.5 percent sodium hypochlorite solution, or bleach.

Reviewed by Ronald Nath, M.D.

FURTHER READING

Andreoli, Thomas E., et al., eds. *Andreoli and Carpenter's Cecil Essentials of Medicine.* 8th ed. Philadelphia: Saunders/Elsevier, 2010.

"Botulinum Toxin as a Biological Weapon: Medical and Public Health Management." *Journal of the American Medical Association* 285, no. 8 (2001).

Klein, Arnold W., ed. *The Clinical Use of Botulinum Toxin.* Philadelphia: W. B. Saunders, 2004.

Mandell, Gerald L., John E. Bennett, and Raphael Dolin, eds. *Mandell, Douglas, and Bennett's Principles and Practice of Infectious Diseases.* 7th ed. New York: Churchill Livingstone/Elsevier, 2010.

National Research Council. Committee on Advances in Technology and the Prevention of Their Application to Next Generation Biowarfare Threats. *Globalization, Biosecurity, and the Future of the Life Sciences.* Washington, D.C.: National Academies Press, 2006.

Novick, Lloyd F., and John S. Marr. *Public Health Issues in Disaster Preparedness: Focus on Bioterrorism.* Sudbury, Mass.: Jones and Bartlett, 2003.

Center for Biosecurity
http://www.upmc-biosecurity.org

Centers for Disease Control and Prevention, Emergency
Preparedness and Response
http://emergency.cdc.gov

National Library of Medicine
http://www.nlm.nih.gov

Public Health Agency of Canada
http://www.phac-aspc.gc.ca

See also: Airborne illness and disease; Anthrax; Anthrax vaccine; Bacterial infections; Biological weapons; Bioterrorism; Botulism; Bubonic plague; *Clostridium*; Food-borne illness and disease; Glanders; Plague; Respiratory route of transmission; SARS.

Botulism

CATEGORY: Diseases and conditions
ANATOMY OR SYSTEM AFFECTED: All

DEFINITION

Botulism is a potentially deadly illness that is caused by a toxin produced by the bacterium *Clostridium botulinum*. This bacterium is found in the soil and at the bottom of streams, lakes, and oceans. The intestinal tracts of fish, mammals, crabs, and other shellfish may contain *C. botulinum* and its spores. The bacterium's spores can survive in improperly prepared foods.

CAUSES

A small amount of the botulinum toxin can cause illness. People come in contact with this toxin in one of three ways. First, food can be contaminated with the bacterium and its toxin. It is the toxin produced by *C. botulinum*—not *C. botulinum* itself—that causes botulism in humans. Food that may be contaminated with the toxin include home-canned goods, sausage, other meat products, seafood, canned vegetables, and honey.

Second, an infant could swallow *C. botulinum* spores, leading the spores to grow in the baby's body and pro-

duce the toxin. Unlike adults and older children, infants become sick from toxin produced by bacteria growing in their own intestines. Honey is a prime source of infant botulism. Other sources include soil and dust.

Third, and rarely in the United States, a wound can become infected with bacteria. The toxin then travels to other parts of the body through the bloodstream. In some cases, the source of the bacterium is unknown. Botulinum toxin is also a potential bioterrorism agent.

RISK FACTORS

Risk factors for botulism include eating improperly canned foods and (rarely) using intravenous drugs. For infants, consuming honey is a risk factor.

SYMPTOMS

Symptoms begin in the face and eyes and progress down both sides of the body. If the disease is left untreated, muscles in the arms, legs, and torso, and those used in breathing, become paralyzed. Death can occur.

Symptoms in adults can range from mild to severe and include muscle weakness, dizziness, double or blurred vision, droopy eyelids, trouble swallowing, dry mouth, sore throat, slurred speech, difficulty breathing, and constipation. In babies, the symptoms include constipation, not eating or sucking, little energy, poor muscle tone, and a feeble cry.

When food is the cause of botulism, symptoms usually start within thirty-six hours of eating the contaminated food. Some people notice symptoms within a few hours, but others may not develop symptoms for several days. Some people experience nausea, vomiting, and diarrhea. When a wound is the cause of botulism, symptoms start within four to fourteen days.

SCREENING AND DIAGNOSIS

A doctor will ask about symptoms and medical history and will perform a physical exam. Blood, stool, and stomach contents will be tested for the toxin. In infants too, stool will be tested for *C. botulinum*. If available, samples of questionable food may also be tested for the toxin and bacteria. A wound culture will be done if wound botulism is suspected.

Tests to rule out other medical conditions include blood tests, a magnetic resonance imaging (MRI) scan (a scan that uses radio waves and a powerful magnet to produce detailed computer images), spinal fluid analysis, and nerve conduction tests.

TREATMENT AND THERAPY

The most serious complication is respiratory failure. Treatment aims to maintain adequate oxygen supply, which may require a ventilator and close monitoring in an intensive care unit. Feeding through a tube may also be necessary.

If treatment begins early, an antitoxin can stop the paralysis from progressing and may shorten the duration of symptoms. It does not, however, reverse the disease process. Methods to eliminate the toxin include enemas, suctioning of stomach contents, medication to stimulate vomiting, surgery to clean a wound, and antibiotics to treat a wound infection. High temperatures can destroy botulinum toxin.

PREVENTION AND OUTCOMES

Strategies to prevent botulism include the following: Avoid feeding honey to children who are younger than one year of age; refrigerate oils that contain garlic or herbs; bake potatoes without foil (if potatoes are wrapped in foil, keep them hot until served or refrigerate them); avoid tasting foods that appear spoiled; avoid eating food from a can that is bulging; boil home-canned foods for ten to twenty minutes before eating; practice good hygiene when canning; seek medical care for wounds and return to the doctor if the wounds look infected (exhibits redness, warmth, pus, or tenderness); and avoid injecting illicit drugs.

Debra Wood, R.N.;
reviewed by David L. Horn, M.D., FACP

FURTHER READING

Abrutyn, E. "Botulism." In *Harrison's Principles of Internal Medicine*, edited by Anthony Fauci et al. 17th ed. New York: McGraw-Hill, 2008.

Andreoli, Thomas E., et al., eds. *Andreoli and Carpenter's Cecil Essentials of Medicine.* 8th ed. Philadelphia: Saunders/Elsevier, 2010.

Behrman, Richard E., Robert M. Kliegman, and Hal B. Jenson, eds. *Nelson Textbook of Pediatrics.* 18th ed. Philadelphia: Saunders/Elsevier, 2007.

"Botulinum Toxin as a Biological Weapon: Medical and Public Health Management." *Journal of the American Medical Association* 285, no. 8 (2001).

Brachman, Philip S., and Elias Abrutyn, eds. *Bacterial Infections of Humans: Epidemiology and Control.* 4th ed. New York: Springer Science, 2009.

Mandell, Gerald L., John E. Bennett, and Raphael Dolin, eds. *Mandell, Douglas, and Bennett's Principles and Practice of Infectious Diseases.* 7th ed. New York: Churchill Livingstone/Elsevier, 2010.

Pickering, Larry K., et al., eds. *Red Book: 2009 Report of the Committee on Infectious Diseases.* 28th ed. Elk Grove Village, Ill.: American Academy of Pediatrics, 2009.

Pommerville, Jeffery C. *Alcamo's Fundamentals of Microbiology.* 9th ed. Sudbury, Mass.: Jones and Bartlett, 2010.

WEB SITES OF INTEREST

Canadian Partnership for Consumer Food Safety Education
http://www.canfightbac.org

Center for Food Safety and Applied Nutrition
http://www.fda.gov/food

Centers for Disease Control and Prevention, Emergency Preparedness and Response
http://emergency.cdc.gov

Infant Botulism Treatment and Prevention Program
http://www.infantbotulism.org

National Center for Home Food Preservation
http://www.uga.edu/nchfp

Public Health Agency of Canada
http://www.phac-aspc.gc.ca

See also: Airborne illness and disease; Anthrax; Anthrax vaccine; Bacterial infections; Biological weapons; Bioterrorism; Botulinum toxin infection; Children and infectious disease; *Clostridium*; Croup; Food-borne illness and disease; Glanders; Intestinal and stomach infections; Leptospirosis; Respiratory route of transmission; SARS; Soilborne illness and disease; Tetanus; Tularemia; Wound infections.

Breast infection. *See* Mastitis.

Breast milk and infectious disease

CATEGORY: Transmission

DEFINITION

The female breast is a "factory" of milk production. It is composed of milk-producing mammary glands and lactiferous ducts that carry milk to the nipple, which is surrounded by fatty tissue. Breast milk provides ideal nutrition for a growing newborn and offers significant advantages for the baby's immune system. It has been known for some time that breast-fed infants contract fewer infections than those who are formula-fed, but only lately have experts come to understand and identify the specific immune components that are transferred to the infant in breast milk.

Breast milk also contains microorganisms, a few of which can be passed to the infant, leading to infection and clinical disease. Rarely, the considerable benefits of breast-feeding must be weighed against the risk of transmitting infection.

Breast-feeding can also be a source of infection in the breast. Mastitis (infection of the breast tissue) is commonly seen between one and three months of delivery and may cause pain, fever, and malaise in the mother, which makes care of the newborn difficult. In almost all cases, it is recommended that a woman with mastitis continue to breast-feed.

IMMUNITY

During the first months of life, the infant's immune system is immature and unable to make the proteins and cells necessary to respond to "foreign" invaders. Breast milk helps to offer protection in a number of ways. During pregnancy immunoglobulins cross the placenta to help protect the fetus from infections. Some types of antibodies can cross the placenta. IgM, the first antibody to fight acute infection, does not cross the placenta.

All five major antibody types—IgG, IgA, IgM, IgD, and IgE—have been found in human breast milk and are active when ingested by the nursing infant. The most abundant is the type known as secretory IgA, which binds with potential pathogens, preventing them from invading the infant's system. All antibody types are specific for only one pathogen and do not attack irrelevant or commensal (good) organisms.

Other important immune molecules are present in breast milk too. Oligosaccharides (chains of sugars) and mucins (large molecules made of protein and carbohydrates) are able to clump together with invading bacteria, making them harmless.

White blood cells (leukocytes) are abundant in breast milk; most notably in colostrum, the milky fluid that precedes the flow of milk. Neutrophils, macrophages, and lymphocytes are all present and play a role in protecting the infant from disease. In addition, studies suggest that some hormones and other factors in breast milk may induce the infant's own immune system to mature more rapidly, allowing breast-fed infants to protect themselves sooner than formula-fed infants.

INFECTION TRANSMISSION

Few organisms are passed readily by breast milk to cause clinical infection, and it may be difficult to accurately determine the mode of transmission, because breast-feeding requires close contact between mother and infant. Some infections that are spread during the breast-feeding period pass by other means, such as airborne droplets or skin contact. Concern about infection rarely leads to a recommendation against breast-feeding.

Three viruses can be transmitted through breast milk and are of greatest clinical concern. These include cytomegalovirus (CMV), human immunodeficiency virus (HIV), which causes acquired immunodeficiency syndrome or AIDS, and human T-lymphotrophic virus (HTLV). It is thought that transmission occurs through exposure to small amounts of virus for several feedings each day during the prolonged period of breast-feeding.

CMV is a common cause of congenital infection. Most women are infected before becoming pregnant and develop antibodies that cross the placenta to protect the growing fetus and breast-feeding infant. However, if the woman experiences primary infection during pregnancy or breast-feeding, inadequate immune resources and infection can result.

Breast-feeding by an HIV-positive mother increases transmission risk up to 25 percent, in addition to the risk of perinatal transmission. There is no adequate immune protection for mother or infant. HIV-positive mothers should avoid breast-feeding to prevent mother-to-child transmission.

HTLV is a cause of adult leukemia and other chronic

conditions, and it is endemic to several regions of the world. Transmission occurs more often in breast-fed than in formula-fed infants. Mother-to-child transmission can be avoided by not breast-feeding.

Bacterial and other infections are rarely passed to infants through breast milk. Some infections, including having gonorrhea, group B strep, syphilis, or tuberculosis, could lead to an interruption of breast-feeding for a brief time, while the mother or the mother and infant begin antimicrobial therapy. One should not necessarily stop breast-feeding if using antibiotics.

INFECTION IN THE LACTATING BREAST

Mastitis can occur when bacteria from the infant's mouth or the mother's skin enter a duct through a sore, cracked nipple and multiply in breast milk, which is an ideal growth medium. This condition may lead to a localized, minor infection or a more serious deep-breast abscess. Symptoms include tenderness and swelling of the breast, fever, chills, and other flulike symptoms.

Breast infections require treatment with antibiotics. Prevention includes good hygiene and handwashing and proper breast-feeding technique to avoid cracked nipples. Most women with mastitis should continue to breast-feed; doing so does not harm the infant. Also, emptying the breast through feeding speeds healing.

IMPACT

Breast-feeding provides important protection against disease. The immunologic benefits are well documented and beyond question. For those few circumstances where disease transmission is of concern, more work is needed to develop vaccines and other interventions.

Rachel Zahn, M.D.

FURTHER READING

Barbosa-Cesnik, C., K. Schwartz, and B. Foxman. "Lactation Mastitis." *Journal of the American Medical Association* 289 (2003): 1609-1612.

Huggins, Kathleen. *The Nursing Mother's Companion.* 5th ed. Boston: Harvard Common Press, 2005.

Jackson, Kelly M., and Andrea M. Nazar. "Breast-feeding, the Immune Response, and Long-Term Health." *Journal of the American Osteopathic Association* 106, no. 4 (2006): 203-207.

Lawrence, Robert, and Ruth Lawrence, eds. *Breast-feeding: A Guide for the Medical Profession.* St. Louis, Mo.: Mosby, 1999.

Mestecky, Jim, et al., eds. *Immunology of Milk and the Neonate.* New York: Plenum Press 1991.

Riordan, Jan, ed. *Breastfeeding and Human Lactation.* 4th ed. Sudbury, Mass.: Jones and Bartlett, 2010.

WEB SITES OF INTEREST

American Congress of Obstetricians and Gynecologists
http://www.acog.org

BreastFeeding.com
http://www.breastfeeding.com

Healthy Child Healthy World
http://www.healthychild.org

La Leche League International
http://www.llli.org

Women's Health Matters
http://www.womenshealthmatters.ca

Women's Health.gov
http://www.womenshealth.gov

See also: Abscesses; Antibodies; Brucellosis; Children and infectious disease; Cytomegalovirus infection; Food-borne illness and disease; HIV; Immunity; Mastitis; Methicillin-resistant staph infection; Pregnancy and infectious disease; Skin infections; Staphylococcal infections; Transmission routes; Vertical disease transmission; Women and infectious disease.

Bronchiolitis

CATEGORY: Diseases and conditions
ANATOMY OR SYSTEM AFFECTED: Lungs, respiratory system

DEFINITION

Bronchiolitis is most often a childhood disease that affects the lungs. It occurs when a virus enters the respiratory system. The virus causes the tiny airways in the lungs to become swollen. As a result, a thick fluid called mucus collects in the airways, making it difficult for air to flow freely in the lungs.

Usually, the infection goes away after seven to ten days. Some children show mild symptoms. In others, the disease can be severe. Older children are less at risk. If they get bronchiolitis, they do not get as sick as younger children.

Causes

This infection is caused by several kinds of viruses. It easily spreads from person to person in the same way a common cold does. This most often happens when an infected person coughs or sneezes. Droplets of moisture are released into the air, and an uninfected person can become infected by breathing that air.

Risk Factors

Bronchiolitis can affect anyone, but it most often strikes children under the age of two years, especially between three and six months of age, and most often during the winter months. Adults most at risk are those who are immunocompromised or are exposed to toxic fumes. Children most at risk are those who were never breast-fed or were born prematurely, those exposed to tobacco smoke, those who are often in groups of children (as in day care), and those who are living in crowded conditions.

Symptoms

Symptoms of bronchiolitis occur in two stages. During the first two to three days, the child will probably have a runny or stuffy nose and a slight fever. During the next two to three days, the symptoms will increase to include a cough (dry), fever, sneezing, rash, red eyes, fast rate of breathing, difficulty breathing, wheezing (making a whistling noise during breathing), bluish color in the skin (especially around the lips or nails), poor feeding, and restlessness.

Screening and Diagnosis

To diagnose bronchiolitis, the doctor may listen to the child's lungs to check for abnormal breathing, such as wheezing; order a chest X ray to check for swelling in the airways and signs of pneumonia (in severe cases); obtain sample mucus from the nose or throat to test for the virus that may be causing the infection; and test the blood to determine the level of oxygen in the blood and to obtain a complete blood count.

Treatment and Therapy

There is no medication to cure viral infections. Doctors sometimes prescribe corticosteroids. This may help to reduce swelling and mucus in the airways, but there is limited evidence showing their benefits.

The infection usually clears on its own after a week or ten days. There are several ways to make the child more comfortable while he or she is experiencing symptoms: having the child drink clear liquids, and using a vaporizer in the child's bedroom; when the child is coughing or having difficulty breathing, steaming the bathroom using hot water from the shower (and sitting in the bathroom with the child); not smoking in front of child; and using acetaminophen (such as children's or infant's Tylenol) if a fever is present.

In severe cases, medical treatment may be needed. The doctor will check for dehydration and pneumonia and will make sure the child is getting enough oxygen. Medications may be prescribed.

One should consult a doctor if the sick child is vomiting and cannot keep liquids down; is breathing fast (more than forty breaths in one minute); has bluish skin, especially around the lips or on the fingertips; has to sit up to breathe; was born prematurely or has a history of heart disease; or appears dehydrated.

Prevention and Outcomes

Bronchiolitis can spread easily from one person to another. To prevent giving the infection to others, children should be kept home until they are no longer sick.

There is no vaccine to prevent bronchiolitis. There are medications that may lessen the risk of infection by respiratory syncytial virus (RSV), a virus that causes more than one-half of all cases of bronchiolitis. This medication is usually given to high-risk babies.

Proper handwashing habits can help to prevent the spread of illness. Family members should wash their hands before touching a baby or after being in contact with an infected child.

Julie J. Martin, M.S.; reviewed by Christine Colpitts, M.A., CRT

Further Reading

American Academy of Family Physicians. "Bronchiolitis and Your Child." Available at http://familydoctor. org.

Corneli, H. M., et al. "A Multicenter, Randomized, Controlled Trial of Dexamethasone for Bronchiolitis." *New England Journal of Medicine* 357 (2007): 331-339.

Gadomski, A. M., and A. L. Bhasale. "Bronchodilators for Bronchiolitis." *Cochrane Database of Systematic Reviews* (2006): CD001266. Available through *EBSCO DynaMed Systematic Literature Surveillance* at http://www.ebscohost.com/dynamed.

Mason, Robert J., et al., eds. *Murray and Nadel's Textbook of Respiratory Medicine.* 5th ed. Philadelphia: Saunders/Elsevier, 2010.

Myers, Adam. *Respiratory System.* Philadelphia: Mosby/Elsevier, 2006.

National Library of Medicine. "Bronchiolitis." Available at http://www.nlm.nih.gov/medlineplus/ency/article/000975.htm.

Panickar, J., et al. "Oral Prednisolone for Preschool Children with Acute Virus-Induced Wheezing." *New England Journal of Medicine* 360 (2009): 329-338. Available through *EBSCO DynaMed Systematic Literature Surveillance* at http://www.ebscohost.com/dynamed.

Porter, Robert S., et al., eds. *The Merck Manual Home Health Handbook.* 3d ed. Whitehouse Station, N.J.: Merck Research Laboratories, 2009.

Smyth, R. L., and P. J. Openshaw. "Bronchiolitis." *The Lancet* 368 (2006): 312-322.

Steiner, R. W. P. "Treating Acute Bronchiolitis Associated with RSV." *American Family Physician* 69 (2004): 325-330.

WEB SITES OF INTEREST

American Academy of Family Physicians
http://familydoctor.org

American Lung Association
http://www.lungusa.org

Canadian Lung Association
http://www.lung.ca

National Library of Medicine
http://www.nlm.nih.gov

See also: Airborne illness and disease; Allergic bronchopulmonary aspergillosis; *Aspergillus*; Atypical pneumonia; Bronchitis; Children and infectious disease; Common cold; Contagious diseases; Croup; Diphtheria; Histoplasmosis; Influenza; Legionnaires' disease; Pneumonia; Respiratory route of transmission; Respiratory syncytial virus infections; Viral infections; Viral upper respiratory infections; Whooping cough.

Bronchitis

CATEGORY: Diseases and conditions
ANATOMY OR SYSTEM AFFECTED: Lungs, respiratory system, throat
ALSO KNOWN AS: Lower respiratory tract infection, upper respiratory tract infection

DEFINITION

The bronchi are air passages of the lungs. Bronchitis is inflammation of the bronchi. The condition can make breathing difficult and can also be painful. The different types of bronchitis are acute bronchitis (a sudden onset of symptoms) that lasts a short time. There is full recovery of lung function.

Another type is chronic bronchitis, a long-term, serious condition that causes obstruction and erosion of the lungs. It is often the result of many years of cigarette smoking. It is a type of chronic obstructive pulmonary disease (COPD). Another type is asthmatic bronchitis, which occurs in people with asthma and during an asthma attack. Asthmatic bronchitis is most common with allergies. Bronchitis is caused by frequent contact with certain irritants, especially at a person's workplace. Irritative bronchitis is also known as industrial or environmental bronchitis.

CAUSES

Bronchi inflammation may be caused by bacterial and viral infections, smoking (cigarettes or marijuana), and inhalation of respiratory irritants such as ammonia, chlorine, minerals, or vegetable dusts, usually in work settings.

RISK FACTORS

Risk factors for bronchitis include smoking, exposure to secondhand smoke, contact with a person infected with bronchitis, viral upper-respiratory-tract infection (cold or influenza), asthma, chronic sinusitis, occupational exposures to respiratory inhalants, smog (in susceptible persons), enlarged tonsils or adenoids (or both), and malnutrition.

SYMPTOMS

Symptoms will depend on the type of bronchitis. In acute bronchitis, the symptoms are runny nose; malaise; slight fever; back and muscle pain; sore throat; a cough, initially dry, that produces mucus that may be thick, yellow, green, or blood-streaked; and wheezing. In chronic bronchitis, the symptoms include a cough that brings up yellow-green mucus, often worse in the morning; difficulty breathing; bluish tint to lips and skin (in severe cases); and swelling of the feet (in end-stage cases).

SCREENING AND DIAGNOSIS

A doctor will ask about symptoms and medical history and will perform a physical exam. For acute bronchitis, tests are rare. However, the following may be recommended for severe or questionable cases: a blood test; chest X rays, to rule out pneumonia, which is a complication of bronchitis; pulse oximetry, to measure the amount of oxygen in the blood; and a bronchoscopy to obtain sputum for a culture.

For chronic bronchitis, tests may include a blood test; chest X rays; pulmonary function tests or spirometry (to evaluate lung function); sputum culture; arterial blood gas (to test for levels of oxygen, carbon dioxide, and acid in the blood); pulse oximetry; and a bronchoscopy to obtain sputum for a culture.

TREATMENT AND THERAPY

For acute bronchitis, treatment is aimed at relieving the symptoms. Treatment includes aspirin or acetaminophen to treat pain and fever, expectorants or cough suppressants, increased fluid intake, cool-mist humidification, and herbs and supplements (pelargonium sidoides extract may help resolve symptoms in persons with acute bronchitis). Antibiotics will not be helpful if the infection is viral.

There are some concerns about the safety of over-the-counter cough and cold products. The concern is highest for children under two years of age. It is best to avoid these, especially in young children. A doctor should be consulted about medication options.

For chronic bronchitis, treatment is based on age, overall health, extent of the disease, and past response to treatments. Treatment may include oral antibiotics and bronchodilators, particularly clarithromycin. If the patient has chronic bronchitis and mild-to-moderate COPD, he or she may not need antibiotics. A study found that shorter antibiotic treatment (five days or less) is as effective as longer treatment (more than five days).

Treatment for chronic bronchitis also includes bronchodilators, oral or intravenous corticosteroid medications, inhaled bronchodilators or corticosteroids, expectorants to loosen secretions, mucolytics, supplemental oxygen, cool-mist humidification, lung reduction surgery (removal of the most damaged part of the lungs, in severe cases), and lung transplant (in end-stage cases).

PREVENTION AND OUTCOMES

To reduce the chance of getting bronchitis, one should stop smoking, avoid passive (secondhand) smoke, avoid exposure to respiratory irritants, and avoid contact with people who have bronchitis.

Jill Shuman, M.S., RD, ELS; reviewed by Christine Colpitts, M.A., CRT

FURTHER READING

Bishai, W. R. "Macrolide Immunomodulatory Effects and Symptom Resolution in Acute Exacerbation of Chronic Bronchitis and Acute Maxillary Sinusitis: A Focus on Clarithromycin." *Expert Review of Anti-Infective Therapy* 4 (2006): 405-416.

El Moussaoui, R., et al. "Short-Course Antibiotic Treatment in Acute Exacerbations of Chronic Bronchitis and COPD." *Thorax* 63 (2008): 415-422. Available through *EBSCO DynaMed Systematic Literature Surveillance* at http://www.ebscohost.com/dynamed.

Mason, Robert J., et al., eds. *Murray and Nadel's Textbook of Respiratory Medicine*. 5th ed. Philadelphia: Saunders/Elsevier, 2010.

Myers, Adam. *Respiratory System*. Philadelphia: Mosby/Elsevier, 2006.

Smith, S., et al. "Antibiotics for Acute Bronchitis." *Cochrane Database of Systematic Reviews* (2009): CD000245. Available through *EBSCO DynaMed Systematic Literature Surveillance* at http://www.ebscohost.com/dynamed.

Timmer, A., et al. "Pelargonium Sidoides Extract for Acute Respiratory Tract Infections." *Cochrane Database of Systematic Reviews* (2008): CD006323. Available through *EBSCO DynaMed Systematic Literature Surveillance* at http://www.ebscohost.com/dynamed.

U.S. Food and Drug Administration. "Public Health Advisory: FDA Recommends that Over-the-Counter (OTC) Cough and Cold Products Not Be Used for

Infants and Children Under Two Years of Age." Available at http://www.fda.gov/safety/medwatch.

WEB SITES OF INTEREST

American Lung Association
http://www.lungusa.org

Canadian Lung Association
http://www.lung.ca

National Heart, Lung, and Blood Institute
http://www.nhlbi.nih.gov

See also: Airborne illness and disease; Allergic bronchopulmonary aspergillosis; *Aspergillus*; Atypical pneumonia; Bronchiolitis; Common cold; Coronavirus infections; Histoplasmosis; Influenza; Legionnaires' disease; Pneumonia; Respiratory route of transmission; Sinusitis; Viral infections; Viral upper respiratory infections; Whooping cough.

Brucella

CATEGORY: Pathogen
TRANSMISSION ROUTE: Direct contact, ingestion, inhalation

DEFINITION

Brucella are gram-negative, nonmotile, non-spore-forming, nonencapsulated, small coccobacilli of worldwide distribution. They are pathogenic in animals, including humans.

NATURAL HABITAT AND FEATURES

The taxonomy of the genus *Brucella* has gone through several changes. By 1986, there were six recognized species, but scientists believed that not enough genetic difference existed among them and thus suggested that all be combined as *B. melitensis*, with the old species names listed as a subspecies. In 2010, the International Committee on Systematics of Prokaryotes, subcommittee on the taxonomy of *Brucella*, unanimously agreed to reinstate the original six species and to add four additional species.

Each of the ten species has a different host range and has some metabolic differences. Two species that

---

Taxonomic Classification for *Brucella*

Kingdom: Bacteria
Phylum: Proteobacteria
Class: Alphaproteobacteria
Order: Rhizobiales
Family: Brucelliaceae
Genus: *Brucella*
Species:
  B. abortus
  B. canis
  B. ceti
  B. inopinata
  B. melitensis
  B. microti
  B. neotomae
  B. ovis
  B. pinnipedialis
  B. suis

---

have been most studied and whose DNA (deoxyribonucleic acid) has been sequenced, *melitensis* and *abortus*, have two circular chromosomes, one with just more than 2 million base pairs and one with just more than 1 million base pairs.

Brucella spp. are small, gram-negative coccobacilli, approximately 0.5 micrometers (µm) in diameter and 0.6 to 1.5 µm in length. With the exception of *microti*, they are slow-growing in culture, often taking several days to weeks to show growth. Nutritionally, they are considered to be fastidious and require several vitamins and amino acids.

Both *abortus* and *melitensis* grow best when erythritol is added to the medium as a carbon source. They are considered facultative intracellular parasites and can survive for long periods in soil and water. They have worldwide distribution and reservoirs in several domestic and nondomestic mammal species. Studies with *microti* suggest that, in addition to its normal vole reservoir, soil could serve as a reservoir for this species. In their animal reservoirs, there is often a high concentration of bacteria in the reproductive organs; these bacteria are transferred during sex, by licking of the external genitalia, and by contact with the placenta and fluids released during birth. Carnivores can sometimes become infected when they eat an infected animal.

PATHOGENICITY AND CLINICAL SIGNIFICANCE

Each *Brucella* species has a small group of mammals that can serve as hosts. For example, *abortus* affects cattle, bison, buffalo, elk, camels, and yaks; *melitensis* affects sheep, goats, and camels; *suis* affects swine; and *canis* infects dogs. Immunizations and the slaughter of infected animals have eradicated or nearly eradicated brucellosis in many parts of the industrialized world. In the United States, *abortus* infection in domestic cattle has been almost extirpated; however, a reservoir of the bacteria exist in bison and elk in and around Yellowstone National Park. Humans are accidental hosts when they ingest infected meat or unpasteurized dairy products or come in contact with infected body fluids from one of the usual host animals.

In the United States, human brucellosis is rare, causing fewer than one hundred cases per year. It is much more common in the countries bordering the Mediterranean, in countries of the Arabian Peninsula, in India, and in Latin America. In humans, *abortus*, *melitensis*, *canis*, and *suis* can all cause classical brucellosis, while *ceti* and *pinnepedialis* have been associated with neural brucellosis.

Brucellosis, also known as undulant fever, Mediterranean fever, Malta fever, and Crimean fever, has varied, nonspecific, flulike symptoms such as fever, malaise, joint pain, headache, and fatigue. In humans, *melitensis* infections are the most common and cause the most severe symptoms, which can, on rare occasions, lead to death. *Suis* infections are also quite severe and can lead to prolonged illness, often with pus-forming lesions. *Abortus* and *canis* infections are often mild and self-limiting.

Brucellosis can be acute or chronic, with chronic infection being associated with severe debility and increased morbidity. In addition, relapsing brucellosis is difficult to distinguish from reinfection. Subclinical infections are also seen in high-risk occupations, such as veterinarians and workers on the kill-floor of slaughterhouses. In these subclinical infections, the person is asymptomatic but shows *Brucella* infection after serologic screening.

DRUG SUSCEPTIBILITY

Because of high relapse rates with single drug therapy, most treatment regimens are based on two drugs. For adults, recommended drugs are oral doxycycline or ciprofloxacin for six weeks, with either oral rifampin for six weeks or intramuscular streptomycin or gentamicin for three weeks. The streptomycin or gentamicin treatment leads to fewer relapses, and gentamicin has fewer side effects. For children under eight years of age, doxycycline is not recommended. Instead, a regimen using rifampin and trimethoprim-sulfamethoxazole is the standard. Although immunizations have been developed for several species of domestic animals, there is no human immunization against brucellosis.

Richard W. Cheney, Jr., Ph.D.

FURTHER READING

Corbel, Michael J. *Brucellosis in Humans and Animals.* Geneva: World Health Organization Press, 2006. This volume covers both animal and human *Brucella* infections and includes their epidemiology, diagnoses, and prevention.

Krieg, Noel R., et al., eds. *Bergey's Manual of Systematic Bacteriology.* 2d ed. New York: Springer, 2010. Volume 2 of this multivolume work describes the Proteobacteria in detail.

Lopez-Goni, Ignacio, and Ignacio Moriyon, eds. *Brucella: Molecular and Cellular Biology.* Wymondhan, England: Horizon Bioscience, 2004. A comprehensive review of the genus *Brucella* and its varied species.

Madigan, Michael T., and John M. Martinko. *Brock Biology of Microorganisms.* 12th ed. Upper Saddle River, N.J.: Pearson/Prentice Hall, 2010. This text outlines many common bacteria and describes their natural history, pathogenicity, and other characteristics.

Romich, Janet A. *Understanding Zoonotic Diseases.* Clifton Park, N.Y.: Thomson Delmar, 2008. A good introduction to zoonotic diseases, including those caused by *Brucella* species.

WEB SITES OF INTEREST

Centers for Disease Control and Prevention
http://www.cdc.gov/nczved/divisions/dfbmd/diseases/brucellosis

Todar's Online Textbook of Bacteriology
http://www.textbookofbacteriology.net

U.S. Department of Agriculture
http://www.usda.gov

See also: Bacteria: Classification and types; Bacteriology; Brucellosis; Brucellosis vaccine; Fever; Foodborne illness and disease; Zoonotic diseases.

Brucellosis

CATEGORY: Diseases and conditions
ANATOMY OR SYSTEM AFFECTED: All
ALSO KNOWN AS: Bang's disease, Malta fever, undulant fever

DEFINITION

Brucellosis, a rare bacterial disease that causes intermittent fevers, is primarily passed among animals, but people can acquire this disease from domesticated and farm animals. The disease results in flulike symptoms and may cause long-lasting symptoms. Only about one hundred to two hundred reported cases of brucellosis in humans are reported in the United States each year.

CAUSES

Brucellosis is caused by the bacterium *Brucella*. This bacterium primarily infects domesticated animals, but it can be spread to humans in a number of ways, including by consuming unpasteurized milk and dairy foods from infected cows, sheep, or goats; through direct contact with the secretions, excretions, or carcasses of infected animals; by inhaling the bacterium; by breast-feeding (passed from mother to infant); by sex; and by tissue transplantation.

RISK FACTORS

Risk factors for brucellosis include eating or drinking unpasteurized dairy foods, especially when traveling, and working with domesticated animals and livestock, especially sheep, goats, cattle, deer, elk, and pigs, and working with their excretions, secretions, or carcasses. Boys and men are at higher risk, likely because of occupational exposure in male-dominated jobs, including farming, ranching, veterinary medicine, tannery work, and slaughterhouse work.

SYMPTOMS

Symptoms of brucellosis, which usually appear within two weeks of infection, also can appear from five days to several months after infection. In the early stage, symptoms may include malaise, lethargy, headache, muscle pain, fever, chills, severe headache and backache, nausea, vomiting, and diarrhea. As it progresses, brucellosis causes a severe fever (104° to 105° Fahrenheit). This fever occurs in the evening and includes severe sweating. It becomes normal or near normal in the morning and usually begins again at night.

This intermittent fever usually lasts one to five weeks, after which symptoms usually subside or disappear for two days to two weeks. Then the fever recurs. In some patients, the fever recurs only once. In others, the disease becomes chronic, and the fever recurs, subsides, and then recurs repeatedly over months or years.

In later stages, brucellosis can cause loss of appetite, weight loss, abdominal pains, headache, backache, joint pain, weakness, irritability, and insomnia. Patients usually recover within two to five weeks. Rarely, complications can develop. These complications may include abscesses within the liver or spleen; enlargement of the liver, spleen, or lymph nodes; and inflammation and infection of organs in the body, such as the heart (endocarditis), brain and brain lining (meningitis), and bones (osteomyelitis), especially the spine. Brucellosis is also believed to cause a high rate of miscarriage during early pregnancy in infected women.

SCREENING AND DIAGNOSIS

A doctor will ask about symptoms and medical history and will perform a physical exam. Tests may include blood, urine, bone marrow, or tissue tests to look for *Brucella* bacteria; a blood test to look for antibodies against the bacteria; and imaging tests (X ray; computed tomography, or CT, scan; and magnetic resonance imaging, or MRI, scan) to reveal abscesses, calcifications, or enlargement of the liver, spleen, or vertebrae.

TREATMENT AND THERAPY

Many persons recover from brucellosis on their own. However, early diagnosis and treatment can reduce the risk of complications and infection. Treatment options include antibiotics, which a doctor may prescribe. One or more antibiotics (usually doxycycline and rifampin) could be prescribed to control and prevent relapses of brucellosis. Antibiotics are given for up to six weeks.

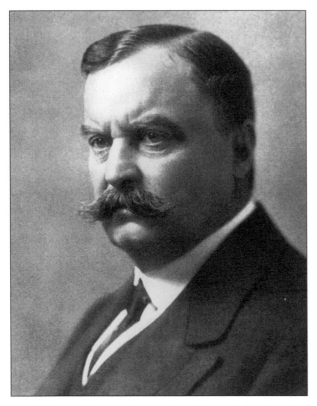

In 1887, Scottish microbiologist David Bruce isolated the bacterium that causes brucellosis.

PREVENTION AND OUTCOMES

To help reduce the chance of getting brucellosis, one should take the following steps: Avoid eating or drinking unpasteurized milk and dairy foods. If one is unsure that a dairy product is pasteurized, avoid consuming that product. One should wear rubber gloves and goggles; securely cover open wounds when handling domesticated animals, including their secretions, excretions, or carcasses; and wear a protective mask when dealing with brucellosis cultures in the laboratory.

One should also vaccinate cattle and bison that live in areas heavily infected with brucellosis. An accredited veterinarian or government health official (the vaccine contains a live virus and is dangerous to humans) can vaccinate animals. For best results, calves should be vaccinated when they are between the age of four and six months. There is no brucellosis vaccine for humans.

Krisha McCoy, M.S.;
reviewed by David L. Horn, M.D., FACP

FURTHER READING

Centers for Disease Control and Prevention. Division of Bacterial and Mycotic Diseases. "Brucellosis." Available at http://www.cdc.gov/ncidod/dbmd/diseaseinfo/brucellosis_g.htm.

Franco, M. P., et al. "Human Brucellosis." *Lancet Infectious Diseases* 7 (2007): 775.

Mackowiak, Philip A., ed. *Fever: Basic Mechanisms and Management.* 2d ed. Philadelphia: Lippincott-Raven, 1997.

Porter, Robert S., et al., eds. *The Merck Manual Home Health Handbook.* 3d ed. Whitehouse Station, N.J.: Merck Research Laboratories, 2009.

Purwar, S. "Human Brucellosis: A Burden of a Half-Million Cases per Year." *Southern Medical Journal* 100 (2007): 1074.

WEB SITES OF INTEREST

Centers for Disease Control and Prevention
http://www.cdc.gov/nczved/divisions/dfbmd/diseases/brucellosis

Communicable Disease Control
http://www.gov.mb.ca/health/publichealth/cdc

National Foundation for Infectious Diseases
http://www.nfid.org

U.S. Department of Agriculture
http://www.usda.gov

See also: Airborne illness and disease; Asplenia; Breast milk and infectious disease; *Brucella*; Brucellosis vaccine; Cat scratch fever; Fever; Food-borne illness and disease; Influenza; Mastitis; Pigs and infectious disease; Q fever; Rat-bite fever; Rocky Mountain spotted fever; Tularemia; Zoonotic diseases.

Brucellosis vaccine

CATEGORY: Prevention
ALSO KNOWN AS: *Brucella abortus* RB51 vaccine

DEFINITION

The brucellosis vaccine (also known as the *Brucella abortus* RB51 vaccine) is an attenuated live bacterial vaccine for cattle. There is no brucellosis vaccine for humans.

The vaccine, which was licensed conditionally by the U.S. Food and Drug Administration in 1996 for cattle, is a strain of live bacterium. RB51 is preferred because it is less likely to cause severe disease in cattle or humans than are other strains of *B. abortus*. *B. abortus* distinguishes serologically vaccinated animals from infected animals and does not cause false-positive reactions on standard brucellosis serologic tests.

IMMUNIZATION

Cattle immunizations against brucellosis started in 1941. The RB51 immunization denotes a safer immunization both for cattle and for the veterinarians administering it. The vaccine received full approval in 2003. *B. abortus* RB51 vaccine is used in forty-nine states and in Puerto Rico and the U.S. Virgin Islands.

PATHOLOGY

Brucellosis is a zoonotic infectious disease caused by the bacteria of the genus *Brucella*. Although it is mostly a disease among livestock, it can be transmitted from animals to humans through human ingestion of undercooked meat and unpasteurized dairy products from infected animals, and through handling infected animal tissue. Three species of *Brucella* cause the most concern: *B. abortus*, principally affecting cattle and bison; *B. suis*, principally affecting swine and reindeer but also cattle and bison; and *B. melitensis*, principally affecting goats but not present in the United States.

PATHOGENICITY

Brucellae are aerobic gram-negative coccobacilli that produce urease and that catalyze nitrite to nitrate. They have a lipopolysaccharide coat that is much less pyrogenic than other gram-negative organisms, which accounts for the rare presence of high fever in brucellosis. Brucellae can enter the human body through breaks in the skin and through mucous membranes, conjunctiva, and the respiratory and gastrointestinal tracts. Ingestion most often occurs by way of contact with or by ingestion of unpasteurized milk; meat products often have a low bacterial load. Percutaneous needle-stick exposure, conjunctival exposure through eye splash, and inhalation are the most common transmission routes in the United States.

Various *Brucella* species affect sheep, goats, cattle, deer, elk, pigs, dogs, and several other animals. Humans become infected by coming in contact with animals or animal products that are contaminated with the *Brucella* bacterium.

IMPACT

The RB51 vaccine was developed as a less pathogenic strain, but it retains pathogenicity for humans; exposure can still pose a human health risk. Identified forms of exposure include needle sticks, eye and wound splashes, and exposure to infected material. In a series of exposures reported to the Centers for Disease Control and Prevention, persons developed local symptoms of brucellosis infection; of those who became ill, most exhibited some systemic symptoms.

Routine serologic testing for brucellosis is not effective in monitoring for infection. Broader symptoms resulting from exposure to RB51 should be passively monitored for six months from the last exposure.

Acute symptoms of infection include fever, chills, headache, low back pain, joint pain, malaise, and occasional diarrhea. Subacute symptoms include malaise, muscle pain, headache, neck pain, fever, and sweating. Chronic symptoms include anorexia, weight loss, abdominal pain, joint pain, headache, backache, weakness, irritability, insomnia, depression, and constipation. Persons who believe they have been exposed to RB51 and who develop symptoms should consult a doctor or other health care provider.

Camillia King, M.P.H.

FURTHER READING

Ashford, David A., et al. "Adverse Events in Humans Associated with Accidental Exposure to the Livestock Brucellosis Vaccine RB51." *Vaccine* 3, no. 22 (September 3, 2004): 3435-3439.

Berkelman, Ruth L. "Human Illness Associated with Use of Veterinary Vaccines." *Clinical Infectious Diseases* 37, no. 3 (August 1, 2003): 407-414.

Centers for Disease Control and Prevention. Division of Bacterial and Mycotic Diseases. "Brucellosis." Available at http://www.cdc.gov/ncidod/dbmd/diseaseinfo/brucellosis_g.htm.

Franco, M. P., et al. "Human Brucellosis." *Lancet Infectious Diseases* 7 (2007): 775.

Web Sites of Interest

Centers for Disease Control and Prevention
http://www.cdc.gov/nczved/divisions/dfbmd/
diseases/brucellosis

U.S. Department of Agriculture
http://www.usda.gov

See also: Airborne illness and disease; Bacteria: Classification and types; Bacterial infections; Breast milk and infectious disease; *Brucella*; Food-borne illness and disease; Pasteurellosis; Pigs and infectious disease; Vaccines: Types; Zoonotic diseases.

Bubonic plague

Category: Diseases and conditions
Anatomy or system affected: Glands, lymphatic system, skin
Also known as: Black Death, plague

Definition

Bubonic plague is a severe bacterial infection characterized by acute, local, necrotizing lymphadenitis (infection of the lymph glands). Bacteremia rapidly follows then spreads to the spleen, liver, and other organs. Bubonic plague is the most common form of plague and has a mortality rate of 50 to 90 percent if not treated. If treated promptly and appropriately, the mortality rate is 5 to 15 percent.

Bubonic plague is one of the oldest diseases known and has been one of the most devastating in human history. It is widely regarded as a disease of mainly historical importance because it is now rare in developed countries and affects mainly poor and remote populations. However, reports of incidence have increased once again.

In Algeria and Madagascar, bubonic plague is re-emerging as a significant health concern. Adding to the new incidence rate is the discovery of antibiotic-resistant strains of the plague bacterium. A few human cases develop each year in the western United States (especially in New Mexico, Arizona, and Colorado). The following countries have reported the most cases of humans infected with the plague since 1979 (in order of most reported cases): Tanzania, Vietnam, Zaire, Peru, Madagascar, Burma, Brazil, Uganda, China, and the United States. The World Health Organization (WHO) concedes that official data on the plague do not truly reflect incidence of plague, mainly because of a reluctance to report plague cases but also because of inadequate surveillance capabilities.

Causes

Bubonic plague is caused by the bacterium *Yersinia pestis* (formerly called *Pasteurella pestis*). Alexandre Yersin isolated the bacterium (germ) that causes plague. (The bacterium was named *Y. pesti* for Yersin.) He developed a treatment (an antiserum) to combat the disease and was the first to suggest that fleas and rats may have spread plague in the epidemic of 1894. *Y. pestis* is a nonmotile, non-acid-fast, non-spore-forming, gram-negative coccobacillus (bacterium) measuring 1.5 by 0.75 microns. The bacterium can be killed in less than ten minutes with sunlight, high temperatures, desiccation, ordinary disinfectants, and preparations containing chlorine.

Y. pestis is primarily an internal parasite of wild rodents. It is transmitted by rat fleas from wild rodents to domestic rats (*Rattus norvegicus* and especially *R. rattus*) and then to humans (or directly from wild rodent to human). *Y. pestis* reproduces rapidly in the wild rodent, which may then be overcome with sepsis. A vector transmits it to a human from the wild rodent. The vector is usually a rat flea of the species *Xenopsylla cheopis*, *X. ramesis*, or *X. nubica*, although thirty different flea species have been identified as carriers of plague; other vectors include ticks and human lice.

The vector takes a blood meal from the rodent, sucks up large amounts of *Y. pestis* bacteria, and then establishes a colony in the stomachs and esophagi of some of these fleas. As a result, the flea cannot fit blood into its stomach and thus becomes extremely hungry. This extreme hunger drives the flea into intense blood-sucking (hematophagia). To avoid starvation, it will seek a blood meal from any nearby host, such as a human, rather than seek out a preferred rodent. This "blocked" flea will suck voraciously until it involuntarily regurgitates some of the blood it is sucking and some of the bacilli. As the flea feeds, it also defecates and thus excretes bacilli onto the human skin. The person scratches at the flea bite and thus deposits *Y. pestis* into his or her bloodstream.

As soon as a rodent that is infected with plague dies, its fleas leave for living hosts, humans often being the only nearby alternative. Under optimal conditions, vector fleas can live for six weeks, but they probably can transmit plague for about two weeks only. *X. cheopis*, the flea species most likely to transmit plague, flourishes in a dry, warm environment of about 60° to 77° Fahrenheit (20° to 25° Celsius). Bubonic plague can persist in relatively small rodent populations from which occasional human epidemics then arise.

Y. pestis probably evolved from the Central Asiatic plateau, the swathe of desert that reaches across Central Asia, the Middle East, and North Africa. It is rich with rodents and fleas that harbor and transmit plague. It is possible that these animals transferred *Y. pestis* from Central Asia to North Africa and subsequently to Central Africa.

The human flea (*Pulex irritans*) may be a transmitter of plague in some areas of Africa. However, human-to-human transmission of bubonic plague is uncommon because *Y. pestis* rarely produces in humans the level of sepsis needed for a flea to become blocked and thereby become a vector for bubonic plague.

Transmission can also occur when a person inhales plague-infected organisms that have been released into the air. The inhalation form of the plague can be aerosolized and used in acts of bioterrorism.

RISK FACTORS

The main risk factor for bubonic plague is contact with rodents carrying infected fleas. This may occur through occupational or environmental exposure to rats, ferrets, rabbits, squirrels, marmots, gerbils, birds, prairie dogs, bobcats, and coyotes. More than two hundred different rodents and other species can serve as hosts. Recent flea bites and scratches or bites from infected domestic cats are also risk factors.

Risk factors may be heightened by environmental and cultural conditions. For example, the Alur ethnic group in the West Nile region store grain and livestock in the same structure where people sleep because of the possibility of theft. This, coupled with the cultural practice of gathering and sleeping in the home of a deceased for three or four days (as dictated by the belief that the deceased spirit lingers and should be recognized by surviving relatives and friends), may increase the risk of contracting plague. An unusually prolonged drought is another risk factor because it may force field rodents to seek food in buildings. Poverty, poor sanitation, and poor food-

storage practices are also risk factors. Late diagnosis is a risk factor for the spread of bubonic plague because it limits the effectiveness of control measures.

SYMPTOMS

The classic symptom of bubonic plague appears usually two to five days after exposure as a smooth and painful lymph gland swelling known as a bubo. A bubo is most commonly found in the groin but is also found in the armpits and neck. A bubo usually occurs at the site of the initial flea bite or scratch. Pain may occur at the site before the bubo appears. If the infected person survives, the bubo usually suppurates in one to two weeks because of secondary infection with pyogenic bacteria. It may then burst and leave a deep ulcer. Other symptoms of bubonic plague are malaise (a general ill feeling), myalgia (muscle aches and pain), high fever, chills, severe headache, nausea, vomiting, seizures, and prostration. Petechiae (purplish spots caused by small hemorrhages); ecchymoses (purple discoloration from ruptured blood vessels); bleeding into the tissues, which turns the tissue black; and bleeding from the gastrointestinal tract may also present. In its mild form, however, bubonic plague may not even confine a person to bed.

SCREENING AND DIAGNOSIS

A doctor will ask the patient about symptoms and medical history and will perform a physical examination. Diagnostic tests may include blood and urine samples, sputum samples, a chest X ray, a computed tomography (CT) scan, a magnetic resonance imaging (MRI) scan, and a bronchoscopy, in which a thin scope is used to look into the lungs. Laboratory confirmation includes cultures from samples of blood, sputum, and fluid from the bubo. Cultures require more than forty-eight hours to produce definitive results. If plague infection is discovered, an infectious disease specialist should be contacted for assistance.

TREATMENT AND THERAPY

One should immediately treat suspected bubonic plague with antibiotics and then initiate confirmatory laboratory work. Without prompt treatment, *Y. pestis* can multiply in the bloodstream or spread to the lungs so rapidly that it may lead to the more serious pneumonic plague. Persons with bubonic plague are often hospitalized and placed in isolation, however.

The standard treatment for bubonic plague is intramuscular streptomycin (1 gram twice daily for ten days). Less severe cases can be treated with 500 milligrams (mg) of oral tetracycline, four times daily. Chloramphenicol is a suitable alternative and is administered in divided doses of 50 mg per kilogram per day, either parenterally or, if tolerated, orally for ten days. Gentamycin is the preferred antibiotic for treatment during pregnancy because it is safe, because it can be administered either intravenously or intramuscularly, and because its concentrations in the blood can be monitored.

The three most effective drugs have potentially serious adverse events associated with use during pregnancy: streptomycin may be ototoxic and nephrotoxic to the fetus, tetracycline has an adverse effect on the developing teeth and bones of the fetus, and chloramphenicol carries a risk, albeit low, of gray baby syndrome or bone-marrow suppression. Sulfonamides have been used extensively in plague treatment; however, some studies have shown higher mortality, increased complications, and longer duration of fever with its use compared with treatment with streptomycin, tetracycline, or chloramphenicol.

PREVENTION AND OUTCOMES

Killed bacteria have been used in plague vaccines since 1896. However, the vaccine licensed for use in the United States is a whole-cell bacterial vaccine, inactivated with formaldehyde and preserved in phenol. The primary series consists of three doses: the first dose at the initial visit, the second dose one to three months later, and the third dose five or six months later. Booster doses can be given at six-month intervals if exposure continues. Common side effects include mild pain, erythema (redness), and induration (hardening) at the injection site. Fever, headache, and malaise are more common and more severe following repeated doses. Rare side effects include difficulty in breathing or swallowing; hives; itching, especially of soles or palms; reddening of skin, especially around ears; swelling of eyes, face, or inside of nose; and unusual, sudden, and severe tiredness or weakness.

In 2000, the United States began working with Great Britain and Canada in sharing information about plague vaccine. In 2005, the three countries agreed to pool their resources to create a vaccine that combines the existing vaccine for the bubonic plague with a new kind of protection from the pneumonic plague, which attacks the lungs. It is hoped the vaccine will be available in 2015. In 2008, researchers from the Pasteur Institute in Paris used the less virulent ancestor to *Y. pestis*, *Y. pseudotuberculosis*, to develop a potentially safer, more efficient, and less expensive live oral vaccine.

Because human plague is rare in most parts of the world, there is no need to vaccinate anyone other than those at particularly high risk of exposure, namely, laboratory and field personnel working with or in proximity to *Y. pestis*. This intramuscular vaccine is not indicated for most travelers to countries reporting cases, particularly those traveling only to urban areas with modern hotel accommodations.

If a person is diagnosed with plague, most countries require that a governmental health agency be notified. The person is usually kept under strict quarantine until the disease is controlled with antibiotics. It is imperative that those who have been in close contact with an infected person be traced, identified, and evaluated. Infected persons might also be put under observation or given preventive antibiotic therapy (with a tetracycline, chloramphenicol, or one of the effective sulfonamides), depending on the degree and timing of contact. Antibiotics can also be given for a brief period to people who have been exposed to the bites of potentially infected rodent fleas or who have handled an animal known to be infected. People who must be present in an area where a plague outbreak is occurring can protect themselves for two to three weeks by taking antibiotics.

Many cities, especially in the United States, have instituted rodent-control programs because rodents also carry rabies and other deadly diseases. In rural areas, eliminating wild-rodent harborage and food sources and clearing brush, rock piles, and junk puts distance between rodents and the home. Ridding pet dogs and cats of fleas regularly prevents the fleas from jumping to other pets. Applying insect repellents, if available, to clothing and skin to prevent flea bites is advisable, as is wearing gloves when handling potentially infected animals. Keeping floors clean and occasionally pouring boiling water on a dirt floor and not sleeping on it is helpful.

In Africa, plague control is often reactive, not proactive, because of a lack of resources for surveillance. Plague control that targets rodents in Africa has focused on trapping, burning homes, and dusting homes and rodent burrows with powdered insecticide or other poisons such as dichloro-diphenyl-trichloro-ethane (DDT) powder followed by anticoagulant bait. Many countries employ rigorous disinfection routines for ships, docks, and aircraft because transportation of infected rodents aboard transcontinental vehicles has led to earlier pandemics.

Stephanie Eckenrode, B.A.

FURTHER READING

Bahmanyar, M., and D. C. Cavanaugh. *Plague Manual.* Geneva: World Health Organization, 1999. Explains in detail the epidemiology, distribution, surveillance, and control of all types of plague.

Borchert, Jeff N., Jeff J. Mach, and Timothy J. Linder. "Invasive Rats and Bubonic Plague in Northwest Uganda." In *Managing Vertebrate Invasive Species*, edited by G. W. Witmer, W. C. Pitt, and K. A. Fagerstone. Fort Collins, Colo.: National Wildlife Research Center, 2007. Provides a history of the entry of bubonic plague into North Africa. Includes an overview of incidence in the twenty-first century.

Cook, Gordon C., and Alimuddin I. Zumla, eds. *Manson's Tropical Diseases.* 22d ed. Philadelphia: Saunders/Elsevier, 2009. Offers an extensive discussion of plague and includes a complete list of rodent reservoirs by country.

Findlay, John, and Drew Shrewsbury. *A History of Bubonic Plague in the British Isles.* New York: Cambridge University Press, 2005. Discusses the effects of bubonic plague on populations and on social and economic life in the British Isles. Also examines the harsh regulations made in vain to control plague and the collapse of law and order during its great epidemics.

Jong, Elaine C., and Russell McMullen, eds. *Travel and Tropical Medicine Manual.* 4th ed. Philadelphia: Saunders/Elsevier, 2008. A useful reference manual with advice on preventing, evaluating, and managing diseases that can be acquired in tropical environments and countries outside the United States.

Mandell, Gerald L., John E. Bennett, and Raphael Dolin, eds. *Mandell, Douglas, and Bennett's Principles and Practice of Infectious Diseases.* 7th ed. New York: Churchill Livingstone/Elsevier, 2010. A standard reference textbook of infectious diseases with a chapter on plague that includes maps and illustrations.

Marquardt, William C., ed. *Biology of Disease Vectors.* 2d ed. New York: Academic Press/Elsevier, 2005. This biology textbook on disease vectors, including fleas, is directed toward graduate students and researchers but is accessible to advanced general readers.

WEB SITES OF INTEREST

Center for Biosecurity
http://www.upmc-biosecurity.org

Centers for Disease Control and Prevention
http://www.cdc.gov/ncidod/dvbid/plague

Emerging and Reemerging Infectious Diseases Resource Center
http://www.medscape.com/resource/infections

World Health Organization
http://www.who.int/topics/plague

See also: Arthropod-borne illness and disease; Bacterial infections; *Bartonella* infections; Biological weapons; Biosurveillance; Botulinum toxin infection; Botulism; Brucellosis; Cat scratch fever; Cats and infectious disease; Colorado tick fever; Developing countries and infectious disease; Dogs and infectious disease; Emerging and reemerging infectious diseases; Fleas and infectious disease; Flies and infectious disease; Hantavirus infection; Lassa fever; Lyme disease; Lymphadenitis; Rat-bite fever; Respiratory route of transmission; Rocky Mountain spotted fever; Rodents and infectious disease; SARS; Tropical medicine; Tularemia; Vectors and vector control; *Yersinia*; *Yersinia pseudotuberculosis*; Zoonotic diseases.

Bubonic plague vaccine

CATEGORY: Prevention

DEFINITION

The bubonic plague vaccine is used to prevent infection with the bacterium *Yersinia pestis*, which causes plague.

EARLY DEVELOPMENTS

In 1897, Waldemar Mordecai Haffkine developed the first effective plague vaccine, a bacterial suspension of killed *Y. pestis* that was injected as a preventive, during a plague epidemic in Bombay (now Mumbai), India. The Haffkine vaccine was not perfect, but it led to a drop in plague mortality by 20 to 30 percent. However, it had numerous unpleasant side effects.

In the 1930's, scientists in Madagascar and Java produced a vaccine based on a live attenuated strain of *Y. pestis*. Both vaccines continued to be used; the United States relied on the Haffkine vaccine while the French, Russians, and Chinese relied on the attenuated strain for vaccination.

Both the Haffkine and the EV (from the initials of the person from whose body it was isolated) attenuated vaccines have problems. Neither provides full protection against bubonic or pneumonic plague. Both have unpleasant side effects (and can be fatal), although recent techniques for administration have decreased these side effects. Both require several booster shots to be effective.

U.S. health officials discontinued administering plague vaccine in 1999 except in special cases. The EV vaccine has shown potential to be lethal in laboratory animals, calling its use into question in countries that had adopted it.

NEW GENERATION VACCINES

Because of difficulties with both early vaccines, scientists have been trying to find vaccines that overcome the health problems of the earlier vaccines, that are easier to administer, and that convey immunity against pneumonic plague too. Because pneumonic plague (unlike bubonic plague) is difficult to treat with antibiotics, scientists consider essential the development of a vaccine that is effective against both types of plague.

Most work has concentrated on developing subunit and live attenuated vaccines. A subunit vaccine (using subunits of the bacteria) in development was effective against both bubonic and pneumonic plague. This vaccine is based on the F1 and V antigens, both of which induce protective responses in persons. When combined, these proteins have shown an additional protective effect.

Other work is concentrating on developing a vaccine using attenuated forms of the bacteria. It is expected that this form of the vaccine, essentially a fourth generation form, will provide greater protection against *Y. pestis* than the subunit form.

IMPACT

Plague vaccines have always been considered effective in dealing with the plague because they prevent the disease rather than, like antibiotics, simply treat it. The first and second generation vaccines helped to reduce plague deaths, but they had several problems, and their use has largely been discontinued. Finally, because some strains of plague have developed antibiotic resistance, it is crucial to develop newer and more effective forms of plague vaccine.

John M. Theilmann, Ph.D.

FURTHER READING

Cornelius, C., et al. "Protective Immunity Against Plague." In *The Genus "Yersinia,"* edited by Robert D. Perry and Jacqueline D. Featherstone. New York: Springer Science, 2007.

Gregg, Charles T., *Plague.* Rev. ed. Albuquerque: University of New Mexico Press, 1985.

Mandell, Gerald L., John E. Bennett, and Raphael Dolin, eds. *Mandell, Douglas, and Bennett's Principles and Practice of Infectious Diseases.* 7th ed. New York: Churchill Livingstone/Elsevier, 2010.

Marquardt, William C., ed. *Biology of Disease Vectors.* 2d ed. New York: Academic Press/Elsevier, 2005.

Plotkin, Stanley A., Walter A. Orenstein, and Paul A. Offit. *Vaccines.* 5th ed. Philadelphia: Saunders/Elsevier, 2008.

Titball, Richard W., and E. Diane Williamson. "Vaccination Against Bubonic and Pneumonic Plague." *Vaccine* 19 (2001): 4175-4184.

WEB SITES OF INTEREST

Centers for Disease Control and Prevention
http://www.cdc.gov/ncidod/dvbid/plague

World Health Organization
http://www.who.int/topics/plague

See also: Arthropod-borne illness and disease; Bacterial infections; Bubonic plague; Developing countries and infectious disease; Fleas and infectious disease; Lassa fever; Lyme disease; Lymphadenitis; Plague; Respiratory route of transmission; Rodents and infectious disease; Vaccines: Types; Vectors and vector control; *Yersinia*; Yersiniosis; Zoonotic diseases.

Burkholderia

CATEGORY: Pathogen
TRANSMISSION ROUTE: Direct contact, ingestion, inhalation

DEFINITION

Burkholderia are gram-negative, motile, non-spore-forming, obligately aerobic rods, some of which can be pathogenic in animals and plants. They have worldwide distribution in soils and in groundwater.

**Taxonomic Classification
for *Burkholderia***

Kingdom: Bacteria
Phylum: Proteobacteria
Class: Betaproteobacteria
Order: Burkholderiales
Family: Burkholderiaceae
Genus: *Burkholderia*
Species:
  B. ambifaria
  B. anthina
  B. cenocepacia
  B. cepacia
  B. dolosa
  B. fungorum
  B. mallei
  B. multivorans
  B. phymatum
  B. pseudomallei
  B. pyrrocinia
  B. stabilis
  B. thailandensis
  B. vietnamiensis
  B. xenovorans

NATURAL HABITAT AND FEATURES

The genus *Burkholderia* was named for plant pathologist and microbiologist Walter Burkholder in 1992. Before this date, most members of this genus were classified as *Pseudomonas* spp.

All *Burkholderia* spp. are gram-negative, motile, non-spore-forming, obligately aerobic rods. Although usually nonencapsulated, they do form polysaccharide capsules at low pH (acidity). They are distributed from the Arctic to the tropics, and are especially common in damp soils, ground water, and stagnant pools. The genus contains animal and plant pathogens and saprobic species, some of which can be opportunistic pathogens. They are easily grown on most common laboratory media, although many strains need forty-eight to seventy-two hours before growth is visible on agar.

Burkholderia have the largest genomes of any known soil bacterium, with three chromosomes and a minimum of one large plasmid. Various strains, especially of *xenovorans*, have diverse metabolic pathways that allow the bacteria to degrade polycyclic aromatic compounds such as naphthalene, halogenated hydrocarbons such as trichloroethylene and polychlorinated biphenyls (PCBs), and chloroorganic pesticides such as 2,4-D.

Nonpathogenic strains have been engineered by knocking out genes needed for pathogenicity. These strains are used for bioremediation of sites contaminated with PCBs and other organics. Several studies have been carried out to see how this degradative ability can be enhanced in situ and in laboratory-based bioreactors. Many *cepacia* strains secrete antimicrobials and antifungals. These strains have been used as biocontrols of plant diseases, although pathogenicity has limited their use.

Pathogenic strains of *Burkholderia* were among the first bioweapons used in modern warfare when Germany attempted to use *mallei*, the equine pathogen that causes glanders, in an attempt to destroy the horses on which enemy cavalries depended in World War I. Both *mallei* and *pseudomallei* are considered possible biowarfare and bioterrorism agents. In the 1980's, the Soviet Union was thought to have produced more than two thousand tons of dried *mallei* preparation, which could be used in biological weapons.

PATHOGENICITY AND CLINICAL SIGNIFICANCE

Several *Burkholderia* spp. can infect humans. *Mallei* primarily causes glanders in equids, but humans and other animals can serve as accidental hosts. In humans, symptoms vary but often include skin and respiratory mucosal lesions, pneumonia, spleen and liver abscesses, muscle aches, and general malaise. Even when treated, mortality approaches 50 percent. In the United States, human glanders is now only seen among those who work with the bacteria, but in other parts of the world, especially tropical regions of Asia, human infections are more common and can be contracted directly from infected animals. Human-to-human transfer is rare.

Pseudomallei causes melioidosis, also called Whitmore's disease, in humans and other animals. It is usually transmitted through direct contact with contaminated soil or water through abrasions, inhalation, or ingestion. The disease is mainly found in tropical areas and is endemic to southeastern Asia and northern Australia. The most common symptoms are respiratory and can range from mild bronchitis to severe pneumonia. Localized skin infections are also seen when the route of entry is through an abrasion.

Although rare in healthy adults, systemic and disseminated melioidosis can occur in debilitated and immune compromised persons. It is also more common in those with diabetes mellitus. The disease can become chronic and lead to multiple abscesses on internal organs or on the skin. Untreated, the disease has 100 percent mortality; among those treated, mortality is 40 percent. Because many of the symptoms mimic other diseases, melioidosis is not always diagnosed immediately and, thus, has a chance to become more serious.

Members of the *cepacia* complex, a group of nine similar species including *multivorans, cenocepacia, stabilis, vietnamiensis, dolosa, ambifaria, anthina,* and *pyrrocinia,* have a very low pathogenicity in healthy humans, but they are significant pathogens in persons with cystic fibrosis and in those who are immune compromised. Unlike *mallei* and *pseudomallei,* these strains are usually transmitted by direct human-to-human contact. *Multivorans,* however, seems to be most commonly acquired from an environmental source. The most common symptom of a *cepacia* complex infection is pneumonia, although urogenital, surgical-wound, and catheter-related hospital infections are known to occur.

DRUG SUSCEPTIBILITY

Many antibiotics, including ceftazidime, imipenem, meropenem, doxycycline, penicillin, piperacillin, amoxicillin-clavulonic acid, amiloride, tobramycin, and aztreonam, have been used to treat *Burkholderia* infections. In all cases, ten to fourteen days of intravenous (IV) antibiotic infusion is usually followed by three to six months of oral antibiotic therapy.

For severe cases, the oral therapy can include a combination of antibiotics and can last up to one year.

In disseminated infections, the surgical removal of abscesses is sometimes necessary. Persons with cystic fibrosis who have a *cepacia* complex infection will need three to six months of aerosolized antibiotics, often a combination of amiloride and tobramycin. This regimen is usually preceded by an IV antibiotic infusion comprising tobramycin, meropenem, and ceftazidime. Many strains of *mallei* are more susceptible to antibiotics than are strains of *pseudomallei* or *cepacia* complex and, thus, do not need lengthy antibiotic treatment.

Richard W. Cheney, Jr., Ph.D.

FURTHER READING

Coenye, Tom, and Peter Vandamme, eds. *Burkholderia: Molecular Microbiology and Genomics.* Wymondhan, England: Horizon Bioscience, 2006. The first two chapters give a comprehensive review of the genus. Later chapters look at the genus from the perspective of biochemistry and genetics.

Krieg, Noel R., et al., eds. *Bergey's Manual of Systematic Bacteriology.* 2d ed. New York: Springer, 2010. Volume 2 of this multivolume work describes the Proteobacteria in detail.

Madigan, Michael T., and John M. Martinko. *Brock Biology of Microorganisms.* 12th ed. Upper Saddle River, N.J.: Pearson/Prentice Hall, 2010. This text outlines many common bacteria and describes their natural history, pathogenicity, and other characteristics.

Romich, Janet A. *Understanding Zoonotic Diseases.* Clifton Park, N.Y.: Thomson Delmar, 2008. A good introduction to zoonotic diseases, including glanders and melioidosis.

WEB SITES OF INTEREST

Center for Biosecurity
http://www.upmc-biosecurity.org

Centers for Disease Control and Prevention, Division of Foodborne, Bacterial, and Mycotic Diseases
http://www.cdc.gov/nczved/divisions/dfbmd

Todar's Online Textbook of Bacteriology
http://www.textbookofbacteriology.net

See also: Biological weapons; Glanders; Melioidosis; Microbiology; Skin infections; Soilborne illness and disease; Waterborne illness and disease.

C

Caliciviridae

CATEGORY: Pathogen
TRANSMISSION ROUTE: Direct contact, inhalation

DEFINITION

The caliciviridae family comprises positive-sense viruses with nonsegmented single-stranded RNA. The virus has a simple construction with a nonenveloped hexagonal shape. The fact that it is not enveloped makes the virus especially resistant to temperature changes for extended periods. Additionally, this characteristic makes the virus hard to kill with common detergents.

Caliciviruses are responsible for the majority of acute attacks of nonlethal gastroenteritis worldwide. The virus can infect a variety of life-forms, ranging from mammals to marine life to reptiles and amphibians.

NATURAL HABITAT AND FEATURES

The appearance of the virus is simple, with a diameter of 35 to 39 nanometers (nm) and cup-shaped dimensions on the surface. (In Latin, *calyx* means "cup" or "goblet.") In addition to lacking an envelope, which allows the Caliciviridae to flourish in harsh conditions, it does not grow in culture or in an animal model, which makes research difficult.

In general, Caliciviridae viruses spread in closed environments. For example, a the Norovirus can spread on a cruise ship or in a nursing home, and the Sapporo virus can spread in a day-care center. Feline calicivirus spreads in animal shelters, and rabbit hemorrhagic fever spreads on farms. One of the key features of the calicivirus is that it is transmitted through close contact. Also, incubation times are short, and sick animals will shred the virus if they recover or die.

PATHOGENICITY AND CLINICAL SIGNIFICANCE

Norovirus, known colloquially as the stomach flu, accounts for 90 percent of nonbacterial gastroenteritis epidemics worldwide, mainly because few particles of

---

Taxonomic Classification for Caliciviridae

Order: Unassigned
Family: Caliciviridae
Genera: *Norovirus, Sapovirus*
Species:
Norwalk virus
Sapporo virus

---

this highly contagious virus are needed to spread illness. The onset of illness is twenty-four to forty-eight hours after infection, and the infection lasts twenty-four to sixty days in a healthy person.

The virus multiplies in the small intestine. Most cases involve vomiting, diarrhea, and abdominal pain, but symptoms also can include low-grade fever and malaise. Dehydration is always a risk; however, only vulnerable groups, such as the elderly and immunocompromised, may need hospitalization.

Sapporo virus has similar clinical features, with a few exceptions. It is usually milder and tends to infect children under five years of age; therefore, child-care and day-care facilities and kindergarten and primary schools are high risk areas for transmission. It is possible for adults to get a mild version of the virus, but most people develop antibodies to the Sapporo virus by five years of age.

Caliciviruses are found throughout the animal world, but one of the most common forms of the virus, rabbit hemorrhagic fever, has had a widespread influence on both the wild and domestic rabbit population of the common species *Oryctologus cuniculus.* The fever is extremely infectious and can kill rapidly; infected animals rarely recover unless they have been vaccinated.

DRUG SUSCEPTIBILITY

No drugs are available to eradicate the caliciviruses. Most persons with a Norovirus infection or infection with the milder Sapporo virus will never need a vaccination. It is believed that most people on average will be infected with a Norovirus four to five times during their lifetime. It is likely that an antiviral medication will be developed to treat calcivirus infections.

S. M. Willis, M.S., M.A.

FURTHER READING

Hutson, Anne M., Robert L. Atmar and Mary Estes. "Norovirus Disease: Changing Epidemiology and Host Susceptibility Factors." *Trends in Microbiology* 12 (2004): 279-287.

Norkin, Leonard. Virology: Molecular Biology and Pathogenesis. Washington, D.C.: ASM Press, 2010.

"Norwalk Virus Family." In *The Bad Bug Book: Food-borne Pathogenic Microorganisms and Natural Toxins Handbook.* U.S. Food and Drug Administration, Center for Food Safety and Applied Nutrition. Available at http://www.fda.gov/food/foodsafety/foodborneillness.

WEB SITES OF INTEREST

Centers for Disease Control and Prevention, Division of Viral Diseases
http://www.cdc.gov/ncidod/dvrd/revb/gastro/norovirus.htm

Virus Pathogen Database and Analysis Resource
http://www.viprbrc.org/brc

See also: Food-borne illness and disease; Microbiology; Viruses: Structure and life cycle; Viruses: Types.

Campylobacter

CATEGORY: Pathogen
TRANSMISSION ROUTE: Direct contact, ingestion

DEFINITION

Campylobacter is a slender, curved-rod, gram-negative bacterium. The genus *Campylobacter* was first proposed in 1963, and at that time it included only *C. fetus* and *C. bululus* (later renamed *C. sputorum*). *Campylobacter*, the leading cause of bacterial gastroenteritis worldwide, has a corkscrew appearance. The pathogen propels itself with one or two flagella, depending on

> **Taxonomic Classification for *Campylobacter***
>
> **Kingdom:** Bacteria
> **Phylum:** Proteobacteria
> **Order:** Campylobacterales
> **Family:** Campylobacterales
> **Genus:** *Campylobacter*
> **Species:**
> *C. coli*
> *C. fetus*
> *C. helveticus*
> *C. jejuni*
> *C. sputorum*

the subspecies. It thrives best in a nonacidic environment that is 3 to 5 percent oxygen and 2 to 10 percent carbon dioxide. It is sometimes found in nonchlorinated bodies of water, such as ponds and streams.

The primary source of infection with campylobacteriosis in humans is *C. jejuni,* which represents about 90 percent of all infections caused by *Campylobacter* worldwide and up to 99 percent of *Campylobacter* infections in the United States. The highest rate of infection with *Campylobacter* is seen in New Zealand, with 396 cases per 100,000 persons in 2005, compared with a far lower rate of 12.7 per 100,000 people in the United States in 2005. The reasons for the high rate in New Zealand are unknown.

Humans are infected through the consumption of contaminated food, such as raw or undercooked meat, especially chicken; through the consumption of unpasteurized milk; by drinking contaminated water; and by physical contact with fecal material expelled from infected humans or animals.

It is estimated that about two million people experience symptomatic *Campylobacter* infections each year in the United States. The incidence of such infections is as much as six times greater in rural areas. This higher incidence may occur because people in rural locations are believed to be more likely to drink unpasteurized (raw) milk than are persons in urban settings.

NATURAL HABITAT AND FEATURES

Campylobacter colonizes the intestinal tract, the urogenital tract, or the oral cavity of healthy and sick animals, particularly chickens. It is also found in the intestinal tract of humans. *C. jejuni* is found in human and bovine (cow) feces, while *C. coli* is commonly found in the feces of pigs, humans, and chickens and in contaminated water. *C. helveticus* is found in the feces of cats and dogs.

The acidity of the human stomach kills most ingested *Campylobacter*, but some of the bacteria survive and attach themselves to the intestinal epithelial cells or the mucus on these cells. They then reproduce and proliferate within the intestines. Some people do not react symptomatically to this colonization, while others develop severe diarrhea. The diarrhea may be caused by an inflammatory response that occurs in the intestine as a result of the bacterial presence, or it may result from toxins that are produced by *Campylobacter*, which affect fluid resorption and cause diarrhea. In most cases, *Campylobacter* remains in the intestine of humans; rarely, it migrates to the bloodstream or to the lymphatic system. Such a migration is unusual in persons with normal immune systems.

PATHOGENICITY AND CLINICAL SIGNIFICANCE

The illness caused by *Campylobacter* has an incubation period of two to five days, and the illness lasts up to ten days. It is believed that fewer than five hundred organisms are required to cause an infection in the host. This is equivalent to about one drop of juice from an infected chicken.

An estimated 1 in 1,000 persons who are infected with *Campylobacter* develop Guillain-Barré syndrome (GBS), a neurological disorder and a leading cause of acute paralysis in the United States. Most infected persons recover in six to twelve months, but some never recover. According to the Centers for Disease Control and Prevention, up to 40 percent of all cases of GBS in the United States may be caused by infection with *Campylobacter*. When it occurs, GBS develops within two to four weeks after infection.

Persons with the acquired immunodeficiency syndrome (AIDS) have an incidence of *Campylobacter* that is about forty times greater than those without AIDS. Some persons without AIDS have an immune deficiency in immunoglobulin A (IgA), thus increasing their risk for infection with *Campylobacter*. Breast-fed babies have a reduced risk for infection with *Campylobacter*, probably because of the lactating woman's transfer of maternal substances, particularly secretory IgA.

DRUG SUSCEPTIBILITY

An increasing, worldwide resistance of the *Campylobacter* pathogen to drugs in the fluoroquinolone class has been noted since the late 1990's. Largely responsible for this resistance is the treatment of animals with fluoroquinolone drugs to promote their growth. As a result, erythromycin is now the recommended treatment drug for those with *Campylobacter* infection. There is some resistance to erythromycin, but it is much lower than the resistance to fluoroquinolone drugs such as ciprofloxacin. Newer macrolide drugs, such as azithromycin and clarithromycin, are also effective against *Campylobacter* infections.

Some studies have shown that *Campylobacter* infections acquired during travel are more resistant to antibiotics than those acquired at home. For example, in one study in the Netherlands, resistance to fluoroquinolone antibiotics was 54 percent in travel-related infections while the rate of resistance was a significantly lower 33 percent in infections in the study subject's native area.

Christine Adamec, M.B.A.

FURTHER READING

Alfredson, David A., and Victoria Korolik. "Antibiotic Resistance and Resistance Mechanisms in Campylobacter jejuni and Campylobacter coli." *Federation of European Microbiological Societies Letter* 277 (2007): 123-132. This article describes C. jejuni and C. coli, their increasing resistance to antibiotics worldwide, and the reasons for this resistance.

Ang, Jocelyn Y., and Sharon Nachman. "Campylobacter Infections." This article provides basic overview information on Campylobacter. Available at http://emedicine.medscape.com/article970552-overview.

Janssen, Riny, et al. "Host-Pathogen Interactions in Campylobacter Infections: The Host Perspective." *Clinical Microbiology Reviews* 21, no. 3 (2008): 505-518. An extensive discussion of how Campylobacter causes infection, of worldwide rates of infection, and of those persons most prone to becoming infected with this pathogen.

Minocha, Anil, and Christine Adamec. *The Encyclopedia of the Digestive System and Digestive Disorders.* New York: Facts On File, 2011. This reference book includes broad information on Campylobacter and on other causes of infectious digestive diseases and digestive disorders.

Nachamkin, Irving, Christine M. Szymanski, and Martin J. Blaser, eds. *Campylobacter.* 3d ed. Washington, D.C.: ASM Press, 2008. A text examining the bacterium.

Van Hees, B. C., et al. "Regional and Seasonal Differences in Incidence and Antibiotic Resistance of Campylobacter from a Nationwide Surveillance Study in The Netherlands: An Overview of 2000-2004." *Clinical Microbiology and Infectious Diseases* 13 (2007): 305-310. This article describes a study of infection with Campylobacter and the differences between infections acquired in one's own country versus those acquired abroad.

WEB SITES OF INTEREST

American College of Gastroenterology
http://www.acg.gi.org

Centers for Disease Control and Prevention, Division of Foodborne, Bacterial, and Mycotic Diseases
http://www.cdc.gov/nczved/divisions/dfbmd

See also: Amebic dysentery; Antibiotic-associated colitis; Ascariasis; Bacterial infections; Campylobacteriosis; Cholera; Cryptosporidiosis; Enteritis; Escherichia; Fecal-oral route of transmission; Food-borne illness and disease; Giardiasis; Intestinal and stomach infections; Salmonella; Shigella; Travelers' diarrhea; Waterborne illness and disease; Yersinia.

Campylobacteriosis

CATEGORY: Diseases and conditions
ANATOMY OR SYSTEM AFFECTED: Blood, gastrointestinal system,
ALSO KNOWN AS: Campylobacter infection

DEFINITION

Campylobacteriosis is a common infectious disease that is transmitted to humans through contact with animals or animal products. It often manifests as a food-borne illness and is a principal cause of diarrheal disease. Its causative agents are *CampylobacterCampylobacter* organisms that infect the gastrointestinal tract and, more rarely, the bloodstream.

CAUSES

The bacteria responsible for campylobacteriosis belong to the *Campylobacter* genus and include *C. jejuni*, the strain associated with most human infections, and *C. coli*, among other species. *Campylobacter* organisms are widely distributed, live in the intestines of many food and domestic animals, and pass to the environment through feces. Campylobacteriosis is usually caused by handling or consuming raw or undercooked poultry or meat, by drinking unpasteurized milk or untreated water, and through contact with feces of infected animals.

RISK FACTORS

Although anyone can contract campylobacteriosis, the following groups are at higher risk for this food-borne illness: persons with occupational exposure to cattle and other farm animals; young children; pregnant women; older adults; and persons with kidney disease, diabetes, and compromised immune systems (such as persons with acquired immunodeficiency syndrome or persons who have had organ transplants).

SYMPTOMS

Campylobacter organisms can live in the intestinal tract of humans without causing illness, but even low bacterial concentrations can cause disease, with symptoms manifesting two to ten days after exposure. Symptoms typically last one week and include fever, abdominal pain, diarrhea, headache, nausea, and vomiting. Complications may include infections of the blood, liver, and urinary tract; meningitis; arthritis; and, rarely, Guillain-Barré syndrome, a form of paralysis. Although most people recover completely, some cases of campylobacteriosis can be fatal.

SCREENING AND DIAGNOSIS

Presumptive diagnosis can be established when microscopic examination and a Gram-staining test of a stool sample reveal the presence of *Campylobacter* bacteria. More definitive diagnosis requires a culture of a stool specimen to detect the growth of *Campylobacter* bacteria among normal fecal organisms.

TREATMENT AND THERAPY

Because campylobacteriosis is usually self-limiting, treatment generally consists of supportive measures such as electrolyte replacement and rehydration. Antimicrobial treatment with antibiotics is indicated for patients whose symptoms persist for more than one week or who have bloodstream infections or compromised immune systems.

PREVENTION AND OUTCOMES

Reduction of campylobacteriosis requires control measures in the agricultural setting and in the commercial manufacturing of food. In the household kitchen, food, especially poultry and meat, should be handled safely with frequent washing of utensils, cutting boards, counter tops, and hands with soapy water. Because *Campylobacter* bacteria are readily destroyed by heat, all foods should be cooked to a safe minimum internal temperature. Other preventive measures include drinking only treated water and pasteurized milk.

Anna Binda, Ph.D.

FURTHER READING

Bell, Chris, and Alec Kyriakides. *Campylobacter: A Practical Approach to the Organism and Its Control in Foods.* Malden, Mass.: Wiley-Blackwell, 2009.

Blaser, Martin J. "Infections Due to Campylobacter and Related Species." In *Harrison's Principles of Internal Medicine,* edited by Joan Butterton. 17th ed. New York: McGraw-Hill, 2008.

Humphrey, Tom, Sarah O'Brien, and Mogens Madsen. "Campylobacters as Zoonotic Pathogens: A Food Production Perspective." *International Journal of Food Microbiology* 117 (2007): 237-257.

Johnson, Leonard R., ed. *Gastrointestinal Physiology.* 7th ed. Philadelphia: Mosby/Elsevier, 2007.

Nachamkin, Irving, Christine M. Szymanski, and Martin J. Blaser, eds. *Campylobacter.* 3d ed. Washington, D.C.: ASM Press, 2008.

Newell, Diane G., Julian M. Ketley, and Roger A. Feldman, eds. *Campylobacters, Helicobacters, and Related Organisms.* New York: Springer, 1997.

WEB SITES OF INTEREST

American College of Gastroenterology
http://www.acg.gi.org

Centers for Disease Control and Prevention
http://www.cdc.gov

National Center for Emerging and Zoonotic Infectious Diseases
http://www.cdc.gov/ncezid

See also: Amebic dysentery; Antibiotic-associated colitis; Ascariasis; Bacterial infections; Balantidiasis; Campylobacter; Cholera; Cryptosporidiosis; Developing countries and infectious disease; Fecal-oral route of transmission; Food-borne illness and disease; Giardiasis; Intestinal and stomach infections; Reiter's syndrome; Travelers' diarrhea; Waterborne illness and disease; Worm infections; Zoonotic diseases.

Cancer and infectious disease

CATEGORY: Epidemiology

DEFINITION

Infectious diseases caused by viruses, bacteria, and parasites have been linked to cancer, an uncontrolled growth of cells in the body. Globally, an estimated 20 percent of cancers are linked to some type of infectious disease. The incidence is less common in developed countries, with approximately 10 percent of cancers linked to an infectious disease.

CAUSES

Infection with viruses, bacteria, or parasites stimulates production of white blood cells and other immune responses, which ultimately cause inflammation. This inflammatory response is necessary to kill the foreign organisms. The substances that white blood cells produce, however, also damage deoxyribonucleic acid (DNA), proteins, and other cells. Also, inflammation causes cells to divide at a faster rate than normal. With chronic infection, inflammation may also become chronic, which suggests continued cell damage that could lead to the development of mutated cells and cancer.

Foreign organisms, particularly viruses, can enter human cells and directly interact with DNA. This interaction can activate genes that promote tumor growth or can inactivate genes that prevent tumors from growing. These organisms may prevent the body from destroying damaged cells. These cells can then continue to grow and may become cancerous through a process called oncogenesis. Some viruses, such as the human immunodeficiency virus (HIV), prevent the immune system from recognizing cancer cells or cells infected with cancer-causing viruses.

An estimated 40 percent of persons in the United

States are infected with *Helicobacter pylori* at any given time. *H. pylori* is a screw-shaped bacterium that burrows into the stomach lining and causes chronic inflammation and cell proliferation. An estimated 20 percent of persons infected with *H. pylori* will develop peptic ulcers and 5 percent will develop stomach cancer. Infection with *H. pylori* increases the risk of developing stomach cancer eightfold.

There are more than one hundred types of human papillomavirus (HPV). Infection with certain types of these viruses can cause warts or benign tumors called papillomas. Some types of HPV cause common warts on hands and feet, while other types cause warts in the genital area. Most of these infections are self-limited (they resolve without treatment); however, for some persons, infection can last many years and may or may not lead to cancer. HPV can interfere with human proteins that keep tumors from growing, and persistent HPV infection is associated with cervical cancer. Other cancers associated with HPV include cancer of the anus, vulva, vagina, and penis.

Infection with hepatitis B virus causes inflammation of the liver. Infection is usually acute, lasting no more than six months. Persons who develop the chronic form of hepatitis B, which lasts for more than six months, are at high risk for cirrhosis and for liver cancer. Chronic infection with the hepatitis C virus leads to permanent scarring of the liver (referred to as cirrhosis) and, in some persons, liver cancer.

HIV infection is associated with Kaposi's sarcoma, non-Hodgkin's lymphoma, cervical cancer, anal cancer, Hodgkin's lymphoma, liver cancer, and lung cancer. The association between HIV and certain cancers is unclear, however, but it is believed that because the virus severely weakens the body's immune system, the body is made more susceptible to cancer. Persons infected with HIV are also more likely to be infected with other viruses that increase the risk of certain cancers.

The Epstein-Barr virus (EBV) causes infectious mononucleosis. EBV infection is associated with about one-third of Hodgkin's lymphoma cases and with developing non-Hodgkin's lymphoma. EBV is detected in tumors, and the EBV genome (hereditary information) is detected in the cancer cells.

Infections with parasites that cause cancer are more common in underdeveloped and developing countries. Parasites, such as blood flukes, can cause schistosomiasis, which is associated with bladder cancer, and liver flukes can cause an infection with *Opisthorchis viverrini*, which is associated with cancer of the bile duct and other types of liver cancer.

RISK FACTORS

H. pylori is acquired by consuming contaminated food or water or by direct oral contact. In many cases, it is first acquired during childhood. Living in crowded, unhealthful conditions and having a lower socioeconomic status (which often precipitates poor living conditions) are risk factors for *H. pylori* infection.

HPV, HIV, and hepatitis B and C viruses can be spread by sex with an infected partner; by using shared, contaminated hypodermic needles; and by getting an unsterile tattoo, body piercing, or surgical procedure. Having many sexual partners increases the likelihood of acquiring these infections. Having received a blood transfusion before 1992 is also a risk factor for HIV and hepatitis C virus infection. Health care workers are at risk for acquiring HIV or hepatitis B or C from patients, and infants are at risk of acquiring any of these viruses from his or her infected mother.

Many persons are infected with EBV by the time they reach adulthood. The virus is transmitted by contact with an infected person's saliva through kissing, coughing, or sneezing. Sharing food or beverages from the container or utensil of an infected person also can transfer the virus. Up to 80 percent of people who develop mononucleosis and recover will continue to secrete EBV in their saliva for years and are believed to be a primary source for spreading the virus.

SYMPTOMS

H. pylori infection is associated with aching or burning pain in the abdomen and with nausea, vomiting, frequent burping, bloating, and weight loss.

HPV infection can occur without symptoms, however, some persons can develop genital warts with an HPV infection. The warts may be raised, flat, pink, or flesh-colored; large or small; or shaped like cauliflower. Single or multiple warts may appear on the anus, cervix, scrotum, groin, thigh, or penis.

Infection with hepatitis B or C virus may be asymptomatic. However, some persons may complain of right upper quadrant abdominal pain, ascites (fluid collection in the abdomen), bleeding varices (dilated veins in the esophagus), dark urine, fatigue, fever, generalized itching, jaundice (yellowing of the skin), anorexia (loss of appetite), nausea, light-colored stools, and vomiting.

When persons first become infected with HIV, many are without symptoms; some get a flulike illness within three to six weeks of exposure. These persons may complain of fever, headache, tiredness, nausea, diarrhea, and enlarged lymph nodes, which can last one to four weeks. For a period of time, the body's immune response keeps the virus in check. Eventually, however, the virus load rises to high levels. Over time, the immune system is weakened and the infected person becomes more susceptible to opportunistic infections and cancer.

Symptoms of infection with EBV include a fever, malaise (feeling very tired), swollen lymph nodes, and a sore throat.

SCREENING AND DIAGNOSIS

Screening and early diagnosis of infection can increase the likelihood of treatment and subsequently reduce the risk of developing an associated cancer. With infections that are asymptomatic, screening and early diagnosis of the cancer may improve the chance of early treatment and cure.

H. pylori testing is routinely done for persons diagnosed with a peptic ulcer. In addition, patients with a family history of stomach cancer should be tested for *H. pylori* infection. Testing includes a blood test to check for *H. pylori* antibodies; a urea breath test, which is positive if *H. pylori* is present; and a stool antigen test, which checks for *H. pylori* antigens in the person's stool. A biopsy to check for *H. pylori* may also be obtained through endoscopy.

The Pap test (or smear) is part of a gynecological exam that checks for changes in the cells of the cervix. A test to check for types of HPV that are high risk for cancer in cervical cells is done as part of the Pap test.

Hepatitis B and C are diagnosed using blood tests that check for virus antibodies and virus levels (also called viral load). In addition, liver function tests, albumin level, and prothrombin time are checked to assess the effects of the virus on the liver.

Two tests are used in combination to check for HIV antibodies and to increase testing accuracy. If antibodies are detected by the ELISA (enzyme-linked immunoabsorbent assay) method, then a second test using the Western blot procedure confirms the diagnosis. Persons who are diagnosed with a sexually trans-

mitted disease or have other risk factors for acquiring HIV should be tested. Other tests include a viral load and a CD4 count.

Antigens for EBV are done to determine if a person has been infected with the virus. EBV can cause mononucleosis, which is diagnosed when a person has an elevated monocyte (type of white blood cell) count.

TREATMENT AND THERAPY

Treatment of infection may prevent cancer from developing, if the infection is cured. In many cases, however, the infection cannot be cured but its severity can be reduced, helping to lessen damage to the immune system and body and reducing the likelihood of developing cancer.

H. pylori infection is treatable. Persons with peptic ulcers caused by *H. pylori* are treated with antibiotics and medications, such as proton pump inhibitors, histamine 2 receptor blockers, or bismuth subsalicylate, that block the production of stomach acid.

There is no cure for HPV infection; however, the warts that develop with the infection can be treated with cryosurgery (freezing that destroys tissue), loop electrosurgical excision procedure (removal of tissue using a hot wire loop), and conventional surgical removal.

No cure exists for hepatitis B infection, but medications may suppress the virus production and reduce the damage to the liver. No medications exist that can prevent acute hepatitis B from becoming a chronic infection. Acute hepatitis B infection is usually a self-limiting infection and resolves within a few weeks. Hepatitis B immunoglobulin may be given within twenty-four hours of exposure to the virus to protect the person from developing chronic hepatitis B infection. Several medications have been approved by the U.S. Food and Drug Administration for the management of chronic hepatitis B virus infection. These medications include interferon, lamivudine, telbivudine, tenofovir, adefovir, and entecavir.

No cure for hepatitis C infection has been developed, but medications may suppress virus production and reduce damage to the liver. No medications exist that can prevent acute hepatitis C from becoming a chronic infection. Management of hepatitis C infection includes pegylated interferon and ribavirin, which may be given for up to forty-eight weeks.

No cure exists for HIV; however, based on the person's viral load and CD4 count, antiretroviral treatment is recommended. HIV treatments have dramatically improved since first introduced. Newer, more effective medications and older proven medications can be taken less frequently with reduced adverse effects. Highly active antiretroviral therapy, or HAART, includes a drug combination that targets different aspects of virus replication or growth to control the infection. A paradigm shift is occurring in the treatment of HIV. Many persons now consider HIV to be a chronic disease rather than a progressive, fatal infection.

There is no cure for mononucleosis. Persons infected with EBV may have symptoms for several months, however, the infection is usually self-limiting. In general, antiviral medications are not effective, and supportive care (plenty of oral fluids to prevent dehydration, acetaminophen for fever, and bed rest) is recommended to manage the symptoms of the infection.

Prevention and Outcomes

If infection with the offending organism is prevented, then the associated cancer will likely be avoided. The efficacy of vaccines that prevent chronic infection with these organisms is based on this premise. Minimizing the exposure of infected persons to other persons also can decrease the risk of spreading infections.

One can reduce the spread of viruses, bacteria, and parasites through good handwashing technique and covering the mouth and nose when coughing or sneezing. One should also eat food that has been washed well or cooked properly and should drink water from a clean source. Eating a nutritious diet and exercising regularly also decrease the risk of developing cancer. Routine doctor visits allow early screening and diagnosis, and follow-up on abnormal test results may prevent cancer.

To reduce the risk of infection with HIV or hepatitis B or C virus, persons should avoid contact with blood or blood products whenever possible. Sexual transmission of infectious diseases is low among monogamous couples. Persons should not inject illicit drugs or share needles and should not share razors, toothbrushes, or nail clippers in households with an infected person.

There is no vaccine for the prevention of hepatitis C infection; however, there is a vaccine for hepatitis B. The hepatitis B vaccine should be given to newborns, children who were not previously vaccinated, and adults in high-risk groups. There is no vaccine for the prevention of HIV; however, condom use minimizes the risk of acquiring and spreading HIV.

Avoiding genital contact with another can prevent infection with HPV. For those who choose to be sexually active, a long-term, mutually monogamous relationship with an uninfected partner reduces the risk of infection. However, it is difficult to determine if a partner who has been sexually active in the past is currently infected. HPV infection can occur in both male and female genital areas that are covered or protected by a latex condom, and in areas that are not covered. Vaccines that prevent HPV infection are available.

There is no vaccine to prevent infection with EBV. Avoiding persons infected with the virus is difficult because many who carry the virus do not know they are infected. However, general good hygiene and being cautious if a person's immune system is suppressed or not functioning properly can help reduce the risk of contracting the infection.

Beatriz Manzor Mitrzyk, Pharm.D.

Further Reading

Alberts, Bruce, et al. *Molecular Biology of the Cell.* 5th ed. New York: Garland, 2008. Describes the evolution of cells and introduces cell structure and function. The text is aimed at the college level and is illustrated by numerous diagrams and photographs.

Broomall, E. M., S. M. Reynolds, and R. M. Jacobson. "Epidemiology, Clinical Manifestations, and Recent Advances in Vaccination Against Human Papillomavirus." *Postgraduate Medicine* 122, no. 2 (2010): 121-129. An updated article on the HPV vaccine.

Fuccio, L., et al. "Meta-analysis: Can Helicobacter pylori Eradication Treatment Reduce the Risk for Gastric Cancer?" *Annals of Internal Medicine* 151, no. 2 (2009): 121-128. A journal article exploring the question of reducing the risk of gastric cancer through the eradication of H. pylori.

Gisbert, J. P., et al. "Prevalence of Hepatitis C Virus Infection in B-Cell Non-Hodgkin's Lymphoma" *Gastroenterology* 125, no. 6 (2003): 1723-1732. An analysis of the connections between hepatitis C infection and non-Hodgkin's lymphoma.

Krueger, Hans, et al. *HPV and Other Infectious Agents in Cancer: Opportunities for Prevention and Public Health.* New York: Oxford University Press, 2010. Includes a helpful introduction to cancer and infectious agents and chapters on HPV, H. pylori, hepatitis viruses, and others.

McKinnell, Robert Gilmore, ed. *The Biological Basis of Cancer.* 2d ed. New York: Cambridge University Press, 2006. This text is designed to be used for undergraduate courses on cancer. It covers everything from the molecular to the clinical aspects of the subject and includes a lengthy bibliography.

Murphy, Kenneth, Paul Travers, and Mark Walport. *Janeway's Immunobiology.* 7th ed. New York: Garland Science, 2008. An excellent text that provides a lucid and comprehensive examination of the immune system, covering such topics as immunobiology and innate immunity, the recognition of antigen, the development of mature lymphocyte receptor repertoires, the adaptive immune response, and the evolution of the immune system.

National Digestive Diseases Information Clearinghouse. "H. pylori and Peptic Ulcers." Available at http://digestive.niddk.nih.gov/ddiseases/pubs/hpylori. A good introduction to the role of H. pylori in the development of peptic ulcers.

Stern, Peter L., Peter C. L. Beverley, and Miles W. Carroll, eds. *Cancer Vaccines and Immunotherapy.* New York: Cambridge University Press, 2000. This book covers the rationale, development, and implementation of vaccines in human cancer treatment, with a review of target identification, delivery vectors, and clinical trial design.

WEB SITES OF INTEREST

American Cancer Society
http://www.cancer.org

National Cancer Institute
http://www.cancer.gov/iib

See also: Bacteria: Classification and types; Cancer vaccines; Cervical cancer; Epstein-Barr virus infection; Epstein-Barr virus vaccine; Flukes; Helicobacter; Hepatitis A; Hepatitis B; Hepatitis C; Hepatitis vaccines; HIV; HIV vaccine; Human papillomavirus (HPV) infections; Human papillomavirus (HPV) vaccine; Infection; Inflammation; Kaposi's sarcoma; Liver cancer; Parasitic diseases; Peptic ulcer; Viruses: Structure and life cycle; Viruses: Types.

Cancer vaccines

CATEGORY: Prevention

DEFINITION

Cancer vaccines are either preventive or therapeutic. Preventive, or prophylactic, vaccines prevent cancer from developing in healthy persons. Therapeutic, or treatment, vaccines treat existing cancer by strengthening the body's immune response against the malignancy.

IMMUNOTHERAPY

Vaccines are commonly known for their benefits in preventing or fighting infectious diseases such as polio, tetanus, or measles. Vaccines, as a form of immunotherapy, promote immunity, the body's defense against pathogens and injured or abnormal cells, such as cancer cells. The immune system, which can deliver its effector components to different locations in the body, is such a highly specific system that it can isolate one cancer cell from a vast amount of other healthy cells and destroy that cancer cell.

Utilizing basic principles of infectious disease vaccines, a new type of vaccine is being developed to target one of the most critical public health concerns: cancer. Although some advances have been made, cancer is still the leading cause of death in persons younger than age eighty-five years in the United States.

Cancer is a group of diseases characterized by abnormal and uncontrolled cell growth, invasion, and sometimes metastasis. In a healthy body, cells grow, die, and are replaced in a regulated fashion. Damage or change in the genetic material of cells by internal or environmental factors sometimes results in immortal cells, which continue to multiply until a mass of cancer cells, or a tumor, develops. Most cancer-related deaths are caused by metastasis, in which malignant cells make their way into the bloodstream and establish colonies in other parts of the body. Cancer immunotherapy manipulates the immune system to overcome self-tolerance and to recognize cancer cells.

Like the traditional vaccines that present inactivated, attenuated, or subunit pathogens to the immune system, cancer vaccines present the right cancer antigen in combination with the right adjuvant to generate the right type of immune response. This response, whether humoral or cellular, ideally should destroy the cancer only and leave healthy cells untouched. Cancer

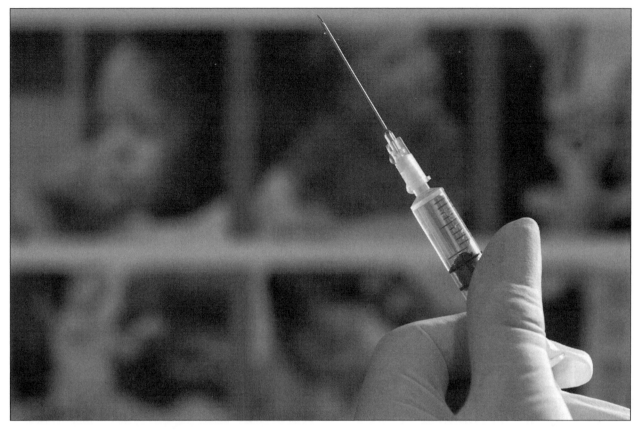

A syringe with Gardasil, a vaccine effective against human papillomaviruses, which can cause cervical and other genital cancers. (AP/Wide World Photos)

cells are different from normal healthy cells. As such, they are recognized by the immune system as being different. Proteins expressed by cancer cells are different from normal proteins or are absent in normal differentiated cells. These proteins can be immunogenic when presented in the context of a cancer vaccine.

The vaccine is made from cancer-specific proteins or proteins that are found predominantly in cancer cells. Because of the associated immunologic memory, the risk of recurrence is reduced compared with traditional treatments. Rather than compromise the immune system, as many chemotherapy treatments do, cancer vaccines train the immune system to target those specific malignant cells. Consequently, some cancer vaccines are safer and do not have the traditional side effects associated with chemotherapy or radiation therapy. Depending on the specific vaccine, cancer vaccines might be stand-alone therapies or may be used with other conventional cancer therapies.

Every cancer, and its vaccine, is different. Personalized medicine is critical to the development of vaccines that must be tailor-made to each person.

PASSIVE AND ACTIVE IMMUNOTHERAPY

Cancer vaccines are characterized as either active or passive immunotherapies. While the active type aims to elicit the host immune system to fight the disease, the passive type does not depend on the body's defenses to start the attack. Instead, it uses administered medicines (antibodies or T cell therapy) to destroy the tumor. Passive immunotherapy has no immunologic memory associated with the treatment. Any of these therapies can be targeted to one type of tumor cell or antigen (specific immunotherapies) or can generally stimulate the immune system (nonspecific immunotherapies).

Cancer vaccines are either therapeutic or preventive. Therapeutic vaccines treat persons at early stages of the disease or with minimal residual disease after removal of the main tumor. In some cases, advanced disease may be treated with a vaccine. Preventive vaccines include the human papillomavirus (HPV) vaccine, which can prevent cervical, vaginal, and vulvar cancers. The hepatitis B virus (HBV) vaccine lowers the risk of developing liver cancer. The *Helicobacter pylori* vaccine targets the bacterium *H. pylori*, which is associated with stomach cancer. Hence, the HPV, HBV, and *H. pylori* vaccines do not target cancer cells; rather, they are specific to the viruses or bacteria that give rise to these cancers.

VACCINE STRATEGIES

Cancer vaccines target malignancies such as melanoma, leukemia, and non-Hodgkin's lymphoma, and cancers of the lung, breast, kidney, ovary, pancreas, prostate, and colorectal area. The unique complex strategies used in cancer vaccine design depend on various considerations particular to the specific cancer process, the optimum level of immunity that can potentially be achieved, and a person's health status.

In whole cancer-cell vaccines, cancer cells are irradiated before they are returned to the treated person's body through injection. These vaccines contain thousands of potential antigens expressed in the whole tumor. Antigen vaccines, however, use only one antigen (or a few), whereas peptide vaccines present short fragments of the tumor protein.

Dendritic cell vaccines use specialized antigen-presenting cells that are efficient in presenting tumor antigens and tumor peptides to the immune system. Dendritic cells break down cancer proteins into small fragments and then present these antigens to T cells, thus improving immunologic antigen recognition and, eventually, cancer destruction. Nucleic acid vaccines use the genetic code that codes for cancer protein antigens so that the host cells make the cancer antigen continuously while keeping the immune response stimulated and strong.

Viral and bacterial, vector-based, vaccines can deliver antigens or genes encoding the tumor proteins or peptides to make the host's immune system more apt to respond. Because bacterial and viral components on these vector vaccines represent pathogen danger signals, they may trigger additional immune responses that might benefit the overall response, making it more robust and longer lasting.

Anti-idiotype vaccines can act passively against B-cell lymphomas or actively by mimicking cancer antigens. In the latter case, these vaccines work through antibody cascades. Some of these vaccines contain adjuvants to amplify either the humoral or the cell-mediated (or both) immune responses to an antigen and break self-tolerance. Adjuvants have been developed to enhance immunogenicity when mixed with proteins, peptides, or deoxyribonucleic acid (DNA). Tumor peptide-MHC (major histocompatibility complex) complexes are important for the recognition of tumor cells by the immune system because tumor peptides are recognized only if they are joined to the MHC complex. Cytotoxic T cells are the killer cells that recognize the peptide-MHC complexes on the tumor cells and destroy the cancer cells.

IMPACT

Cancer vaccines have the potential to treat cancers in line with treatments such as surgery or radiation therapy. Cancer vaccines are mostly experimental, although some have already entered the drug market after receiving U.S. Food and Drug Administration approval. Some vaccines have shown promise in clinical trials, while others have advanced through late-stage clinical studies.

Using cancer vaccines after the removal of the main tumor by traditional means helps lead the body's own immune system to destroy any remaining cancer cells and to target metastasis. Immunotherapy has the potential to strengthen the body's natural defenses, despite cancers that might have already developed, and it can prevent new growth of existing cancers, hamper recurrence of treated cancers, and destroy cancer cells not previously eliminated by other treatments.

When cancer is controlled or cured, cachexia usually stops. During cachexia, there is wasting of adipose and skeletal muscle. Persons with pancreatic and gastric cancer, for example, suffer from acute cachexia. Those with cachexia suffer from poor functional performance, depressed chemotherapy response, and greater mortality. Therefore, the success of cancer vaccine development may benefit persons with cachexia enormously.

Immunotherapies themselves are costly, but in the long term, they reduce overall medical costs by reducing fees for patient care, management, hospitalization, and death. The pursuit and development of safe and effective cancer vaccines can greatly benefit immunologists, oncologists, molecular biologists, chemists, public health workers, and society in general. Above all, they help persons with cancer.

Ana Maria Rodriguez-Rojas, M.S.

FURTHER READING

Finn, O. J. "Cancer Vaccines: Between the Idea and the Reality." *Nature Reviews Immunology* 3, no. 8 (2003): 630-641. A review that addresses unique and common challenges to cancer vaccines and the progress that has been made in meeting those challenges.

Jemal, A., et al. "Cancer Statistics, 2010." *CA: A Cancer Journal for Clinicians* 60, no. 5 (2010): 277-300. This clinical report examines cancer incidence, mortality, and survival based on incidence data.

Murphy, J. F. "Trends in Cancer Immunotherapy." *Clinical Medicine Insights: Oncology* 4 (July 14, 2010): 67-80. Discusses the attempts of cancer immunotherapy to redirect the power and specificity of the immune system toward effectively and safely treating malignancy.

Plotkin, Stanley A., Walter A. Orenstein, and Paul A. Offit. *Vaccines.* 5th ed. Philadelphia: Saunders/Elsevier, 2008. A comprehensive vaccination textbook covering the topics of development, production, safety and efficacy, morbidity, and mortality.

Raez, L. E., and E. S Santos. "Cancer Vaccines: A New Therapeutic Alternative for Lung Cancer Therapy?" *Immunotherapy* 1, no. 5 (2009): 727-728. An editorial that discusses challenges for lung cancer vaccine development and clinical activities.

Rosenberg, S. A., J. C. Yang, and N. P. Restifo. "Cancer Immunotherapy: Moving Beyond Current Vaccines." *Nature Medicine* 10, no. 9 (2004): 909-915. Review of a cancer vaccine trial that highlights secondary strategies that facilitate cancer regression in preclinical and clinical models.

Schlom, J., P. M. Arlen, and J. L. Gulley. "Cancer Vaccines: Moving Beyond Current Paradigms." *Clinical Cancer Research* 13, no. 1 (2007): 3776-3782. Reviews several different cancer-vaccine clinical trials and respective patient response and survival outcomes.

The Scientist.com. "Immune System Versus Cancer." Available at http://www.the-scientist.com/2009/11/1/36/1. Article that underscores the role of the immune system in cancer within the context of immune surveillance.

Sonpavde, G., et al. "Emerging Vaccine Therapy Approaches for Prostate Cancer." *Reviews in Urology* 12, no. 1 (2010): 25-34. Explores different prostate vaccine approaches with selecting proper patient populations, discovering optimal doses, and routes of administration for better outcomes.

WEB SITES OF INTEREST

American Cancer Society
http://www.cancer.org

Cancer Research Institute
http://www.cancerresearch.org

National Cancer Institute
http://www.cancer.gov

See also: Cancer and infectious disease; Cervical cancer; Immunity; Immunization; Kaposi's sarcoma; Liver cancer; Vaccines: Experimental; Vaccines: History; Vaccines: Types.

Candida

CATEGORY: Pathogen
TRANSMISSION ROUTE: Direct contact

DEFINITION

Candida is a genus of often polymorphic yeasts that are endosymbionts of many other organisms. They can move from being commensal to parasitic in humans, especially in persons with an compromised immune system.

NATURAL HABITAT AND FEATURES

Many species of *Candida* have been isolated from the guts or body surfaces of mammals and insects. They are so common that 75 percent of humans support commensal *Candida* spp. on their skin and exposed mucous membranes, and virtually all human guts are host to a minimum of one species of *Candida*; most humans host several. Fourteen different species have been found in cow's milk.

Some *Candida* spp. can move from their commensal site and invade underlying tissue, where they can form a parasitic relationship. Most species, however, do not cause problems because the host's immune system

Taxonomic Classification for *Candida*

Kingdom: Fungi
Phylum: Ascomycota
Subphylum: Saccharomycotina
Class: Saccharomycetes (Hemiascomycetes)
Order: Saccharomycetales
Family: Saccharomycetaceae
Genus: *Candida*
Species:
C. albicans
C. antarctica
C. castellii
C. dublinensis
C. glabrata
C. guilliermondii
C. krusei
C. oleophila
C. parapsilosis
C. tropicalis

can recognize and remove them before parasitism is established.

All *Candida* spp. can exist in the yeast form, but many can form hyphae, which are branched multicellular vegetative structures, or pseudohyphae, which are multinucleate branches that have not separated into individual cells. *C. albicans* and *tropicalis* are examples of species that can exist in all three forms, and *krusei* and *parapsilosis* can exist as yeasts and pseudohyphae. *Guilliermondii* and *parapsilosis* are common commensals on human skin, and *albicans, glabrata, krusei, kefyr, tropicalis, intermedia,* and many others, are more commonly symbionts in the human gut. Cell-wall carbohydrates are usually phosphorylated mannans and glucans, with small amounts of chitin possible. Polypeptides and enzymatic proteins are also found in the cell wall.

Deoxyribonucleic acid sequence comparisons suggest that the pathogenic *Candida* fall within three genetically related groups, or clades. Clade 1 contains *albicans* and most other pathogenic *Candida* spp. Clade 2 contains *guilliermondii* and the *Debaryomyces* spp. The more distantly related clade 3 includes *castellii, glabrata,* and their close relative, *Saccharomyces cerevisiae,* the familiar baker's or brewer's yeast. Of seventy-eight *Candida* spp. tested, sixty-seven used CUG as an mRNA (messenger ribonucleic acid) code for

serine instead of the normal leucine. This was probably not caused by a single mutation because members of different clades show this change; within a clade, both CUG codes are present.

The genomes of *Candida* spp. differ, as does their reproduction. *Albicans* and its close relatives are usually diploid organisms, although both haploid and tetraploid forms have been discovered, often in the same species. They usually reproduce asexually, although modified sexual reproduction without normal meiosis has been shown in this clade. *Guilliermondi* is always haploid, and only asexual reproduction has been observed in this species. A few other *Candida* spp. that usually reproduce asexually can go through a normal fungal sexual cycle with meiosis.

PATHOGENICITY AND CLINICAL SIGNIFICANCE

Candida spp. are opportunistic pathogens and, most of the time, live symbiotically with their hosts as commensals. *Albicans,* followed by *glabrata* and *tropicalis,* are the three most common human pathogens, although more than 160 *Candida* spp. can cause opportunistic infection. All have the ability to adhere to epithelial cells and to secrete digestive enzymes, both of which these commensals need to scavenge nutrients from the epithelium. However, this could lead to parasitism under the proper circumstances.

Fungal populations are usually held in check on the skin and in the digestive and reproductive systems by the many competing bacteria. Two common human candidiases—vulvovaginitis, a vaginal yeast infection, and thrush, an oral yeast infection—often occur when this bacterial competition is lessened. The most common cause of this lowered competition is antibiotic therapy, which reduces bacterial numbers and allows the yeast to overgrow and cause damage.

Suppressed immune systems also allow overgrowth of the fungi. Persons who have acquired immunodeficiency syndrome, who have taken immunosuppressive drugs after transplants, and who have genetically depressed immune systems are all susceptible to opportunistic candidiasis. Superficial infections can occur in the epithelium of the digestive or reproductive tract, but infections are more serious when the fungi migrate into underlying tissue and become systemic. Untreated, systemic infections lead to 100 percent mortality. In immune suppressed persons, all areas of the body are susceptible to fungal infection. Although it was once though that the yeast had to

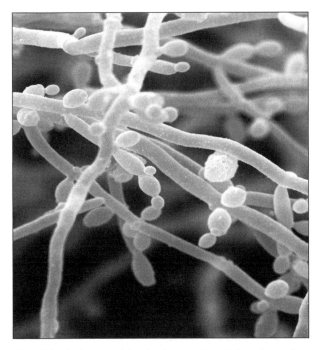

Candidiasis is caused by the fungus Candida, *shown here in a micrograph.*

convert to the hyphal form to infect its host, both the yeast and hyphal forms of *Candida* are infective in some strains.

DRUG SUSCEPTIBILITY

Oral amphotericin B is a very effective fungicide that can be used against systemic and oral *Candida* infections, but it is being supplanted because of its many toxic side effects. The echinocandins, such as anidulafungin, caspofungin, and micafungin, can also be taken orally and are effective against oral and systemic infections. They are fairly nontoxic because they target the fungal cell-wall carbohydrates, which have no counterparts in human cells. Oral azole antifungals, fluconozole (narrow spectrum, which kills *glabrata* but not *albicans*), posaconozole, and voriconazole are also used against systemic infections. Topical applications of micononozole and imidazole can be used for cutaneous and vaginal infections, although oral antifungals are better for hard-to-treat infections. In severe infections, intravenous administration of the antifungal is the preferred route.

Richard W. Cheney, Jr., Ph.D.

FURTHER READING

Alby, Kevin, and Richard J. Bennet. "Sexual Reproduction in the Candida Clade: Cryptic Cycles, Diverse Mechanisms, and Alternate Functions." *Cellular and Molecular Life Sciences* 67 (2010): 3275-3285.

Anaissie, Elias J., Michael R. McGinness, and Michael A Pfaller, eds. *Clinical Mycology.* 2d ed. New York: Churchill Livingstone/Elsevier, 2009.

Dietzman, Stephanie, et al. "Phylogeny and Evolution of Medical Species of Candida and Related Taxa." *Journal of Clinical Microbiology* 42 (2004): 5624-5635.

Gullo, Antonio. "Invasive Fungal Infections." *Drugs* 69 (2009): 65-73.

Winn, Washington C., Jr., et al. *Koneman's Color Atlas and Textbook of Diagnostic Microbiology.* 6th ed. Philadelphia: Lippincott Williams & Wilkins, 2006.

WEB SITES OF INTEREST

Microbiology and Immunology On-line: Mycology
http://pathmicro.med.sc.edu/book/mycol-sta.htm

National Candida Center
http://www.nationalcandidacenter.com

See also: AIDS; Antifungal drugs: Types; Bacterial vaginosis; Candidiasis; Fungi: Classification and types; Mouth infections; Oral transmission; Pathogens; Pelvic inflammatory disease; Skin infections; Thrush; Trichomonas; Urinary tract infections; Vaginal yeast infection; Women and infectious disease.

Candidiasis

CATEGORY: Diseases and conditions
ANATOMY OR SYSTEM AFFECTED: Gastrointestinal system, genitalia, intestines, mouth, skin
ALSO KNOWN AS: Moniliasis, thrush, yeast infection

DEFINITION

Candidiasis is a yeast infection caused by the *Candida* fungi. *C. albicans* is the most common of about twenty types of *Candida*.

CAUSES

Candida fungi coexist with bacteria normally occurring in the human intestine, mouth, vagina, bowels, and skin. Usually the immune system maintains a balance in these organisms. An imbalance leads to an overgrowth of *Candida* and the development of candidiasis.

The use of antibiotics and steroids can disturb this balance by suppressing the normal bacteria flora that keep *Candida* in check. The *Candida* fungi multiply and flourish, causing a yeast infection. Factors that contribute to vaginal candidiasis include taking birth control pills, being pregnant, and having diabetes. Spermicidal foams can change the balance of bacteria in the vagina. Any factor that suppresses the immune system can contribute to candidiasis.

Candida thrives in warm, moist places. A cutaneous candidiasis may present as a rash on various parts of the body, including the groin, underarms, and under the female breast. *Candida* also is often the cause of diaper rash.

RISK FACTORS

Persons at risk for candidiasis include those with chronic diseases who are on long-term, broad-spectrum antibiotic therapy. However, some persons may experience candidiasis while taking antibiotics for a short time. Others at risk include people with compromised immune systems or who have autoimmune diseases (such as cancer and human immunodeficiency virus, or HIV, infection). Diabetics may be more susceptible to candidiasis because of the growth of fungus in the presence of sugar. High-stress lifestyles can lower immune-system function and predispose a person to candidiasis. Persons with urinary catheters or persons who use intravenous drugs may be prone to candidiasis. A break in the skin can result in a life-threatening blood infection known as systemic candidiasis.

SYMPTOMS

Symptoms of a candidiasis depend on the location of the infection. A woman who has vaginal candidiasis will likely experience burning during urination and itching of the vulva. Sexual intercourse may be painful because of irritation and swelling of the female organs. A vaginal discharge will present as either thick, white, and clumpy (like cottage cheese) or thin and watery with a characteristic yeast odor.

The infant or toddler with a diaper rash may have red, itchy bumps or papules or a raw, painful rash. If the yeast infection occurs in the mouth or throat to become thrush, white patches will likely appear on the tongue and oral mucosa. Oral yeast can form around dentures. The affected person or infant with oral thrush may experience difficulty swallowing.

Cutaneous candidiasis may present as pimples at the base of hair follicles or as a rash under the arms or breasts or around the genital area, groin, or folds of skin. The infected skin may become inflamed with intense itching.

Candidiasis can affect the internal organs in persons with a suppressed immune system. A person undergoing chemotherapy or a person who has acquired immunodeficiency syndrome (AIDS) may experience oral candidiasis that spreads down the throat, causing esophagitis, or spreads into the stomach and the rest of the gastrointestinal system. These persons tend to become dehydrated and show symptoms such as fever, rash, or chills, indicating possible extensive disease involvement. One should seek immediate treatment if these symptoms appear.

SCREENING AND DIAGNOSIS

A health care provider can diagnosis candidiasis by physical examination. To diagnosis oral candidiasis or thrush, the provider examines the mucous membranes of the mouth for white patches that look like milk curds that cannot be wiped off. Cutaneous candidiasis can be diagnosed by inspecting the affected skin and collecting scrapings for microscopic review. Vaginal candidiasis can be diagnosed by the appearance and yeastlike odor of the discharge and by a culture obtained during a pelvic exam. Internal organ disease may require computed tomography (CT) or magnetic resonance imaging (MRI) scans or a biopsy for definitive diagnosis. Systemic candidiasis infections may be detected with blood sample testing. Undiagnosed immune deficiency diseases, such as leukemia or AIDS, can be discovered secondary to diagnosis of candidiasis.

TREATMENT AND THERAPY

Candidiasis is treated based on the location and severity of the infection. Cutaneous skin infections require the use of a topical antifungal medication. Diaper rash can be treated with over-the-counter powders or creams such as Mycostatin. Vaginal yeast infections require intravaginal antifungal creams or suppositories such as miconazole (Monistat) or an oral antifungal medication such as fluconazole (Diflucan), or both. For thrush, an oral antifungal mouth rinse such as nystatin or a medicated oral lozenge may be recommended. If the infection is systemic or life-threatening, intravenous antifungal medications such as amphotericin B may be prescribed.

Complementary or natural therapy practitioners recommend taking dietary supplements such as garlic, digestive enzymes, psyllium husk and seed powder, and homeopathic tinctures. A diet designed to starve the yeast would limit the intake of sugar, alcohol, and refined and processed foods. Acupuncture may be used to boost the immune system.

PREVENTION AND OUTCOMES

To prevent candidiasis, some practitioners pre-scribe probiotics and yogurt to prevent growth of *Candida* and to return the balance of healthy normal flora. Avoiding the overuse of antibiotics can help maintain balance between *Candida* and normal bacteria

Though not considered a sexually transmitted disease, candidiasis should keep an infected person from having sexual intercourse until symptoms are gone. Also, one should avoid any contact with substances that can change the balance of normal flora bacteria of the vagina; these substances include douches, vaginal deodorants, and bubble bath.

Yeast thrives in warm, dark, and moist areas such as the groin, so wearing loose-fitting cotton under-garments may decrease the incidence of infection. Avoiding tight pantyhose (or nylons) in warm or hot weather is recommended as well. One should also practice good personal hygiene and keep the skin clean and dry. Babies and toddlers should be kept clean and dry with frequent diaper changes. Other preventive measures include eating a healthy, well-balanced diet and drinking adequate fluids to pro-mote a healthy immune system; restricting one's intake of sugar, alcohol, and processed foods; maintaining control of blood sugar levels (especially persons with diabetes); and losing weight.

Marylane Wade Koch, M.S.N., R.N.

FURTHER READING

Mandell, Gerald L., John E. Bennett, and Raphael Dolin, eds. *Mandell, Douglas, and Bennett's Principles and Practice of Infectious Diseases.* 7th ed. New York: Churchill Livingstone/Elsevier, 2010. An out-standing textbook on infectious diseases, with chapters on the various diseases caused by Can-dida, illnesses and conditions associated with this fungus, and antifungal agents.

Margolis, Simon. *Johns Hopkins Complete Home Guide to Symptoms and Remedies.* New York: Black Dog and Leventhal, 2004. Provides insights on more than five hundred conditions, including candidiasis, with advice by leading specialists at Johns Hopkins Medical Center.

National Library of Medicine. "Cutaneous Candi-diasis." Available at http://www.nlm.nih.gov/medlineplus/ency/article/000880.htm.

Parker, James N., and Philip M. Parker, eds. *The Official Patient's Sourcebook on Genital Candidiasis.* San Diego, Calif.: Icon Health, 2002. Draws from public, academic, government, and peer-reviewed research to provide a wide-ranging handbook for persons with candidiasis.

Quick Access Patient Information on Conditions, Herbs, and Supplements. New York: Thieme, 2000. Provides information on common health conditions, in-cluding candidiasis, and alternative approaches for treatment. Includes reviews by physicians at noted universities and hospitals.

Winn, Washington C., Jr., et al. *Koneman's Color Atlas and Textbook of Diagnostic Microbiology.* 6th ed. Phila-delphia: Lippincott Williams & Wilkins, 2006. A practical text with excellent tables, charts, and pho-tographs of microorganisms, including Candida.

WEB SITES OF INTEREST

American Congress of Obstetricians and Gynecologists
http://www.acog.org

National Candida Center
http://www.nationalcandidacenter.com

National Women's Health Information Center
http://www.womenshealth.gov

See also: Alternative therapies; Antibiotics: Types; An-tifungal drugs: Types; Bacterial vaginosis; Candida; Cervical cancer; Fungal infections; Fungi: Classifica-tion and types; Intestinal and stomach infections; Mouth infections; Oral transmission; Pelvic inflamma-tory disease; Skin infections; Thrush; Trichomonas; Urinary tract infections; Vaginal yeast infection; Women and infectious disease.

Capillariasis

CATEGORY: Diseases and conditions
ANATOMY OR SYSTEM AFFECTED: Gastrointestinal system, intestines, liver, lungs, respiratory system

DEFINITION

Capillariasis is a disease of the intestines, lungs, or liver caused by nematodes (roundworms) belonging to the genus *Capillaria*.

CAUSES

There are three causes of human capillariasis: *C. philippinensis*, which causes intestinal capillariasis; *C. hepatica*, which causes hepatic capillariasis; and *C. aerophila*, which causes pulmonary capillariasis.

Humans become infected with intestinal capillariasis when they ingest raw and undercooked fish containing the *C. philippinensis* nematodes. These worms live in the small intestine and burrow into the mucosa. Female worms deposit unembryonated (noninfectious) eggs, some of which can become embryonated and can thus release larvae. Autoinfection with the larvae can result in hyperinfection with massive numbers of adult nematodes.

Infection with *C. hepatica* results from consuming food, water, or soil that has been contaminated with feces containing embryonated eggs. The infective eggs hatch in the intestine and release larvae. The larvae migrate to the liver, mature into adults, mate, and lay hundreds of unembryonated eggs that remain in the liver until the infected person dies. Eggs, subsequently eaten by a internal predator or scavenger, are passed in the feces into the environment, where they can then become embryonated.

Female *C. aerophila* deposit unembryonated eggs in the lungs of many domestic and wild animals. The eggs are coughed up, swallowed, and passed in the animal's feces. Under favorable conditions, the eggs become embryonated in the soil, are ingested by earthworms, and hatch inside earthworms. Other animals become infected when they ingest the earthworms. Human infection results from ingestion of embryonated eggs in contaminated soil (such as through the consumption of vegetables not sufficiently washed). Once in the human host, the larvae migrate to the lungs and invade the mucosa.

RISK FACTORS

Eating raw or undercooked fish is a risk factor for intestinal capillariasis. The bite of an urban rodent is a risk factor for hepatic capillariasis because these rodents harbor *C. hepatica* eggs in their liver, which are natural reservoirs of the nematodes. Another risk factor for both hepatic and pulmonary capillariasis is consuming undercooked food, untreated water, or unwashed fruits and vegetables. In addition, increasing numbers of foxes and stray dogs and cats living in urban areas may increase the risk for pulmonary capillariasis.

SYMPTOMS

The symptoms of intestinal capillariasis include watery diarrhea, abdominal pain, edema, weight loss, borborygmus (stomach growling), and decreased potassium and albumin levels in the blood. Hepatic capillariasis causes severe symptoms that mimic acute hepatitis. The clinical symptoms of pulmonary capillariasis are bronchitis, coughing, mucoid or blood-tinged sputum, fever, dyspnea, and eosinophilia.

SCREENING AND DIAGNOSIS

The diagnosis of human capillariasis usually involves finding the eggs or adults of *C. philippinensis* in stool samples. Hepatic capillariasis is diagnosed by the finding of the eggs or adult of *C. hepatica* in biopsy or autopsy specimens. Bronchial biopsies and sputum containing *C. aerophila* eggs or adults is helpful in the diagnosis of pulmonary capillariasis.

TREATMENT AND THERAPY

Capillariasis is treated with anthelmintics such as mebendazole and albendazole.

PREVENTION AND OUTCOMES

Capillariasis can be prevented by avoiding the consumption of raw or undercooked fish and other foods, by avoiding drinking untreated water, and by cleaning fruits and vegetables thoroughly before eating.

Diep Koly, M.D.

FURTHER READING

Berger, Stephen A., and John S. Marr. *Human Parasitic Diseases Sourcebook*. Sudbury, Mass.: Jones and Bartlett, 2006.

Icon Health. *Roundworms: A Medical Dictionary, Bibliog-*

raphy, and Annotated Research Guide to Internet References. San Diego, Calif.: Author, 2004.

Roberts, Larry S., and John Janovy, Jr. *Gerald D. Schmidt
and Larry S. Roberts' Foundations of Parasitology.* 8th
ed. Boston: McGraw-Hill, 2009.

Weller, P. F., and T. B. Nutman. "Intestinal Nematodes."
In Harrison's Principles of Internal Medicine, ed-
ited by Joan Butterton. 17th ed. New York: Mc-
Graw-Hill, 2008.

WEB SITES OF INTEREST

Centers for Disease Control and Prevention
http://www.cdc.gov/parasites

Microbiology and Immunology On-line: Parasitology
http://pathmicro.med.sc.edu/book/parasit-sta.htm

See also: Amebic dysentery; Ascariasis; Cryptosporidiosis; Diverticulitis; Elephantiasis; Fecal-oral route of
transmission; Food-borne illness and disease; Giardiasis; Hookworms; Intestinal and stomach infections;
Norovirus infection; Parasites: Classification and types;
Parasitic diseases; Peritonitis; Pinworms; Roundworms;
Strongyloidiasis; Travelers' diarrhea; Tropical medicine; Waterborne illness and disease; Whipworm infection; Worm infections.

Capnocytophaga infections

CATEGORY: Diseases and conditions
ANATOMY OR SYSTEM AFFECTED: All

DEFINITION

Capnocytophaga infections are caused by the bacterium *Capnocytophaga,* a slender, fusiform-shaped, gram-
negative rod that requires a carbon-dioxide-enriched
environment to grow. *Capnocytophaga* is an opportunistic pathogen.

There are seven species of *Capnocytophaga: cani-
morsus* and *cynodegmi* are part of the oropharyngeal
flora of dogs and cats; *ochracea, sputigena, gingivalis,
granulosa,* and *haemolytica* are part of the oropharyngeal flora in humans.

CAUSES

Capnocytophaga possesses virulence factors that degrade tissue, inhibit macrophage activity, and increase
inflammation. *Capnocytophaga* species can enter the
bloodstream in the immunocompromised person
through ulcers in the mouth, leading to sepsis and endocarditis.

An infection caused by a human, dog, or cat *Capnocytophaga* bite can develop into cellulitis. *Capnocytophaga* species has been isolated from dental plaque
and is a cause of juvenile gingivitis and periodontal
disease.

RISK FACTORS

The following factors increase the risk of developing a *Capnocytophaga* infection: poor dental hygiene, leukemia, multiple myeloma, cirrhosis of the
liver caused by alcoholism, splenectomy, use of corticosteroids, and chemotherapy. Another risk factor is
contact with dogs and cats.

SYMPTOMS

Symptoms are not specific for *Capnocytophaga* infection and will vary depending on the site of infection. The symptoms range from fever, cellulitis, and
sinusitis to abscesses, skin lesions, and renal failure.

SCREENING AND DIAGNOSIS

A physician will consider *Capnocytophaga* infection
in immunocompromised persons and in persons who
have been bitten by a dog, a cat, or another person.
Diagnosis involves isolating one of the *Capnocytophaga*
species from clinical specimens. The type of specimens submitted for culture depends on the site of the
infection and include blood, an aspirate from an infected wound, sputum if pneumonia is present, and
spinal fluid if meningitis is suspected. *Capnocytophaga*
species are all slow-growing; they require a minimum
of forty-eight hours of incubation to develop their
characteristic morphology.

TREATMENT AND THERAPY

In serious infections, one should start empiric
therapy based on the clinical findings and the patient's history. *Capnocytophaga* species are susceptible
to the antibiotics erythromycin, clindamycin, tetracycline, and imipenem/cilastatin. Penicillin-resistant
strains are being isolated, so testing for beta-lactamase
using the nitrocefin test can help direct therapy. For
beta-lactamase-positive strains, the use of amoxicillin/
clavulanate is effective. The fluoroquinolones (ciprofloxacin) have also shown resistance. Abscesses need

to be drained, and the patient needs treatment with antibiotics.

PREVENTION AND OUTCOMES

Preventing *Capnocytophaga* infections requires treatment of any underlying diseases, maintaining good dental health, the administration of prophylactic antibiotics before dental work for persons at risk, and thorough handwashing after contact with cats and dogs.

Carol Ann Suda, B.S., MT(ASCP)SM

FURTHER READING

Engelkirk, Paul G., and Janet Duben-Engelkirk. *Laboratory Diagnosis of Infectious Diseases: Essentials of Diagnostic Microbiology.* Baltimore: Lippincott Williams & Wilkins 2008.

Gomez-Garces, Jose-Luis, et al. "Bacteremia by Multidrug-Resistant Capnocytophaga sputigena." *Journal of Clinical Microbiology* 32, no. 4 (April, 1994): 1067-1069.

Winn, Washington C., Jr., et al. *Koneman's Color Atlas and Textbook of Diagnostic Microbiology.* 6th ed. Philadelphia: Lippincott Williams & Wilkins, 2006.

WEB SITES OF INTEREST

American Dental Association
http://www.ada.org

Centers for Disease Control and Prevention
http://www.cdc.gov

See also: Antibiotics: Types; Bacteria: Classification and types; Bacterial infections; Cat scratch fever; Cats and infectious disease; Cellulitis; Dogs and infectious disease; Endocarditis; Gingivitis; Mouth infections; Nasopharyngeal infections; Sepsis; Thrush.

Carriers

CATEGORY: Transmission
ALSO KNOWN AS: Vectors

DEFINITION

A carrier is an intermediary, usually an insect or an arthropod, that transfers pathogenic microbes from an infected host to another living thing, including a human. For example, a mosquito or tick may be carrying bacteria or viruses (pathogens) from a sick bird or rodent. When the mosquito or tick bites someone, the pathogens enter the body through the break in the skin. These pathogenic microbes cause infection in the recipient, but they do not make the carrier ill.

VECTOR-BORNE DISEASES

The most commonly reported vector-borne disease in the United States is Lyme disease, which is caused by the bacterial spirochete *Borrelia burgdorferi.* Humans acquire it by being bitten by an infected black-legged tick. Other varieties of ticks are carriers of Rocky Mountain spotted fever, caused by the bacterium *Rickettsia rickettsii.*

Mosquitoes may carry the *Plasmodium* protozoan and introduce it into humans through bites, thus causing malaria in those persons. Similarly, mosquitoes may carry the yellow fever virus and several encephalitis viruses. Transmission of these diseases to humans typically occurs in tropical regions of Africa, South Asia, and parts of South America. In the United States, mosquitoes may transmit West Nile Virus to humans after the insects have fed on infected birds.

Tularemia, caused by the bacterium *Francisella tularensis,* is transmitted to humans who are bitten by infected ticks and deer flies. People may also acquire tularemia from handling infected rabbits and rodents, drinking contaminated water, and inhaling contaminated dust.

PREVENTION AND OUTCOMES

Vector-borne diseases may be prevented by limiting exposure to mosquitoes, ticks, flies, and fleas. People working or playing outdoors should use insect repellent; wear long-sleeved shirts, long pants, and socks in wooded areas; remove ticks promptly; wear gloves when handling sick or dead animals; and avoid mowing over dead animals. Mosquito populations may be controlled by limiting areas of stagnant water. Screens in windows and doors should be installed and maintained. In malaria-prone tropical areas, one should sleep in an enclosure of mosquito netting (a sleeping net) sprayed with insecticide.

IMPACT

The World Health Organization estimates that 250 million cases of malaria appear annually worldwide,

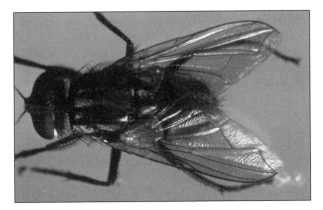

Flies, such as Musca domestica, are common carriers of infectious disease. (CDC)

and that malaria causes 1 million deaths each year, predominantly in children younger than five years of age. In the United States, about 1,500 cases of malaria are diagnosed each year, mainly in travelers and immigrants who had been in countries where malaria is readily transmitted. Such cases may be treated with antimalarial drugs such as chloroquine. Vector-borne diseases from bacterial agents may be treated with antibiotics such as doxycycline and amoxicillin; those diseases caused by viral agents often require hospitalization.

Bethany Thivierge, M.P.H.

FURTHER READING

Goddard, Jerome. *Infectious Diseases and Arthropods.* Totowa, N.J.: Humana Press, 2008.

Higgs, Steve. "Vector-Borne and Zoonotic Diseases Circa 2010: A Brave New World." *Vector-Borne and Zoonotic Diseases,* January/February, 2010, 1-2.

Marquardt, William C., ed. *Biology of Disease Vectors.* 2d ed. New York: Academic Press/Elsevier, 2005.

Schmidt, Laurie J. "Genetically Engineered Mosquitoes Are 100 Percent Resistant to Malaria Parasite." *Popular Science,* July 15, 2010.

WEB SITES OF INTEREST

Centers for Disease Control and Prevention, Division of Vector Borne Infectious Diseases
http://www.cdc.gov/ncidod/dvbid

U.S. Geological Survey, Patuxent Wildlife Research Center
http://www.pwrc.usgs.gov/resshow/ginsberg

See also: Arthropod-borne illness and disease; Bats and infectious disease; Birds and infectious disease; Blood-borne illness and disease; Developing countries and infectious disease; Fleas and infectious disease; Flies and infectious disease; Hosts; Insect-borne illness and disease; Lyme disease; Malaria; Mites and chiggers and infectious disease; Mosquitoes and infectious disease; Sleeping nets; Ticks and infectious disease; Transmission routes; Tropical medicine; Vectors and vector control.

Cat scratch fever

CATEGORY: Diseases and conditions
ANATOMY OR SYSTEM AFFECTED: All
ALSO KNOWN AS: Cat scratch disease

DEFINITION

Cat scratch fever is a bacterial infection caused by a scratch or bite from a cat or kitten (and sometimes from a dog). The infection usually heals without treatment, but it can become a potentially serious condition that requires care from a doctor.

CAUSES

The bacteria that cause cat scratch fever are found in fleas and are passed to cats through flea bites, then to humans through a cat scratch or bite. Children age ten years and younger are most often affected because they are most often bitten or scratched by a cat during play.

RISK FACTORS

Factors that increase the chance of getting cat scratch fever include a recent bite or scratch from a cat or kitten and a weakened immune system, which increases the chance of getting serious complications of the disease. People with weakened immune systems include babies, the elderly, those who have human immunodeficiency virus (HIV) infection or acquired immunodeficiency syndrome (AIDS), those who have had organ transplants, and those who have cancer.

SYMPTOMS

Symptoms of cat scratch fever include a crusting sore or blister that develops over the scratch or bite site; swollen, painful lymph nodes; low-grade fever;

and flulike symptoms, such as weakness, nausea, chills, loss of appetite, and headache. If the patient does not begin to get well within a few days, he or she may develop complications, such as a high fever or pneumonia. Severe cases have caused infections of the brain (encephalitis), hepatitis, and even death.

SCREENING AND DIAGNOSIS

A doctor will ask about symptoms and medical history and will perform a physical exam. The doctor will probably be able to diagnose the disease based on the patient's knowledge of being bitten or scratched and of getting painful, swollen lymph nodes. The doctor may order a blood test, especially if the diagnosis is not clear from the exam and medical history.

TREATMENT AND THERAPY

Treatment options include rest and nonprescription pain relievers, such as acetaminophen, and lymph node drainage. If a lymph node is swollen or painful, the doctor may drain it to relieve pain and help it heal. To do this, the doctor will put a hypodermic needle into the swollen node. Fluid inside the node will then drain out through the needle.

Cat scratch fever usually clears up without treatment, but if the lymph nodes stay painful and swollen for more than two or three weeks, or if the patient gets very ill, the doctor may prescribe antibiotics for treatment. Antibiotics may also be prescribed for those with HIV infection or other immunocompromising diseases.

PREVENTION AND OUTCOMES

The best prevention against cat scratch fever is to keep from getting scratched or bitten by a cat or dog. If bitten or scratched, one should wash the bite or scratch immediately with antiseptic soap and hot water. Also, one should keep pets free of fleas.

Nathalie Smith, M.S.N., R.N.;
reviewed by David L. Horn, M.D., FACP

FURTHER READING

Chomel, B. B. "Cat-Scratch Disease." *Revue Scientifique et Technique* 19, no. 1 (2000): 136-150.

Conrad, D. A. "Treatment of Cat-Scratch Disease." *Current Opinion in Pediatrics* 13, no. 1 (2001): 56-59.

Lamps, L. W., and M. A. Scott. "Cat-Scratch Disease: Historic, Clinical, and Pathologic Perspectives." *American Journal of Clinical Pathology* 121, suppl. (2004): S71-80.

Reynolds, M. G., et al. "Epidemiology of Cat-Scratch Disease Hospitalizations Among Children in the United States." *Pediatric Infectious Disease Journal* 24, no. 8 (August, 2005): 700-704.

Windsor, J. J. "Cat-Scratch Disease: Epidemiology, Aetiology, and Treatment." *British Journal of Biomedical Science* 58, no. 2 (2001): 101-110.

WEB SITES OF INTEREST

Companion Animal Parasite Council
http://www.capcvet.org

National Center for Emerging and Zoonotic Infectious Diseases
http://www.cdc.gov/healthypets/diseases/catscratch.htm

Winn Feline Foundation
http://www.winnfelinehealth.org

See also: Arthropod-borne illness and disease; Bacterial infections; Bartonella infections; Brucellosis; Bubonic plague; Cats and infectious disease; Colorado tick fever; Dogs and infectious disease; Fleas and infectious disease; Lyme disease; Lymphadenitis; Pasteurellosis; Plague; Rocky Mountain spotted fever; Tularemia; Vectors and vector control; Wound infections; Zoonotic diseases.

Cats and infectious disease

CATEGORY: Transmission

DEFINITION

Feline-to-human infections are zoonotic diseases that are transmitted through bites and scratches, through contact with shared vectors (such as ticks, fleas, or mosquitoes), through shared environments (such as contaminated soil), and through direct contact with infected skin.

Bites and scratches. About 1 percent of emergency room visits are attributed to injuries caused by animal bites. Out of those cases, the majority (85 to 90 percent) involves dog bites and a small minority (5 to 10 percent) involves cat bites. Despite the disparities, few dog-related bites result in infectious complications; 50 to 80 percent of cat bites (depending on the source) become infected. Although a dog can exert 450 pounds of pressure per inch when biting, canine teeth are relatively dull. A feline's long and sharp teeth, in contrast, can penetrate human skin, create deep puncture wounds, and penetrate tissue surrounding bones. Consequently, a cat-related bite wound is more likely to result in an infection.

Pasteurella multocida is a gram-negative bacteria found in the mouths of most cats. The bacteria are very common and can be transmitted through cat scratches, bites, or saliva (by licking). The first signs of infection (pain, swelling, and redness) usually occur within two to twelve hours of being bitten. Pasteurellosis, the disease caused by the bite, can spread quickly through the body from the wound site, so one should seek medical attention immediately. Bites to the hand require special attention. If left untreated, the infection can cause complications, such as upper respiratory problems, pneumonia, prosthetic-valve endocarditis, and, less often, meningitis and brain abscesses.

Shared vectors. Cat scratch fever (CSF), or bartonellosis, is transmitted through cat scratches and bites. Between twenty thousand and twenty-five thousand people in the United States are diagnosed with this infection every year, but the disease is most prevalent in warm, humid climates where fleas thrive. Although 30 to 40 percent of healthy looking cats may be carriers, kittens most often transmit CSF. When fleas bite an infected cat, the bacteria are spread through flea excretions onto the cat's skin and, ultimately, to the cat's claws or saliva.

CSF is more common among persons with suppressed immune systems (persons with HIV or who are undergoing chemotherapy) and with children because their immunity is less developed and because they are more likely to roughhouse with cats. Symptoms include a rash or blister at the wound site; swollen lymph nodes around the head, neck, and upper limbs; fever; headache; and sore muscles and joints. The infection usually disappears in four to eight weeks. In immunosuppressed persons, however, complications, often severe, include high fever, sweats, chills, vomiting, and weight loss. Flea control is the key to preventing this disease, so one should consult a veterinarian.

Shared environment. Salmonellosis is a common bacterial disease of the intestinal tract of many animals. It usually is contracted by eating undercooked meat and eggs or contaminated vegetables. When cats eat raw meat or wild prey, they are more likely to contract this bacteria and transmit it through contaminated stools. Salmonellosis is one of the few infections that can be passed from humans to cats and back to humans.

Following a twelve- to thirty-six-hour incubation period, symptoms include headache, fever, diarrhea, nausea, and dehydration. The best prevention is to feed cats processed foods and to wash hands thoroughly after cleaning litter boxes. Also, a person who has a cat as a pet should be extra vigilant if the cat has diarrhea.

Another form of transmission in a shared environment is contact with cat feces contaminated with *Toxoplasma gondii*, a single-celled protozoal organism that infects animals and birds. Only in the cat, however, does this organism find an ideal host to reproduce and complete its life cycle. Cats become targets when they ingest contaminated prey or raw meat, or infected soil. Once ingested, the bacteria burrow into the cat's intestine, and early-stage cells, called oocytes, are eliminated in cat feces. The bacteria can also foul soil, water, gardens, sand boxes, or any location where an infected cat defecates. Because toxoplasma oocysts require one to four days to incubate to become infective, it is important to empty litter daily and dispose of waste properly to prevent this serious parasitic disease.

Typically, symptoms include body aches, swollen lymph nodes, headaches, fever, fatigue, and eye infections. However, in immunosuppressed persons or in pregnant women, complications can be serious. Pregnant women who contract toxoplasmosis have a 30 percent chance of passing this infection to their fetus, which can result in stillborn births or miscarriage. Even children who survive may develop complications, such as seizures, an enlarged spleen, jaundice, and eye infections. Additionally, research has linked toxoplasma to mental illness such as schizophrenia and bipolar disorder in adults.

Pregnant or immunocompromised persons should ask another person to change a litter box daily, and those who clean the litter box should wear gloves and wash hands thoroughly afterward. Cat owners can limit exposure by keeping cats indoors.

Direct contact. Ringworm is a fungal infection, whose manifestation in cats includes, most commonly, *Microsporum canis*; *Trichophyton*, through rodent contact; and *M. gypseum*, through contact with contaminated soil. Ringworm is highly contagious and is spread through direct contact with an infected animal or through spores shed in carpets, furniture, bedding, and air filters. Spores can last eighteen months, so treatment must include thorough house cleaning. Most common among kittens, the resulting ringworm lesions consist of localized hair loss, scaling, and crusting, although some cats are asymptomatic carriers. Treating cats with medication is highly recommended. To reduce environmental contamination, infected cats should be confined to one room until they are ringworm free and until the household can be disinfected.

IMPACT

Although there are thirty or more zoonotic infectious diseases, people are more likely to contract infections from other people than from cats. Also, the principal cause of certain common infections, such as those caused by *Salmonella* and *T. gondii*, is not a cat scratch or bite; instead, *Salmonella* and *T. gondii* are spread most often through contaminated food and soil and through undercooked meat.

Most cat-to-human infections can be prevented by keeping cats indoors and by practicing good hygiene, which includes washing hands after handling pets, disinfecting contaminated areas, wearing rubber gloves when disposing of cat litter, and following recommended practices, such as regular veterinary checkups, rabies vaccinations, and flea control. Lastly, because kittens are more likely to harbor certain bacteria and to engage in play-stalk behavior, which can result in bites or scratches, immunocompromised persons who want a pet cat should adopt or otherwise obtain an adult cat and not a kitten.

Adriane Bishko, M.A.

FURTHER READING

Lacasse, Alexandre, et al. "Pasteurella multocida Infection." Available at http://emedicine.medscape.com/article/224920-overview. Discusses the frequency, mortality rates, and clinical assessments of pasteurellosis.

Lamps, L. W., and M. A. Scott. "Cat-Scratch Disease: Historic, Clinical, and Pathologic Perspectives." *American Journal of Clinical Pathology* 121, suppl. (2004): S71-S80. A multidisciplinary look at cat scratch fever.

Regnery, Russell, and John Tappero. "Unraveling Mysteries Associated with Cat-Scratch Disease, Bacillary Angiomatosis, and Related Syndromes." Atlanta: Centers for Disease Control and Prevention, January-March, 1995. Discusses the transmission of Bartonella henselae infection.

Reynolds, M. G., et al. "Epidemiology of Cat-Scratch Disease Hospitalizations Among Children in the United States." *Pediatric Infectious Disease Journal* 24, no. 8 (August, 2005): 700-704. A study of cat scratch disease incidence rates and patterns in children.

Talan, D. A., et al. "Bacteriologic Analysis of Infected Dog and Cat Bites." *New England Journal of Medicine* 340 (1999): 85-92. Discusses the particular dangers of cat bites and dog bites.

WEB SITES OF INTEREST

Centers for Disease Control and Prevention: Healthy Pets Healthy People
http://www.cdc.gov/healthypets/diseases/catscratch.htm

Companion Animal Parasite Council
http://www.capcvet.org

Winn Feline Foundation
http://www.winnfelinehealth.org

See also: Bacterial infections; Bartonella infections; Brucellosis; Bubonic plague; Cat scratch fever; Children and infectious disease; Dogs and infectious disease; Fecal-oral route of transmission; Fleas and infectious disease; Food-borne illness and disease; Microsporum; Pasteurellosis; Rabies; Rabies vaccine; Toxocariasis; Toxoplasmosis; Transmission routes; Trichophyton; Vectors and vector control; Wound infections; Zoonotic diseases.

CDC. *See* Centers for Disease Control and Prevention (CDC).

Cellulitis

CATEGORY: Diseases and conditions
ANATOMY OR SYSTEM AFFECTED: Skin, tissue
ALSO KNOWN AS: Bacterial skin infection

DEFINITION

Cellulitis is a bacterial infection of deep skin tissues. Bacteria enter the skin through cuts, insect bites, and sores. Persons who are debilitated, such as older adults, diabetics, or persons unable to fight infection, may develop cellulitis without a break in the skin.

CAUSES

Streptococcal and staphylococcal bacteria are the most common causes of cellulitis. Methicillin-resistant *Staphylococcus aureus* (MRSA) infections that lead to cellulitis are often obtained in hospitals. Although bacteria are normally found on the skin, they do not cause problems unless there is a break in the skin.

RISK FACTORS

Any exposure to bacteria may lead to cellulitis. People who work in gardens or other outdoor areas without gloves may get bacteria from the soil. Handling poultry, fish, or meat without gloves or without careful handwashing also exposes a person to bacteria. Any break in the skin from, for example, surgery, liposuction, eczema, illegal drug use, or athlete's foot may allow cellulitis to develop. Athletic events, athletic facilities, day care, and other crowded areas are also sources for infections, including infections with MRSA. Swelling in the legs (edema) from diseases such as peripheral artery disease, even without a break in the skin, may lead to cellulitis.

SYMPTOMS

Redness, tightness, and a glossy look to the skin are symptoms of cellulitis. The area may grow in size and be painful and tender. Fever, chills, and muscle aches may indicate infection. Another symptom is a skin rash that appears suddenly and spreads.

SCREENING AND DIAGNOSIS

There is no screening for cellulitis. A physician usually makes the diagnosis by observing the area of redness. In rare cases, radiology tests such as ultrasound, magnetic resonance imaging, or a computed tomography scan may be used to rule out other problems.

TREATMENT AND THERAPY

The primary therapy for cellulitis is antibiotics, drugs that are prescribed to fight infections. A doctor will carefully monitor the initial response to antibi-otics to be sure the infected area gets better with treatment. If the cellulitis does not improve, the doctor may take blood samples to determine what bacteria are involved in the infection and thus to find a more appropriate antibiotic. In rare cases, sepsis (bacteria in the bloodstream) may occur, leading to the need for additional laboratory blood work. Antibiotics may be given by mouth (orally). For cases in which the infection is more severe or does not respond to oral antibiotics, intravenous antibiotics (administered directly into the bloodstream using a needle) may be indicated; admission to a hospital is likely too. Local treatment of the infected area may include elevating the area and applying moist dressings. If not treated, cellulitis can cause more serious problems, including meningitis, infection in the bone, and gangrene (tissue death).

PREVENTION AND OUTCOMES

Preventing cellulitis means taking care of the skin. Cleanliness; wearing gloves when needed; treating cuts, scrapes, and bites promptly; and treating any skin infections such as athlete's foot immediately are important preventive measures. Persons with risk factors for cellulitis should discuss with their doctor the ways to prevent its development, including taking antibiotics on a regular basis.

Patricia Stanfill Edens, R.N., Ph.D., FACHE

FURTHER READING

Archer, G. L. "Staphylococcal Infections." In *Andreoli and Carpenter's Cecil Essentials of Medicine*, edited by Thomas E. Andreoli et al. 8th ed. Philadelphia: Saunders/Elsevier, 2010.

Hall, John C. *Sauer's Manual of Skin Diseases*. 9th ed. Philadelphia: Lippincott Williams & Wilkins, 2006.

Stevens, Dennis L. "Infections of the Skin, Muscle, and Soft Tissues." In *Harrison's Principles of Internal Medicine*, edited by Joan Butterton. 17th ed. New York: McGraw-Hill, 2008.

Swartz, Morton N., and Mark S. Pasternack. "Cellulitis and Subcutaneous Tissue Infection." In *Mandell, Douglas, and Bennett's Principles and Practice of Infectious Diseases*, edited by Gerald L. Mandell, John E. Bennett, and Raphael Dolin. 7th ed. New York: Churchill Livingstone/Elsevier, 2010.

Turkington, Carol, and Jeffrey S. Dover. *The Encyclopedia of Skin and Skin Disorders*. New York: Facts On File, 2002.

WEB SITES OF INTEREST

American Academy of Dermatology
http://www.aad.org

*National Arthritis and Musculoskeletal and Skin Diseases
    Information Clearinghouse*
http://www.niams.nih.gov

See also: Bacterial infections; Elephantiasis; Erysipelas; Erythema nodosum; Eye infections; Fasciitis; Gangrene; Impetigo; Leprosy; Skin infections; Streptococcal infections; Streptococcus; Wound infections.

Centers for Disease Control and Prevention (CDC)

CATEGORY: Epidemiology

DEFINITION

The Centers for Disease Control and Prevention (CDC), a branch of the U.S. , Department of Health and Human Services (DHHS), is the major agency in the United States for monitoring infectious diseases and other threats to public health and safety.

HISTORY AND ORGANIZATIONAL STRUCTURE

The CDC grew out of an organization called Malaria Control in War Areas (MCWA), which was formed in 1942 as a branch of the U.S. Public Health Service (PHS). Because malaria was common in southern states at the time, the MCWA's headquarters was in Atlanta. The organization's mission was to control malaria around military bases. Following World War II, under the leadership of Joseph W. Mountin, the MCWA was transformed on July 1, 1946, into the Communicable Disease Center, remaining as a division of the PHS. Most of the early activities of the CDC, as it came to be known, remained focused on mosquito control.

With the control and eradication of malaria in the United States, the CDC shifted focus and assumed responsibility for all communicable diseases in the United States, except sexually transmitted diseases, or STDs (formerly called venereal diseases, or VD), and tuberculosis, which were handled by other agencies.

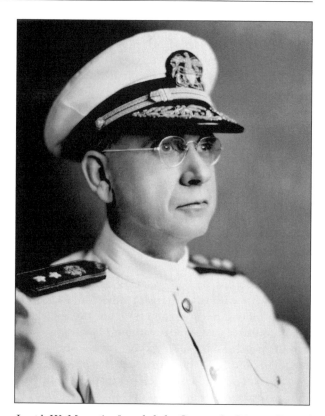

Joseph W. Mountin founded the Centers for Disease Control and Prevention in 1946. (CDC)

Beginning in 1949 under the leadership of Alexander Langmuir, the CDC also became an important center for epidemiology. Additionally, in its attempt to control illness, the organization continued as a strong advocate of immunization programs. In 1955, careful surveillance work by the CDC allowed polio immunizations to be resumed after they had been stopped because of fears that the vaccine was causing the disease. Contamination was traced to a particular laboratory, the problem was corrected, and the program was resumed. The credibility of CDC was strengthened by this successful detective work, and in the following years, PHS oversight of STDs and tuberculosis was transferred to the CDC, in 1957 and 1960, respectively. In subsequent years, more programs were moved to the CDC, expanding the organization and bringing in knowledge resources.

As the responsibility of the CDC increased over the years, the mission expanded from focusing only on communicable diseases to other types of illnesses, and even to nondisease threats to health. Among the programs transferred to the CDC was the National Institute for Occupational Safety and Health. In 1970, officials determined that the word "communicable" did not adequately describe the work of the CDC, and the name was changed to the Center for Disease Control, retaining the well-known initials "CDC." In 1981, with continued growth, the organization was reconfigured, and the name was changed again to reflect the new structure, changing "Center" to "Centers." Since 1992, the even-broader work of the CDC was acknowledged with another name change, this time to Centers for Disease Control and Prevention. The initials "CDC" were retained because of their familiarity.

The CDC is one of eleven operating divisions of the DHHS. The CDC itself is subdivided into an institute, centers, and offices. The major divisions are National Institute for Occupational Safety and Health; the National Center for Health Statistics; Offices of Surveillance, Epidemiology, Informatics, Laboratory Science, and Career Development; National Center on Birth Defects and Developmental Disabilities; National Center for Chronic Disease Prevention and Health Promotion; National Center for Environmental Health/Agency for Toxic Substances and Disease Registry; National Center for Injury Prevention and Control; National Center for Immunization and Respiratory Diseases; National Center for Emerging and Zoonotic Infectious Diseases; National Center for HIV/AIDS, Viral Hepatitis, STD, and TB Prevention; and Center for Global Health.

The headquarters of the CDC remains Atlanta, on land acquired from Emory University. Other than the main headquarters, the CDC has locations in Anchorage, Alaska; Cincinnati, Ohio; Fort Collins, Colorado; Hyattsville, Maryland; Morgantown, West Virginia; Pittsburgh, Pennsylvania; Research Triangle Park, North Carolina; San Juan, Puerto Rico; Spokane, Washington; and Washington, D.C. Researchers from the CDC will travel wherever a potential threat to health requires their expertise, including to many locations around the world.

The CDC also includes a separate foundation—the CDC Foundation—which is a nonprofit organization created by the U.S. Congress in 1995. The CDC Foundation is not part of the CDC, but it does coordinate nongovernmental resources with the CDC to aid a variety of CDC programs.

EPIDEMIOLOGY AND INFECTIOUS DISEASES

In 1951, Alexander Langmuir created a class to train physicians for the newly formed Epidemic Intelligence Service (EIS). That first course was taught by experts recruited by Langmuir to turn EIS officers into disease "detectives." From the beginning, the course emphasized the use of statistics, which laid a quantitative, mathematical foundation under the epistemological work of the CDC. Because the EIS was formed during the Korean War out of fear of biological warfare, the original emphasis of epidemiological work was on infectious diseases. Later, as the CDC mission grew, other sections of the CDC began to use epidemiological investigations for noninfectious diseases as well, including chronic illnesses such as diabetes and heart disease.

From the first class of the EIS, Langmuir insisted that officers engage in "shoe leather" work, that is, going into the field to investigate and collect evidence anywhere there was evidence of a possible epidemic; EIS officers continue to fill this role. Epidemiology is so integral to the work of the CDC that many divisions have their own epidemiology branches. CDC investigators have helped to pinpoint the cause of new diseases, including Legionnaires' disease and toxic shock syndrome. Among the cases handled by EIS officers have been investigations of H1N1 flu in various states, *Staphylococcus aureus* in West Virginia, rabies from a bat in Montana, *Salmonella* infections in various states, and monkeypox in the Democratic Republic of the Congo. In addition to work in the United States, epidemiologists from the CDC now travel the world to work with local health practitioners. Biological materials are sent back to CDC headquarters for identification.

Since the 1960's, the CDC has worked to control diseases in other countries, in part through disease surveillance and vaccination programs. One of the great successes of the CDC was to help develop techniques that led to the eradication of smallpox in 1977. CDC investigators working abroad have also helped to identify and treat Ebola, HIV/AIDS, Lassa fever, and other diseases.

Attempts to control three longstanding serious diseases illustrate the variety of approaches used by the CDC in dealing with infectious diseases. A great deal of attention has been given to HIV/AIDS since an article on the first diagnosis of what would later be termed "AIDS" was published in the CDC's *Morbidity and Mortality Weekly Report* in 1981. As an example of the changing work of the CDC since its inception, part of its strategy for fighting AIDS is to promote prevention—to influence people to change their behaviors and not become infected. The CDC has a Division of HIV/AIDS Prevention, itself containing sections dealing with prevention, epidemiology and surveillance, intervention, and research. In addition, a number of other branches of the CDC have sections that deal with HIV/AIDS. These sections include the Global AIDS Program, which helps with prevention and treatment in other countries; the National Center for Infectious Diseases, which has a division to help control the spread of HIV in health care settings; the National Center for Chronic Disease Prevention and Health Promotion, which supports education programs for young people; and the National Center for Environmental Health, which supports quality assurance for laboratories that test the blood of newborns. Sections of the CDC also collect and analyze statistics to create more effective programs.

The HIV/AIDS pandemic's association with tuberculosis (TB) has increased attention given to TB, which had already been a concern of the CDC since 1960. Internationally, TB is one of the leading causes of death in people with HIV infection. CDC guidelines have been published with recommendations on avoiding exposure to TB and with information for travelers who may be exposed in high-risk settings overseas, such as in prisons or in homeless shelters. As with other diseases, TB rates are closely tracked in the United States. Through surveillance, the CDC notes that there are higher rates of TB among particular population groups or in certain settings, information that aids in attempts to control the disease by prevention. The Division of Tuberculosis Elimination has a laboratory branch that performs genotyping on samples sent in by local health departments. In addition, the division has established the Tuberculosis Epidemiologic Studies Consortium to coordinate efforts among many organizations and researchers.

Another infectious disease that has had great attention from the CDC is influenza (flu), in its various strains. One of the early surveillance successes of the CDC was tracking an influenza outbreak in 1957, helping lead to guidelines for using influenza vaccines. The CDC refers to the use of vaccines to reduce infectious diseases as "the greatest success story in public health," and in February, 2010, a CDC advisory committee even recommended that every person in

the United States get a flu shot. The CDC also provides information specifically for vaccine makers. Patient information on the topic of flu vaccination is considered important enough that it is made available on the CDC Web site in many languages, and special information is provided for people with diabetes, asthma, and cancer. Besides informing the public, the CDC addresses flu prevention and treatment by providing physicians and public-health workers with both information and training. As part of the epidemiological work of the CDC, close surveillance is conducted of viral types found around the United States, and of patient illness and mortality.

NONINFECTIOUS DISEASES AND THREATS TO HEALTH AND SAFETY

The CDC has gone far beyond its original focus on communicable diseases, and the agency now gives attention to any issue in the United States or the world that might pose a threat to health or safety. Within this broad view, issues receiving attention include those, such as gun violence, that are far removed from infectious diseases.

As an example of CDC interest in noninfectious diseases, the CDC created an arthritis program that worked with other agencies to write a National Arthritis Action Plan. According to the CDC, the plan was "a landmark document that put arthritis on the public health map." Other noninfectious diseases addressed by the CDC are heart disease and cancer. The Division for Heart Disease and Stroke Prevention works with and helps to fund several programs fighting heart disease. For cancer control, the Division of Cancer Prevention and Control engages in monitoring, research, and education. In addition, the CDC seeks to educate the public about changing behaviors, focusing on issues such as obesity and exercise.

While continuing its focus on health, the mission of the CDC also includes a focus on safety. General safety concerns include driving, boating, injuries at home, and domestic violence. In attending to workplace safety, the CDC looks at such factors as exposure to asbestos or carbon monoxide, danger from falls, and the environmental quality of the workplace. Food safety concerns include food contamination and the use of antibiotics in animals raised for food. Other examples of work done by the CDC not related to infectious diseases is the agency's recognition of the connection between aspirin use in young people and the development of Reye's syndrome; also the CDC recognized the dangers of lead in gasoline.

The concern for safety and well-being also has led the CDC to focus on a need for emergency preparedness at the national level and the local levels. Terrorism is a threat that can come in the form of biological attack (such as with anthrax or other biological agent). Other threats are industrial chemical accidents, radiation emergencies, natural disasters such as tornadoes and earthquakes, human-made disasters such as oil spills, and outbreaks of food poisoning. For each scenario, the CDC has prepared educational materials for the general public and for emergency responders.

IMPACT

The CDC has made achievements in areas of public health once deemed impossible to reach, including completely eradicating diseases. The CDC was instrumental in eradicating malaria in the United States by 1951, and it was a major partner in ridding the world of smallpox. Because of CDC efforts, other diseases, in the United States and abroad, have been identified. The CDC has also ensured that vaccination programs in the United States are now routine and widely accepted.

Given the size and extensive activities of the CDC, its impact too has been far-reaching. The organization is now recognized in the United States as the main provider of information on disease occurrence, and through the EIS, the CDC often leads the way in fighting diseases. The application of careful surveillance and epidemiological techniques to track diseases has proven effective, and the CDC has made these techniques a basic part of fighting disease. The work has been so effective that it is now applied to noninfectious diseases, such as heart disease.

The CDC's focus on disease prevention also affects the national approach to health care, an approach that has implemented measures to avoid infection and to influence public behavior. Part of the influence of the CDC comes from the strong voice its has among physicians and other health workers with its publication *Morbidity and Mortality Weekly Report*, which summarizes health data from around the United States.

The CDC will continue to have a major impact on health care through disease surveillance and through research. Also, the increasingly broad CDC concerns with health and safety have greatly influenced health and safety discourse in the United States. Future national discussions about health care will likely include the topics of accidents, safety, and emergency preparedness for terrorist threats or natural disasters.

David Hutto, Ph.D.

FURTHER READING

Etheridge, Elizabeth W. *Sentinel for Health: A History of the Centers for Disease Control.* Berkeley: University of California Press, 1992. Details the development of the CDC from its early fight against malaria to its role in fighting infections in Africa and helping to identify the HIV/AIDS epidemic.

Giesecke, Johan. *Modern Infectious Disease Epidemiology.* 2d ed. New York: Oxford University Press, 2002. Divided into two sections, the first covers the tools and principles of epidemiology from an infectious disease perspective. The second covers topics such as infectivity, incubation periods, seroepidemiology, and immunity.

Institute of Medicine. *An Assessment of the CDC Anthrax Vaccine Safety and Efficacy Research Program.* Washington, D.C.: National Academy Press, 2003. This is a representative example of independently contracted evaluations of DHHS agency projects' effectiveness.

Lee, Philip R., and Carroll L. Estes, eds. *The Nation's Health.* 7th ed. Sudbury, Mass.: Jones and Bartlett, 2003. A compendium of articles compiled by two preeminent American health policy analysts. Chapters discuss the complex web of issues, policies, controversies, and proposed solutions that surround health policy, public health, community health, and health care in the United States.

McCormick, Joseph B., Susan Fisher-Hoch, and Leslie Alan Horvitz. *Level 4: Virus Hunters of the CDC.* Rev ed. New York: Barnes & Noble, 1999. A popular account of the role of the CDC in identifying, tracking, and containing viruses. Discusses the experiences of CDC epidemiologists in identifying the most dangerous known viruses.

Marienau, Karen J., et al. "Tuberculosis Investigations Associated with Air Travel: U.S. Centers for Disease Control and Prevention, January, 2007-June, 2008." *Travel Medicine and Infectious Disease* 8, no. 2 (2010): 104-112. Discusses a CDC study of Americans who contracted tuberculosis, and who had also traveled by air, to try to ascertain the danger of contracting TB during air travel.

Meyerson, Beth E., Fred A. Martich, and Gerald P. Naehr. *Ready to Go: The History and Contributions of U.S. Public Health Advisors.* Research Triangle Park, N.C.: American Social Health Association, 2008. A history of the role of public health advisors, including those of the CDC, that includes the topics of "humanitarian disasters such as floods, nuclear disasters, [and] the fall of Saigon," and "smallpox eradication, hantavirus discovery, and health work in unimaginable conditions" around the world.

Pendergrast, Mark. *Inside the Outbreaks: The Elite Medical Detectives of the Epidemic Intelligence Service.* Boston: Houghton Mifflin Harcourt, 2010. The story of the Epidemic Intelligence Service, founded in Atlanta in 1951 under the auspices of the Centers for Disease Control and Prevention to train disease "detectives" to address global epidemics.

Regis, Edward. *Virus Ground Zero: Stalking the Killer Viruses with the Centers for Disease Control.* New York: Pocket Books, 1996. Relates the CDC's role in the containment of an outbreak of the Ebola virus in Kikwit, Zaire, in 1995.

Shroff, Sunil. "Update on Emerging Infections: News from the Centers for Disease Control and Prevention." *Annals of Emergency Medicine* 55, no. 3 (2010): 280-282. Discusses the results of a CDC surveillance report for infections by body and head lice.

WEB SITES OF INTEREST

Association for Professionals in Infection Control and Epidemiology
http://www.knowledgeisinfectious.org

CDC Foundation
http://www.cdcfoundation.org

Centers for Disease Control and Prevention
http://www.cdc.gov

Clean Hands Coalition
http://www.cleanhandscoalition.org

Public Health Foundation
http://www.phf.org

See also: Biosurveillance; Bioterrorism; Developing countries and infectious disease; Disease eradication campaigns; Emerging and reemerging infectious diseases; Emerging Infections Network; Epidemic Intelligence Service; Epidemics and pandemics: Causes and management; Epidemiology; Infectious disease specialists; Koch's postulates; National Institute of Allergy and Infectious Diseases; National Institutes of Health; Outbreaks; Public health; Social effects of infectious disease; U.S. Army Medical Research Institute of Infectious Diseases; World Health Organization (WHO).

Cephalosporin antibiotics

CATEGORY: Treatment

DEFINITION

Cephalosporins are a major subclass of beta-lactam antibiotics. The initial cephalosporin isolated from the fungus *Cephalosporium acremonium* was not active enough for clinical use, and it took substantial modifications to yield a useful antibiotic. The fermentation process required to produce cephalosporins is inefficient; when chemists developed a method of converting penicillins to cephalosporins, the class of drugs became financially viable and substantial research was put into developing more drugs in this class.

Cephalosporins are less associated with drug allergy than are penicillins, and the allergies are typically less severe. They may be given to persons with mild or delayed penicillin allergy, but caution should be used. They should not be given to persons with severe penicillin allergy.

MECHANISM OF ACTION

The beta-lactam ring is responsible for the antibacterial actions of the cephalosporins. They are believed to act like penicillins and prevent the formation of peptidoglycan, a substance crucial to the structural stability of bacteria cell walls. The weakened cell walls eventually lyse, or break apart, leading to cell death.

DRUGS IN THIS CLASS

Cephalosporins are classified as first, second, third, and fourth generation agents. Generally, a higher generation implies a broader spectrum of activity. As gram-negative spectrum increases, however, activity against gram-positive bacteria decreases. Adverse effects are generally mild (nausea, vomiting, diarrhea), but rare cases of life-threatening pseudomembranous colitis and aplastic anemia have been recorded.

Most drugs in this class are relatively unstable in solution; injectable preparations should either be prepared just before using or be frozen until needed. Because cephalosporins are carboxylic acids, they form water-soluble sodium salts; the free acid form is relatively insoluble. If the free acid is used for an injectable formulation, it typically includes sodium bicarbonate to aid dissolution.

Unlike penicillins, cephalosporins are penicillinase resistant. They are not, however, resistant to all beta-lactamases. The first-generation cephalosporins (cefazolin and cephalexin) have a similar spectrum to penicillinase-resistant bacteria, plus activity against Enterobacteriaceae.

Second generation agents (cefoxitin and cefaclor) are resistant to some of the beta-lactamases that inactivate the first-generation drugs. They have greater activity against Enterobacteriaceae, plus activity against some anaerobes, including *Bacteriodes fragilis*.

Third generation agents have a wider spectrum of activity, particularly against gram-negative bacteria. They also are highly potent and have low toxicity. This makes third generation agents (including ceftriaxone, cefotaxime, and ceftazidime) preferred in life-threatening conditions without an isolated causative agent. Ceftazidime is the only drug in this generation to show consistent activity against *Pseudomonas aeroginosa*. Ceftriaxone and cefotaxime show higher activity against the major causative agents of childhood meningitis and are the drugs of choice for that indication. Most are available as injections only.

Fourth generation cephalosporins have greater beta-lactamase resistance and improved ability to cross gram-negative bacterial membranes. Cefepime is a semisynthetic injectable agent with improved activity against staphylococci and an even broader range of activity against gram-negative bacteria than the third generation drugs.

Impact

Although few cephalosporins can be given by mouth, this class has come to dominate the beta-lactam category of antibiotics. They have a broad spectrum of activity, including effectiveness against a wide range of life-threatening bacteria. Only some of the available agents have been listed, and it is likely that new agents will continue to be introduced.

Karen M. Nagel, Ph.D.

Further Reading

"Antibiotics and Antimicrobial Agents." In *Foye's Principles of Medicinal Chemistry,* edited by Thomas L. Lemke et al. 6th ed. Philadelphia: Lippincott Williams & Wilkins, 2008.

Murray, Patrick R., Ken S. Rosenthal, and Michael A. Pfaller. "Antibacterial Agents." In *Medical Microbiology.* 6th ed. Philadelphia: Mosby/Elsevier, 2009.

Sanford, Jay P., et al. *The Sanford Guide to Antimicrobial Therapy.* 18th ed. Sperryville, Va.: Antimicrobial Therapy, 2010.

Tortora, Gerard J., Berdell R. Funke, and Christine L. Case. "Antimicrobial Drugs." In *Microbiology: An Introduction.* 10th ed. San Francisco: Benjamin Cummings, 2010.

Van Bambeke, Françoise, et al. "Antibiotics That Act on the Cell Wall." In *Cohen and Powderly Infectious Diseases,* edited by Jonathan Cohen, Steven M. Opal, and William G. Powderly. 3d ed. Philadelphia: Mosby/Elsevier, 2010.

Web Sites of Interest

Alliance for the Prudent Use of Antibiotics
http://www.tufts.edu/med/apua

eMedicineHealth: Antibiotics
http://www.emedicinehealth.com/antibiotics

See also: Alliance for the Prudent Use of Antibiotics; Antibiotic-associated colitis; Antibiotics: Types; Bacteria: Classification and types; Bacterial infections; *Clostridium difficile* infection; Drug resistance; Enterobacter; Penicillin antibiotics; Prevention of bacterial infections; Pseudomonas; Pseudomonas infections; Treatment of bacterial infections.

Cervical cancer

CATEGORY: Diseases and conditions
ANATOMY OR SYSTEM AFFECTED: Cervix, reproductive system, uterus

Definition

Cervical cancer is a disease in which cancer cells grow in the cervix. The cervix is the lower, narrow part of the uterus that connects the uterus with the vagina.

It is the outlet of the uterus through which menses flow and infants are delivered.

Staging System Used to Classify Cancer of the Cervix

Stage 0: The abnormal cells are found only in the first layer of cells lining the uterus.

Stage I: The cancer involves the cervix but remains in the uterus. This stage has six levels, depending on the size of the cancer: levels IA, IA1, IA2, IB, IB1, and IB2.

Stage II: The cancer has spread to nearby areas but is still inside the pelvic area. This stage has two levels, depending on whether the cancer has spread to the upper two-thirds of the vagina (IIA) or into the pelvis (IIB).

Stage III: The cancer has spread throughout the pelvic area. This stage has two levels, depending on whether the cancer has spread to the lower-third of the vagina (IIIA) or more broadly into the pelvic sidewall (IIIB).

Stage IV: The cancer has spread to other parts of the body. This stage has two levels, depending on what organs the cancer has spread to: level IVA (involving the bladder, rectum, or both) and level IVB, involving more distant organs.

CAUSES

Normally, the cells of the cervix divide in a regulated manner. If cells keep dividing in an unregulated manner, a mass of tissue forms. This mass is called a tumor, and it can be benign or malignant. Squamous cell carcinoma (cancer) can arise either from the squamous cells that line the outer surface of the cervix or, in the case of adenocarcinoma, the glandular cells that are found in the channel that connects to the rest of the womb.

A benign tumor is not cancerous. It will not spread to other parts of the body. A malignant tumor is cancerous, and its cells divide and damage tissue around them. The cells can enter the bloodstream and spread to other parts of the body to become a life-threatening condition.

Pap tests (or smears) are largely responsible for the significant decline in deaths from cervical cancer. Despite this success, more than eleven thousand women in the United States each year are diagnosed with cervical cancer.

Squamous cell carcinoma is more common than adenocarcinoma. Many cases of squamous cancer are associated with a viral infection (such as with the human papillomavirus, or HPV), which, in addition to increasing the risk for cervical cancer, causes tell-tale changes in the cells of the cervix. These changes can be detected by a Pap test and indicate an increased risk for developing cervical cancer. A vaccine has been developed to protect against infection by some (but not all) of the HPV strains associated with cervical cancer.

RISK FACTORS

It is possible to develop cervical cancer with or without the risk factors of HPV infection, sexual history, history of not having Pap tests, history of diethylstilbestrol (hormone) use by one's mother, a weakened immune system, and poor nutrition. Other persons at high risk in the United States are African Americans, Hispanics, and American Indians; those without ready access to adequate health care services; smokers; and women age twenty-five years and older. However, the more risk factors, the greater the likelihood of developing cervical cancer.

Risk factors include HPV infection of the cervix. HPV infection is a sexually transmitted disease (STD) and is the primary risk factor for cervical cancer. There are more than seventy types of papillomaviruses. Certain HPV types can cause warts on the female and male genital organs and on the anus. HPV is passed from one person to another during sexual contact. Large studies have found a particular type of HPV (HPV C, with types HPV 16, 18, 31, and 45C) in more than 93 percent of cervical cancer cases. A vaccine has been developed to protect against infection by the most common types of HPV associated with cervical cancer, but the vaccine must be given before infection to be effective.

After age twenty-five years, the risk of developing cervical cancer begins to increase, but this cancer, or its precancerous changes, can be diagnosed in young women in their early twenties and their teenage years. After the age of forty years, the risk of developing cervical cancer remains stable. The risk of dying from cervical cancer increases as women get older.

Women who had sexual intercourse at an early age or women who have had many sexual partners are at an increased risk of cervical cancer. If a woman is with a partner who has had many sexual partners, this also increases her risk.

Women who have never had a Pap test or who have not had one for several years have a higher-than-average risk of developing cervical cancer. This screening tool is quite effective for catching abnormal cell growth early, before it progresses to cancer.

By smoking, a person exposes her or his body to many cancer-causing chemicals. Tobacco by-products have been found in the cervical mucus in women who smoke. The risk appears to increase with the number of cigarettes smoked per day and the number of years a woman has smoked. Smokers are about twice as likely as nonsmokers to get cervical cancer.

Between 1940 and 1971, doctors prescribed diethylstilbestrol (DES), a hormone, to pregnant women who were thought to be at an increased risk for miscarriage. About 1 of every 1,000 women whose mother took DES when pregnant with them will develop cancer of the cervix or vagina. Almost all these women who develop cervical cancer because of DES have an early cellular pattern change in the cervix that can be detected. Women born between 1940 and 1972 who have been exposed to DES, or who are uncertain about their exposure history, should discuss with their doctor how to determine their risk and the best screening measures.

Several reports have shown that women with weakened immune systems, such as those with human immunodeficiency virus (HIV) infection or those taking immune-suppressing drugs after a transplant, are more likely to develop cervical cancer. HIV damages the body's immune system; this makes a woman more susceptible to HPV infection, which may increase the risk of cervical cancer. In someone with a weakened immune system a cervical precancer may develop into an invasive cancer faster than it normally would in a woman without a weakened immune system.

Poor nutrition is also a factor in the development of cervical cancer. For example, diets low in fruits and vegetables are associated with an increased risk.

In the United States, several racial and ethnic groups have higher cervical cancer death rates. Among African Americans, the death rate from cervical cancer is more than twice the national average. Hispanics and American Indians also have death rates above the average.

Also, experts believe that women with low socioeconomic status are at an increased risk because they lack ready access to adequate health care, which may keep women from getting the necessary screening needed to diagnose and treat cervical cancer in its early stages.

Symptoms

There are no obvious signs or symptoms of cervical cancer in its beginning stages. The precancerous changes happening in the cervix usually do not cause pain or other symptoms. Most cervical cancers are detected through a routine pelvic exam and Pap test. Because of this, women should have regular Pap tests.

When the abnormal cells become cancerous, accumulate to a sufficient size, and begin to invade nearby tissues, signs and symptoms may appear. These symptoms include abnormal bleeding, the most common symptom, indicated by bleeding between regular menstrual periods, menstrual bleeding that is heavier or lasts longer than usual, and bleeding after sexual intercourse, douching, a pelvic exam, and menopause. Other symptoms of cervical cancer include increased vaginal discharge and pain during sexual intercourse or in the lower pelvic region.

The foregoing symptoms can be caused by other, less serious conditions, so having these symptoms does not necessarily mean that one has cervical cancer. One should consult a doctor if any of these symptoms occur. Because cervical cancer does not produce symptoms in its earliest and most curable stages, a regular examination by a doctor and regular Pap tests remain the best ways to diagnose this disease in its earliest stages.

Screening and Diagnosis

The number of new cases and deaths caused by cervical cancer is decreasing each year. Experts agree that this is the case because of rising rates of early detection and treatment. Early detection and treatment are possible because of the widespread availability and use of cervical-cancer screening methods, namely the pelvic exam and the Pap test.

The diagnosis of cervical cancer usually begins in a doctor's office during a routine pelvic exam, which includes a Pap test. The doctor may complete other aspects of a physical exam first, including examining the woman's thyroid gland, heart, lungs, breasts, and abdomen. Part of the pelvic exam includes an examination of external genitalia for redness and signs of infection. The doctor will next perform a Pap and other tests to check for STDs such as chlamydia or gonorrhea.

The Pap test involves collecting a sample of cells from the outer cervix and its canal. These cells are placed on a slide or suspended in an aqueous solution and sent to a laboratory for evaluation. If the Pap test shows abnormal changes or unhealthy cell growth in the cervix, the doctor will need to perform further testing to determine if the woman has cancer, an infection, or some other condition.

If it is determined that the woman has cervical cancer, additional diagnostic tests are necessary to determine the precise type, location, and extent of the tumor to plan effective treatment. Diagnostic tests will determine the nature of the abnormal cell growth of the cervix. Diagnostic tests include a colposcopy, in which a colposcope (an instrument that shines a light on the cervix and magnifies the view) is used to closely examine the genitals, vagina, and cervix. First, the doctor places the speculum into the vagina and opens it slightly to see the cervix. A vinegar solution is swabbed onto the cervix and vagina. This solution makes abnormal tissue turn white, helping the doctor identify the areas that need to be evaluated. If abnormal cells are found during a colposcopy, the doctor may do a biopsy.

During a biopsy, the doctor removes a small amount of cervical tissue for examination. There are several procedures used to obtain biopsies, including a cone biopsy (also known as cold cone biopsy or cold knife cone biopsy), a procedure that uses a laser or a surgical scalpel to remove tissue; a loop electrosurgical excision procedure (LEEP), which uses an electric wire loop to slice off a thin, round piece of tissue; and an endocervical curettage, which uses a small, spoon-shaped instrument called a curette to scrape tissue from inside the cervical opening.

If the area of abnormal cell growth is small, these biopsy procedures may be able to remove all the affected area. The tissue removed during biopsy is sent to a laboratory to be analyzed. If cancer is found, the patient's prognosis and treatment depend on the location, size, and stage of the cancer and on the patient's general health.

Staging is a careful attempt to determine if the cancer has spread and, if it has, what body parts are affected. The higher the stage, the more advanced the cancer and the greater the need for more aggressive therapy. Cure rates decline as the stage of the tumor increases. Additional tests to determine staging may include urine and blood tests; an additional physical exam, including another pelvic exam under anesthesia in surgery; X rays of various parts of the body, including the lungs, bladder, kidneys, and lymph nodes; a barium enema, to check the intestines and rectum with an X ray of the gastrointestinal tract; a CT or CAT scan (a series of X rays that make detailed pictures of areas inside the body); an ultrasonography, in which sound waves are bounced off tissues and the echoes produce a picture; and an MRI, in which a magnet linked to a computer is used to create detailed pictures of areas inside the body.

TREATMENT AND THERAPY

The type of treatment for and management of cervical cancer depends on the location and size of the tumor, the stage of the cancer, the patient's age and general health, and other factors. Cervical cancer treatment most often involves surgery and radiation therapy, and sometimes chemotherapy or biological therapy. Other treatments include lifestyle changes, medications, and alternative and complementary therapies.

PREVENTION AND OUTCOMES

A risk factor increases one's chance of developing a disease. Risk factors for many diseases have been identified. Some risk factors, such as smoking, can be avoided. Other risk factors, such as genetic predisposition, are out of a person's control. Having a certain risk factor does not mean that a person will definitely get a certain disease, but if it is a controllable risk factor, and the person changes it, the risk can be reduced. This is true for cervical cancer too. Several risk factors can be modified by having Pap tests, by practicing safer sex, by considering vaccination, by avoiding smoking, and by eating a balanced diet.

Pap tests. Early detection and treatment of precancerous tissue remain the most effective ways of preventing cervical cancer. Because cervical cancer rarely produces symptoms in its early stages, the best way to detect it is to have pelvic exams and Pap tests. In November, 2009, the American Congress of Obstetricians and Gynecologists updated its guidelines for Pap tests. These guidelines recommend that women age twenty-one to twenty-nine years have a Pap test every two years and women age thirty years or older, every three years. Women age sixty-five years and older may be able to stop having the Pap tests done if they have had normal results for the previous three Pap tests and have had no abnormal results for the previous ten years. However, regular, more frequent Pap tests are recommended for all women who have had abnormal results or have certain conditions, such as a suppressed immune system or a history of cervical dysplasia or cervical cancer.

Safer sex. Infection with the human papillomavirus (HPV), an STD, is the primary risk factor for cervical cancer. Women who have had multiple sex partners or who began having sex before the age of sixteen years are at greater risk of exposure to HPV infection and of developing cervical cancer.

To decrease the risk of getting an STD or cervical cancer, one should maintain a monogamous relationship. However, if a woman is not in a monogamous relationship, she should insist on the use of a condom during sexual intercourse. Although it is always wise to use a condom to prevent some STDs, a condom will not prevent an HPV infection because the virus can be transmitted by perianal contact.

Vaccination. Two vaccines, Gardasil and Cervarix, have been approved to prevent infection by some, but not all, HPV strains that cause cervical cancer. The vaccines reduce the risk of infection from two HPV strains (16 and 18) that account for more than 70 percent of HPV infections that lead to cancer. Gardasil also protects against two additional HPV strains that cause genital warts.

For both vaccines, three injections are required in a period of six months. It is not known how frequently boosters will be required or the degree to which the vaccine will be effective in the long term because of changes in antibody titers through time. In addition, the vaccines ideally should be given before sexual activity begins, as vaccination after exposure to the strains of HPV in the vaccine is ineffective. Gardasil is approved for use in females and males nine to twenty-six years of age, and Cervarix is approved for use in females ten to twenty-five years of age.

Smoking. Smoking exposes the body to many cancer-causing chemicals. Smokers are about twice as likely as nonsmokers to develop cervical cancer, so stopping will greatly reduce the risk of cervical cancer.

Balanced diet. Good nutrition is essential for health and well being. Women with poor diets may be at an increased risk for cervical cancer. Studies have found an association between diets low in fruits and vegetables and an increased risk of cervical cancer.

Mary Calvagna, M.S.

FURTHER READING

American Congress of Obstetricians and Gynecologists. "First Cervical Cancer Screening Delayed Until Age Twenty-one: Less Frequent Pap Tests Recommended." Available at http://www.acog.org.

Berek, Jonathan S., ed. *Berek and Novak's Gynecology.* 14th ed. Philadelphia: Lippincott Williams & Wilkins, 2007.

Dollinger, Malin, et al. *Everyone's Guide to Cancer Therapy.* 5th ed. Kansas City, Mo.: Andrews McMeel, 2008.

Dunne, E. F., and L. E. Markowitz. "Genital Human Papillomavirus Infection." *Clinical Infectious Diseases* 43 (2006): 624.

Henderson, Gregory, and Batya Swift Yasgur. *Women at Risk: The HPV Epidemic and Your Cervical Health.* New York: Putnam, 2002.

Hoskins, William J., et al., eds. *Principles and Practice of Gynecologic Oncology.* 4th ed. Philadelphia: Lippincott Williams & Wilkins, 2005.

Kerr, Shelly K., and Robin M. Mathy. *Preventive Health Measures for Lesbian and Bisexual Women.* New York: Haworth Medical Press, 2006.

"Quadrivalent Vaccine Against Human Papillomavirus to Prevent High-Grade Cervical Lesions." *New England Journal of Medicine* 356 (2007): 1915-1927.

Rushing, Lynda, and Nancy Joste. *Abnormal Pap Smears: What Every Woman Needs to Know.* Rev. ed. Amherst, N.Y.: Prometheus Books, 2008.

Sarg, Michael J., and Ann D. Gross. *The Cancer Dictionary.* 3d ed. New York: Checkmark Books, 2007.

Schottenfeld, David, and Joseph F. Fraumeni, Jr., eds. *Cancer Epidemiology and Prevention.* 3d ed. New York: Oxford University Press, 2006.

Weinberg, Robert. *The Biology of Cancer.* New York: Garland Science, 2007.

WEB SITES OF INTEREST

American Cancer Society
http://www.cancer.org

American Congress of Obstetricians and Gynecologists
http://www.acog.org

National Cancer Institute
http://www.nci.nih.gov

National Cervical Cancer Coalition
http://www.nccc-online.org

National Women's Health Information Center
http://www.womenshealth.gov

Our Bodies Ourselves
http://www.obos.org

Women's Health Matters
http://www.womenshealthmatters.ca

See also: Bacterial vaginosis; Cancer and infectious disease; Cancer vaccines; Endometritis; Genital herpes; Genital warts; HIV; Human papillomavirus (HPV) infections; Pelvic inflammatory disease; Pregnancy and infectious disease; Sexually transmitted diseases (STDs); Trichomonas; Urinary tract infections; Vaginal yeast infection; Women and infectious disease.

Chagas' disease

CATEGORY: Diseases and conditions
ANATOMY OR SYSTEM AFFECTED: All
ALSO KNOWN AS: American trypanosomiasis

DEFINITION

Chagas' disease is caused by the protozoan parasite *Trypanosoma cruzi* and occurs in rural areas of Mexico, Central America, and South America. Some cases have occurred in the United States (Louisiana and Arizona). The parasite is commonly spread by a blood-sucking (hematophagous) insect from the family Reduviidae. Less often, it is spread from human to human through childbirth, blood transfusion, organ transplant, contaminated food, and laboratory exposure to bodily fluids. Chagas' disease has acute and chronic phases.

CAUSES

Chagas' disease is usually transmitted by an insect from subfamily Triatominae and the species *rubida*, *protracta*, *recurva*, *triatomona*, *rhodnius*, and *panstron-*

gylus. Triatomine bugs pick up *T. cruzi* from infected persons or animals. These insects are known as kissing bugs because they usually bite the human face. They live in cracks in the walls of thatch, adobe, and mud huts and houses and bite sleeping persons at night. After the bug bites, it defecates on the bite, introducing the parasites, which are in the bug's feces. The parasites enter the person's body when the person scratches the bite.

RISK FACTORS

The primary risk factor is living in homes that have Reduviidae bugs. Another risk factor is living in a tropical area. Chagas' disease is more common in children.

SYMPTOMS

Symptoms include a red, swollen bug bite; fever; fatigue; rash; body aches; headache; loss of appetite; nausea; vomiting; diarrhea; swollen glands; enlargement of the liver or spleen; and swelling of the eye nearest the bug bite. After eight weeks, Chagas' disease goes into remission.

Symptoms may not reappear for ten to twenty years. Chronic Chagas' disease damages the muscular walls of the heart and the gastrointestinal tract, leading to dilation of these organs. This causes irregular heartbeat, congestive heart failure, sudden cardiac arrest, enlarged heart, weight loss, constipation, abdominal pain, and difficulty swallowing. Some persons develop pain or numbness in their hands or feet, encephalopathy, stroke, motor deficits, dementia, and confusion. Infected pregnant women may deliver a stillborn baby. Rarely, persons with Chagas' disease can die in the acute phase because of inflammation of the heart or brain.

SCREENING AND DIAGNOSIS

Most countries screen all blood donors and organ transplant donors for Chagas' disease. It is diagnosed by blood cultures that demonstrate the presence of *T. cruzi*, which resembles a moving, slender worm. Tests are performed to diagnose complications. These tests include an electrocardiogram, a chest X ray, and echocardiogram, abdominal X rays, and endoscopy of the esophagus.

TREATMENT AND THERAPY

Chagas' disease is treated with antiparasitic medications, which cure 60 to 90 percent of acute cases.

The drugs are less effective in the chronic phase. At this time, heart problems are treated with cardiac medications or a pacemaker, and gastrointestinal tract problems are treated with diet change, medication, and, if necessary, surgery.

PREVENTION AND OUTCOMES

Chagas' disease can be prevented by using insecticide sprays; by not sleeping in mud, thatch, or adobe huts or houses; and by using a sleeping net.

Christine M. Carroll, R.N.

FURTHER READING

Jong, Elaine C., and Russell McMullen, eds. *Travel and Tropical Medicine* Manual. 4th ed. Philadelphia: Saunders/Elsevier, 2008.

Mascola, L., et al. "Chagas' Disease After Organ Transplantation—Los Angeles, California, 2006." *Morbidity and Mortality Weekly Report* 55, no. 29 (July 28, 2006): 798-800.

Reisenman, Carolina E., et al. "Infection of Kissing Bugs with Trypanosoma cruzi, Tucson, Arizona, U.S.A." *Emerging Infectious Diseases* 16, no. 3 (March, 2010). Available at http://www.cdc.gov/eid/content/16/3/400.htm.

Rottenberg, Martín E., and Anders Örn. "Chagas' Disease." In *Encyclopedia of Immunology,* edited by Peter Delves and Ivan Roitt. 2d ed. Boston: Elsevier, 2004.

Seguraa, E. L., and S. Sosa-Estani. "Protozoan Diseases: Chagas' Disease." In *International Encyclopedia of Public Health,* edited by Stella Quah and Kris Heggenhougen. Boston: Academic Press/Elsevier, 2008.

WEB SITES OF INTEREST

American Society of Tropical Medicine and Hygiene
http://www.astmh.org

Centers for Disease Control and Prevention
http://www.cdc.gov/parasites

Emerging and Reemerging Infectious Diseases Resource Center
http://www.medscape.com/resource/infections

See also: Antiparasitic drugs: Types; Children and infectious disease; Developing countries and infectious disease; Emerging and reemerging infectious diseases; Encephalitis; Fleas and infectious disease; Flies and infectious disease; Insect-borne illness and disease; Insecticides and topical repellants; Intestinal and stomach infections; Myocarditis; Parasitic diseases; Parasitology; Tropical medicine; Trypanosoma; Trypanosomiasis; Vectors and vector control.

Chancroid

CATEGORY: Diseases and conditions
ANATOMY OR SYSTEM AFFECTED: Genitalia, skin
ALSO KNOWN AS: Soft chancre, ulcus molle

DEFINITION

Chancroid is a sexually transmitted disease (STD) caused by the bacterium *Haemophilus ducreyi*. The disease, which causes painful sores on the genitalia, is most common in developing countries. Chancroid increases the risk of infection by other sexually transmitted pathogens, including the human immunodeficiency virus.

CAUSES

Chancroid is caused by *H. ducreyi*, a sexually transmitted, gram-negative, facultatively anaerobic, coccobacillus. The bacterium grows in chains and requires hemin for growth. The bacterium needs breaks in the host's epidermal layer to initiate infection.

RISK FACTORS

Chancroid is more common in uncircumcised males and in persons who have sex with sex workers in developing countries.

SYMPTOMS

The initial appearance after infection is a reddened, raised lesion on the genitalia three to five days after exposure, although the infection can appear in as little as one day or in as many as fourteen days. Within twenty-four hours, the lesion converts to a painful, soft-edged ulcer with irregular borders that often secrete pus. Men often have a single ulcer and women usually have four or more.

Swollen, painful lymph nodes are also present in approximately one-half of cases. These swollen nodes, called buboes, may rupture and form abscesses that drain pus. Women tend to have milder symptoms than men, and more than 50 percent of infected women are asymptomatic. Self-inoculation with the fingers can transfer the bacteria, so that chancroid ulcers appear at other locations on the body, especially on the conjunctiva, a membrane that covers the eye and lines the inner surface of the eyelid.

SCREENING AND DIAGNOSIS

Chancroid can be confused with the hard chancre of syphilis, but chancre, unlike chancroid, is usually painless, does not exude pus, and heals on its own within six weeks. Samples from a skin ulcer can also be looked at with dark-field microscopy; a lack of visible spirochetes indicates chancroid rather than a syphilitic chancre. Definitive diagnosis depends on isolating the bacteria and growing it on one of three specialized media, although this test is only 80 percent effective in diagnosis.

TREATMENT AND THERAPY

Chancroid responds well to antibiotics. The most common regimen is a single dose of azithromycin. Other possible treatments include a single intramuscular injection of ceftriaxone, oral ciprofloxacin twice daily for three days, or erythromycin four times a day for a week. Infections in uncircumcised males are more resistant to antibiotic therapy. Sex partners of infected persons are also treated, even if they show no signs of chancroid.

PREVENTION AND OUTCOMES

The use of latex condoms decreases the likelihood of infection. Infection does not cause lasting immunity, and no effective immunizations have been developed.

Richard W. Cheney, Jr., Ph.D.

FURTHER READING

Klausner, Jeffrey D., and Edward W. Hook III. *Current Diagnosis and Treatment of Sexually Transmitted Diseases.* New York: McGraw-Hill, 2007.

Larsen, Laura. *Sexually Transmitted Diseases Sourcebook.* Detroit: Omnigraphics, 2009.

Murphy, T. F. "Haemophilis Infections." In *Mandell, Douglas, and Bennett's Principles and Practice of Infectious Diseases,* edited by Gerald L. Mandell, John E Bennett, and Raphael Dolin. 7th ed. New York: Churchill Livingstone/Elsevier, 2010.

Spinola, Stanley M., Margaret E. Bauer, and Robert S. Munson, Jr. "Immunopathenogenesis of Haemophilus ducreyi Infection (Chancroid)." *Infection and Immunity* 70 (2002): 1667-1676.

Workowski, Kimberly A., and Stuart M. Berman. "Diseases Characterized by Genital Ulcers." *Morbidity and Mortality Weekly Report* 55 (2006): 14-30.

WEB SITES OF INTEREST

American Social Health Association
http://www.ashastd.org

Centers for Disease Control and Prevention
http://www.cdc.gov/std

See also: Bacterial vaginosis; Chlamydia; Conjunctivitis; Contagious diseases; Genital herpes; Genital warts; Gonorrhea; Haemophilus; Herpes simplex infection; HIV; Human papillomavirus (HPV) infections; Pelvic inflammatory disease; Sexually transmitted diseases (STDs); Syphilis; Trichomonas; Urethritis; Vaginal yeast infection.

Chemical germicides

CATEGORY: Treatment

DEFINITION

Germicides are chemical agents that, as antiseptics, kill microorganisms (bacteria, viruses, and fungi) on the surface of skin or other living tissues and as disinfectants kill microorganisms on nonliving surfaces.

APPLICATION

The following is a list of the effectiveness of germicidal chemicals against pathogens, in descending order: lipid or medium-sized viruses, vegetative bacteria, fungi, nonlipid or small viruses, mycobacteria, and bacterial spores. Unlike antibiotics, chemical germicides typically target multiple sites within the microorganism when used at sufficiently high concentrations. For that reason, microorganisms tend to develop tolerance to germicides more slowly than develop resistance to an antibiotic.

EFFICACY

The agent's effectiveness depends on several factors, including its chemical composition, temperature, the amount of organic matter and microbes on the object that needs to be treated, and the amount of time the germicide is left on the object's surface. In most cases, higher concentrations increase germicidal activity and rapidity of action, but organic matter (such as blood or fecal material) decreases activity. Germicidal strength is classified as being of high, medium, or low level activity.

TYPES

Chemicals used as germicides include chlorine compounds, phenolics, alcohols, aldehydes, hydrogen peroxide, iodophors, peracetic acid, and quaternary ammonium compounds. These compounds are not interchangeable because no single germicide is effective against all pathogens and because the agents vary widely according to rapidity of action.

Chlorine compounds. Hypochlorites are oxidizing agents that are widely used to disinfect floors, laundry, and water distribution systems, and to decontaminate small blood spills and medical laboratory waste. They include sodium hypochlorite (bleach), which has broad-spectrum antimicrobial activity but is less effective against fungi. Its advantages are its low cost and rapid action, but it can be corrosive to metal and is inactivated by organic matter. Although relatively nontoxic, mixing sodium hypochlorite with ammonia or acid releases a toxic chlorine or chloramine gas. Other hypochlorites include calcium hypochlorite, sodium dichloroisocyanurate, and chloramine.

Phenolics. Phenol has been used as a germicide since the nineteenth century, and numerous derivatives (phenolics) have developed. Phenolics are medium-to-high level germicides used on environmental surfaces and noncritical medical devices. Exposure to these compounds can cause hyperbilirubinemia in infants; therefore, if used on objects such as infant bassinets and incubators, these surfaces should be rinsed thoroughly with water and dried before use.

Alcohols. Ethyl alcohol (ethanol) and isopropyl alcohol (isopropanol) are traditional disinfectants that are often combined or are mixed with formaldehyde or sodium hypochlorite to increase potency. Alcohols are medium-level germicides that are generally ineffective against bacterial spores and fungi, and they show variable activity against nonlipid viruses. Alcohols are used for equipment such as stethoscopes, scissors, rubber stoppers of medication vials, and the external surfaces of medical equipment.

Aldehydes. The two most commonly used aldehyde disinfectants are formaldehyde and glutaraldehyde. Formaldehyde is active against all organisms at low temperatures; however, it is a potential carcinogen and can irritate the skin and respiratory system, which limits its use. Glutaraldehyde is considered a high-level disinfectant with excellent germicidal activity against all types of microorganisms. Sodium bicarbonate activates glutaraldehyde; it is not sporicidal when acidic. It is commonly used in health care settings for medical equipment because it is not corrosive to metal, rubber, or plastic, and it is not inactivated by organic matter. Ortho-phthalaldehyde has a mechanism of action similar to that of glutaraldehyde, but is more stable, appears to have higher germicidal activity, and does not need to be activated with sodium bicarbonate. However, if not rinsed thoroughly from medical equipment, the residue can stain unprotected skin and mucous membranes.

Hydrogen peroxide. Hydrogen peroxide is a relatively stable and safe compound that exerts medium-to-high level activity. Its mechanism of action involves the release of hydroxyl free radicals, which damage microbial cells. In the hospital, hydrogen peroxide-based products are used to clean equipment and instruments such as endoscopes and ventilators.

Iodophors. Iodophors are solutions or tinctures of iodine complexed to a solubilizing agent or carrier that gradually releases free iodine. The most commonly used iodophor is povidone-iodine. Iodophors are relatively nontoxic medium-level germicides traditionally used as antiseptics. Unlike other germicides, iodophors are diluted to increase bactericidal action. The iodine rapidly penetrates microorganisms, where they appear to damage proteins and nucleic acids and inhibit their synthesis. They are also used to disinfect various types of medical equipment, but they can damage silicone tubing.

Peracetic acid. Peracetic acid is a fast-acting medium-level germicide that effectively inactivates pathogens, even in the presence of organic material. Because it does not leave a residue, it is useful for disinfecting medical instruments. The combination of peracetic acid and hydrogen peroxide is used to disinfect hemodialyzers for reuse in dialysis centers.

Quaternary ammonium compounds. Quaternary ammonium compounds are low-level disinfectants that appear to exert their effects in microorganisms by denaturing proteins, inactivating energy-producing

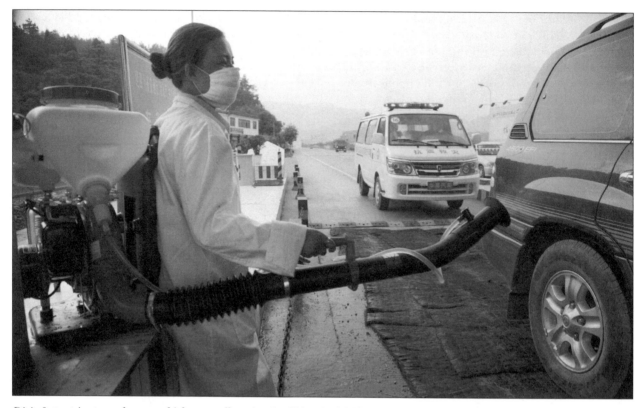

Disinfectant is sprayed on a vehicle at a toll station in China in 2008 to prevent the spread of infectious diseases following a strong earthquake in the region. (AP/Wide World Photos)

enzymes, and disrupting the cell membrane. They are not effective against spores and tend not to be active against nonlipid viruses and mycobacteria. Accordingly, these compounds are used to disinfect noncritical surfaces such as floors, furniture, and walls.

Nonchemical germicides. Nonchemical germicides include ozone, a colorless pungent gas that is a powerful oxidizing agent. Because it leaves no residues or toxic compounds, ozone is safe for treating drinking water, food, food containers, and food storage rooms. Certain metals (such as copper, silver, and iron) exert germicidal activity and are therefore incorporated into medical devices and the environments of hospitals and laboratories. Ultraviolet light is also used to inactivate pathogens on surfaces and in the air.

Impact

A variety of germicidal agents are used as antiseptics and disinfectants in health care settings. Germicides are effective against most emerging pathogens, including *Cryptosporidium parvum, Escherichia coli*

O157:H7, avian influenza virus, and multidrug-resistant bacteria such as vancomycin-resistant *Enterococcus* and methicillin-resistant *Staphylococcus aureus.* Germicides are also increasing used, and perhaps overused, in the home. Their overuse does appear to be a factor in the development of antibiotic-resistant pathogens.

Kathleen LaPoint, M.S.

Further Reading

Block, Seymour S., ed. *Disinfection, Sterilization, and Preservation.* 5th ed. Philadelphia: Lippincott Williams & Wilkins, 2001. Extensively covers the prevention of infection with disinfectants. Includes detailed descriptions of each class of disinfectant, their regulation and testing, and special applications.

Rutala, William A., et al. Centers for Disease Control and Prevention: Guideline for Disinfection and Sterilization in Healthcare Facilities, 2008. Available at http://www.cdc.gov/hicpac/disinfection_sterilization/toc.html. This guideline discusses the use of germicides and similar products in the home, in hospitals, and in other health care settings.

Sanford, Jay P., et al. *The Sanford Guide to Antimicrobial Therapy*. 18th ed. Sperryville, Va.: Antimicrobial Therapy, 2010. A comprehensive guide to antimicrobial agents.

Weber, David J., et al. "Role of Hospital Surfaces in the Transmission of Emerging Health Care-Associated Pathogens: Norovirus, Clostridium difficile, and Acinetobacter Species." *American Journal of Infection Control* 38 (2010): S25-S33. Explores the role of hospitals in the spread of pathogens and discusses current guidelines for surface disinfection and hand hygiene.

Westin, Debbie. *Infection Prevention and Control: Theory and Practice for Healthcare Professionals*. Hoboken, N.J.: John Wiley & Sons, 2008. Includes background information to support the rationale behind basic principles of infection control and how to apply them using evidence-based recommendations on infection control management.

WEB SITES OF INTEREST

Association for Professionals in Infection Control and Epidemiology
http://www.knowledgeisinfectious.org

Clean Hands Coalition
http://www.cleanhandscoalition.org

Healthcare Infection Control Practices Advisory Committee
http://www.cdc.gov/hicpac

See also: Antibiotics: Types; Aseptic technique; Bacterial infections; Bloodstream infections; Contagious diseases; Decontamination; Disinfectants and sanitizers; Drug resistance; Epidemiology; Hospitals and infectious disease; Hygiene; Iatrogenic infections; Infection; Insecticides and topical repellants; Methicillin-resistant staph infection; Opportunistic infections; Prevention of bacterial infections; Prevention of viral infections; Public health; Superbacteria; Transmission routes; Vancomycin-resistant enterococci infection; Viral infections; Wound infections.

Chemical weapons. See Biological weapons; Bioterrorism.

Chickenpox

CATEGORY: Diseases and conditions
ANATOMY OR SYSTEM AFFECTED: All
ALSO KNOWN AS: Varicella

DEFINITION

Chickenpox is a highly contagious viral infection that produces a widespread itchy rash and crusting.

CAUSES

Chickenpox is caused by the varicella zoster virus (VZV), which can spread from person to person through airborne droplets of moisture containing VZV and through direct contact with fluid from a chickenpox rash. The virus is most contagious for one to two days before the rash erupts and during the first day or so after the rash has broken out. The infection remains contagious until all the blisters have crusted.

Because of an extensive vaccination program, the incidence of chickenpox has declined greatly in the United States. The majority of cases (about 90 percent) occur in infants, children, and adolescents age fourteen years and younger. The incidence among adults age twenty years or older is low (approximately 5 percent of cases). When contracted during childhood, chickenpox is usually not serious. Serious complications are more common when the infection occurs in adolescents, adults, newborns, or people with suppressed immune systems. These complications, which usually occur in adults or older children, can include pneumonia; liver or kidney inflammation; central nervous system complications, including aseptic meningitis, acute cerebellar ataxia (most common), encephalitis, transverse myelitis, Guillain-Barré syndrome, and Reye's syndrome (generally only in children and teenagers); bleeding problems because of low platelet counts; and bacterial infections from group A *Streptococcus* and *Staphylococcus aureus*, which lead to infections in the skin (cellulitis) and to toxic shock syndrome, bacteremia, arteritis, gangrene, osteomyelitis, and pericarditis.

If a susceptible woman gets chickenpox while pregnant, injury to the fetus may occasionally result. Some associated birth disorders include poor growth of arms or legs, skin scarring, a small head, and perhaps mental disability (retardation) or other abnormalities of the nervous system.

Another complication of chickenpox is shingles. This can occur years after the chickenpox infection.

RISK FACTORS

If a person is not immune to chickenpox, factors that will increase the risk of contracting the disease include coming in direct contact with someone infected with chickenpox and sharing eating utensils or other personal items with someone who has chickenpox. Some populations are at a higher risk for chickenpox, including persons of any age who have neither had chickenpox in the past nor been immunized against chickenpox (with varicella vaccine); newborns, especially those born prematurely, less than one month old, or whose mothers had never contracted chickenpox before pregnancy; people with a weakened immune system (from chemotherapy, human immunodeficiency virus [HIV] infection, acquired immunodeficiency syndrome [AIDS], or congenital or acquired immunodeficiencies); people with cancer; pregnant women; people who are taking immunosuppressant drugs (such as high-dose steroids); people who are moderately or severely ill and are not yet fully recovered; and people who have certain disorders affecting the blood, bone marrow, or the lymphatic system.

If one is not immune to chickenpox, traveling abroad can increase the risk of contracting chickenpox. The disease is much more prevalent outside the United States because of much lower rates of vaccination.

SYMPTOMS

Symptoms usually occur ten to twenty-one days after contact with the chickenpox virus. Initial symptoms include headache, fever, a general feeling of malaise, and loss of appetite. Within one to two days after the initial symptoms, a rash develops. Characteristics of the rash include, initially, small, flat, red spots. The spots become raised and form clusters of round, itchy, fluid-filled blisters on a red base. The blisters develop in clusters, with new clusters forming in five or six days.

Once the rash develops, a variety of spots are almost always visible. These spots include flat red areas, blisters with clear fluid, blisters with cloudy fluid, and open blisters. This variety helps doctors determine that the rash is from chickenpox.

The rash usually develops on the skin above the waist, including the scalp. Exposed areas are often most significantly affected. The rash may sometimes appear on the inside of the eyelids and in the mouth, nose, throat, upper airway, larynx (voice box), rectum, or vagina. In healthy children, the rash usually crusts over by day six or seven. The crusts disappear within three weeks, usually without scarring. Adults and im-

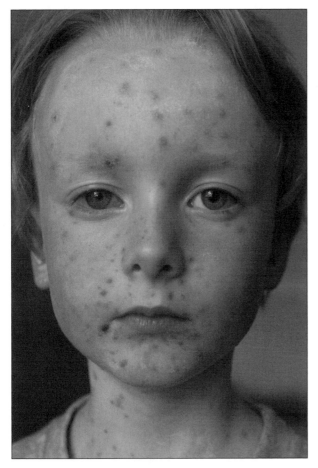

A child with chickenpox, a common childhood infectious disease. (AP/Wide World Photos)

munocompromised persons may have more severe cases of chickenpox that last longer than the norm.

SCREENING AND DIAGNOSIS

Screening tests include blood and laboratory tests, including a skin smear to infer the presence of chickenpox virus by staining, a skin smear to detect chickenpox viral proteins using immunofluorescence, and a blood test to detect the presence and measure the amounts of antibodies to chickenpox virus.

TREATMENT AND THERAPY

In most children, chickenpox is mild and will naturally run its course and disappear on its own. In these cases, treatment focuses on relieving the symptoms through medications. There are no surgical options, however.

PREVENTION AND OUTCOMES

To avoid getting chickenpox, one should avoid contact with people who have the infection and should avoid sharing personal items with infected persons. Also, one should get a chickenpox vaccination if he or she has not already done so. The National Immunization Program of the Centers for Disease Control and Prevention (CDC) recommends that those persons who are unsure if they have had chickenpox or if they have been vaccinated should consult a doctor about getting a blood test to determine immunity. A negative test result means the person is not immune.

People who have had chickenpox are unlikely to get it a second time. However, because the chickenpox virus remains in the body (by hiding in spinal nerve cells), some adults will develop a localized recurrence of chickenpox known as herpes zoster or shingles.

The CDC and the American Academy of Family Physicians recommend that all healthy people (especially adults and infants age one year and older) who have not had chickenpox receive the vaccination. However, those who should not receive the varicella vaccine include persons who are severely allergic to neomycin or gelatin; are recovering from a recent illness and not yet fully recovered; are recent recipients of certain kinds of blood or plasma transfusions (in the preceding five months); are immunocompromised because of HIV, immunosuppression (such as after a kidney transplant), or a congenital condition; are living with a person who is immunocompromised and who cannot leave the living arrangement for three weeks following immunization in case the newly immunized person develops a rash; are affected by disorders of the blood, bone marrow, or the lymphatic system; are pregnant or might become pregnant within the next month (according to the CDC, women should avoid becoming pregnant for one month following varicella vaccination); are taking relatively large doses of corticosteroids or are on other immunosuppressant drugs; or are currently taking aspirin. Because of the association between aspirin and Reye's syndrome in children and teens with chickenpox, the resumption of aspirin should ideally be delayed for six weeks after a chickenpox vaccination. Where this is not feasible, one should carefully discuss risks and benefits with a doctor.

Persons who have been exposed to VZV and who cannot receive the varicella vaccine might be able to receive immunoglobulin instead. Immunoglobulin is a blood product that contains antibodies to the chickenpox virus. As a form of prevention, immunoglobulin is given by injection immediately after exposure to VZV (within ninety-six hours) and is only given, most usually, to people who are at very high risk for severe complications from the disease. These persons include adults (including pregnant women), newborns whose mothers have chickenpox, and people who are immunosuppressed or very ill.

Rick Allen; reviewed by David L. Horn, M.D., FACP

FURTHER READING

Crossley, Kent B., Kimberly K. Jefferson, and Gordon L. Archer, eds. *Staphylococci in Human Disease.* Hoboken, N.J.: John Wiley & Sons, 2009.

Daley, A. J., S. Thorpe, and S. M. Garland. "Varicella and the Pregnant Woman: Prevention and Management." *Australian and New Zealand Journal of Obstetrics and Gynaecology* 48 (2008): 26-33.

Galil, K., et al. "Hospitalizations for Varicella in the United States, 1988 to 1999." *Pediatric Infectious Disease Journal* 10 (2002): 931-935.

Levin, M. J. "Varicella Vaccination of Immunocompromised Children." *Journal of Infectious Diseases* 197 (2008): S200-206.

McCarter-Spaulding, D. E. "Varicella Infection in Pregnancy." *Journal of Obstetric, Gynecologic, and Neonatal Nursing* 30, no. 6 (2001): 667-673.

Memish, Z. A., et al. "The Cost-Saving Potential of Prevaccination Antibody Tests When Implementing a Mass Immunization Program." *Military Medicine* 166, no. 1 (2001): 11-13.

Niederhauser, V. P. "Varicella: The Vaccine and the Public Health Debate." *Nurse Practitioner* 3 (1999): 74-76, 79, 83-84.

Long, Sarah S., Larry K. Pickering, and Charles G. Prober, eds. *Principles and Practice of Pediatric Infectious Diseases.* 3d ed. Philadelphia: Churchill Livingstone/Elsevier, 2008.

Ratner, A. J. "Varicella-Related Hospitalizations in the Vaccine Era." *Pediatric Infectious Disease Journal* 10 (2002): 927-931.

Ronan, K., and M. R. Wallace. "The Utility of Serologic Testing for Varicella in an Adolescent Population." *Vaccine* 19, no. 32 (2001): 4700-4702.

Weller, T. H. "Varicella: Historical Perspective and Clinical Overview." *Journal of Infectious Diseases* 174 (1996): S306-309.

WEB SITES OF INTEREST

About Kids Health
http://www.aboutkidshealth.ca

American Academy of Family Physicians
http://familydoctor.org

Centers for Disease Control and Prevention
http://www.cdc.gov

National Immunization Program
http://www.cdc.gov/nip

National Shingles Foundation
http://www.vzvfoundation.org

See also: Airborne illness and disease; Chickenpox vaccine; Children and infectious disease; Contagious diseases; Herpes zoster infection; Herpesviridae; Herpesvirus infections; Immunity; Immunization; Postherpetic neuralgia; Pregnancy and infectious disease; Schools and infectious disease; Shingles; Skin infections; Vaccines: Types; Viral infections.

Chickenpox vaccine

CATEGORY: Prevention
ALSO KNOWN AS: Varicella zoster vaccine

DEFINITION

The chickenpox vaccine is a live, attenuated vaccine producing CD4 and CD8 effector and memory T cell antibody immunity to the varicella zoster virus (VZV), which causes chickenpox.

PATHOGENICITY AND CLINICAL SIGNIFICANCE

Varicella is a highly contagious viral illness caused by VZV, a human herpesvirus of the Alphaherpesvirinae subfamily. Transmission is by respiratory droplets or by direct contact with the virus-containing vesicle fluid. Household transmission rates approach 90 percent.

During the ensuing week, the virus spreads to various parts of the body, including the skin, liver, central nervous system, lymphatic system, and spleen. The majority of affected persons have symptoms that include fever, malaise, and inflamed, pruritic vesicles, which resolve in two to three weeks.

Approximately 1 in 50 persons exhibit complications that include encephalitis, pneumonia, and hepatitis. Secondary bacterial skin infections can occur as open skin lesions provide an entry portal. Varicella virus can be transmitted through the placenta to the fetus if the disease is acquired by the pregnant girl or woman during pregnancy. The fetus may be born with congenital varicella syndrome and demonstrate skin, extremity, ocular, and brain abnormalities.

Herpesvirus remains dormant in the spinal and cranial sensory ganglia. It reactivates typically in later life as the person's antibody level wanes or the person experiences immune suppression, like that seen in cancer. Reemergence of the herpesvirus is called shingles and can lead to extremely painful postherpetic neuralgia, which lasts from weeks to years.

DISEASE PREVENTION

The vaccine Varivax was licensed in the United States in 1995. In 1996, the Advisory Committee on Immunization Practices of the Centers for Disease Control and Prevention recommended Varivax as part of routine childhood immunizations. Initially a single dose, a second dose was added in 2006. The combination vaccine ProQuad, which contains mumps, measles, rubella, and varicella antigens, was approved in 2005. The vaccine Zostavax has been effective in boosting cell-mediated immunity (antibody production) and in providing partial immunity. It is approved for use in persons at age sixty years.

The most common side effects of varicella vaccine include fever, injection-site complaints, and a varicella-like rash. The vaccine is not recommended for persons with hypersensitivity to its ingredients, which include gelatin and neomycin; for persons with immunosuppression or with active tuberculosis; or for women or girls who are pregnant.

POSTEXPOSURE VACCINE

Post-varicella-exposure vaccination in children has shown some effectiveness in preventing disease if administered within three days of exposure. Protection has not been demonstrated in adolescents and adults.

IMPACT

Before the development of a chickenpox vaccine, four million people in the United States acquired var-

icella annually, leading to ten thousand hospitalizations and one hundred deaths. After the development of a vaccine, these numbers were reduced by 85 to 90 percent. The initial vaccine dose reduced varicella infection by 64 percent, and the second dose further reduced infection by 90 percent. Research has shown that the administration of varicella vaccine in childhood reduces the incidence of herpes zoster in adulthood as well.

Wanda Bradshaw, M.S.N., R.N., NNP-BC, PNP, CCRN

FURTHER READING

Campos-Outcalt, Doug. "ACIP Immunization Update." *Journal of Family Practice* 59, no. 3 (2010): 155-158.

Centers for Disease Control and Prevention. "Recommended Immunization Schedules for Persons Aged 0-18 Years—United States, 2008." *Morbidity and Mortality Weekly Report* 57 (2008): Q1-Q4. Available at http://www.cdc.gov/mmwr/preview/mmwrhtml/mm5701a8.htm.

_____. "Varicella (Chickenpox) Vaccination." Available at http://www.cdc.gov/vaccines/vpd-vac/varicella.

Macartney, K., and P. McIntryre. "Vaccines for Postexposure Prophylaxis Against Varicella (Chickenpox) in Children and Adults." *Cochrane Database of Systematic Reviews* (2008): CD001833. Available through EBSCO DynaMed Systematic Literature Surveillance at http://www.ebscohost.com/dynamed.

Marin, M., H. C. Meissner, and J. F. Seward. "Varicella Prevention in the United States." *Pediatrics* 122 (2008): 744-751.

Roush, Sandra, et al. "Historical Comparisons of Morbidity and Mortality for Vaccine-Preventable Diseases in the United States." *Journal of the American Medical Association* 298, no. 18 (2007): 2155-2163

Smith, Candace, and Ann Arvin. "Varicella in the Fetus and Newborn." *Seminars in Fetal and Neonatal Medicine* 14 (2009): 209-217.

Tyring, S. K. "Management of Herpes Zoster and Postherpetic Neuralgia." *Journal of the American Academy of Dermatology* 57, no. 6 (December, 2007): S136-S142.

Ward, Mark A. "Varicella." In *Conn's Current Therapy 2011*, edited by Robert E. Rakel, Edward T. Bope, and Rick D. Kellerman. Philadelphia: Saunders/Elsevier, 2010.

Whitley, Richard J. "Varicella-Zoster Virus." In *Mandell, Douglas, and Bennett's Principles and Practice of Infectious Diseases,* edited by Gerald L. Mandell, John F. Bennett, and Raphael Dolin. 7th ed. New York: Churchill Livingstone/Elsevier, 2010.

WEB SITES OF INTEREST

About Kids Health
http://www.aboutkidshealth.ca

American Academy of Family Physicians
http://familydoctor.org

American Academy of Pediatrics
http://www.healthychildren.org

Centers for Disease Control and Prevention
http://www.cdc.gov/vaccines/vpd-vac/varicella

National Shingles Foundation
http://www.vzvfoundation.org

See also: Airborne illness and disease; Chickenpox; Children and infectious disease; Contagious diseases; Herpes zoster infection; Herpesviridae; Herpesvirus infections; Immunity; Immunization; Postherpetic neuralgia; Pregnancy and infectious disease; Shingles; Skin infections; Vaccines: Types; Viral infections.

Chiggers. *See* Mites and chiggers and infectious disease.

Chikungunya

CATEGORY: Diseases and conditions
ANATOMY OR SYSTEM AFFECTED: All

DEFINITION

Chikungunya is a relatively rare form of viral fever caused by an alphavirus infection spread by mosquito bites. It is a debilitating but generally nonfatal viral illness, with some reported deaths in parts of Africa, Asia, Australia, and Europe.

CAUSES

Chikungunya is transmitted primarily through infected *Aedes aegypti* and *A. albopictus* mosquitoes. The mosquitoes become infected when they feed on an infected person during the viraemic period (within five days from the onset of the mosquito bites and symptoms) and then transmit the virus to other humans.

RISK FACTORS

The only known risk factor for Chikungunya is an initial exposure to the virus through bites from infected mosquitoes.

SYMPTOMS

The clinical symptoms of the disease appear in two to twelve days after the initial infection. Symptoms include fever, debilitating joint pains, swelling and stiffness of joints, muscular pain, headache, fatigue, nausea, vomiting, and rash. Many of the clinical symptoms are short in duration, but joint pain can continue for some time, as much as two years, after initial infection. Other nonspecific symptoms include conjunctival infection and slight photophobia. Infection with the virus, whether clinically symptomatic or silent, confers lifelong immunity.

SCREENING AND DIAGNOSIS

The common screening and diagnostic confirmation tests for the viral infection include detection of antigens or antibodies in the blood. The common laboratory tests for Chikungunya are virus isolation, specific reverse transcriptase-polymerase chain reaction (RT-PCR), and serological tests. The virus isolation test provides the most definitive diagnosis. This technique involves exposing specific cell lines to whole blood samples and identifying Chikungunya virus-specific responses. The RT-PCR uses nested primer pairs to intensify several Chikungunya-specific genes from whole blood while the serological diagnosis uses an enzyme-linked immunoabsorbent assay to measure anti-Chikungunya antibody levels of immunoglobulin M and immunoglobulin G.

TREATMENT AND THERAPY

There are no specific antiviral treatments or vaccines available for the treatment of Chikungunya fever. Treatments include rest, fluids, and drugs to relieve the symptoms of fever and aching. Commonly used medications include ibuprofen, naproxen, acetaminophen, paracetamol, aspirin, nonsteroidal anti-inflammatory (NSAID) drugs, and chloroquine phosphate. Some reports have discouraged the use of aspirin, ibuprofen, naproxen, and other NSAIDs that are recommended for arthritic pain and fever.

Homeopathic medicines have also been used in the treatment and prevention of Chikungunya. Homeopathic remedies such as *Lycopodium, Colchicum, Ledum palustre, Arnica, Eupatorium perfoliatum,* and *Ruta* are known to relieve fever symptoms.

PREVENTION AND OUTCOMES

Prevention of Chikungunya is through effective control of the environmental-host-agent (EHA) and epidemiological triad factors that inhibit the spread of mosquitoes (as disease vectors), and through the use of chemicals. EHA control consists of ridding the environment of mosquito breeding sites (such as stagnant water), avoiding mosquito bites, and using screens on windows and doors to keep mosquitoes out of the house. Other preventive measures include the use of insect repellants on exposed skin and wearing bite-proof long sleeves and trousers. Another preventive concept that has been proposed and tried is the use of homeopathy, which claims to boost cellular and humoral immunity and, thereby, render the virus ineffective.

Olalekan E. Odeleye, Ph.D.

FURTHER READING

Peters, C. J. "Infections Caused by Arthropod- and Rodent-Borne Viruses." In *Harrison's Principles of Internal Medicine,* edited by Joan Butterton. 17th ed. New York: McGraw-Hill, 2008.

Simon, Fabrice, Elodie Vivier, and Philippe Parola. "Chikungunya: An Emerging Disease in Travelers." In *Tropical Diseases in Travelers,* edited by Eli Schwartz. Hoboken, N.J.: Wiley-Blackwell, 2009.

Tolle, Michael A. "Mosquito-Borne Diseases." *Current Problems in Pediatric and Adolescent Health Care* 39 (2009): 97-140.

WEB SITES OF INTEREST

American Society of Tropical Medicine and Hygiene
http://www.astmh.org

Centers for Disease Control and Prevention
http://www.cdc.gov/ncidod/dvbid/chikungunya

Microbiology and Immunology On-line: Parasitology
http://pathmicro.med.sc.edu/book/parasit-sta.htm

World Health Organization
http://www.who.int/mediacentre/factsheets/fs327

See also: Arthropod-borne illness and disease; Chagas' disease; Dengue fever; Developing countries and infectious disease; Emerging and reemerging infectious diseases; Encephalitis; Insect-borne illness and disease; Malaria; Mosquito-borne viral encephalitis; Mosquitoes and infectious disease; Parasitic diseases; Pathogens; Tropical medicine; Vectors and vector control; Viral infections; West Nile virus; Yellow fever.

Childbirth and infectious disease

CATEGORY: Epidemiology

DEFINITION

Pregnancy and childbirth present unique challenges to the physiology of both the pregnant woman and her fetus (or newborn after birth) and significantly affect the body's immune system's ability to combat infection. The immune system considers a growing fetus to be a foreign object. To prevent an "attack" by this "object," the pregnant woman's immune system self-modulates, resulting in a condition of immunosuppression that exposes her and her fetus to infections that would not pose a threat to healthy, nonpregnant women.

In addition, the developing immunity of the fetus does not effectively protect against disease. Maternal IgG antibodies (proteins that fight infection, also called immunoglobulins) cross the placenta to provide protection, but IgM (immunoglobulin M) antibodies do not. The function of disease-fighting white blood cells and complement-protein activity (another form of immune protection) are decreased. Threats to the fetus include bacterial, viral, and other pathogens inside and outside the genital tract. Some of these cause serious infection in both the pregnant woman and the fetus, while others threaten only the pregnant women or only the fetus. Modes of transmission vary too.

Congenital infections, which occur during pregnancy, cross the placenta to infect a growing fetus and may result in abnormal development, fetal disease, or fetal death. These include the TORCH agents, an acronym that has been used to describe the most common congenital infections. Intrapartum infections are passed during labor and delivery as the fetus travels through the infected birth canal. Examples of these infections include many of the sexually transmitted diseases and group B *Streptococcus*. Postpartum infections occur after delivery and most often involve the genitourinary tract of the mother. In the past, these infections were known as childbirth fever and were once leading causes of morbidity and mortality. However, with the widespread use of improved sterile techniques and of antibiotics, incidence has decreased dramatically. In addition, some microbes (such as human immunodeficiency virus and cytomegalovirus) can infect the newborn through breastfeeding; other infections are acquired during the postdelivery hospital stay, an infection known as nosocomial.

THREATS TO THE FETUS AND THE NEWBORN

Many infectious agents are able to cross the placenta during pregnancy and cause congenital infection, whether these agents originate in the genitourinary system or elsewhere in the body. Some organisms that cause little or no clinical illness in the pregnant woman can present significant danger to the developing fetus; these organisms are teratogenic (they cause birth defects). In utero transmission of infection can occur at any time before birth, and the period of greatest risk varies by organism. TORCH is the acronym that has been used for these common organisms in the past, but as more and more organisms belonging to the "other" category are identified, the term has lost favor. The original purpose of the TORCH designation was to group infections with similar patterns of transmission and presentation. TORCH includes *Toxoplasma*, coxsackie virus, human parvovirus, hepatitis B, syphilis, Epstein-Barr virus, varicella zoster virus (or chickenpox; a primary infection during pregnancy is considered a medical emergency), LCMV (lymphocytic choriomeningitis), parvovirus B19, rubella virus, cytomegalovirus (CMV), HIV, and herpes simplex virus.

The agents responsible for congenital infection carry significant risk of morbidity and mortality and can cause neurological damage, blindness, deafness, cardiac defects, intrauterine growth restriction, skin lesions, and a host of other abnormalities. HIV, one of the congenital agents recently added to the foregoing list, is now known to be a major cause of infant mortality worldwide. Influenza, including H1N1 (swine flu), is a growing significant threat. Many of these organisms can also be transmitted during passage through the birth canal if they are present at the time of delivery.

Routine maternal screening for serologic evidence of organisms causing congenital infection during pregnancy is commonplace in many parts of the world, but its use as a diagnostic tool is controversial in the United States because of overuse and a lack of consistent interpretation of results. Screening is limited to cases in which exposure is known or suspected or in which symptoms are present. (Syphilis is a notable exception, and it is routinely screened for.)

Symptoms of infection in the newborn cover a broad range and are often nonspecific. Fever, hypothermia, vomiting, rash, and decreased muscle tone may indicate infectious illness, and many congenital infections acquired during gestation are accompanied by abnormalities specific to the organism involved. When a diagnosis is confirmed, the organism identified determines the availability of treatment for mother and newborn. Antiviral medications, intravenous gammaglobulin (IVIg), and antibiotics are mainstays of treatment.

Listeriosis is a less common but devastating cause of fetal infection. Maternal infection comes from eating contaminated food. The organism crosses the placenta to cause amnionitis (infection of the amniotic sac); the infant mortality rate for this infection is almost 50 percent. Prevention through avoidance of high-risk foods is the mainstay treatment, but infection can sometimes be treated with antibiotics (with limited success).

The most common cause of life-threatening infection in the newborn is group B *Streptococcus* (GBS), which affects both mother and child. GBS is a beta-hemolytic gram-positive coccus that is often found in normal vaginal flora. Intrapartum transmission to the newborn occurs during delivery and can be the result of ascending infection after the rupture of membranes or of direct contact in the vaginal canal. Infection can cause severe illness and death.

Infants with GBS infection will present with either early-onset or late-onset disease, depending on the time between delivery and onset of symptoms. Early-

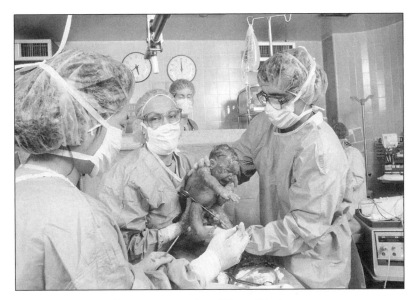

A newborn delivered by cesarean section. (PhotoDisc)

woman, bacteria including gram-positives, gram-negatives, aerobes, and anaerobes, can overgrow and cause infection of the fetus or newborn; these bacteria can also cause preterm labor and delivery. The index of suspicion required to seek diagnosis and treatment should be low.

The degree of risk associated with congenital, intrapartum, and postpartum infections in the newborn is highly correlated with gestational age. The immune function of premature infants is less mature than that of term infants, with decreased white-cell function, antibody production, and complement activity. Premature infants spend more time in the hospital and undergo invasive procedures, exposing them to nosocomial (hospital acquired) infection.

THREATS DURING AND AFTER PREGNANCY

In spite of the immune suppression that is a hallmark of forty weeks of pregnancy, the most serious infectious disease dangers for the pregnant woman-mother are from intrapartum and postpartum events (during and immediately following birth). Historically, childbirth fever from genital tract infection following delivery has been a leading cause of maternal morbidity and mortality. The traumatic nature of vaginal or cesarean delivery predisposes to the local spread of colonized bacteria, and though the incidence has decreased significantly with the widespread use of improved hygiene and of antibiotics, obstetric infection still accounts for more than 12 percent of maternal deaths.

Puerperal or postpartum infection is a bacterial infection that occurs during or after childbirth. Most of these infections begin in the genitourinary tract and infect the uterus and surrounding areas soon after delivery. In some cases, however, organisms may be carried through the blood to seed other parts of the body or may occur through breast-feeding. Vaginal delivery carries an infection risk of 1 to 3 percent, while the risk after cesarean delivery may be as high as 20 percent. Other factors making infection more likely include repeated vaginal examinations during labor, early rupture of membranes and early internal fetal

onset disease occurs before seven days of age and includes symptoms of sepsis, pneumonia, or meningitis. Newborns who become ill between age seven and eighty-nine days have late-onset disease, which typically manifests as generalized bacteremia and meningitis. Common sequelae for those who survive the infection are vision loss, neurologic damage, and developmental delay.

Up to 30 percent of pregnant girls and women are colonized with GBS, but less than 1 percent of these cases have symptoms of disease. Therefore, the Centers for Disease Control and Prevention (CDC) recommends GBS screening by vaginal and rectal cultures for all pregnant females who are between thirty-five and thirty-seven weeks gestation. New mothers with positive or unknown culture results are treated with antibiotic prophylaxis (most often with penicillin G), and their newborns are closely observed for signs and symptoms of disease. The incidence of early-onset disease has decreased dramatically since screening and prophylaxis became routine, but the frequency of late-onset disease remains stable.

Other causes of intrapartum disease transmission include sexually transmitted organisms such as chlamydia and gonorrhea, so the CDC recommends routine screening of all women early in pregnancy. Antibiotic treatment can prevent infant disease. Bacteria colonizing the vagina and rectum of the pregnant monitoring, postpartum hemorrhage, retained placental fragments, prolonged labor, young age, and low socioeconomic group.

Postpartum infection is typically diagnosed when a fever greater than 100.4° Fahrenheit (38° Celsius) is present for two of ten days following delivery. Endometritis (infection of the uterine lining) is the most common site, followed by postcesarean wound infections, perineal cellulitis (infection of perineal tissue), mastitis (breast infection), urinary tract infections (UTIs), and septic phlebitis (infection of pelvic blood clots). Maternal death rates because of infection are approximately 0.6 deaths per 100,000 live births.

Symptoms may include fever, low abdominal and uterine pain, heavy malodorous lochia (bloody discharge that follows delivery), chills, and general malaise. Those with a UTI may have pain on voiding and nausea and vomiting. Those who received general anesthesia for cesarean delivery may present with symptoms of pneumonia, and wound infections may develop swelling and drainage. Breast infection, which can occur when nipples become sore and cracked, allowing bacteria to enter, manifests as a breast that appears red, warm, swollen, and painful (often after the immediate postpartum period but before six weeks after delivery).

Diagnosis is based on observation of symptoms, physical examination, and the results of bacterial cultures and blood studies. If left untreated, severe complications of postpartum infection can occur and include peritonitis (infection of the abdominal lining), septic embolism (infected blood clots that travel to lungs and other areas of the body), and septic shock. Treatment generally includes intravenous antibiotics for forty-eight hours or more, sometimes followed by a course of oral medication after hospital discharge.

Colonization with group B *Streptococcus* during pregnancy is a cause of maternal UTI, amnionitis, endometritis, and fetal loss. Rarely, it can cause pelvic abscess, meningitis, and endocarditis. Clinical diagnosis of infection is difficult because few pregnant women who carry GBS develop signs and symptoms of disease. The current screening and treatment approach, which is delayed until thirty-five to thirty-seven weeks gestation, just before delivery, does not address the incidence of maternal GBS disease during pregnancy. Several vaccines to prevent GBS colonization and disease are in development; routine vaccination would decrease risk significantly.

UTI is a common problem for women, and the risk is exacerbated during pregnancy. The proximity of the (short) urethra to the vagina and anus, compounded by (in the pregnant woman) a weakened immune system and by stasis caused by a growing fetus crowding the urinary system, make frequent UTIs a common complaint. Responsible organisms include *Escherichia coli, Klebsiella, Enterobacter, Enterococcus*, GBS, staph species, and *Proteus*.

Infection may be symptomatic or asymptomatic, and both are clinically important to the health of the mother and newborn. Asymptomatic infection is more likely to lead to acute pyelonephritis (kidney infection), which is a common reason for hospitalization in pregnant women. The severity of infection varies, but it can progress to generalized urosepsis and is associated with low neonatal birth weight and prematurity. Because so many of these infections are asymptomatic, it is recommended that all pregnant women be screened by urine culture during early pregnancy and treated with antibiotics if indicated.

Bacterial vaginosis is a condition caused by the overgrowth of colonizing bacteria of the vagina. Normal vaginal flora varies depending on the pH of the vagina, and overgrowth is polymicrobial. It may be asymptomatic or may present with burning and discharge. The organisms can ascend and infect the amniotic membranes, causing premature labor. It is estimated that 40 percent of these pregnancies will go on to have preterm labor. Therefore, the CDC recommends that females at risk for premature labor (prior preterm delivery or high-risk pregnancy) be screened for bacterial vaginosis and treated if indicated.

All antimicrobial medications cross the placenta and expose the fetus to possible adverse effects, so they should be used with caution. Most commonly prescribed antibiotics are safe for use during pregnancy and include penicillins, cephalosporins, nitrofurantoin, and macrolides, but some have been associated with birth defects and disorders (tetracyclines) and increased toxicity (sulfonamides).

IMPACT

Infections associated with childbirth affect pregnant girls and women and their fetuses and newborns worldwide. Infections can occur from the time the fertilized egg is implanted up to and beyond the moment of delivery, sometimes with devastating results. Expanded prenatal care, improved hygiene, aseptic technique, and the use of antibiotics have made death from childbed fever rare in the developed world, but congenital and perinatal infections continue to take a toll, especially in developing countries.

Infection is understood to be a major cause of preterm birth and may account for 25 to 40 percent of events that result in maternal and fetal (and newborn) morbidity and mortality; infections also add to the rapidly rising cost of health care. The development of vaccines to protect newborns and mothers from disease is ongoing.

Rachel Zahn, M.D.

FURTHER READING

Campos, Bonnie C., and Jennifer Brown. *Protect Your Pregnancy.* New York: McGraw-Hill, 2003. A pregnancy guide with a special focus on at-risk pregnancies. Reviews how to recognize signs and symptoms of pregnancy complications and explores preexisting and developing medical conditions that can lead to premature delivery, among other topics.

Cunningham, F. Gary, et al. *Williams Obstetrics.* 23d ed. New York: McGraw-Hill, 2010. The bible of obstetrics theory and practice.

Forsgren, M. "Prevention of Congenital and Perinatal Infections." *Eurosurveillance* 14 (2009). Available at http://www.eurosurveillance.org/viewarticle.aspx?articleid=19131. A scholarly look at what can be done to prevent infection, now and in the future.

Newell, Marie-Louise, and James McIntyre. *Congenital and Perinatal Infections: Prevention, Diagnosis, and Treatment.* New York: Cambridge University Press, 2000. A comprehensive examination of infections associated with childbirth for medical professionals and educated general readers.

Thornton, C. A. "Immunology of Pregnancy." *Proceedings of the Nutrition Society* 69 (2010): 357-365. An advanced article on the significance of maternal diet and nutrition in healthy fetal development.

WEB SITES OF INTEREST

International Birth Defects Information Systems
http://www.ibis-birthdefects.org

KidsHealth
http://www.kidshealth.org

March of Dimes
http://www.modimes.org

Pediatric Infectious Diseases Society
http://www.pids.org

See also: Bacterial infections; Breast milk and infectious disease; Children and infectious disease; Developing countries and infectious disease; Hospitals and infectious disease; Immunity; Immunization; Pregnancy and infectious disease; Public health; Schools and infections disease; Transmission routes; Vaccines: Types; Vertical disease transmission; Vertical disease transmission; Viral infections; Women and infectious disease.

Children and infectious disease

CATEGORY: Epidemiology

DEFINITION

Infectious diseases are an unavoidable fact of life. Infections are caused by microorganisms that are found in the environment or that are passed from one person to another, and children are particularly susceptible to these organisms for a number of reasons. Most of these infections are mild, resolving with the help of the child's immune system and, in some cases, treatment with antimicrobial medications, such as antibiotics.

Not all microbes (bacteria, viruses, fungi, and parasites) cause disease. Many are normal inhabitants (called normal flora) and coexist on the skin and inside the body of children and adults. Microbes serve important functions, such as preventing the growth of dangerous pathogens (organisms that cause illness) and manufacturing essential vitamins, such as vitamin K, which are not produced by the human body.

At birth, the immune system of the child is immature and cannot work at full strength. While in utero, the growing fetus depends on the pregnant woman (or girl) for much of its immune function. Antibodies and other immune factors cross the placenta to provide protection and are boosted during breastfeeding. The newborn immune system will not catch up for several months and will not be fully mature until the child is fourteen years of age.

The small child is immunologically naïve, and repeated exposure to microbes, including pathogens (disease-causing organisms), helps the child build a strong immune system; this exposure also makes infection a frequent cause of visits to the family doctor or pediatrician. Risk of infection is also increased for young children because babies and toddlers tend to put things in their mouths and pay little, if any, attention to hygiene. Children in group settings, such as child care and school, easily pass infection to other children.

Childhood infections, whether caused by bacteria, viruses, or other organisms, take many forms and can affect many parts of the body. Among the most classic infections are those, such as rubella and measles, that cause skin rash and fever. Others, like the common cold, which can occur an average of six to eight times per year in the young child, affect the respiratory tract and other body systems.

The prevention of childhood infection is based in part on the development of vaccines and immunization. Many diseases that were once considered major killers of children are now well controlled. Some of these diseases remain significant threats in developing countries. Recurrent outbreaks of vaccine-preventable illnesses point to the ongoing and critical need for widespread immunization.

Other ways to provide a boost to the immune system include good nutrition, adequate sleep, and careful hygiene and food preparation practices. The overuse of antibiotics is a serious concern too, as overuse leads to new strains of antibiotic-resistant organisms and, thus, weakened immunity.

THE IMMUNE SYSTEM

Immunity is the ability of the body to resist infection. The child's immune system will develop to become an intricate system of organs, cells, and proteins that work to protect against foreign invaders such as bacteria, viruses, fungi, and parasites. The immune system is unique in that its parts are not physically connected to each other and are scattered through the body. The system includes the thymus gland, the spleen, the appendix, lymphoid tissue and lymph nodes, and bone marrow. The job of this loosely connected system is to produce white blood cells, antibodies, and other factors that seek out and destroy organisms and abnormal cells that cause disease, and to do so without harming the body's healthy tissue.

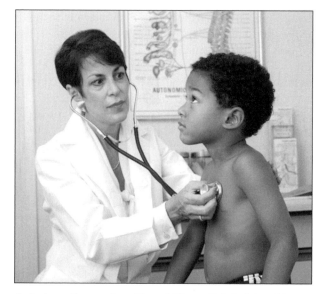

Infectious disease also affects children. (Digital Stock)

Critical cells of the immune system include neutrophils, monocytes, macrophages, T lymphocytes, and B lymphocytes. These cells develop from stem cells in the growing embryo beginning at about five weeks gestation. By birth, the cells are getting ready to respond to foreign invaders, but this response will still be developing. The newborn depends on passive immunity that is acquired from the pregnant female through the placenta or through breast-feeding after birth. This type of immunity lasts six to eight months only and then begins to wane.

Infants begin to make their own antibodies at an increased rate soon after birth, when their environment presents many new antigens (molecules that induce the production of antibodies). The serum concentration of antibodies reaches adult levels by the end of the child's first year and peaks at age seven or eight years.

The immune system works by responding to an organism or substance that enters the body. The cells "see" the invader and produce specific antibodies and proteins to attack it. Later, if the body is presented with the same invader, it is primed to prevent illness. In this case, the child (or adult) has developed active immunity.

Active immunity may arise naturally or through immunization. For example, when a child contracts an infection such as chickenpox, which is caused by the varicella virus, the immune system develops anti-

Children's Vaccination Schedule

The following vaccination schedule, by age and type of vaccine or vaccines, is recommended by the American Academy of Pediatrics. The schedule is updated frequently.

Age	Vaccine or vaccines
Birth	Hepatitis B (HepB)
1 to 2 months	HepB (second dose)
2 to 4 months	DTaP (diphtheria, tetanus, pertussis), Hib (*Haemophilus influenzae* type b), IPV (inactivated poliovirus), PCV (pneumococcal), Rota (rotavirus)
6 months	DTaP, Hib, IPV, PCV, Rota, Seasonal influenza (Inf)
6 to 18 months	HepB, Inf, IPV
12 to 15 months	Hib, Inf, MMR, PCV, varicella (chickenpox)
12 to 23 months	HepA (hepatitis A; two doses)
15 to 18 months	DTaP
4 to 6 years	DTaP, Inf, IPV, MMR, varicella
7 to 10 years	Inf (and start of catch-up schedule): HepB series, IPV series, MMR series, varicella series
11 to 12 years	HPV (human papilloma virus), Inf, MCV4 (meningococcal), Tdap (DTaP booster), and continued catch-up schedule: HepB, IPV, MMR, varicella
13 to 18 years	Catch-up schedule: HepB, IPV, MMR, varicella, and Tdap, HPV series, MCV4

Note: This schedule only supplements the more detailed schedule available from one's health care provider.

bodies to fight it. After several days of illness, the virus is defeated and the child recovers. The primed immune cells and antibodies specific to varicella remain, and if the child is exposed again, no illness will result.

A vaccine that protects against chickenpox exists. It consists of an attenuated (weakened) form of the virus that cannot cause full-blown disease and that tricks the body into mounting an immune response. Later exposure to the live virus will not cause disease. This is the basic mechanism of childhood immunization.

Conditions can sometimes place added burdens on the immune system, making the job of fighting infection much more difficult. Some children are born with immune deficiencies or acquire them after birth. These children cannot mount a normal immune response and may be more susceptible to common infections. Children treated with cancer or organ transplant medications, and those on steroids, may become immune suppressed. Medical devices such as catheters and tubes that enter the body provide a direct path for invaders and often lead to infection. Over-prescription of antibiotics can kill normal protective flora and leave room for the overgrowth of pathogenic species that may become resistant to antibiotics.

COMMON INFECTIONS

As soon as a child is born, his or her body is exposed to microbes that can cause infection. Some of these cause illness, while others do not, and the reasons are not always known. It is clear, however, that infection is a normal part of childhood, and most children will have several infections each year. These infections include colds and other respiratory infections, ear infections, infections of the gastrointestinal tract, and nonspecific viral infections that cause a fever and rash.

The incubation period is the time it takes for a child to become ill after infection. The incubation period can be as short as one day for the common cold or for viral diarrhea or as long as two weeks for chickenpox. It typically takes several years for the human immunodeficiency virus (HIV) to cause disease (such as those related to acquired immunodeficiency syndrome, or AIDS).

Not all infections are contagious (spread from child to child). Ear infections and bladder infections are caused by microbes that gain access to collections of fluid (mucus and urine, respectively) and are not passed from one child to another. Diarrhea and colds, on the other hand, can spread quickly. When and for how long a child is contagious varies with the infection and the child. Young children may be contagious for a longer period than older children.

It is useful to categorize common childhood infections by the part of the body affected. Respiratory infections can cause a wide range of symptoms. Some are mild (such as runny nose, sneezing, and cough) while others are more severe and include wheezing and respiratory distress. Severity may depend on the age and health of the child and on the virulence of the organism. Some of these more severe respiratory infections include bronchiolitis (infection of the small airways), croup, the common cold, flu, pneumonia, and whooping cough.

The primary symptom of a skin infection is a rash, which is the result of the organism's direct invasion of the skin itself. These infections can be caused by viruses, bacteria, fungi, and parasites and include yeast diaper rash, ringworm, scabies, cold sores, impetigo, warts, and head lice.

Intestinal infections cause nausea and vomiting, diarrhea, and cramping pain. They are either food-borne or are transmitted through direct contact between children. These infections include (by organism) rotavirus, *Clostridium difficile*, *Cryptosporidium*, pinworm, *Escherichia coli*, *Salmonella*, and *Staphylococcus* species. Infectious diarrhea is the primary cause of child morbidity and mortality in the developing world.

Head, ear, nose, and throat infections cause diverse symptoms depending on the area of the body affected. Ear infections are second only to the common cold in causing a visit to a doctor. Pinkeye, thrush (yeast infection of the mouth), strep throat, and mononucleosis are common and easily treatable. Meningitis is an infection of the tissues surrounding the brain. Symptoms can be serious and difficult to treat.

Urinary tract infections are more common in girls than in boys because of the anatomy of the female urinary tract. The short urethra, in proximity to the bacteria of the vagina and anus, makes infection more likely. Cystitis is an infection of the bladder and is the most common type of urinary tract infection. Pyelonephritis is an infection of the kidneys and can be more serious.

Childhood infections can also be organized by the type of organism involved.

Viral infections. Viral infections are the most common cause of childhood illness. Many of the classic childhood infections are viral, including measles (rubeola), rubella, chickenpox (varicella), croup (parainflu-enza), hand, foot, and mouth disease (enterovirus), respiratory syncytial virus infection, roseola, the cold, and the flu. Some of these are preventable with vaccines and others resolve on their own without treatment. Antibiotics do not treat viral infections.

Bacterial infections. Bacteria causes many infections, including those of the ear and the urinary tract, some pneumonias, some forms of meningitis, sinusitis, impetigo, strep throat, tetanus, whooping cough (pertussis), and cat scratch fever. Bacterial infections can be treated with antibiotics. Antibiotic-resistant strains of several types of bacteria have emerged because of the over-prescription of antibiotics and because of its overuse in the food supply.

Yeast and other fungi. Yeast and other fungi are microbes that commonly infect the skin, hair, and nails. Fungal infections can be more serious in children who are immunosuppressed. Thrush (yeast), ringworm (tinea), and athlete's foot (tinea) are types of fungal infection. They can be treated with topical or systemic antifungal medications (or both).

Parasitic infections. Parasitic infections are quite common worldwide. They cause life-threatening diarrheal and blood diseases (cryptosporidiosis, giardiasis, and malaria) in the developing world and more superficial infections (scabies and pinworm) elsewhere. They can be treated with antimicrobial medications when available.

PREVENTING INFECTION

Many of the important infections of childhood are preventable with immunization and with improved hygiene. Vaccines used in immunization stimulate the immune system to respond to small doses of a killed or weakened microbe as if it were a real infection, thus helping the body develop immunity to the disease. Vaccines have been so effective at controlling disease, particularly in the developed world, that it is easy to forget the harm caused by the infections they prevent. Many of these diseases are still present, especially in the developing world, and outbreaks are common. Unvaccinated children are at risk of catching preventable disease, and they also put others at risk.

An example of an outbreak in the developed world is the 2010 epidemic of pertussis infection (whooping cough) in the United States. Thousands of cases were identified nationwide, and several children died in California alone. It is believed that infants who were not immunized or who were under-immunized were infected by their adult caretakers and by older children, who tend to get a milder form of the disease. The Centers for Disease Control and Prevention (CDC) recommends that persons who are frequently around young children, especially infants, receive boosters.

The concept of community (or herd) immunity is important in health policy. Children who are not immunized are partially protected against vaccine-preventable disease by being surrounded by immunized people. This community immunity is especially important in the protection of children who have immune deficiencies or who are immunosuppressed and cannot receive vaccinations.

Some parents have concerns about vaccine safety, causing them to delay or deny immunization for their children. While no vaccine is 100 percent safe (or 100 percent effective), and all medicines have risks and side effects, serious physical reactions to vaccination are rare. Preventable childhood infection is a greater risk.

The widespread use of improved hygiene also lowers the risk of infection. Respiratory hygiene, including using tissues or coughing or sneezing into one's elbow; isolation during respiratory illness; and frequent, thorough handwashing can help limit the spread of colds and the flu. Other preventive measures include careful food preparation that includes the washing of fruits and vegetables, disinfectant use on preparation surfaces and utensils, and thorough cooking of raw foods, particularly meats and eggs, to a temperature high enough to kill microbes. These measures are essential to the prevention of food-borne illnesses and diseases.

IMPACT

Infection is the leading cause of death in children worldwide and the leading cause of childhood illness in the United States. Public health policy aimed at reducing infant and childhood mortality will depend on increased attention to the prevention and control of infection, particularly in the developing world, where HIV infection, AIDS, diarrheal disease, and malaria account for almost one-half of all deaths. Ongoing research into new vaccines to prevent these diseases will play a critical role in the prevention of childhood (and adult) diseases.

Rachel Zahn, M.D.

FURTHER READING

Behrman, Richard E., Robert M. Kliegman, and Hal B. Jenson, eds. *Nelson Textbook of Pediatrics.* 18th ed. Philadelphia: Saunders/Elsevier, 2007. Text covering all disorders in children with authoritative information on genetics, endocrinology, etiology, epidemiology, pathology, pathophysiology, clinical manifestations, diagnosis, prevention, treatment, and prognosis.

Fisher, Margaret C. *Immunizations and Infectious Diseases: An Informed Parent's Guide.* American Academy of Pediatrics, 2006. A pediatrician explains childhood infection and its prevention.

Kimball, Chad T. *Childhood Diseases and Disorders Sourcebook: Basic Consumer Health Information About Medical Problems Often Encountered in Pre-adolescent Children.* Detroit: Omnigraphics, 2003. Offers basic facts about common illnesses, serious diseases, and chronic conditions in children. Discusses frequently used diagnostic tests, surgeries, and medications. Also examines long-term care for seriously ill children.

Long, Sarah S., Larry K. Pickering, and Charles G. Prober, eds. *Principles and Practice of Pediatric Infectious Diseases.* 3d ed. Philadelphia: Churchill Livingstone/Elsevier, 2008. An excellent text focusing on children and infectious diseases and conditions.

Martin, Richard J., Avroy A. Fanaroff, and Michele C. Walsh, eds. *Fanaroff and Martin's Neonatal-Perinatal Medicine: Diseases of the Fetus and Infant.* 2 vols. 8th ed. Philadelphia: Mosby/Elsevier, 2006. This classic reference work includes discussions of the practice of neonatal-perinatal medicine and the development and disorder of organ systems.

Murphy, Kenneth, Paul Travers, and Mark Walport. *Janeway's Immunobiology.* 7th ed. New York: Garland Science, 2008. A thorough and comprehensive review of the human immune system.

Pickering, Larry K., et al., eds. *Red Book: 2009 Report of the Committee on Infectious Diseases.* 28th ed. Elk Grove Village, Ill.: American Academy of Pediatrics, 2009. The bible on infections of children and the official source for American Academy of Pediatrics policy.

Plotkin, Stanley A., Walter A. Orenstein, and Paul A. Offit. *Vaccines.* 5th ed. Philadelphia: Saunders/Elsevier, 2008. An excellent discussion of the role of vaccines in the prevention of disease. The book begins with a history of immunization practices, and each subsequent chapter deals with a specific disease and the role and history of vaccine production in its prevention.

WEB SITES OF INTEREST

About Kids Health
http://www.aboutkidshealth.ca

American Academy of Family Physicians
http://familydoctor.org

American Academy of Pediatrics
http://www.healthychildren.org

Centers for Disease Control and Prevention
http://www.cdc.gov

Clean Hands Coalition
http://www.cleanhandscoalition.org

Global Health Council
http://www.globalhealth.org/infectious_diseases

KidsHealth
http://www.kidshealth.org

Pediatric Infectious Diseases Society
http://www.pids.org

See also: Bacterial infections; Biosurveillance; Childbirth and infectious disease; Developing countries and infectious disease; Emerging and reemerging infectious diseases; Endemic infections; Epidemiology; Fungal infections; Globalization and infectious disease; Horizontal disease transmission; Parasitic diseases; Pregnancy and infectious disease; Public health; Rotavirus infection; Schools and infectious disease; Social effects of infectious disease; Tropical medicine; Vaccines: Types; Viral infections.

Chlamydia

CATEGORY: Diseases and conditions
ANATOMY OR SYSTEM AFFECTED: Eyes, genitalia, lungs, reproductive system, respiratory system, skin, vision

ALSO KNOWN AS: Inclusion blenorrhea, inclusion conjunctivitis, lymphogranuloma venereum, nongonococcal urethritis, trachoma

DEFINITION

The disease known as chlamydia is an infection with the bacterium *Chlamydia trachomatis*, which is not capable of surviving on its own. The bacteria can grow only inside other living cells, such as viruses. Outside living cells, *Chlamydia* is dormant, like a spore. In its dormant form, *Chlamydia* can travel from one person or animal to another.

There are several different species of *Chlamydia*. A number of strains within each species are responsible for a variety of diseases in birds, humans, and other mammals. The most common appearance of these diseases is the sexually transmitted genital infection called chlamydia, or nongonococcal urethritis.

Chlamydia is one of the most common sexually transmitted diseases (STDs) in the United States, especially among sexually active teenagers and young adults. More than 1.2 million cases were reported to the Centers for Disease Control and Prevention (CDC) in 2008. This particular strain also causes Reiter's syndrome and can cause neonatal infections, such as pneumonia or conjunctivitis (pinkeye), when passed from a pregnant girl or woman who is infected.

Other types of chlamydia can cause another less common STD known as lymphogranuloma venereum. Other strains can cause lung, heart, and intestinal infections, and an eye infection called trachoma, or Egyptian ophthalmia, which leads to millions of cases of blindness in developing countries around the world. This latter infection is known in developed countries as inclusion conjunctivitis or inclusion blenorrhea.

CAUSES

Genital chlamydial infections are caused by the transmission of *C. trachomatis* during oral, vaginal, or anal sex with an infected partner. Other forms of chlamydia can be transmitted by nonsexual contact, such as by flies, dirty hands, or other contaminated objects, and through inhalation and childbirth.

RISK FACTORS

Each chlamydial infection has a different set of risk factors and can be considered a separate disease entity.

Speaking with a Healthcare Provider About Chlamydia

SPECIFIC QUESTIONS TO ASK ABOUT CHLAMYDIA
What is my diagnosis?
How serious is my condition?
Do I have other conditions that might interact unfavorably with this condition?

SPECIFIC QUESTIONS ABOUT THE RISK OF DEVELOPING CHLAMYDIA
Based on my medical history, lifestyle, and family background, am I at risk for chlamydial infections?
How can I prevent them?

SPECIFIC QUESTIONS ABOUT TREATMENT OPTIONS
What medications are available to help me?
What are the benefits and side effects of these medications?
Will these medications interact with other medications, over-the-counter products, or dietary and herbal supplements?
What time of day should I take my medications?
Is timing of meals relevant to my medication?
What should I do if I forget to take a dose?
Are there any alternative or complementary therapies I should consider?

SPECIFIC QUESTIONS ABOUT LIFESTYLE CHANGES
Just how risky is my lifestyle?
By how much will I reduce my risk by using condoms?
Are there any other risk reduction measures I can take besides abstinence?

SPECIFIC QUESTIONS ABOUT YOUR TREATMENT GOALS
Will the treatment cure me, or will there be residual effects?
How do I know if I am cured?
How often should I be rechecked by a doctor?

Sexually transmitted chlamydia. Sexually transmitted chlamydial infections are transferred from one person to another by direct contact with genital tissues. Risk factors include the following: age fifteen to twenty-five years for *C. trachomatis* in girls and women and age fifteen to twenty-five years for *L. venereum* in boys and men; having multiple sex partners; having sex without

a condom; and having a history of sexually transmitted diseases.

Neonatal chlamydia. Neonatal chlamydia is the same organism transmitted in childbirth from an infected woman to her fetus. It accounts for 30 to 50 percent of newborn conjunctivitis and is so common that every newborn in the United States is treated to prevent it. Infants born to infected women are at risk of developing chlamydial conjunctivitis (in 25 percent of cases) and chlamydial pneumonia (in 16 percent of cases).

Respiratory chlamydia. Chlamydia bacteria that infect the respiratory system are a different species and enter the body when they are inhaled. These germs in spore form are wafted into the air from infected birds. The risk is limited to those in contact with infected birds, especially psittacines (parrots, parakeets, budgies) but also barnyard birds (ducks, chickens, and turkeys), pigeons, and most other kinds.

Ocular chlamydia (trachoma). Trachoma is yet another chlamydial infection by a different strain of this group of germs. Trachoma causes ocular chlamydia. The germ is carried from one person to another by direct contact or by inanimate objects known as fomites. The risk of acquiring trachoma is high in endemic areas such as Africa, India, Southeast Asia, and the Middle East, and is especially high for children. Risk factors include flies in developing countries; objects that can transmit germs, such as towels and wash cloths; and contaminated fingers.

SYMPTOMS

Genital infections. It is possible to have a chlamydial infection and have no symptoms. This happens in about 70 percent of cases. Many people who do not know they are infected carry the infection for years. They can transmit it to others and can slowly scar their own genital organs. In these cases, infected people may have nonspecific symptoms, such as vague back or pelvic pain, bowel trouble, painful intercourse, or loss of energy. If recognizable symptoms do occur, they usually appear within one to three weeks of exposure. Symptoms in men are purulent (made up of pus) discharge from the penis; burning, itchy, or painful sensation while urinating; and swollen or tender testicles. Symptoms in women are increased or abnormal vaginal discharge, strong vaginal odor, vaginal redness or irritation, painful and frequent urination, unusual vaginal bleeding (for example, between periods), pain or bleeding during or after sex, and abdominal pain.

An untreated chlamydial STD can have serious results, including the following in men: epididymitis, a painful swelling and inflammation of the testicles that may lead to infertility. The inside of the urethra may become inflamed (urethritis), which will cause burning when passing urine and can lead to scarring. This can cause difficulty passing urine and even urine flow blockage. Chlamydia also may cause inflammation of the prostate gland (prostatitis). Symptoms include pain in and around the groin and pelvis, discomfort when urinating, and perhaps flulike symptoms (fever, chills, aching-all-over, lethargy). Chlamydia also may cause joint pain, which is just one symptom in a collection of conditions called Reiter's syndrome, which also includes urethritis, arthritis, and conjunctivitis (pinkeye).

In women, an untreated chlamydial STD can lead to pelvic inflammatory disease (PID), a serious infection that in turn can lead to infertility, even in women who never have symptoms. If symptoms do occur, they are usually pelvic pain and pain with intercourse. PID causes scar tissue to form in the Fallopian tubes and may even produce an abscess in a Fallopian tube. Scarring also increases the risk of a tubal pregnancy and of infertility. A tubal pregnancy occurs when a fertilized egg cannot reach the uterus (womb) because of scarring in the Fallopian tube. The result can be disastrous if an abscess or a tubal pregnancy is not removed surgically. Either one can rupture and cause bleeding or infection inside the abdomen, leading to a surgical emergency.

Chlamydia and gonorrhea can both cause inflammation inside the abdomen, not only around the reproductive organs but also around the appendix or the liver. When the liver is involved, the symptoms resemble gallbladder disease (fever and pain under the right ribs). This condition is called Fitz-Hugh-Curtis syndrome. There also may be vaginal discharge or bleeding because of the involvement of the cervix, or there may be swelling and pain in small (Bartholin's) glands in the external genitals.

An untreated chlamydial STD, in both women and men, can spread to the rectum or begin there after anal intercourse. Infection in this area causes pain, anal discharge and bleeding, and lower abdominal cramping. Oral sexual contact can lead to a chlamydial infection in the throat that resembles strep throat. Another infection is lymphogranuloma venereum, which usually begins with a small and transient blister, lump, or ulcer in the genitals. This lesion usually goes unnoticed. Two to six weeks later, regional lymph nodes begin to swell and reach alarming proportions, and some may form abscesses that drain pus. Other common symptoms include fever, painful urination, and pain in the low back, abdomen, or the groin area. The most obvious site is in the groin. Untreated, the swollen nodes eventually resolve, leaving behind scars or lumps of scar tissue.

Eye infections. Trachoma begins like a mild case of pinkeye or an allergic reaction in the eye. Slowly, the upper eyelid becomes scarred and retracted, drawing the eyelashes into contact with the cornea then scratching it. A fogging of the cornea develops and eventually clouds over and obscures vision. An estimated eighty-four million people in the world have trachoma.

Lung infections. Chlamydial infections of the lungs may cause acute pneumonia with fever, chills, headache, cough, nosebleeds, and light sensitivity. In some cases, the illness can resemble bronchitis. It may also involve other organs in the chest, such as the heart or the lung linings.

Neonatal chlamydia. Pregnant women can transmit chlamydia to their fetuses during birth. This may cause conjunctivitis (pinkeye) or pneumonia in the newborn.

SCREENING AND DIAGNOSIS

Screening tests are usually administered to people without current symptoms but also to those at high risk for certain diseases or conditions. Screening for chlamydia is done only for sexually transmitted forms and is especially important for pregnant women to prevent neonatal infections.

Anyone can contract chlamydia after unprotected sexual contact with a person who is infected. All pregnant women, and persons with an STD, could have a chlamydial infection. All those who are not treated routinely should be screened.

The symptoms of common chlamydial STD and gonorrhea are similar, so accurate diagnosis can be important; although, in practice, it is standard to treat for both and not bother with the expensive testing often necessary to prove the diagnosis. A swab test from the discharge of the penis or the cervix is the most reliable method for detecting chlamydia. A urine sample also may be used. Persons also may be tested for other STDs, including human immunodeficiency virus (HIV) infection.

Diagnosing other forms of chlamydial infection depends on a combination of a person's medical history (such as exposure to birds, the health of sexual partners, and history of foreign travel), a physical examination, and a collection of lab tests. In some cases, making the diagnosis can be quite difficult.

The diagnosis of psittacosis is difficult when an obvious history of exposure to birds is not present. There is a lab test that identifies antibodies to the germ and is performed by the Centers for Disease Control and Prevention. Trachoma is diagnosed by culturing a swab from the conjunctiva, examining cells scraped from the conjunctiva, and doing an eye exam in later stages of the infection. The diagnosis of Reiter's syndrome depends entirely upon symptoms. Because the symptoms may take time to appear, the diagnosis may be delayed for several months.

Definitive diagnosis involves many different techniques. These may include taking specimens from infected areas, identifying molecules associated with the germ or antibodies to the germ, and recognizing strands of nucleic acid unique to the germ. The latter is done by using the most up-to-date methods of molecular biology.

TREATMENT AND THERAPY

Treatment for chlamydia may include medications and lifestyle changes. For persons with chlamydia, and their partners, it is important to be treated with medication before resuming sex. Persons who still have symptoms may need to be tested again. Those who have no symptoms are encouraged to return after treatment to be retested, as drug resistance or reactions, reinfection, or infection of other organs is possible.

It is standard practice to test for multiple STDs after identifying one, and it also is standard practice to treat for chlamydia if gonorrhea is identified. The likelihood of both being present is high.

The scarring from PID may require surgery to restore fertility or to remove chronically infected tissue. The scarring caused by trachoma may require eyelid surgery or corneal transplant. Reiter's syndrome does not respond completely to antibiotics because the disease is an immune reaction to the infection. Treatment resembles that for rheumatoid arthritis.

PREVENTION AND OUTCOMES

One can prevent chlamydia by abstaining from sex or by having a mutually monogamous relationship. Furthermore, one can reduce the risk of acquiring STDs or of developing their long-term consequences by taking the following measures: Always use a latex condom throughout sexual activity and according to directions; get checked regularly for STDs, especially if younger than age twenty-five years; get immunized for preventable STDs; and use other barrier methods of contraception, such as a diaphragm, which may partially protect against chlamydial infection. (These methods, however, are not as reliable as using a condom.)

Persons who already have chlamydia can prevent transmission by ensuring that all sexual partners are tested and treated and by refraining from sexual activity until the infection disappears. One can reduce the risk of getting infected again by helping partners get treatment.

Other forms of chlamydia may be prevented by avoiding close contact with birds in endemic areas and by getting regular prenatal checkups, including testing for STDs. Every newborn is routinely treated to prevent neonatal chlamydia or gonorrhea.

Ricker Polsdorfer, M.D.

FURTHER READING

Centers for Disease Control and Prevention. "Sexually Transmitted Diseases: Chlamydia." Available at http://www.cdc.gov/std/chlamydia. An informative government agency guide to chlamydia as an STD.

Cook, R. L., et al. "Systematic Review: Noninvasive Testing for Chlamydia trachomatis and Neisseria gonorrhoeae." *Annals of Internal Medicine* 142 (2005): 914-925. Scholarly journal article on testing procedures for the two infectious bacteria.

Golden, M. R., et al. "Effect of Expedited Treatment of Sex Partners on Recurrent or Persistent Gonorrhea or Chlamydial Infection." *New England Journal of Medicine* 352 (2005): 676-685. Argues for the timely treatment of sex partners of persons infected.

Hollblad-Fadiman, K., and S. M. Goldman. "American College of Preventive Medicine Practice Policy Statement: Screening for Chlamydia trachomatis." *American Journal of Preventive Medicine* 24 (2003): 287-292. Presents screening guidelines for Chlamydia trachomatis.

Khare, Manjiri. "Infectious Disease in Pregnancy." *Current Obstetrics and Gynaecology* 15 (2005): 149-156. An overview of the many infectious diseases of pregnancy and childbirth, including chlamydia, with discussion of their impact.

Miller, K. E. "Diagnosis and Treatment of Chlamydia trachomatis Infection." *American Family Physician* 73 (2006): 1411-1416. A guide for the clinician.

National Library of Medicine. "Chlamydia Infections in Women." Available at http://www.nlm.nih.gov/medlineplus/ency/article/000660.htm. A Web-based article examining chlamydia and its effects on women.

Trelle, Sven, et al. "Improved Effectiveness of Partner Notification for Patients with Sexually Transmitted Infections: Systematic Review." *British Medical Journal* 334 (January, 2007): 354. Discusses partner notification as a means to help stop the spread of STD infection.

WEB SITES OF INTEREST

American Social Health Association
http://www.ashastd.org

Centers for Disease Control and Prevention
http://www.cdc.gov/std

International Trachoma Initiative
http://www.trachoma.org

National Institute of Allergy and Infectious Diseases
http://www.niaid.nih.gov

National Women's Health Information Center
http://www.womenshealth.gov

World Health Organization
http://www.who.int/blindness/causes/priority

See also: Acute cystitis; Bacteria: Classification and types; Bacterial infections; Bacterial vaginosis; Chancroid; Childbirth and infectious disease; Chlamydia; Chlamydophila; Conjunctivitis; Cytomegalovirus infection; Endometritis; Epididymitis; Gonorrhea; Herpes simplex infection; HIV; Insect-borne illness and disease; Ophthalmia neonatorum; Pelvic inflammatory disease; Pregnancy and infectious disease; Prostatitis; Reiter's syndrome; Respiratory route of transmission; Sexually transmitted diseases (STDs); Trachoma; Trichomonas; Urethritis; Vaginal yeast infection.

Chlamydia

CATEGORY: Pathogen
TRANSMISSION ROUTE: Direct contact

DEFINITION

Chlamydia is a gram-negative, aerobic, obligate, intracellular parasite with a reduced genome and limited metabolism.

**Taxonomic Classification
for *Chlamydia***

Kingdom: Bacteria
Phylum: Chlamydiae
Class: Chlamydiae
Order: Chlamydiales
Family: Chlamydiaceae
Genus: *Chlamydia*
Species:
C. muridarum
C. suis
C. trachomatis

NATURAL HABITAT AND FEATURES

The three species of *Chlamydia* are host specific: *C. trachomatis* to humans, *C. suis* to pigs, and *C. muridarum* to mice and related small rodents. All are obligate intracellular parasites that exist in two phases, the elementary body and the reticulate body. The elementary bodies are small, spore-like, nonreplicating, infectious particles with a diameter of about 0.3 micrometers (μm). They have a strong cell wall but one that lacks the peptidoglycan seen in most bacterial cell walls. Instead, the protective wall contains lipopolysaccharides and unique cysteine-rich proteins. Upon contact with a host cell, elementary bodies induce their own endocytosis. Once inside the cell, elementary bodies convert to larger, replicating, noninfectious reticulate bodies with diameters more than 0.5 μm.

Reticulate bodies lack a cell wall and are able to

divide every two to three hours. After multiple divisions, reticulate bodies can covert to elementary bodies that are released from the cell through exocytosis. The genomes of *Chlamydia* spp. are quite small: approximately 0.5 to 1.0 megabases (Mb) compared with the 4.6 (Mb) in *Escherichia coli*, for example.

The genome of *C. trachomatis* has been sequenced and contains 1,042,519 base pairs (approximately six hundred genes), and most strains also contain a large plasmid with 7,498 base pairs. Some *C. trachomatis* genes are more homologous to eukaryotic than bacterial genes and were probably obtained from host genomes. The bacteria are quite capable of this recombination because the genome contains all of the expected deoxyribonucleic acid (DNA) replication and repair genes needed. Genes coding for enzymes in other metabolic pathways, however, are missing. Because of the lack of certain enzymes, metabolism is incomplete.

Electron transport proteins are present, but *Chlamydia* spp. have only limited abilities to produce adenosine triphosphate (ATP), usually by substrate-level phosphorylation, and so must obtain most of their ATP from the host cell. In addition, pathways to produce many amino acids and other cellular building blocks are incomplete or missing, so that these too must be obtained from the host. Glucose can be broken down by a modified glycolytic pathway, but the tricarboxylic acid (TCA) cycle is incomplete. A primary carbon source for these bacteria is glutamate, which can feed into the TCA cycle after a missing enzymatic step. Although they lack an ability to use fats for ATP production or as carbon sources, these bacteria have extensive lipid synthetic pathways to produce their complex cell walls. They can also store and break down glycogen.

Pathogenicity and Clinical Significance

C. trachomatis is the only *Chlamydia* species that affects humans. Two related species (*psittaci* and *pneumoniae*) that can be pathogenic to humans were moved from the genus *Chlamydia* to the new genus *Chlamydophila* in 1999. Also, four related nonhuman pathogens were moved from *Chlamydia* to *Chlamydophila*.

Depending on the site of infection, *C. trachomatis* can cause ocular or genital infections. A *C. trachomatis* infection of the eye is called trachoma. Infection can be transmitted through contact with eye discharges on skin, inanimate objects, or eye-seeking flies. Infection also can be transmitted during birth, as the fetus passes through the birth canal of an infected woman. In trachoma, the inside of the eyelid becomes scarred and, after repeated infection, can cause scarring of the cornea, which eventually leads to blindness. About 84 million people worldwide have trachoma, and the disease is responsible for 3 percent of all blindness, down from 15 percent in 1996.

C. trachomatis infection can also be transmitted sexually and is the most common sexually transmitted disease (STD). Its exact prevalence is not known because it is asymptomatic in 60 to 75 percent of infected women and in 25 to 50 percent of infected men. The most common symptom in women is pelvic inflammatory disease (PID), which may not be apparent until several years after the initial infection. PID can lead to scarring in the reproductive tract, which causes chronic pelvic pain, vaginal bleeding, painful urination, ectopic pregnancy, and difficulty or impossibility in becoming pregnant. Chronic infection also can lead to spontaneous abortion and premature birth. Also, women with chlamydial infections are five times more likely to be infected with the human immunodeficiency virus if exposed to that virus.

In men, the most common symptom is urethritis, which leads to painful urination, purulent discharge from the penis, and swollen or tender genitalia. It is possible for the bacteria to spread farther through the reproductive tract and cause prostatitis and epididymitis. Other problems that can be caused by *C. trachomatis* are reactive arthritis, which is more common in men, and lymphogranuloma venereum, an inflammation of the lymphatic system, especially in the groin area, which may lead to ulceration of the genitalia.

Drug Susceptibility

Once detected, *C. trachomatis* infection is easily cured with the appropriate antibiotic regimen. The Centers for Disease Control and Prevention guidelines suggest either a single dose of azithromycin or twice-daily doses of doxycycline for seven to fourteen days. Tetracycline and erythromycin are also effective, and ciprofloxacin also has been used. Penicillin and other beta-lactam antibiotics are ineffective because they are chlamydiostatic only, not chlamydiocidal. Sex partners of infected persons are also treated with antichlamydials, as are persons with other STDs, because many persons infected with gonorrhea and syphilis also have "silent" chlamydial infections.

Richard W. Cheney, Jr., Ph.D.

FURTHER READING

Krieg, Noel R., et al., eds. *Bergey's Manual of Systematic Bacteriology*. 2d ed. New York: Springer, 2010. Volume four of this multivolume set describes Chlamydia species in detail.

Madigan, Michael T., and John M. Martinko. *Brock Biology of Microorganisms*. 12th ed. Upper Saddle River, N.J.: Pearson/Prentice Hall, 2010. This text outlines many common bacteria, describing their natural history, pathogenicity, and more.

Ojgius, David M., Toni Darville, and Patrik Bavoil. "Can Chlamydia be Stopped?" *Scientific American* 292 (2005): 72-79. This article describes chlamydial pathogenesis and possibilities for decreasing infections worldwide.

Stephens, Richard S., et al. "Genome Sequence of an Obligate Intracellular Pathogen of Humans: Chlamydia trachomatis." *Science* 282 (1998): 754-759. This article provides much information on the C. trachomatis genome and the bacterium's metabolism.

WEB SITES OF INTEREST

American Social Health Association
http://www.ashastd.org

Centers for Disease Control and Prevention
http://www.cdc.gov

See also: Bacterial infections; Childbirth and infectious disease; Chlamydia; Chlamydophila; Gonorrhea; Herpes simplex infection; HIV; Horizontal disease transmission; Pathogens; Pelvic inflammatory disease; Prostatitis; Sexually transmitted diseases (STDs); Trachoma; Trichomonas; Urethritis.

Chlamydophila

CATEGORY: Pathogen
TRANSMISSION ROUTE: Direct contact, inhalation

DEFINITION

Chlamydophila is a gram-negative, aerobic, obligate, intracellular parasite with a reduced genome and a limited metabolism.

Taxonomic Classification for *Chlamydophila*

Kingdom: Bacteria
Phylum: Chlamydiae
Class: Chlamydiae
Order: Chlamydiales
Family: Chlamydiaceae
Genus: *Chlamydophila*
Species:
C. abortus
C. felis
C. pneumoniae
C. psittaci

NATURAL HABITAT AND FEATURES

Until the 1990's, all members of the order Chlamydiales were placed in the single family Chlamydiaceae and the single genus *Chlamydia*. Studies on the DNA (deoxyribonucleic acid) and rRNA (ribosomal ribonucleic acid) of several species culminated, in 1999, with the publication of a new taxonomy of the order. Chlamydiales is now thought to contain three families: Chlamydiaceae, Parachlamydiaceae, and Simkaniaceae. Members of Chlamydiaceae have been separated into two monophyletic genera–*Chlamydia* and *Chlamydophila*—mainly by differences in their 23s rRNA and genomic DNA. Because of this change, *Chlamydophila* spp. are often still referred to as *Chlamydia* spp.

Like *Chlamydia* spp., all *Chlamydophila* spp. are obligate intracellular parasites that exist in two phases, the elementary body and the reticulate body. Their cell wall is without a peptidoglycan layer but does contain gram-negative-like lipopolysaccharides and unique cysteine-rich proteins found only in Chlamydiales. They are usually coccobacilli with diameters of 0.1 to 0.2 micrometers (um). The genomes of *Chlamydophila* spp. are quite small: approximately 1.1 million to 1.2 million base pairs compared with 0.5 million to 1.0 million in *Chlamydia* spp. and 4.6 million in *Escherichia coli*.

The genomes of several *Chlamydophila* strains have been sequenced, and most strains also contain a large plasmid of about 7,550 base pairs. This plasmid seems to be involved in virulence because avirulent strains have been found to lack this plasmid. The only exception is *C. abortus*, which has not been found in any strains. Genes coding for enzymes in many metabolic pathways are missing. Because of the lack of various enzymes, metabolism is incomplete. Some electron transport proteins are present, but *Chlamydophila* spp. have only limited abilities to produce adenosine triphosphate (ATP), usually by substrate-level phosphorylation, and so must obtain most of their ATP from the host cell.

In addition, pathways to produce many amino acids and other cellular building blocks are incomplete or missing, so that these too must be obtained from the host. Some carbohydrates can be broken down by a modified glycolytic pathway, but carbohydrate metabolism is incomplete. *Chlamydophila* spp. lack an ability to use fats for ATP production or as carbon sources, but these bacteria have extensive lipid biosynthetic pathways that produce their complex cell wall lipopolysaccharides. Unlike *Chlamydia* spp., they do not produce glycogen.

PATHOGENICITY AND CLINICAL SIGNIFICANCE

Of the six species of *Chlamydophila*, two, *pneumoniae* and *psittaci*, commonly cause human disease. Humans are occasional hosts for two others, *abortus* and *felis*, while the final two, *pecorum* and *caviae*, are not known to infect humans.

In humans, *pneumoniae*, as its name implies, is primarily found in the respiratory tract, where it causes bronchitis and pneumonia. It has also been associated with other chronic respiratory diseases and chronic infections have been implicated in a higher risk of lung cancer. The bacterium had been considered a strictly human parasite, but some strains have been found in koalas, where they are associated with respiratory infections too, and in horses, where they seem to be asymptomatic. Occasionally, strains can be also isolated from the conjunctiva and the urogenital tract.

Although *psittaci* primarily infects birds, humans can become infected by close contact with infected pet birds or infected poultry. In humans, the infection leads to a severe atypical pneumonia called psittacosis (also known as ornithosis and parrot fever). A pandemic of the disease occurred in 1929-1930 following a shipment of infected parrots to various parts of the world.

Abortus, once considered a subspecies of *psittaci*, is associated with placental colonization and abortion in ruminants. These bacteria have been associated with respiratory disease in humans who work with infected animals and associated with abortion in women who work with infected sheep.

Felis usually causes conjunctivitis, rhinitis, and pneumonia in domestic cats. Humans who have close contact with infected cats are occasionally infected, showing many of the same symptoms. *Caviae* is very host specific and is limited to guinea pigs. *Pecorum* has a broader host range and has been found in koalas, ruminants, and swine. In most organisms, it is associated with abortion, conjunctivitis, and respiratory infections. In koalas, it is also a leading cause of infertility and other reproductive diseases.

DRUG SUSCEPTIBILITY

Although *Chlamydophila* spp. are affected by penicillin, the primary antibiotic of choice for *psittaci* infections specifically is tetracycline. A course of a minimum of fourteen days is recommended to prevent relapse. Children and pregnant women can be treated with erythromycin. For *pneumoniae* infections, doxycycline is usually used.

Richard W. Cheney, Jr., Ph.D.

FURTHER READING

Everett, Karen D. E., et al. "Emended Description of the Order Chlamydiales." *International Journal of Systematic Bacteriology* 49 (1999): 415-440. This article gives a detailed description of the taxonomy of the order Chlamydiales, including the genus Chlamydophila and its species.

Krieg, Noel R., et al., eds. *Bergey's Manual of Systematic Bacteriology.* 2d ed. New York: Springer, 2010. Volume 4 of this multivolume work describes Chlamydophila in detail.

Romich, Janet A. *Understanding Zoonotic Diseases.* Clifton Park, N.Y.: Thomson Delmar, 2008. A good introduction to zoonotic diseases, including psittacosis and other Chlamydophila infections.

Schlossberg, D. "Chlamydia psittaci (Psittacosis)." In *Mandell, Douglas, and Bennett's Principles and Practice of Infectious Diseases,* edited by Gerald L. Mandell, John F. Bennett, and Raphael Dolin. 7th ed. New York: Churchill Livingstone/Elsevier, 2010. This two-volume textbook provides background and detailed information about all types of microbes and infectious sources, including Chlamydophila.

WEB SITES OF INTEREST

American Social Health Association
http://www.ashastd.org

Centers for Disease Control and Prevention
http://www.cdc.gov

See also: Atypical pneumonia; Bacteria: Classification and types; Bacteriology; Birds and infectious disease; Cats and infectious disease; Chlamydia; Chlamydophila pneumoniae infection; Microbiology; Ornithosis; Pneumonia; Psittacosis; Respiratory route of transmission; Zoonotic diseases.

Chlamydophila pneumoniae infection

CATEGORY: Diseases and conditions
ANATOMY OR SYSTEM AFFECTED: Lungs, respiratory system

DEFINITION

Chlamydophila pneumoniae infection is caused by the bacterium *Chlamydophila pneumoniae*, which leads to pneumonia, bronchitis, sinusitis, and pharyngitis. There are about 100 cases of infection with *C. pneumoniae* for every 100,000 persons in the United States each year. Infections with *C. pneumoniae* occur year-round.

CAUSES

C. pneumoniae infection causes up to 10 percent of the cases of pneumonia that are acquired outside hospitals and nursing homes. Infection is transmitted through droplets of respiratory secretions in the air.

RISK FACTORS

Persons who are sixty-five to seventy-nine years of age have the greatest risk for infection with *C. pneumoniae*. In addition, persons of all ages who are immunocompromised also have an elevated risk for infection. These persons include those with human immunodeficiency virus (HIV) infection and those with organ transplants and who consequently must take immunosuppressant drugs to avoid the body's rejection of the organ.

SYMPTOMS

Headache is a common symptom of *C. pneumoniae*, as is lethargy. Persons with asthma often experience worsening symptoms, and recurrent infections with this bacterium may lead to the onset of chronic asthma in children and adults. The presence of laryngitis is the most common symptom differentiating persons with infection caused by *C. pneumoniae* versus infection caused by another bacterium. Fever is another common symptom, as are chills and muscle pain (myalgia). Persistent cough is another frequently occurring symptom. However, some persons have no symptoms because the infection is mild.

SCREENING AND DIAGNOSIS

This infection is diagnosed with nasopharyngeal swabs used to obtain samples; these samples are then cultured. A chest X ray will show if a person has pneumonia, although the X ray does not differentiate the type of pneumonia. A sputum culture test can identify *C. pneumoniae*. Deoxyribonucleic acid (DNA) tests such as the polymerase chain reaction-enzyme immunoassay are used to identify the bacterium in some outbreaks, but these tests are not practical in diagnosing a person who is not associated with an outbreak of pneumonia. Diagnosis also is based on clinical symptoms.

TREATMENT AND THERAPY

Antibiotics such as erythromycin, doxycycline, and tetracycline are used for acute infections. For example, tetracycline may be given at 500 milligram (mg) doses, four times daily for fourteen days; doxycycline at 100 mg twice daily for fourteen days; and erythromycin at 500 mg for fourteen days. If cough or malaise continues after a full course of treatment, the doctor may choose to prescribe a second course of treatment.

PREVENTION AND OUTCOMES

Stopping a smoking habit decreases the risk for all forms of pneumonia, including infection with *C. pneumoniae*.

Christine Adamec, M.B.A.

FURTHER READING

Burllo, Almudena, and Bouza, Emilion. "Chlamydophila pneumoniae." *Infectious Disease Clinics of North America* 24 (2010): 61-71.

Krüll, Matthias, and Norbert Suttorp. "Pathogenesis of Chlamydophila pneumoniae Infections: Epidemiology, Immunity, Cell Biology, Virulence Factors." In *Community-Acquired Pneumonia,* edited by Norbert Suttorp, Tobias Welte, and Reinhard Marre. Boston: Birkhäuser, 2007.

Lutfiyya, M. Nawal, et al. "Diagnosis and Treatment of Community-Acquired Pneumonia." *American Family Physician* 73 (2006): 442-450.

National Heart, Lung, and Blood Institute. "Pneumonia." Available at http://www.nhlbi.nih.gov/ health/dci/diseases/pnu/pnu_whatis.html.

Web Sites of Interest

American Lung Association
http://www.lungusa.org

National Heart, Lung, and Blood Institute
http://www.nhlbi.nih.gov

See also: Airborne illness and disease; Allergic bronchopulmonary aspergillosis; Aspergillosis; Aspergillus; Bacterial infections; Bronchiolitis; Bronchitis; Chlamydophila; Legionnaires' disease; Pharyngitis and tonsillopharyngitis; Pneumonia; Respiratory route of transmission; Sinusitis; Tuberculosis (TB); Whooping cough.

Cholecystitis

Category: Diseases and conditions
Anatomy or system affected: Digestive system, gallbladder, gastrointestinal system

Definition

Cholecystitis is an inflammation of the gallbladder, usually caused by the formation of gallstones (cholelithiasis). Research has revealed cholecystitis is often accompanied by a bacterial infection, particularly a form of *Helicobacter.* Cholecystitis may be acute or chronic. If it is acute, pain generated by the inflammation is extremely severe, and most affected persons attempt to see their physicians as soon as possible or go to a hospital emergency room. If cholecystitis is chronic, pain is intermittent and characterized by periodic bouts of exacerbation. Chronic cholecystitis can escalate to acute cholecystitis.

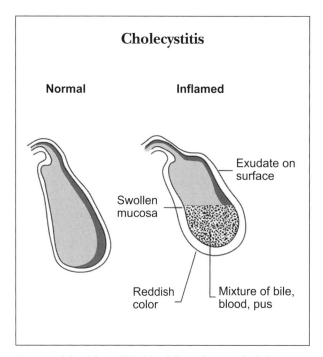

A normal, healthy gallbladder, left, and one with cholecystitis.

Causes

About 90 percent of all cases of cholecystitis involve gallstones, which can cause blockage and inflammation of the gallbladder. About 80 percent of these stones are formed by cholesterol, while others are pigment stones comprising bilirubin or are mixed stones composed of cholesterol and pigment. Gallstones can be as tiny as a grain of sand or may be the size of a golf ball. Affected persons may have one gallstone or hundreds of small stones.

Some persons have acalculous cholecystitis, gallbladder inflammation without gallstones. Up to 15 percent of all cases of acute cholecystitis are cases of acalculous cholecystitis. Various bacteria are known to cause acalculous cholecystitis, most prominently *Helicobacter.* Researchers have found that the bacterial culprits in acalculous cholecystitis are *Escherichia coli, Citrobacter, Klebsiella, Campylobacter,* and *Pseudonomas.*

Some strains of *Helicobacter* are implicated in the formation of cholesterol or mixed cholesterol gallstones (but not pigment gallstones) that lead to cholecystitis. Rapid weight loss, as may occur after elective bariatric surgery chosen by obese persons, may lead to gallstones. Some bariatric surgeons may check the gallbladder before weight loss surgery to ensure against asymptomatic gallstones. In addition, some doctors perform a cholecystectomy, the removal of the gallbladder, during weight loss surgery to avoid the risk of gallstones. Chronic cholecystitis is more likely to occur after a susceptible person eats a large meal or one that is high in fat.

Risk Factors

The following factors increase the chance of developing cholecystitis: obesity, family history of gallstones, rapid weight loss, and type 2 diabetes. Women and girls are at increased risk. In the United States, American Indians have a high rate of gallstones; for example, 70 percent of Pima Indian females develop gallstones before the age of thirty years. Mexican American adults also have a high risk for gallstones and cholecystitis. Age is another risk factor, and adults older than age sixty years have an increased risk for gallstones.

Persons with hepatitis C are at increased risk for gallstones, and persons with Crohn's disease have an elevated risk for cholecystitis.

Acute acalculous cholecystitis is more common in persons who are critically ill, have had heart surgery, experienced extreme trauma, suffered severe burns, or engaged in extended fasting. Persons with autoimmune diseases, cardiovascular disease, acquired immunodeficiency syndrome (AIDS), or complicated diabetes mellitus are more likely to develop this problem. People who take cholesterol-lowering drugs have an elevated risk for cholecystitis because these medications elevate cholesterol secreted into bile.

Few people die from cholecystitis, but the risk for death increases with age. Most people who die from gallbladder inflammation are age sixty-five years and older.

Symptoms

Acute cholecystitis is characterized by severe pain in the right upper part of the abdomen. It is often accompanied by nausea and vomiting and chills and fever. Jaundice, yellowing of skin and eyes, may be present, as may abdominal bloating. The affected person may experience extreme pain from deep breathing. Other symptoms include excessive perspiration and loss of appetite. The pain may extend into the back. Some persons will have clay-colored stools, and diarrhea may be present. With chronic cholecys-

titis, the primary symptoms are pain in the upper right abdomen, nausea, and vomiting.

Screening and Diagnosis

A doctor will take a complete medical history and perform a physical examination. If cholecystitis is suspected, the doctor may refer the affected person to a gastroenterologist, an expert in diseases of the gastrointestinal system. Diagnostic tests may include an abdominal X ray, abdominal ultrasound, or a computed tomography (CT) scan. A hepatobiliary iminodiacetic acid scan of the gallbladder, liver, and small intestine may be ordered. This scan uses an injected radioactive chemical to show the path of the bile as it travels through the body. The scan can help the physician diagnose obstruction of the gallbladder and bile duct. A complete blood count may show an elevated white blood cell count, indicating infection. Other laboratory tests may include a bilirubin count and liver function tests.

Treatment and Therapy

Treatment of acute cholecystitis usually consists of the removal of the gallbladder through cholecystectomy. This surgery can be performed laparoscopically or with a large abdominal incision, although most surgeries are performed laparoscopically.

Medications may also be used to dissolve gallstones, and drugs such as chenodiol (Chenix) and usodiol (Actigall) are most commonly used. Nonsurgical means are more likely to be used in persons who cannot have surgery and are limited to persons with cholesterol stones. Patients may need pain medication, although doctors may initially avoid pain medications until the diagnosis is clear. Antibiotics are often needed to treat associated infections.

Prevention and Outcomes

Weight loss among the obese may decrease the risk for cholecystitis, although people should strive for weight loss of only 2 to 3 pounds per week to avoid elevating the risk for gallstones.

Persons with chronic cholecystitis should avoid fasting, which can increase the risk for gallstones, and should not skip meals. Sedentary behavior increases the risk for gallstones, so regular exercise is recommended. Regular consumption of dietary fiber is believed to decrease the risk for gallstones. Some studies have shown regular consumption of peanuts and other nuts decreases the likelihood of needing a cholecystectomy. In addition, increasing consumption of foods rich in vitamin D may decrease the risk for gallstones and cholecystitis.

Christine Adamec, M.B.A.

FURTHER READING

De Moricz, Andre, et al. "Prevalence of Helicobacter spp. in Chronic Cholecystitis and Correlation with Changes on the Histological Pattern of the Gallbladder." *Acta Cirurgica Brasileira* 25, no. 3 (2010): 218-224.

Everhart, James E. "Gallstones." In *The Burden of Digestive Diseases in the United States,* edited by James E. Everhart. Washington, D.C.: National Institute of Diabetes and Digestive and Kidney Diseases, 2008.

Feldman, Mark, Lawrence S. Friedman, and Lawrence J. Brandt, eds. *Sleisenger and Fordtran's Gastrointestinal and Liver Disease: Pathophysiology, Diagnosis, Management.* New ed. 2 vols. Philadelphia: Saunders/Elsevier, 2010.

Gaby, Alan R. "Nutritional Approaches to Prevention and Treatment of Gallstones."*Alternative Medicine Review* 14, no. 3 (2009): 258-267.

Ganpathi, Iyer Shridhar, et al. "Acute Acalculous Cholecystitis: Challenging the Myths." *HPB: International Journal of the Hepato-Pancreato-Biliary Association* 9 (2007): 131-134.

Lee, Jin-Woo, et al. "Identification of Helicobacter pylori in Gallstones, Bile, and Other Heptatobiliary Tissues of Patients with Cholecystitis." *Gut and Liver* 4, no. 1 (2010): 60-67.

Maurer, Kirk J., Martin C. Carey, and James G. Fox. "Roles of Infection, Inflammation, and the Immune System in Cholesterol Gallstone Formation." *Gastroenterology* 136, no. 2 (2009): 425-440.

Minocha, Anil, and Christine Adamec. *The Encyclopedia of the Digestive System and Digestive Disorders.* 2d ed. New York: Facts On File, 2010.

WEB SITES OF INTEREST

National Digestive Diseases Information Clearinghouse
http://digestive.niddk.gov/ddiseases

National Institute of Diabetes and Digestive and Kidney Diseases
http://niddk.nih.gov

See also: Clonorchiasis; Empyema; Gastritis; Helicobacter; Infection; Inflammation; Intestinal and stomach infections; Pancreatitis; Peritonitis.

Cholera

CATEGORY: Diseases and conditions
ANATOMY OR SYSTEM AFFECTED: Gastrointestinal system, intestines

DEFINITION

Cholera, an infection caused by the *Vibrio cholerae* bacterium, can kill a person within hours if it is left untreated. Contaminated water and food transmit the bacteria. The most dangerous symptom is acute watery diarrhea with severe dehydration.

People with low immunity, such as malnourished children or persons with human immunodeficiency virus (HIV) infection, are much more likely to die if they are infected. The risk of contracting cholera is greatest in urban slums and in camps for refugees and other displaced peoples.

One of the features of cholera is the ease with which the disease spreads, despite the success of treatment with rehydration and antibiotics. In the twenty-first century, cholera remains a threat in Asia, Africa, and parts of Central America and South America.

A child is treated for cholera symptoms in Haiti in late 2010. A cholera epidemic was preceded by months of poor sanitary conditions, including contaminated water, in the wake of the Haitian earthquake of January, 2010. (AP/Wide World Photos)

Cholera in Marine Plankton

Outbreaks of cholera can occur in nonendemic areas when, for example, an infected person travels to another country or when infected water is carried in the ballast of ships to another country. These two processes alone, however, could not explain all of the outbreaks of cholera observed worldwide. In the late 1960's, the bacterium *Vibrio cholerae* was found in the ocean associated with marine plankton. This association, along with climate change, helps to explain the spread of cholera.

Plankton, the small organisms suspended in the ocean's upper layers, can be divided into two groups, phytoplankton (small plants) and zooplankton (small animals). V. cholerae is found associated with the surface and gut of copepods, which are members of the zooplankton group. These small crustaceans act as a reservoir for the cholera bacteria, allowing them to survive in the ocean for long periods of time.

A change in weather that causes the ocean temperature to rise could also cause currents that stir up nutrients from lower layers of the ocean to the upper layers. The numbers of phytoplankton, which live in the upper layers of ocean waters, increase in these periods because of the warmer temperatures and greater availability of nutrients. Zooplankton numbers increase too because of the increase in their main food source, the phytoplankton. Consequently, the number of cholera bacteria increases to a level that can cause the disease. Thus, climate change can result in an outbreak of cholera in a region where cholera is endemic, or, if currents move the plankton to other coastal areas, in a new, nonendemic region. This scenario is believed to explain the 1991 cholera epidemic in Peru, when the oceanic oscillation known as El Niño caused a warming of ocean temperature.

Because of the association of V. cholerae with plankton, scientists hope to be able to track or identify future epidemics with satellite imagery. Increases in phytoplankton turn the ocean from blue to green. Thus, changes in green areas in the ocean on satellite images show where the phytoplankton and, by association, zooplankton and cholera bacteria are relocating or increasing in number.

The association of cholera with zooplankton also has helped reveal a new way to prevent the disease. People get cholera by ingesting several thousand cholera bacteria at one time. A single copepod can harbor ten thousand bacteria; therefore, the ingestion of one infected copepod can cause disease in a person. Researchers have found a simple and inexpensive way to reduce this risk from copepods dramatically. Filtering water through four layers of fabric used to make saris, which are commonly worn in regions plagued by cholera, removes 99 percent of copepods from water that contains high levels of plankton.

Now that the entire genetic sequence of V. cholerae has been determined, scientists have additional genetic data to elucidate the relationship of the bacterium with copepods, which may help scientists and health experts find more ways of controlling the spread of the disease.

Vicki J. Isola, Ph.D.

The incubation period is as little as two to five hours. Each year, 3 million to 5 million people become infected and between 100,000 and 120,000 people die of the disease.

For centuries, it was difficult to convince people that cholera existed, because acute diarrhea is a component of many illnesses. In 1883, German scientist Robert Koch hypothesized that cholera was spread by microbes. He obtained fecal specimens during a cholera outbreak in Egypt and isolated the bacterium, which he named *V. cholerae*.

CAUSES

Cholera is caused by drinking water that is contaminated with feces or by eating food that has been handled by infected persons. Raw or insufficiently cooked shellfish, such as shrimp, lobster, and crabs, can also transmit *V. cholerae*, which is carried in the chitin of the shell.

RISK FACTORS

The risk factors for cholera include eating contaminated food or fluids, eating raw or undercooked shellfish, living or traveling in areas where cholera is present, having blood type O (a ninefold increase in risk), having a compromised immune system, and having low levels of stomach acid. Cholera also is most common in areas with poor sanitation and poor water quality.

SYMPTOMS

Cholera's most prominent symptom is the acute onset of watery diarrhea, often accompanied by vomiting, dehydration, weakness, and abdominal pain. Of people infected with *V. cholerae* bacteria, about 75 percent never develop symptoms. The bacteria remain in infected patients' feces for seven to fourteen days, are excreted into the environment, and can infect other people.

About 25 percent of persons with the disease will experience cholera symptoms. Of this smaller number, about 80 to 90 percent have mild to moderate symptoms only. The remaining symptomatic patients are at risk of death if they do not receive treatment.

SCREENING AND DIAGNOSIS

One should consult a doctor if he or she has recently traveled to areas where cholera is common. If cholera is suspected, the doctor will order stool and blood samples for testing. In response to a 1991 cholera outbreak in South America, three rapid diagnostic tests were developed. These tests can be performed in the field by technicians with limited training, and the results are provided within a few minutes.

TREATMENT AND THERAPY

The rapid loss of fluids and electrolytes can prove fatal, so cholera treatment focuses on oral rehydration therapy, a method that in itself is successful for about 80 percent of infected persons. Some persons are so severely dehydrated that they require intravenous fluids. In serious cases, antibiotics may be given to shorten the course of the illness and to reduce symptoms.

Two oral cholera vaccines are available, and they offer protection to more than 50 percent of vaccinated persons for up to two years. Typically, vaccines are administered for short-term protection, while long-term measures, such as improvements to local water supplies, must be implemented.

The World Health Organization recommends against using antidiarrheal, anti-emetic, antispasmodic, cardiotonic, or corticosteroid drugs for the treatment of cholera. It also deems as unnecessary blood transfusions and plasma volume expanders. Infected persons may resume eating a normal diet as soon as vomiting has stopped. Among those who receive quick treatment, the mortality rate is less than 1 percent.

PREVENTION AND OUTCOMES

The most effective prevention against cholera is proper water treatment and sanitation. The fecal wastewater of infected persons and all contaminated materials, such as clothing and bedding, must be sterilized. Hands that have touched infected persons must be disinfected.

General sewage can be treated with chlorine, ozone, or ultraviolet light, and through sterilization or antimicrobial filtration before it is returned to water supplies or waterways. The same methods should be applied to all water used for drinking, washing, or cooking.

Food safety measures include avoiding raw foods, except when the peel can be removed; cooking food until it is thoroughly heated; and eating cooked food when it is still hot. One should wash and dry cooking and serving utensils after use and should not let cooked food come in contact with uncooked food or unclean utensils. People can also protect themselves with thorough handwashing after defecation, after coming into contact with feces, before preparing food, and before feeding children.

Merrill Evans, M.A.

FURTHER READING

Briggs, Charles L., and Clara Mantini-Briggs. *Stories in the Time of Cholera: Racial Profiling During a Medical Nightmare.* Berkeley: University of California Press, 2003.

EBSCO Publishing. DynaMed: Cholera. Available through http://www.ebscohost.com/dynamed.

Feldman, Mark, Lawrence S. Friedman, and Lawrence J. Brandt, eds. *Sleisenger and Fordtran's Gastrointestinal and Liver Disease: Pathophysiology, Diagnosis, Management.* New ed. 2 vols. Philadelphia: Saunders/Elsevier, 2010.

Joralemon, Donald. *Exploring Medical Anthropology.* Boston: Pearson/Allyn and Bacon, 2006.

Kalluri, P., et al. "Evaluation of Three Rapid Diagnostic Tests for Cholera: Does the Skill Level of the Technician Matter?" *Tropical Medicine in Health,* January 11, 2006, 49-55.

Pennisi, Elizabeth. "Infectious Disease: Cholera Strengthened by Trip Through Gut." *Science* 296 (June, 2002): 1783-1784.

Reidl, Joachim, et al. "Vibrio cholerae and Cholera: Out of the Water and into the Host." *FEMS Microbiological Reviews* 26 (June, 2002): 125-139.

Sack, D. A., et al. "Cholera." *The Lancet* 363 (2004): 223-233.

Sridhar, Saranya. "An Affordable Cholera Vaccine: An Important Step Forward." *The Lancet* 374 (2009): 1658-1660.

WEB SITES OF INTEREST

Centers for Disease Control and Prevention
http://www.cdc.gov

World Health Organization, Global Task Force on Cholera Control
http://www.who.int/cholera

See also: Antibiotic-associated colitis; Ascariasis; Campylobacteriosis; Cholera vaccine; Cryptosporidiosis; Developing countries and infectious disease; Diverticulitis; Fecal-oral route of transmission; Food-borne illness and disease; Giardiasis; Hookworms; Intestinal and stomach infections; Leptospirosis; Parasites: Classification and types; Parasitic diseases; Peritonitis; Shigellosis; Travelers' diarrhea; Tropical medicine; Typhoid fever; Vibrio; Water treatment; Waterborne illness and disease.

Cholera vaccine

CATEGORY: Prevention

DEFINITION

Cholera vaccine can offer up to two years protection for more than 50 percent of the treated population against the sometimes fatal disease cholera. The disease is caused by eating food or water contaminated by the *Vibrio cholerae* bacterium.

Cholera has multiplied during the first decade of the twenty-first century because increased numbers of people are moving from areas at high risk for cholera to other regions, at a pace too fast for local governments and health authorities to provide safe water and sanitation.

Cholera vaccines have been available for more than twenty years. However, many countries have not been able to use them because of high cost, limited supply, and logistical problems in providing two doses.

The World Health Organization (WHO) reports there are three million to five million cases of cholera each year, with an estimated 120,000 to 200,000 of these cases resulting in death.

Data collected by WHO may represent only 5 to 10 percent of actual cases of cholera, because of the difficulty of keeping accurate records in the chaotic conditions in which cholera thrives, such as in natural disasters and civil unrest.

VACCINE ADMINISTRATION

The Durokal vaccine is prequalified by WHO and is licensed in more than sixty countries. It provides short-term protection against *V. cholerae* for up to 90 percent of all age groups, including infants. The Shanchol vaccine provides longer-term protection and is pending WHO prequalification. Its formula is particularly effective in children younger than five years of age.

The Durokal and Shanchol vaccines are administered orally, offering ease of administration and freedom from the risks of needle-borne infection. The vaccines must be administered in two doses, between seven days and six weeks apart. Persons in areas of the world in which cholera is prevalent should receive booster shots every six months. Musocal vaccines are also under development for treatment of cholera.

IMPACT

Vaccines are one facet of cholera eradication. They provide temporary protection while safe water and improved sanitation are secured. Community education on safe practices is also necessary. Persons who survive infection by *V. cholerae* develop a protective immunity.

Merrill Evans, M.A.

FURTHER READING

Ali, Mohammad, et al. "Community Participation in Two Vaccination Trials in Slums of Kolkata, India." *Journal of Health, Population, and Nutrition* 28 (October, 2010): 450-458.

Chatterjee, Patralekha. "High Hopes for Oral Cholera Vaccine." *Bulletin of the World Health Organization* 88 (2010): 165-166.

"Cholera Outbreak—Haiti, October, 2010." *Morbidity and Mortality Weekly* Report 59 (November 5, 2010): 1411.

Plotkin, Stanley A., Walter A. Orenstein, and Paul Offit. *Vaccines*. 5th ed. Philadelphia: Saunders/Elsevier, 2008.

Sridhar, Saranya. "An Affordable Cholera Vaccine: An Important Step Forward." *The Lancet* 374 (2009): 1658-1660.

World Health Organization. "Cholera." Fact Sheet No. 107. Available at http://www.who.int/mediacentre/factsheets/fs107.

WEB SITES OF INTEREST

Centers for Disease Control and Prevention
http://www.cdc.gov

Emerging and Reemerging Infectious Diseases Resource Center
http://www.medscape.com/resource/infections

World Health Organization, Global Task Force on Cholera Control
http://www.who.int/cholera

See also: Bacteria: Classification and types; Bacterial infections; Cholera; Developing countries and infectious disease; Emerging and reemerging infectious diseases; Endemic infections; Fecal-oral route of transmission; Immunity; Public health; Tropical medicine; Vaccines: History; Vaccines: Types; Vibrio; Waterborne illness and disease.

Chromoblastomycosis

CATEGORY: Diseases and conditions
ANATOMY OR SYSTEM AFFECTED: Skin

DEFINITION

Chromoblastomycosis is a chronic fungal infection of the skin caused by a group of dematiaceous, or darkly pigmented, fungi found in soil and decaying vegetation. The incidence of the disease is higher in bare-footed rural populations of tropical and subtropical areas of Africa and South America. This type of infection usually affects the limbs, especially the lower extremities, where the skin is broken.

CAUSES

Several species of dematiaceous fungi cause chromoblastomycosis. These include *Fonsecaea pedrosoi*, and *F. compacta, Phialophora verrucosa*, and *Cladosporium carrionii*. Infection occurs when the fungus is traumatically implanted under the skin through minor injuries such as a cut with a splinter, thorn, or other plant debris. Infected persons rarely seek medical care because the trauma often goes unnoticed and because the progression of the disease is slow.

RISK FACTORS

All ages may be affected by the disease. The majority of reported cases, however, involve healthy males with an outdoor hobby or occupation such as agricultural work. Immunocompromised persons are more likely to have a severe form of the disease.

SYMPTOMS

Chromoblastomycosis initially begins with small, painless, sometimes itchy, bumps on lower extremities at the site of implantation. Lesions may be wartlike, ulcerated, tumorlike, crusted, flat, or raised. Infections are localized and can progress slowly over many years. Satellite lesions may develop on other areas (hands, arms, buttocks, ears, face, and breasts) and coalesce to form a large cauliflower-like rash that gradually covers the extremities. In severe cases, complications can arise; these include elephantiasis and secondary bacterial infections that result in lymphatic stasis (lymph fluid retention) and sepsis (bloodstream infection). Dissemination to the brain known as cerebral chromoblastomycosis may also occur.

SCREENING AND DIAGNOSIS

Chromoblastomycosis is a long-term fungal infection of the skin, sometimes confused with blastomycosis, lobomycosis, paracoccidioidomycosis, or sporotrichosis. Primary care physicians should consult with an infectious disease specialist or pathologist for early diagnosis and treatment. Diagnosis involves isolation, microscopic examination, morphological testing, and culture of infected specimens for characteristic brown-colored, round, thick-walled, sclerotic bodies. These sclerotic bodies resemble copper pennies and are characteristic of the dematiaceous fungi responsible for chromoblastomycosis. Blood analysis and imaging studies are not frequently used for diagnosis.

TREATMENT AND THERAPY

Treatment of chromoblastomycosis is long and difficult. Depending on the extent and severity of the disease, treatment includes surgical excision, heat, electric current, cryosurgery, and antifungal therapy. Intraconazole, terbinafine, and flucytosine are the drugs of choice. A chromoblastomycosis infection is rarely fatal.

PREVENTION AND OUTCOMES

The etiologic agents of chromoblastomycosis are

everywhere. The best form of prevention is to avoid walking barefoot in wooded areas, especially where the fungus is prevalent.

Rose Ciulla-Bohling, Ph.D.

FURTHER READING

Hamza, Sate H., et al. "An Unusual Dematiaceous Fungal Infection of the Skin Caused by Fonsecaea pedrosoi: A Case Report and Review of the Literature." *Journal of Cutaneous Pathology* 30 (2003): 340-343.

Richardson, Malcolm D., and Elizabeth M. Johnson. *Pocket Guide to Fungal Infection.* 2d ed. Malden, Mass.: Wiley-Blackwell, 2006.

St. Georgiev, Vassil. *Opportunistic Infections: Treatment and Prophylaxis.* Totowa, N.J.: Humana Press, 2003.

Schwartz, Robert A., and Eugeniusz Baran. "Chromoblastomycosis." Available at http://emedicine.medscape.com/article/1092695.

WEB SITES OF INTEREST

International Society for Human and Animal Mycology
http://www.isham.org

Mycology Online
http://www.mycology.adelaide.edu.au

New Zealand Dermatological Society
http://dermnetnz.org/fungal/chromoblastomycosis.html

See also: Antifungal drugs: Types; Blastomycosis; Coccidioides; Coccidiosis; Cryptococcosis; Elephantiasis; Fungal infections; Fungi: Classification and types; Fusarium; Histoplasmosis; Mycoses; Pathogens; Ringworm; Sepsis; Skin infections; Soilborne illness and disease; Sporotrichosis; Tropical medicine.

Chronic fatigue syndrome

CATEGORY: Diseases and conditions
ANATOMY OR SYSTEM AFFECTED: All
ALSO KNOWN AS: Chronic fatigue, chronic fatigue immune dysfunction syndrome, myalgic encephalomyelitis, myalgic encephalopathy

DEFINITION

Chronic fatigue syndrome (CFS) is a debilitating disorder. It affects the brain and multiple parts of the body. It causes extreme fatigue and is not relieved by bed rest. Physical or mental fatigue often makes the condition worse. Symptoms last a minimum of six months and are severe enough to interfere with daily activities. CFS is often accompanied by other disorders, such as fibromyalgia, which has many similar symptoms.

Recovery time varies among persons with CFS. One may recover enough to resume work and other activities yet continue to experience various or periodic CFS symptoms. CFS typically follows a cyclical course that alternates between periods of illness and relative well-being. One may also recover completely with time.

CAUSES

There is no specific laboratory test or clinical sign for CFS, and its cause is unknown. The Centers for Disease Control and Prevention estimates that as many as one-half million people in the United States have a condition similar to or diagnosable as CFS.

Doctors have reported seeing illnesses similar to CFS since the nineteenth century. In the 1860's, George Beard named the syndrome neurasthenia, believing it was a nervous disorder accompanied by weakness and fatigue. Experiments in men supported Beard's idea that the brain is somehow involved in CFS.

In the early 1980's, CFS was considered a "yuppie flu" and was especially stigmatized. Primarily upper-middle-class women in their thirties and forties were seeking help for their symptoms. Also in the 1980's, however, health experts began to suggest other explanations for this baffling illness, including the following: various viruses (such as Epstein-Barr virus, enteroviruses, parvovirus B19), the bacterium *Coxiella burnetii*, the bacterium *Chlamydophila pneumoniae*, a malfunction of the hypothalamic-pituitary-adrenal axis, emotional stress, iron-poor blood (anemia), low blood sugar (hypoglycemia), low blood pressure, environmental allergy or toxins, and a body-wide (systemic) yeast infection (candidiasis).

Doctors continue to report seeing the syndrome in people of all ages, races and ethnicities, and social and economic classes. It is also found in people around the world. However, women, still, are more affected than are men (by about 4 to 1).

RISK FACTORS

It is possible to develop CFS with or without the risk factors listed here. However, the more risk factors one has, the greater the likelihood of developing CFS. Risk factors for developing CFS may include one's gender. CFS is diagnosed more often in women than in men. This may be because of biological or psychological influences, or because of social influences (women may be more likely than men to consult a doctor about CFS-like symptoms). However, an increasingly diverse patient group seems to be emerging as more doctors acknowledge CFS to be a "real" medical disorder.

CFS is most common in people between the age of twenty and fifty years but can develop in people of all age groups, including teenagers and young children. Also, research suggests that people who are highly active and achievement-oriented may be more at risk for developing CFS. However, perhaps this personality type increases the risk only after exposure to new mental stresses or to viral infections.

SYMPTOMS

Symptoms of CFS may occur suddenly after a person has a cold, bronchitis, hepatitis, or an intestinal infection. Symptoms may follow a bout of infectious mononucleosis (also known as mono), which is caused by a virus that temporarily depletes one's energy. CFS can also begin after a period of high stress. Sometimes it develops more gradually, with no clear illness or other event noted as a starting point.

Unlike flu symptoms that usually disappear in a few days or weeks, symptoms of CFS persist or recur in cycles for a minimum of six months, 50 percent of the time. CFS symptoms vary from person to person. Since 1994, the guidelines for diagnosing CFS include, in addition to a six-month history of fatigue that is not relieved with bed rest, a minimum of four of the following eight symptoms: muscle aches, joint pain without swelling or redness, headaches, problems with short-term memory or concentration, forgetfulness, confusion, sore throat, tender lymph nodes, trouble sleeping or not feeling rested after sleep, and worsening symptoms twenty-four hours or more after exercise.

In addition to the eight diagnostic symptoms, per-

sons with CFS also experience mood swings, depression, anxiety, dizziness, chronic mononucleosis, fibromyalgia, low blood pressure, and sensitivity to many chemicals.

SCREENING AND DIAGNOSIS

The purpose of screening is early diagnosis and treatment. Screening tests are usually given to people without current symptoms, but who may be at high risk for certain diseases or conditions. There are no screening tests or screening guidelines for CFS, however.

A diagnosis of CFS is based on the following criteria: severe and chronic fatigue that lasts a minimum of six months, 50 percent of the time, and is not caused by another illness; and, at minimum, four of the following eight symptoms: impairment of short-term memory or concentration, sore throat, tender lymph nodes, muscle pain, joint pain without swelling or redness, headaches, sleep that is not refreshing, and prolonged fatigue lasting twenty-four hours or more after exercise.

If a person has these symptoms, the doctor will conduct more tests. These tests include the following standardized lab tests to exclude other causes of fatiguing illness: alanine aminotransferase (ALT; liver test), albumin (liver test), alkaline phosphatase (ALP; bone and liver test), blood urea nitrogen (BUN; kidney test), calcium, complete blood count (white and red cells), creatinine (kidney test), electrolytes (salt and potassium), erythrocyte sedimentation rate (ESR; inflammation test), globulin (liver test), glucose (blood sugar), phosphorus, thyroid stimulating hormone (TSH), total protein, transferrin saturation (iron level), and urinalysis.

If one of the foregoing tests suggest an illness, the doctor may order more tests to confirm an illness other than CFS. Additional tests may include Lyme disease antibody, cytomegalovirus titer, a test for mononucleosis (heterophile test), and tests for *Candida*, viral hepatitis, and human immunodeficiency virus infection.

Psychological and neurological tests may be administered to assess the impact of CFS on certain mental skills, such as concentration, memory, and organization. A personality assessment can help to determine coping abilities and to identify any coexisting affective disorders, such as depression, panic disorder, or other anxiety disorders.

In Her Own Words: Living with Chronic Fatigue Syndrome

Alicia is a fifty-four-year-old mother of two who lives in New York. Having lived with crippling chronic fatigue syndrome (CFS) for more than ten years, she has learned how to get through each day–although some days are much more difficult than others.

What was your first sign that something was wrong? What symptoms did you experience?

In 1990, I was all set to accept a new position in research, hoping it would help to finance my children's college education. Instead, I ended up totally disabled. The onset of my troubles was violent. A virus attacked my bronchial area and it was swollen shut, making it extremely difficult to breathe. I was under the care of a lung specialist for six weeks. I had a bronchioscopy, and they looked for tumors. The virus left me with asthma, a condition that I still have today. Eventually my breathing got better, but I felt that the life was drained out of me.

Aside from tremendous fatigue, I have blurred vision, dizziness, and pain (in my connective tissue, not my joints), mostly in my breast bone and hips. I experienced pressure headaches, orthostatic intolerance (I can't bend over or I feel like I'm going to pass out), low blood volume, irritable bowel syndrome, and loss of short-term memory. I often know what I want to say but I can't think of the word. I have other symptoms too.

What was the diagnosis experience like?

On the day that I was scheduled to start my new job, I literally couldn't get my head off of the pillow in the morning. I went to a medical clinic and saw a young female doctor who said "I think you're depressed." She didn't even know me! But shortly thereafter, depression was ruled out.

Six months lapsed before I had a definitive diagnosis. I went through all kinds of tests. They checked me for cancer, multiple sclerosis (MS), all types of ominous illnesses, even AIDS. And all I got back were negative results from all the tests. Then my cousin went to Toronto and found a magazine article on chronic fatigue syndrome and told me about it. I met all the criteria, but it was a very subjective diagnosis.

My husband went with me to my doctor and told him that I was "very, very ill," and the doctor seemed more willing to listen to me after hearing my husband's testimony. Then I had to deal with trying to get disability. The organization I was dealing with said to me, "Your word means nothing. We'll only listen to a doctor."

What was your initial and then longer-term reaction to the diagnosis?

Well, I wanted to know the truth and find a way to get through it. Being an extremely active person, it was very hard for me to make adjustments. I went through a grieving process. Initially, there was denial–I kept telling myself "This isn't going to stop me." But when you do that, you fall on your face. I went through a period of anger. Then finally acceptance–that's when you start to live more successfully, but as a disabled person. It's very painful. You want to be a productive person, but it's hard.

One of the hardest things for me emotionally is that I don't think that most doctors, or health care institutions, know the truth about this disease. Another difficult thing is that I've lost friends because of this disease. They don't understand. They say to me "Well, I get tired too, but. . . ." My prayer is that one day people will really understand this illness.

How do you manage your disease?

Mostly by listening to my body. When I am feeling ill or tired, I have to take it easy. The disease will only let you do so much before it knocks you out.

Did you have to make any lifestyle or dietary changes in response to CFS?

I have to watch overexertion, even something like walking into a grocery store and trying to do the aisles. It goes beyond what my energy will allow. I'm also like a barometer. I have an especially hard time when it's cold outside, when it's rainy or humid. But the disease runs me, really. I can't do a lot to worsen my condition because it just exhausts me and prevents me from overdoing. Whatever the disease chooses to do to you, it can run your life. It's very frustrating. You save up all your energy to go to a wedding but your body may not cooperate.

I also take vitamins. But many people with this disease are preyed upon by quacks. I feel that you need to know what's going on in your body first. I think it's dangerous to randomly treat this. Some people are so desperate that they spend a fortune on all kinds of "treatments." I believe in getting blood tests and treating aspects of the disease that need to be treated.

(continued on the following page)

In Her Own Words: Living with Chronic Fatigue Syndrome *(continued)*

Did you seek any type of emotional support?

Well, I'm not into organized religion really, but I do have faith in God. I believe that things will ultimately be okay. When I initially became ill, I asked the doctor for a referral to a counselor. My children were ten and thirteen at the time, and I thought we'd have a lot of adjustments. I wanted something that would help everyone in the family. But we did have a bad experience with the psychologist who made a really insensitive comment to me once about how lucky I was to have my family and that without them I'd be living alone and on welfare. I was ready to fire her after that, but she sent a very sincere letter of apology, stating that she had no right to say that. After that, we saw her as needed and she gave us some coping tools. But I'm luckiest because I have such a loving family.

Does CFS have any impact on your family?

Definitely. It puts quite a burden on the healthy spouse.

If I take my daughter shopping, I need to stop and rest all the time. At most I can go to one store, but I can't walk through the whole mall. I need to save up my energy. Usually, I sit and wait for my daughter to shop. I can't go to the grocery store anymore. My family helps out. But many people with this disease who don't have families have to go to a nursing home. It's heartbreaking.

What advice would you give to anyone living with CFS?

First, go to a doctor who knows about the disease and will do the appropriate diagnosis. Unfortunately, I don't think most doctors really understand this disease. Also, listen to your body. You know when you're ill. Write down your symptoms and try to find a knowledgeable doctor.

As told to Amy Scholten, M.P.H.

TREATMENT AND THERAPY

Because no cause for CFS has been identified, the therapies for this disorder are directed at relief of symptoms until the affected person gradually recovers. Ideally, treatment will be based on a combination of therapies and approaches, including lifestyle changes, medications, and alternative and complementary therapies. Also, no surgical procedures exist for the treatment of CFS.

PREVENTION AND OUTCOMES

There are no guidelines for preventing CFS. Research is under way for a better understanding of CFS and for ways to prevent it. However, one can take the following preventive measures: Eat a balanced diet and exercise regularly and avoid the use of the following drugs because they are known to cause fatigue: hypnotics, blood pressure medications, antidepressants, seizure medications, antihistamines, beta-blockers, and tranquilizers.

Amy Scholten, M.P.H.

FURTHER READING

Bennett, R. M. "Fibromyalgia and Chronic Fatigue Syndrome." In *Cecil Textbook of Medicine*, edited by Lee Goldman and Dennis Ausiello. 23d ed. Philadelphia: Saunders/Elsevier, 2007.

Berne, Katrina. *Chronic Fatigue Syndrome, Fibromyalgia, and Other Invisible Illnesses: The Comprehensive Guide.* 3d ed. Alameda, Calif.: Hunter House, 2002.

Bested, Alison, and Alan Logan. *Chronic Fatigue Syndrome and Fibromyalgia.* Nashville: Cumberland House, 2006.

Craig, T., and S. Kakumanu. "Chronic Fatigue Syndrome: Evaluation and Treatment." *American Family Physician* 65 (2002): 1083-1090.

Devanur, L. D., and J. R. Kerr. "Chronic Fatigue Syndrome." *Journal of Clinical Virology* 37 (2006): 139-150.

Engleberg, C. N. "Chronic Fatigue Syndrome." In *Mandell, Douglas, and Bennett's Principles and Practice of Infectious Diseases,* edited by Gerald L. Mandell, John F. Bennett, and Raphael Dolin. 7th ed. New York: Churchill Livingstone/Elsevier, 2010.

Englebienne, Patrick, and Kenny DeMeirleir, eds. *Chronic Fatigue Syndrome: A Biological Approach.* Boca Raton, Fla.: CRC Press, 2002.

Lo, Shyh-Ching, et al. "Detection of MLV-related Virus Gene Sequences in Blood of Patients with Chronic Fatigue Syndrome and Healthy Blood Donors." *Proceedings of the National Academy of Sciences,* August 23, 2010. Available at http://www.pnas.org/content/early/2010/08/16/1006901107.

Patarca-Montero, Roberto. *Chronic Fatigue Syndrome*

and the Body's Immune Defense System. New York: Haworth Medical Press, 2002.

Prins, J. B., J. W. van der Meer, and G. Bleijenberg. "Chronic Fatigue Syndrome." *The Lancet* 367 (2006): 346-355.

Van Houdenhove, B., et al. "Does Hypothalamic-Pituitary-Adrenal Axis Hypofunction in Chronic Fatigue Syndrome Reflect a 'Crash' in the Stress System?" *Medical Hypotheses* 72, no. 6 (2009): 701-705.

WEB SITES OF INTEREST

Centers for Disease Control and Prevention
http://www.cdc.gov/cfs

Chronic Fatigue and Immune Dysfunction Syndrome Association of America
http://www.cfids.org

Trans-NIH Working Group for Research on Chronic Fatigue Syndrome
http://orwh.od.nih.gov/cfs.html

See also: Bacterial infections; Candidiasis; Diagnosis of bacterial infections; Diagnosis of viral infections; Epstein-Barr virus infection; Fever of unknown origin; Immunodeficiency; Mononucleosis; Retroviral infections; Social effects of infectious disease; Viral infections; Women and infectious disease.

CJD. *See* Creutzfeldt-Jakob disease.

Clonorchiasis

CATEGORY: Diseases and conditions
ANATOMY OR SYSTEM AFFECTED: Gastrointestinal system, intestines, liver, stomach

DEFINITION

Clonorchiasis is an infection of the biliary ducts of the liver caused by the parasite *Clonorchis sinensis,* also known as *Opisthorchis sinensis.* Infection with this liver fluke (trematode) is endemic to Asia, particularly in Korea, Japan, Taiwan, China, and Vietnam, but is introduced occasionally in other countries such as the United States through contaminated food imported from Asia.

CAUSES

Humans become infected by *C. sinensis* by eating raw, dried, salted, or pickled fresh-water fish that contain the parasite. Immature flukes are released into the duodenum and ascend the common biliary tract through the ampulla of Vater. The flukes mature to adults in approximately one month and reside in the small- and medium-size intrahepatic ducts. Occasionally, the flukes migrate into the gallbladder and the pancreatic ducts. Adult flukes, which can live for more than twenty years, are 10 to 25 millimeters (mm) long and 3 to 5 mm wide.

RISK FACTORS

The greatest risk factor for contracting clonorchiasis is eating uncooked or undercooked fresh-water fish or crayfish imported from the Far East. Fish from this region should be thoroughly cooked to avoid the liver fluke infection. Clonorchiasis is in turn a known risk factor for the development of cholangiocarcinoma, a neoplasm of the biliary duct system.

SYMPTOMS

Minor liver fluke infections are typically asymptomatic. Higher-level infections can cause fever, chills, abdominal pain, nausea, diarrhea, mild jaundice, and eosinophilia. Bilirubin levels may be elevated. Severe fluke infestation may cause stenosis of the bile ducts and develop into cholangiohepatitis and liver failure. In long-standing infections, cholangitis, choletithiasis, pancreatitis, and cholangiocarcinoma can develop.

SCREENING AND DIAGNOSIS

A medical history should include questions about the person's diet, travel history, and history of regions where the patient has lived. A physical examination should include gentle palpation of the liver. Medical tests often include endoscopy and an examination of stool.

Diagnosis of clonorchiasis typically depends on recovering and identifying the liver fluke's eggs in a stool sample. Abdominal X rays, computed tomography scans, and sonographic assessments may be used to identify diffuse dilatation of small intrahepatic ducts or thickening of the bile duct walls. The adult fluke may also be recovered surgically.

TREATMENT AND THERAPY

The drugs of choice for treating clonorchiasis are praziquantel or albendazole. Praziquantel paralyzes the musculature of the fluke, leading to its death. Albendazole inhibits metabolism in the cells of the fluke, causing immobilization and death. In most cases, only a single dose of either drug is necessary, but for severe infections, longer-term treatment may be required.

PREVENTION AND OUTCOMES

The best way to avoid clonorchiasis is to refrain from eating fish imported from the Far East. If eaten, however, the fish should be thoroughly cooked.

Alvin K. Benson, Ph.D.

FURTHER READING

Berger, Stephen A., and John S. Marr. *Human Parasitic Diseases Sourcebook.* Sudbury, Mass.: Jones and Bartlett, 2005.

Icon Health. *The Official Patient's Sourcebook on Clonorchiasis.* San Diego, Calif.: Author, 2002.

"Intestinal Trematodes" In *Diagnostic Medical Parasitology,* edited by Lynne Shore Garcia. 5th ed. Washington, D.C.: ASM Press, 2007.

"Liver and Lung Trematodes." In *Diagnostic Medical Parasitology,* edited by Lynne Shore Garcia. 5th ed. Washington, D.C.: ASM Press, 2007.

Sithithaworn, Paiboon, et al. "Food-Borne Trematodes." In *Manson's Tropical Diseases,* edited by Gordon C. Cook and Alimuddin I. Zumla. 22d ed. Philadelphia: Saunders/Elsevier, 2009.

WEB SITES OF INTEREST

Centers for Disease Control and Prevention
http://www.cdc.gov/parasites

Microbiology and Immunology On-line: Parasitology
http://pathmicro.med.sc.edu/book/parasit-sta.htm

See also: Cholecystitis; Dracunculiasis; Flukes; Foodborne illness and disease; Hookworms; Intestinal and stomach infections; Pancreatitis; Parasitic diseases; Schistosomiasis; Waterborne illness and disease; Worm infections.

Clostridium

CATEGORY: Pathogen
TRANSMISSION ROUTE: Blood, ingestion, inhalation

DEFINITION

Clostridium is a gram-positive, rod-shaped, spore forming, chiefly anaerobic bacteria that can produce lethal toxins. There are approximately 134 species, 25 to 30 of which are infectious to animals and humans.

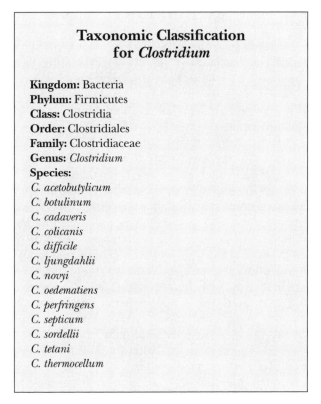

Taxonomic Classification for *Clostridium*

Kingdom: Bacteria
Phylum: Firmicutes
Class: Clostridia
Order: Clostridiales
Family: Clostridiaceae
Genus: *Clostridium*
Species:
C. acetobutylicum
C. botulinum
C. cadaveris
C. colicanis
C. difficile
C. ljungdahlii
C. novyi
C. oedematiens
C. perfringens
C. septicum
C. sordellii
C. tetani
C. thermocellum

NATURAL HABITAT AND FEATURES

Clostridium is found in soil, water, and sewage. It is also found as normal microbial flora in the gastrointestinal tract and in the vagina. It is saprophytic in nature, playing an important role in the degradation of organic materials. Most *Clostridium* species are obligate anaerobes, but a few can grow in the air at atmospheric pressure. Because *Clostridium* cannot use molecular oxygen as a final electron acceptor, it generates energy solely by fermentation. Endospores produced by *Clostridium* are extremely hearty and can survive adverse environmental conditions such as extreme heat and oxygen deprivation.

Clostridium can be seen microscopically, appearing pink to red when stained for gram-positive bacteria. They comprise straight or slightly curved rods that are 0.3 to 1.6 micrometers (μm) wide and 1 to 14 μm long, and they are found singly, in pairs, in short or long chains, or in helical coils. Most are motile with flagella. *Clostridium* grown on agar will appear as a series of flat, round colonies and demonstrate hemolysis. Clinically, *Clostridium* is detected through enzyme immunoassay, cytotoxin assay, polymerase chain reaction (PCR), and tissue sampling.

Clostridium is characterized by its potent and often lethal endotoxins. *C. botulinin* and *C. tetani* produce the most lethal toxins known to affect humans. Most *Clostridium* species are benign to humans, and some play an essential biological role in degrading biological molecules.

PATHOGENICITY AND CLINICAL SIGNIFICANCE

Clostridium infections range from mild food poisoning to life-threatening septic shock. There are four methods of infection with, for example, *C. botulinum,* which leads to botulism: food-borne, wound colonization, intestinal colonization, and inhalation. All these methods of infection are rare; in general, only food-borne and intestinal colonization in infants is fatal if not treated properly. In cases of food poisoning, spores will grow in anaerobic, nonacidic pH, and in low salt and low sugar environments; contaminated food is usually found in canned goods in the home or in fermented, uncooked meat. Wound botulism is almost exclusively found in users of black tar heroin, which is injected under the skin rather than intravenously. These wounds are usually self-limiting with supportive treatment.

Infants with botulism have intestinal colonization of *C. botulinum* because of competition with healthy gut flora; botulism manifests as infant paralysis, also known as floppy infant. An iatrogenic risk also exists for botulism symptoms for persons receiving botulinum toxin injections for either cosmetic or therapeutic purposes.

C. difficile is the most identifiable bacterial cause of diarrhea. Widespread use of broad-spectrum antibiotics such as the fluoroquinolones and third generation cephalosporins is the primary cause, but any antibiotic use, especially long-term use, can cause a *C.*

difficile infection. The symptoms of *C. difficile* include watery diarrhea, pseudomembranous colonitis, fever, fecal leucocytes, cramping, and, if severe, toxic megacolon. *C. difficile* infection is also a high-risk nosocomial (hospital acquired) infectious disease.

C. perfringens can cause a range of illnesses, from food poisoning to toxic shock to gas gangrene. The source of *C. perfringens* food poisoning is meats; gravies; and dried, processed, and inadequately heated foods. Symptoms include vomiting and diarrhea and are usually self-limiting. Clostridial myonecrosis, or gas gangrene, is characterized by gas bubbles under the skin, a distinctive foul odor, and a blackish discoloration of the skin. It usually occurs with injuries, such as severe crushing traumas and penetrating wounds, or at the site of recent surgery. The onset is sudden and dramatic. Persons with existing blood vessel diseases such as diabetes or atherosclerosis are most at risk. Shock, delirium, and renal failure are followed by death. *C. perfringens*, in addition to *C. sordellii*, has also been linked to toxic shock after surgical abortions or spontaneous miscarriages.

C. tetani causes tetanus, or lockjaw, and intermittent spasms of the masseter muscles, which can move into the lower muscles and eventually cause death. The *C. tetani* bacteria can enter the body through a burn, surgical wound, or puncture wound. It can also enter through the uterus (maternal tetanus) and the umbilical cord. *C. tetani* produces an exotoxin called tetanospasmin, which enters the central nervous system and releases an inhibitory neurotransmitter, causing generalized tonic spasticity. Symptoms include jaw stiffening, difficulty swallowing, irritability, tonic spasms, and the characteristic facial expression of a fixed smile with elevated eyebrows (risus sardonis). The patient may be in extreme pain but will be unable to speak, although mental capacity remains intact. Death is caused by asphyxia or cyanosis.

Botulinum toxin has been found to have important therapeutic effects for persons with a range of illnesses including minor nerve spasticity disorders, Tourette's syndrome, cerebral palsy, migraines, and Parkinsonian tremors. Botulinum toxin type A can be injected intramuscularly and prevent the release of acetylcholine, resulting in a temporary paralysis of muscles. Commercially known as Botox, it is also used for cosmetic purposes to freeze facial muscles to give the appearance of youth.

DRUG SUSCEPTIBILITY

Botulism antitoxin is the only treatment for botulism poisoning. Some of the *Clostridium* species can be killed with antimicrobials. Both metronizole and vancomycin are given for *C. difficile* infections. Penicillin G is effective against mild cases of *C. perfringens*; however, metronizole is also effective. Both antibiotics can be given as supportive drugs in cases of tetanus, although the primary treatment is a tetanus antitoxin. A vaccine and regular booster shots can protect against tetanus.

S. M. Willis, M.S., M.A.

FURTHER READING

Abrutyn, E. "Botulism." In *Harrison's Principles of Internal Medicine,* edited by Joan Butterton. 17th ed. New York: McGraw-Hill, 2008. A chapter on botulism in a respected text on internal medicine.

Finsterer, J. "Neuromuscular and Central Nervous System Manifestation of Clostridium perfringens Infections." *Infection* 356 (2007): 396-405. An overview of infectious diseases caused by C. perfringens.

Pickering, Larry K., et al., eds. "Clostridial Infections." *In Red Book: 2009 Report of the Committee on Infectious Diseases.* 28th ed. Elk Grove Village, Ill.: American Academy of Pediatrics, 2009. An overview of clostridial infections and treatments.

Sobel, J. "Botulism." *Food Safety* 41 (2005) 1167-1173. Overview of how botulism can be contracted. Includes symptoms, treatments, and prevention.

Ward, A. B. "Clinical Value of Botulinum Toxin in Neurological Indications." *European Journal of Neurology* 13 (2006) 20-26. Overview of clinical uses for the botulinum toxin for persons with neurological disorders.

WEB SITES OF INTEREST

American College of Gastroenterology
http://www.acg.gi.org

American Lung Association
http://www.lungusa.org

Center for Food Safety and Applied Nutrition
http://www.fda.gov/food

See also: Airborne illness and disease; Amebic dysentery; Anthrax; Bacterial infections; Biological weapons; Bioterrorism; Botulinum toxin infection; *Clostridium difficile* infection; Food-borne illness and disease; Gangrene; Intestinal and stomach infections; Opportunistic infections; Soilborne illness and disease; Tetanus; Wound infections.

Clostridium difficile infection

CATEGORY: Diseases and conditions
ANATOMY OR SYSTEM AFFECTED: Abdomen, colon, gastrointestinal system, intestines
ALSO KNOWN AS: Antibiotic-associated colitis, antibiotic-associated diarrhea, *Clostridium difficile*-induced colitis, infectious colitis

DEFINITION

Clostridium difficile is an anaerobic, gram-positive, spore-forming bacteria that is part of the normal intestinal flora. It can lay dormant and never cause disease, becoming pathogenic only when the balance of bacterial flora shifts, for example, after a person has antimicrobial therapy or immunosuppressive treatment. *C. difficile* is the most identifiable bacterial cause of diarrhea in industrialized countries. It is also one of the most significant; nosocomial pathogens, affecting up to 1.2 percent of all hospitalized persons and causing death to 3.2 percent of those infected.

C. difficile produces toxin A, a potent enterotoxin that combines with toxin B, a potent cytotoxin; toxin A is primarily responsible for the pathogenetic nature of the disease. Another cytotoxin, known as the binary toxin, is believed to be responsible for a newer, more virulent strain of *C. difficile* called NAP1/027.

CAUSES

Since 1978, *C. difficile* has been established as the most significant pathogen of antibiotic-related diarrhea. The widespread use of broad-spectrum antibiotics such as the fluoroquinolones and third generation cephalosporins has been identified as the primary cause, but any antibiotic use, especially long-term use, can initiate an episode of *C. difficile*. *C. difficile* is also a virulent nosocomial disease.

RISK FACTORS

The following are the most common risk factors associated with a *C. difficile* infection: antibiotic use within the past three months, age sixty-five years or older, proton pump inhibitor use, renal insufficiency, gastrointestinal surgery or procedure, nasogastric intubation, prolonged hospital stay, sharing a hospital room with a person infected with *C. difficile*, and working at a health care facility, nursing home, or day-care center. The newer strain of *C. difficile*, NAP1/027, adds a new population of those persons at risk: healthy young adults. It is unknown why this group is vulnerable. *C. difficile* is also a food-borne pathogen; the bacteria and its spores have been found in meat, poultry, and vegetables and are resistant to heat.

SYMPTOMS

Most persons will experience watery diarrhea, colitis, pseudomembranous colonitis, fever, fecal leucocytes, cramping, dehydration, and in severe cases, toxic megacolon. The symptoms of *C. difficile* can be aggravated if the person has a preexisting bowel disorder.

SCREENING AND DIAGNOSIS

Laboratory findings may be nonspecific and may mimic other illnesses, including leukocytosis, hypoalbuminemia, and fecal leukocytosis. A blood draw may show an increase in white blood cells up to 30,000 to 50,000 cubic millimeters. A computed tomography (CT) scan will also mimic other conditions, such as megacolon or perforation of the intestine. An endoscopy or sigmoidoscopy can provide a quick visual diagnosis of pseudomembranous colonitis on the colonic mucosa. Approximately 50 percent of persons with *C. difficile* will have ulceration of the colonic mucosa.

The gold standard of diagnosis of *C. difficile* is a cytotoxin assay, yet most hospitals do not have the equipment to perform the test, which also has the disadvantage of taking three days to receive results. Most institutions use the enzyme immunoassay (EIA) because it is easy to use and because results are reported quickly. However, EIA has sensitivity only up to 75 percent. It is recommended that tests be performed on multiple stool samples.

TREATMENT AND THERAPY

The first treatment step is to discontinue the person's antibiotic therapy (if he or she is undergoing this treatment). Next, the person is hydrated with intravenous fluids. Also, one should avoid using any opiates or antidiarrheal agents because a decrease in intestinal motility can lead to a backup of bacteria in the

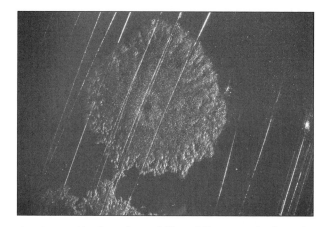

A micrograph of a colony of Clostridium *species bacteria.* (CDC)

colon.

A *C. difficile* infection is, paradoxically, treated with antibiotics. Two antibiotics are used: metronidazole (Flagyl) or vancomycin (Vancocin). Vancomycin may be the preferred choice for persons with a more severe case, although both treatments are equally effective. Probiotics ("helpful" bacteria), especially *Saccharomyces boulardii* and *Lactobacillus rhamnosus*, can be helpful during treatment and taken as a prophylactic to prevent a *C. difficile* infection when taking antibiotics in general. Relapses of *C. difficile* are very common, with first-time relapses occurring 12 to 20 percent of the time after first treatment and 33 to 60 percent of the time after subsequent treatments. Anion binding resins, such as colestipol and cholestyramine, are used concurrently with vancomycin to treat stubborn recurrent infections; intravenous immunoglobulin is another.

An especially innovative treatment is the use of healthy donor feces to repopulate the colon with healthy bacterial flora. Healthy stool sample is transferred to the colon by enema and slurry by nasogastric tube or by colonoscopy. This procedure was first described in 1958 and has had a success rate of more than 90 percent.

Often the last option is the surgical solution: a partial or complete colectomy. This is more common in persons who have a preexisting bowel disease or have a particularly virulent strain of *C. difficile*. This surgery, however, has a high mortality rate, estimated to be 35 to 57 percent.

PREVENTION AND OUTCOMES

Hospitals should isolate persons with *C. difficile* in single rooms with private toilets and should follow infectious-disease protocols. Workers who have been exposed to *C. difficile* should vigorously wash hands with soap and water to disinfect and physically dislodge spores. Alcohol-based gels provide no protection against *C. difficile*. Proper disinfection with the appropriate cleaning agents will also help kill *C. difficile*; one should use a solution of 10 percent sodium hypochlorite or diluted bleach. Ammonia-based cleaners will not kill the spores and even may encourage *C. difficile* growth. Persons who must take antibiotics can take probiotics as a precaution against *C. difficile*.

S. M. Willis, M.S., M.A.

FURTHER READING

Bartlett, J. G. "Narrative Review: The New Epidemic of Clostridium difficile-Associated Enteric Disease." *Annals of Internal Medicine* 145 (2006): 758-764. A history and overview of C. difficile that highlights symptoms and treatment.

EBSCO Publishing. DynaMed: "Clostridium difficile" colitis. A brief outline of C. difficile-related colitis. Available through http://www.ebscohost.com/dynamed.

Feldman, Mark, Lawrence S. Friedman, and Lawrence J. Brandt, eds. *Sleisenger and Fordtran's Gastrointestinal and Liver Disease: Pathophysiology, Diagnosis, Management.* New ed. 2 vols. Philadelphia: Saunders/Elsevier, 2010. An excellent textbook on gastroenterology, intestinal pathology, and treatment protocols.

Issa, M. "Clostridium difficile and Inflammatory Bowel Disease." *Inflammatory Bowel Disease* 14 (2008): 1432-1442. Discussion of the specific dangers of a C. difficile infection for patients with an existing inflammatory bowel disease condition. Also examines treatment and mortality rates.

Van Nod, E., et al. "Struggling with Recurrent Clostridium difficile Infections: Is Donor Faeces the Solution?" *Eurosurveillance* 14 (2009): 1-6. A history and description of the donor feces transplant treatment for recurring C. difficile infections.

Weese, J. S. "Clostridium difficile in Food: Innocent Bystander or Serious Threat?" *European Society of Clinical Microbiology and Infectious Diseases* 16 (2009): 3-10. An overview of the possible threats of food poisoning caused by C. difficile.

WEB SITES OF INTEREST

American College of Gastroenterology
http://www.acg.gi.org

Canadian Association of Gastroenterology
http://www.cag-acg.org

Canadian Digestive Health Foundation
http://www.cdhf.ca

Crohn's and Colitis Foundation of America
http://www.ccfa.org

National Digestive Diseases Information Clearinghouse
http://digestive.niddk.nih.gov

See also: Alliance for the Prudent Use of Antibiotics; Amebic dysentery; Antibiotic-associated colitis; Antibiotics: Types; Bacterial infections; *Clostridium*; Diverticulitis; Enteritis; Hookworms; Infectious colitis; Intestinal and stomach infections; Norovirus infection; Viral gastroenteritis.

Coccidioides

CATEGORY: Pathogen
TRANSMISSION ROUTE: Blood, inhalation

DEFINITION

Pathogenic fungi from the genus *Coccidioides* are soil-based organisms found in particular parts of the southwestern United States, northern Mexico, and several other areas of the Western Hemisphere. These fungi cause coccidioidomycosis, a systemic fungal infection that encompasses a broad spectrum of illness, including asymptomatic, acute, and chronic pneumonia and potentially fatal disseminated disease. The infection can involve any organ in the body.

NATURAL HABITAT AND FEATURES

Members of the genus *Coccidioides* (*C. immitis* and *C. posadasii*) are soilborne fungi that grow in sandy, warm, alkaline soils in low-altitude areas with high summer temperatures and low annual rainfall (five to fifteen inches per year). Although these two fungal species are morphologically indistinguishable, they are genetically distinct and occupy different geographical areas. *C. posadasii* exists in the deserts of the southwestern United States, Mexico, and South America, and *C. immitis* is geographically limited to California's San Joaquin Valley.

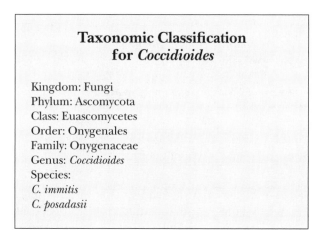

Taxonomic Classification for *Coccidioides*

Kingdom: Fungi
Phylum: Ascomycota
Class: Euascomycetes
Order: Onygenales
Family: Onygenaceae
Genus: *Coccidioides*
Species:
C. immitis
C. posadasii

Both *C. immitis* and *C. posadasii* (*C. immitis/posadasii*) are thermally dimorphic fungi, which means that they vary their growth mode in response to temperature changes. At 77° Fahrenheit (25° Celsius), they grow as extended filaments called hyphae that possess occasional cross-walls (septae). At their tips, some hyphae form barrel-shaped, desiccation-resistant, resting cells called arthroconidia that alternate with empty cells called disjunctor cells.

Arthroconidia (2 to 4 by 3 to 6 micrometers [μm] in size) break apart easily and are readily disseminated by air currents. At 98.6° F (37° C), these fungi grow as large, round, thick-walled structures called spherules. Spherules (20 to 80 μm in diameter) divide by internally partitioning themselves into smaller cells called endospores (2 to 5 μm in diameter) that eventually mature and then rupture the spherule. The liberated endospores then grow into new spherules.

In the laboratory, in addition to a growth temperature of 98.6° to 104° F (37 to 40° C), spherule formation also requires a liquid medium and elevated carbon dioxide levels (up to 20 percent). This has led some researchers to question if *C. immitis/posadasii* are thermally dimorphic fungi because more than just temperature is necessary to induce an alternative growth mode. Nevertheless, mycologists continue to classify *C. immitis/posadasii* with the other thermally dimorphic fungi.

PATHOGENICITY AND CLINICAL SIGNIFICANCE

C. immitis/posadasii cause the systemic fungal infection coccidioidomycosis, which is also known as San Joaquin Valley fever, valley fever, and desert rheumatism. Primary pulmonary coccidioidomycosis begins with the inhalation of arthroconidia. Upon deposition into the lower respiratory system, the arthroconidia transform into spherules and elicit an acute inflammation response in the lungs.

More than 60 percent of infected persons will experience no symptoms (asymptomatic). However, in other cases, one to four weeks after the initial infection, infected persons will have any one or a combination of the following symptoms: fever, chills, cough, chest pain, fatigue, shortness of breath, weight loss, muscle and joint soreness, headache, and night sweats. Some persons (25 percent) may also develop rashes. In the vast majority of people, the disease resolves without intervention.

Between 5 and 8 percent of infected persons develop chronic coccidioidomycosis, in which cavities form in the lungs, but 50 percent of these cases self-resolve within two years. Progressive pulmonary disease occurs in those whose chronic disease does not self-resolve, and in this case the lungs undergo increased and progressive inflammation and scarring, with decreased respiratory capacity.

Less than one percent of all infected persons experience disseminated disease, in which the fungus travels from the lungs, through the bloodstream, and to other organs in the body. Even though disseminated disease can involve any organ in the body, *C. immitis/posadasii* have a predilection for the skin, bone, joints, lymph nodes, adrenal glands, and central nervous system.

People from certain ethnic groups, in particular, Asians, Filipinos, Hispanics, and African Americans, show an increased risk of developing disseminated coccidioidomycosis, as do pregnant women. Likewise at risk are persons with subfunctional immune systems, which includes solid organ transplant recipients undergoing therapies that suppress the immune system and persons with acquired immune deficiency syndrome (AIDS), cancer, or inherited deficiencies of the immune system.

DRUG SUSCEPTIBILITY

People with self-resolving or localized pulmonary infections do not require treatment. However, those with unresolved pulmonary disease, severe pneumonia just after infection, chronic pneumonia, or disseminated disease require antifungal treatment. Specific antifungals for treatment of coccidioidomycosis include amphotericin B and several members of the azole antifungal group, including ketoconazole, itraconazole, and fluconazole.

Though not yet approved by the U.S. Food and Drug Administration for coccidioidomycosis, newer azole antifungal drugs, such as voriconazole, have shown efficacy in specific infected persons. Posaconazole was shown to be effective in a small clinical trial and has been approved by the European Commission for the treatment of refractory coccidioidomycosis. The echinocandin antifungal drug caspofungin has been used with varying success, but it appears mainly to work well in combination with other antifungal drugs.

Because of its superior ability to penetrate the blood-brain barrier, fluconazole is the preferred treatment for coccidioidal meningitis. Even if the infected person improves, relapse is common, so indefinite treatment is necessary. For refractory cases, amphotericin B is given as an intrathecal drug, which means that the drug is introduced into the central nervous system by means of a needle inserted into the subarachnoid space of the spinal cord to bypass the blood-brain barrier.

Experimental drugs that have shown promise in tested animals include sordarins and nikkomycins. For persons with pulmonary, bone, or joint involvement, surgical interventions in combination with antifungal drug therapy are often required.

Michael A. Buratovich, Ph.D.

FURTHER READING

Dismukes, William E., Peter G. Pappas, and Jack D. Sobel, eds. *Clinical Mycology.* New York: Oxford University Press, 2003. A medical mycology textbook with an excellent chapter on coccidioidomycosis.

Galgiani, John, et al. "Coccidioidomycosis." *Clinical Infectious Diseases* 41 (2005): 1217-1223. The guidelines of the Infectious Disease Society of America for the treatment and clinical classification of coccidioidomycosis.

Wright, Patty W., et al. "Donor-Related Coccidioidomycosis in Organ Transplant Recipients." *Clinical Infectious Diseases* 37 (2003): 1265-1269. Case study

of two organ transplant recipients who received organs from a common donor, but later died of rapid, aggressive, coccidioidomycosis. The source of the disease was the organ donor who had active, although unrecognized, coccidioidomycosis at the time of his death.

WEB SITES OF INTEREST

American Lung Association
http://www.lungusa.org

Centers for Disease Control and Prevention
http://www.cdc.gov

Valley Fever Center for Excellence
http://www.vfce.arizona.edu

Systematic Mycology and Microbiology Laboratory
http://www.ars.usda.gov

See also: Airborne illness and disease; Allergic bronchopulmonary aspergillosis; Antifungal drugs: Types; Aspergillosis; Aspergillus; Blastomycosis; Chromoblastomycosis; Coccidiosis; Fungi: Classification and types; Histoplasmosis; Mucormycosis; Mycoses; Paracoccidioides; Respiratory route of transmission; Soilborne illness and disease.

Coccidiosis

CATEGORY: Diseases and conditions
ANATOMY OR SYSTEM AFFECTED: Lungs, respiratory system
ALSO KNOWN AS: California disease, coccidioidomycosis, desert rheumatism, disseminated valley fever, valley fever

DEFINITION

Coccidiosis is a group of diseases caused by the fungi *Coccidioides immitis* or *C. posadasii.*

CAUSES

Residents of California, Arizona, Mexico, and parts of Central America and South America are most likely to acquire coccidiosis. People usually inhale the fungus when soil is disturbed. Occasionally, *Coccidioides* invade lung tissue and blood vessels, leading to infection throughout the body.

RISK FACTORS

Activities that increase exposure to dust in endemic areas increase the risk of coccidiosis. Severe infection can occur in those who are age fifty years and older; in those who have acquired immunodeficiency syndrome, cancer, or diabetes mellitus; and in persons who smoke cigarettes, who are pregnant, or who take medications that suppress the immune system.

SYMPTOMS

Symptoms are nonspecific. Cough, fever, chills, night sweats, joint pain, and fatigue are often mistaken for a viral illness. Most symptoms resolve within several weeks, even without treatment. Occasionally, lung infection leads to pneumonia, manifested as a lung infiltrate on a chest X ray. People with weakened immune systems are more likely to present with infection that spreads to the skin, lymph nodes, joints, bones, or brain.

SCREENING AND DIAGNOSIS

People who have symptoms of valley fever, specifically, should consult a physician for evaluation. A chest X ray may show localized or diffuse lung infiltrates. Positive antibody testing against *Coccidioides* confirms coccidiosis. People with more severe lung infection may require a bronchoscopy, a procedure in which a fiber optic scope is inserted into the airways. The specimens can be sent for culture and histopathology to identify *Coccidioides* on special growth media and to look at lung tissue under the microscope.

TREATMENT AND THERAPY

For most people, coccidiosis resolves spontaneously. People with risk factors for disseminated infection and those with more severe lung infection are more likely to benefit from treatment. Antifungal drugs such as fluconazole or itraconazole are given for three to six months.

PREVENTION AND OUTCOMES

People who live in endemic areas should avoid activities that expose them to dust. There is no vaccine against *Coccidioides*, but one has been in development.
David A. Saunders, M.D., and Steven D. Burdette, M.D.

FURTHER READING

Anstead, Gregory M., and John R. Graybill. "Coccidioidomycosis." *Infectious Disease Clinics of North America* 20, no. 3 (September, 2006): 621-643.

Galgiani, John. "Coccidioides Species." In *Mandell, Douglas, and Bennett's Principles and Practice of Infectious Diseases,* edited by Gerald L. Mandell, John F. Bennett, and Raphael Dolin. 7th ed. New York: Churchill Livingstone/Elsevier, 2010.

Rosenstein, Nancy, et al. "Risk Factors for Severe Pulmonary and Disseminated Coccidioidomycosis: Kern County, California, 1995-1996." *Clinical Infectious Diseases* 32 (2001): 708-715.

Sarosi, George A., and Scott F. Davies, eds. *Fungal Diseases of the Lung.* 3d ed. Philadelphia: Lippincott Williams & Wilkins, 2000. This resource covers a wide range of topics, including coccidiosis, cryptococcosis, blastomycosis, and sporotrichosis.

West, John B. *Pulmonary Pathophysiology: The Essentials.* 7th ed. Philadelphia: Wolters Kluwer/Lippincott Williams & Wilkins, 2008.

WEB SITES OF INTEREST

American Lung Association
http://www.lungusa.org

Centers for Disease Control and Prevention
http://www.cdc.gov

Valley Fever Center for Excellence
http://www.vfce.arizona.edu

Valley Fever Connections
http://www.valley-fever.org

See also: Airborne illness and disease; Allergic bronchopulmonary aspergillosis; Antifungal drugs: Types; Aspergillosis; Blastomycosis; Bordetella; Bronchiolitis; Bronchitis; Chromoblastomycosis; Coccidioides; Cryptococcosis; Fever; Fungal infections; Fungi: Classification and types; Histoplasmosis; Mucormycosis; Paracoccidioidomycosis; Respiratory route of transmission; Soilborne illness and disease; Tuberculosis (TB); Whooping cough.

Cold. See Common cold.

Cold sores

CATEGORY: Diseases and conditions
ANATOMY OR SYSTEM AFFECTED: Genitalia, lips, mouth, nervous system, skin, throat
ALSO KNOWN AS: Canker sores, fever blisters, herpes labialis, herpes simplex virus infection, herpes stomatitis

DEFINITION

Cold sores, or fever blisters, are small, painful, fluid-filled blisters that occur on the lips, mouth, nose, chin, cheeks, and throat.

CAUSES

Cold sores are most commonly caused by the herpes simplex type 1 virus (HSV-1). Less often, they can be caused by herpes simplex type 2 (HSV-2), the virus that most often causes genital herpes. Having a herpes simplex virus infection around the mouth is common. Ninety percent of older adults have been exposed to HSV some time in their lives, but not everyone who is exposed will develop cold sores.

The virus can be spread by contact with the fluid from a cold sore of another person through kissing and other close contact; contact with the eating utensils, razors, towels, or other personal items of a person with active cold sores; sharing food or drink with a person with active cold sores; and contact with saliva containing HSV.

HSV can get on the skin around the mouth and then invade nerves in the area. HSV then remains there, without causing symptoms, usually for two to twenty days, before the first (primary) outbreak occurs. This outbreak can cause blistering across the lips and tongue and inside the mouth. It may be accompanied by a body-wide, flulike illness, consisting of fever, general aches and pains, and swollen lymph glands.

Once this outbreak is over, after about seven to ten days, the virus returns to the nerves, where it remains dormant until it is reactivated, causing another (secondary) outbreak. When this occurs, painful, blistering sores erupt, usually at the border of the colored part of the lip, and can last up to fourteen days. It is impossible to predict when these outbreaks may recur, but typically, stress or illness may bring them on, as will sunlight, immunosuppressants, and menstruation. Some people have outbreaks regularly, while some never have another.

RISK FACTORS

It is possible to develop cold sores with or without the common risk factors. However, the more risk factors, the greater the likelihood a person will develop cold sores.

The viruses that cause cold sores are easily spread. They come out of the skin and are shed from the site of the cold sore for one to two days before the sore appears. Then the viruses exist in the fluid of the cold sore blisters. Although cold sores typically form in response to stress or illness, they can sometimes form without an identifiable trigger.

The risk factors for infection with HSV-1 include close contact (such as kissing) with an infected person and using an infected person's personal items, such as razors, towels, or eating utensils, which may be contaminated with the virus. The virus can also be spread through oral sex. Another risk factor for developing cold sores is exposure to sunlight or other ultraviolet light. Infants and young children (up to the age of three years) have an increased risk of being exposed to HSV-1.

Stress on the body because of illness or excessive exercise can weaken the body's immune system and can lead to an outbreak of cold sores. Common examples of stress or illness include infection, fever, or cold; physical injury; dental surgery; menstruation; medication (such as steroids) or illness (such as human immunodeficiency virus infection) that suppresses the immune system; eczema; and excessive exercise.

Cold sore outbreaks commonly occur during times of emotional stress. The type of stress that activates cold sores is typically negative stress rather than stress from positive or normal life-changing events.

SYMPTOMS

After being exposed to HSV-1 virus for the first time, a person may develop a blistering rash in the mouth or lips, or both, that may be accompanied by a body-wide, flulike illness. This first outbreak of cold sores usually disappears within seven to ten days, but it can last up to twenty days.

The symptoms of the first outbreak are a blistering, painful rash of small ulcerations across the lips, gums, and tongue, and inside the mouth (more common in children); pain and blistering on the soft roof of the mouth, tonsils, and throat (more common in adults); flulike symptoms, including a swollen and sore throat, mouth sores, fever, decreased energy, muscle aches and pains, difficulty breathing, and swollen glands (lymph nodes) in the neck.

After causing these initial symptoms, the virus may remain in the nerves until it is reactivated, typically by stress or illness. Direct sunlight, a weakened immune system, and menstruation can also trigger reactivation. If reactivated, the virus will appear as a cold sore. A few days before this occurs, one may experience some itching, burning, or pain in the area where the cold sore will appear. Some people have outbreaks regularly, and some never have another after the initial infection.

The symptoms of an active cold sore are small, painful, fluid-filled, and red-rimmed blisters. After a few days, the blisters dry and form a scab. The scabs will heal in about five days, usually without scarring or loss of sensation.

SCREENING AND DIAGNOSIS

Because they have recognizable features, cold sores are most often diagnosed by physical exam and by the infected person's medical history. If the doctor is not sure, she or he may take a sample of the fluid or tissue from the blister or a blood sample for testing. Testing may include any of the following:

Viral culture. With a cotton swab, a sample of the fluid from the cold sore blisters is taken as soon as possible after an outbreak begins. The virus is then grown in the laboratory and identified. This test is accurate if the sample is taken while there are still clear blisters.

Tzanck test. The cold sore is lightly scraped to collect cells onto a glass slide. These cells are then examined under a microscope to identify them. This test is quick, but it is accurate in only 50 to 70 percent of cases.

Antibody titer (enzyme-linked immunoabsorbent assay). The body creates antibodies to fight an infection. This blood test measures the level of antibodies, which are created by the body to fight infection, that are battling HSV. The antibody titer is about 85 percent accurate, however, it is not used routinely as the only diagnostic test.

Polymerase chain reaction. This test, also known as PCR, multiplies the number of pieces of HSV in the test fluid, making it easier to detect. PCR is as accurate as a culture, but provides quicker results. It is expensive, however, and not commonly used.

TREATMENT AND THERAPY

The treatment and management of cold sores in-volves medications, behavioral changes, and alternative and complementary therapies. Although treatment can help relieve or reduce outbreaks of cold sores, they cannot be permanently cured. HSV-1 will persist in the nerve tissue once it is infected. Therefore, treatment is focused on preventing cold sore outbreaks and on reducing the severity of symptoms. There are no surgical options for the treatment of cold sores.

PREVENTION AND OUTCOMES

Most people are exposed to HSV as children. Some, however, contract the virus as adults. Once a person has HSV, he or she has it for life. Changing some behaviors can lower the risk of contracting HSV and of having recurrent outbreaks.

To reduce the risks, one should avoid exposure to the virus that causes cold sores, avoid excessive exposure to the sun, reduce physical and emotional stress, practice good hygiene, avoid certain foods, get adequate sleep, and eat a healthful diet.

Avoid exposure to the virus. HSV can be spread by close contact with someone who has a cold sore or by using items contaminated with the virus. One should not kiss, have other close contact with, or share personal items (such as towels, razors, and eating utensils) with a person who has an active cold sore or thinks he or she is about to have one. HSV can also spread to the genital area through oral sex.

Avoid excessive exposure to the sun. Exposure to sunlight is known to cause outbreaks of cold sores. Although it is impossible to avoid all sun exposure, one should use sunscreen on lips and skin to help reduce the sun's effect. Also, one should wear a large-brimmed hat outside in sunny weather to protect the face from ultraviolet rays.

Reduce physical and emotional stress. Physical and emotional stress may reduce the body's ability to fight HSV, and stress may trigger an outbreak of cold sores. Although exercise may actually help to reduce emotional stress, an excessive amount can weaken the body. Relaxation techniques, such as meditation and deep breathing, can help reduce emotional stress.

Practice good hygiene. Good hygiene can prevent the spread of cold sores and help reduce the length and severity of the outbreaks. During an outbreak, one should avoid touching the cold sores, especially open cuts; should wash hands frequently; should keep fingernails clean by scrubbing daily; and should avoid spreading the virus to other parts of the body, such as the eyes and genital area.

Avoid certain foods. Foods that irritate the tissue of the lips and mouth, such as certain fruits or spices, may trigger a cold sore outbreak. These food-related triggers are different for every person.

Get adequate sleep and eat a healthful diet. The body heals fastest when it receives adequate rest and good nutrition.

Reviewed by David L. Horn, M.D., FACP

FURTHER READING

American Academy of Dermatology. "Herpes Simplex." Available at http://www.aad.org. The American Academy of Dermatology provides a brief but comprehensive discussion of the herpes simplex virus and its dermatological manifestations.

Arduino, P. G., and S. R. Porter. "Oral and Perioral Herpes Simplex Virus Type 1 (HSV-1) Infection: Review of Its Management." *Oral Diseases* 12 (2006): 254-270. Examines the medical management of herpes simplex virus in oral disease.

Groves, M. J. "Transmission of Herpes Simplex Virus via Oral Sex." *American Family Physician* 73 (2006): 1153. Discusses how herpes simplex virus infection, including cold sores, is transmissible through oral sex.

"Herpes Simplex." In *Ferri's Clinical Advisor 2011: Instant Diagnosis and Treatment,* edited by Fred F. Ferri. Philadelphia: Mosby/Elsevier, 2011. Provides recommendations on clinical treatments for herpes simplex virus infections.

Langlais, Robert P., and Craig S. Miller. *Color Atlas of Common Oral Diseases.* 4th ed. Philadelphia: Lippincott Williams & Wilkins, 2009. Provides six hundred color photographs of the most commonly seen oral conditions and descriptive text for each condition.

Norkin, Leonard. *Virology: Molecular Biology and Pathogenesis.* Washington, D.C.: ASM Press, 2010. Using the framework of the Baltimore classification scheme, the author provides a detailed account of virus structure and replication and examines the basis for disease pathology.

WEB SITES OF INTEREST

American Academy of Dermatology
http://www.aad.org

American Dental Association
http://www.ada.org

Centers for Disease Control and Prevention
http://www.cdc.gov/std

New Zealand Dermatological Society
http://dermnetnz.org

See also: Abscesses; Contagious diseases; Genital herpes; Herpes simplex infection; Herpesviridae; Herpesvirus infections; Mouth infections; Saliva and infectious disease; Sexually transmitted diseases (STDs); Skin infections; Viral infections.

Colorado tick fever

CATEGORY: Diseases and conditions
ANATOMY OR SYSTEM AFFECTED: All

DEFINITION

Colorado tick fever is an infection that is transmitted to humans by the bite of an infected tick.

CAUSES

Colorado tick fever is caused by the coltivirus, or Colorado tick fever virus. The Rocky Mountain wood tick is the principal carrier of the Colorado tick virus in the United States, and its geographic range is confined to the western United States and areas above five thousand feet in elevation. The virus is also carried by other small mammals, including ground squirrels, porcupines, and chipmunks. There have been reports of rare cases of Colorado tick fever caused by exposure in a laboratory setting and through a blood transfusion.

RISK FACTORS

Living or traveling in mountain forest areas at altitudes above five thousand feet in the Rocky Mountain region, especially between the months of April and July, increases one's chances of developing Colorado tick fever.

SYMPTOMS

Symptoms usually appear four to five days after a tick bite occurs and include high fever, chills, severe

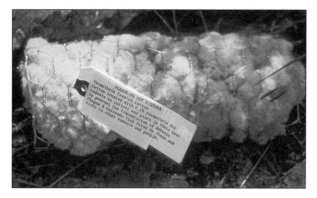

Cotton, treated with the insecticide permethrin, is used by tick-infested rodents as nesting material. Health authorities hope the treated cotton will kill those ticks, which cause Colorado tick fever. (CDC)

headache, pain behind the eyes, sensitivity to light, muscle pain, lethargy, abdominal pain, vomiting, and nausea.

SCREENING AND DIAGNOSIS

A doctor will ask about symptoms and medical history and will perform a physical exam. Tests may include blood tests to identify the virus and tests to identify antibodies for the virus.

TREATMENT AND THERAPY

There is no specific treatment for Colorado tick fever. Complications are extremely rare and include aseptic meningitis, encephalitis, and hemorrhagic fever. The fever and pain may be treated with acetaminophen (such as Tylenol) and other pain-relief medications. Once a person gets Colorado tick fever, it is believed that he or she will have immunity against reinfection.

PREVENTION AND OUTCOMES

To help reduce the chance of getting Colorado tick fever, one should limit exposure to ticks by avoiding tick-infested areas, especially during warmer months; by wearing light-colored clothing; by tucking pants into socks when in tick-infested habitats; by using tick repellents; by regularly inspecting and then removing ticks from the body with fine-tipped tweezers (grasp the tick close to the skin's surface and pull up steadily); and by disinfecting tick bites with soap and water.

Krisha McCoy, M.S.;
reviewed by David L. Horn, M.D., FACP

FURTHER READING

Acute and Communicable Disease Prevention, State of Oregon. "Colorado Tick Fever Fact Sheet." Available at http://www.oregon.gov/dhs/ph/acd/diseases/ctf/facts.shtml.

National Library of Medicine. "Colorado Tick Fever." Available at http://www.nlm.nih.gov/medlineplus/ency/article/000675.htm.

Vanderhoof-Forschner, Karen. *Everything You Need to Know About Lyme Disease and Other Tick-Borne Disorders.* 2d ed. Hoboken, N.J.: John Wiley & Sons, 2003.

Weedon, David. *Skin Pathology.* 3d ed. New York: Churchill Livingstone/Elsevier, 2010.

WEB SITES OF INTEREST

Canadian Cooperative Wildlife Health Centre
http://www.ccwhc.ca

Centers for Disease Control and Prevention
http://www.cdc.gov/ticks

National Institute of Allergy and Infectious Diseases
http://www.niaid.nih.gov

See also: Acariasis; Anaplasmosis; Ehrlichiosis; Encephalitis; Fever; Hemorrhagic fever viral infections; Lyme disease; Mediterranean spotted fever; Mites and chiggers and infectious disease; Reoviridae; Rocky Mountain spotted fever; Rodents and infectious disease; Ticks and infectious disease; Tularemia; Vectors and vector control.

Common cold

CATEGORY: Diseases and conditions
ANATOMY OR SYSTEM AFFECTED: Auditory systemears, eyes, nose, throat, upper respiratory tract
ALSO KNOWN AS: Cold, coronavirus infection, rhinovirus infection, viral rhinitis

DEFINITION

The common cold is a viral infection that irritates the upper respiratory tract, especially the nose and throat.

CAUSES

The common cold is caused by any of two hundred viruses, including rhinovirus, coronavirus, adenovirus, coxsackie virus, paramyxovirus, parainfluenza virus, and respiratory syncytial virus.

RISK FACTORS

Risk factors for getting a cold include being near someone who has a cold; touching one's own nose, mouth, or eyes with virus-contaminated fingers; having allergies (which lengthens the duration of the cold); smoking or being near cigarette smoke; and stress. Also, girls and women are more at risk, especially around the time of their menstrual periods.

SYMPTOMS

Common cold symptoms include a sore or scratchy throat; stuffy nose (hard to breathe through nose); runny nose; sneezing; itchy, stuffed sensation in the ears; watery eyes; slight cough; headache; aches and pains; low energy; and low-grade fever.

SCREENING AND DIAGNOSIS

A doctor will ask about symptoms and medical history. He or she also will conduct a physical examination.

TREATMENT AND THERAPY

A cold usually lasts more than ten days. There are no cures for a cold, but there are treatments that can relieve symptoms. These treatments include the use of pain relievers (for aches and pains and fever) such as acetaminophen (such as Tylenol), ibuprofen (such as Motrin), and aspirin. Aspirin, however, is not recommended for children or teenagers with a current or recent viral infection because of the risk of Reye's syndrome. One should consult a doctor about medicines that are safe for children.

Another treatment for the cold is the use of pills or nasal sprays, which can shrink nasal passages and decrease mucus production. Nasal sprays should be used for two to three days only. If used for a longer period of time, the patient may have increased congestion after using the product.

The U.S. Food and Drug Administration recommends that over-the-counter (OTC) cough and cold products not be used by infants or by children younger than two years of age. Rare but serious side effects have been reported, including rapid heart rates, convulsions, decreased levels of consciousness, and death. OTC cough and cold products for older children and for adults include decongestants, expectorants, antihistamines, and antitussives (cough suppressants).

Another treatment for the common cold is drinking large amounts of fluids. Warm beverages, such as tea, and chicken soup, are soothing and can help reduce congestion. A cool-mist humidifier, cleaned daily, can keep nasal passages moist and can reduce congestion. Saline nasal sprays, too, may provide relief from congestion, and nasal wash may reduce symptoms and help reduce the need for medication.

Researchers are studying whether alternative remedies, such as vitamin C, zinc lozenges, and echinacea, are helpful in preventing colds, reducing symptoms, and lessening the duration of colds. Another natural remedy is honey, which appears to improve nighttime cough and sleep disruption in children. However, one should not give honey to infants younger than twelve months of age because of the risk of infant botulism.

Health experts do not know if herbs work to relieve cold symptoms. Also, some herbal treatments may not be pure. Other treatments for the cold include gargling with warm salt-water, which can help relieve a sore throat, and using throat lozenges as needed every couple of hours, which can help relieve a sore throat and a cough.

PREVENTION AND OUTCOMES

The most important way to keep from getting or spreading a cold is by washing hands, and to do so well and often. Other ways to keep from getting a cold include keeping hands away from one's nose, mouth, and eyes, and avoiding people who have a cold. For those who smoke, stopping or cutting down on smoking can help. Some people take vitamin C and other remedies, such as herbs, to keep from getting a cold, but health care providers are not sure if vitamin C or herbs work.

Rosalyn Carson-DeWitt, M.D.;
reviewed by David L. Horn, M.D., FACP

FURTHER READING

Arruda, E., et al. "Frequency and Natural History of Rhinovirus Infections in Adults During Autumn." *Journal of Clinical Microbiology* 35 (1997): 2864-2868. Available through EBSCO DynaMed Systematic Literature Surveillance at http://www.ebscohost.com/dynamed.

Eccles, Ronald, and Olaf Weber, eds. *Common Cold.* Boston: Birkhäuser, 2009.

Kimball, Chad T. *Colds, Flu, and Other Common Ailments Sourcebook.* Detroit: Omnigraphics, 2001.

National Institute of Allergy and Infectious Diseases. "Common Cold." Available at http://www.niaid.nih.gov/topics/commoncold.

Pappas, D. E., et al. "Symptom Profile of Common Colds in School-Aged Children." *Pediatric Infectious Disease Journal* 27 (2008): 8-11.

Paul, I. M., et al. "Effect of Honey, Dextromethorphan, and No Treatment on Nocturnal Cough and Sleep Quality for Coughing Children and Their Parents." *Archives of Pediatrics and Adolescent Medicine* 161 (2007): 1149-1153. Available through EBSCO DynaMed Systematic Literature Surveillance at http://www.ebscohost.com/dynamed.

Shors, Teri. *Understanding Viruses.* Sudbury, Mass.: Jones and Bartlett, 2008.

Slapak, I., et al. "Efficacy of Isotonic Nasal Wash (Seawater) in the Treatment and Prevention of Rhinitis in Children." *Archives of Otolaryngology—Head and Neck Surgery* 134 (2008): 67-74. Available through EBSCO DynaMed Systematic Literature Surveillance at http://www.ebscohost.com/dynamed.

U.S. Food and Drug Administration. "Public Health Advisory: FDA Recommends that Over-the-Counter (OTC) Cough and Cold Products Not Be Used for Infants and Children Under Two Years of Age." Available at http://www.fda.gov/safety/medwatch.

Wagner, Edward K., and Martinez J. Hewlett. *Basic Virology.* 3d ed. Malden, Mass.: Blackwell Science, 2008.

WEB SITES OF INTEREST

American Academy of Family Physicians
http://familydoctor.org

American Lung Association
http://www.lungusa.org

Centers for Disease Control and Prevention
http://www.cdc.gov

Clean Hands Coalition
http://www.cleanhandscoalition.org

Public Health Agency of Canada
http://www.phac-aspc.gc.ca

See also: Adenovirus infections; Airborne illness and disease; Allergic bronchopulmonary aspergillosis; Alternative therapies; Atypical pneumonia; Bronchiolitis; Bronchitis; Children and infectious disease; Contagious diseases; Coronavirus infections; Coxsackie virus infections; Epiglottitis; Home remedies; Influenza; Laryngitis; Middle-ear infection; Paramyxoviridae; Parvovirus infections; Pharyngitis and tonsillopharyngitis; Pneumonia; Respiratory syncytial virus infections; Rhinovirus infections; Schools and infectious disease; Seasonal influenza; Sinusitis; Strep throat; Viral infections; Viral pharyngitis; Viral upper respiratory infections; Whooping cough.

Communicable diseases. *See* Contagious diseases.

Complementary medicine. *See* Alternative therapies.

Conjunctivitis

CATEGORY: Diseases and conditions
ANATOMY OR SYSTEM AFFECTED: Eyes, vision
ALSO KNOWN AS: Pinkeye

DEFINITION

Conjunctivitis is inflammation of the conjunctiva, a membrane that covers the eye and lines the inner surface of the eyelid. There are many causes of conjunctivitis.

CAUSES

Causes of conjunctivitis include viral infection; bacterial infection, such as that caused by *Staphylococcus* or *Streptococcus*; allergic reaction, usually related to seasonal allergies; and chemical irritation caused by air pollutants, soap, smoke, chlorine, makeup, and other chemicals. Both viral and bacterial conjunctivitis are highly contagious.

RISK FACTORS

Risk factors for conjunctivitis include contact with a person who has conjunctivitis; sharing towels, linens, or other objects with an infected person, and touching doorknobs used by an infected person; exposure to chemical or environmental irritants; wearing contact lenses, particularly if not maintained properly; and seasonal allergies or contact with known allergens. Also, conjunctivitis is more common in children.

SYMPTOMS

Symptoms of conjunctivitis include red, watery eyes; inflamed inner eyelids; scratchy feeling in the eyes; itchy eyes; puslike or watery discharge; sensitivity to light; and swelling of the eyelid. Depending on its cause, conjunctivitis will usually clear up within two to fourteen days. If conjunctivitis is caused by a seasonal allergy, it may continue to occur throughout the season. If it is caused by a nonseasonal allergy, it may continue to occur year-round.

The foregoing symptoms can sometimes indicate a more serious medical problem. If these symptoms or other symptoms are present, one should consult an eye doctor immediately.

SCREENING AND DIAGNOSIS

A doctor will ask about symptoms and medical history and will examine the person's eye. Any discharge from the eye may be tested to determine the cause of the conjunctivitis.

TREATMENT AND THERAPY

Treatment will depend on the cause of the conjunctivitis. If the cause is bacterial infection, a doctor may prescribe antibiotic eye drops or ointment, or both. This will help shorten the course of the infection and the time it is contagious. Wipe away any discharge that accumulates with a clean cotton ball before applying the medication.

There is no medicine to cure a viral infection. However, many doctors will prescribe topical antibiotics if they cannot rule out the possibility of a bacterial infection. Applying warm compresses or "artificial tears" (an over-the-counter medication) may help relieve symptoms. The doctor may also prescribe an anti-inflammatory eye drop, which may help alleviate symptoms.

If allergic or chemical irritation is the cause of the conjunctivitis, one should avoid the cause of the irritation, such as smoke, pollen, and makeup, and should apply cool compresses to the affected area. Furthermore, the doctor may prescribe allergy eye drops to help relieve allergic conjunctivitis.

To prevent further spread of infection, one should avoid touching one's face and rubbing one's eyes; should change pillowcases and towels every night; should avoid sharing pillows, towels, wash cloths, and handkerchiefs; should wash hands frequently and avoid shaking hands with others; should avoid swimming. Also, one should carefully clean away any discharge with warm water and clean cotton (or gauze) and immediately discard the used cotton or gauze.

PREVENTION AND OUTCOMES

Strategies to avoid conjunctivitis include the foregoing measures and the following: Avoid sharing makeup or eye drops; wear watertight goggles when swimming; and clean contact lenses daily and avoid sleeping with them unless doing so is okayed by an eye doctor. In case of allergic conjunctivitis, one should avoid irritants and place allergy-proof covers on pillows and mattress.

Michelle Badash, M.S.;
reviewed by Christopher Cheyer, M.D.

FURTHER READING

American Academy of Ophthalmology. "Conjunctivitis." Available at http://one.aao.org.

Cassel, Gary H., Michael D. Billig, and Harry G. Randall. *The Eye Book: A Complete Guide to Eye Disorders and Health.* Baltimore: Johns Hopkins University Press, 2001.

Ferkat, Sharon, and Jennifer S. Weizer. *All About Your Eyes: A Practical Guide in Plain English from the Physicians at the Duke University Eye Center.* Durham, N.C.: Duke University Press, 2006.

Johnson, Gordon J., et al., eds. The *Epidemiology of Eye Disease.* 2d ed. New York: Oxford University Press, 2003.

Koby, M. "Conjunctivitis." In *Ferri's Clinical Advisor 2011: Instant Diagnosis and Treatment,* edited by Fred F. Ferri. Philadelphia: Mosby/Elsevier, 2011.

Olitzky, S. E., et al. "Disorders of the Conjunctiva." In Nelson Textbook of Pediatrics, edited by Richard E. Behrman, Robert M. Kliegman, and Hal B. Jenson. 18th ed. Philadelphia: Saunders/Elsevier, 2007.

Parker, James N., and Philip M. Parker, eds. *The Official*

Patient's Sourcebook on Conjunctivitis. San Diego, Calif.: Icon Health, 2002.

Riordan-Eva, Paul, and John P. Whitcher. *Vaughan and Asbury's General Ophthalmology.* 17th ed. New York: Lange Medical Books/McGraw-Hill, 2007.

WEB SITES OF INTEREST

American Academy of Family Physicians
http://familydoctor.org

American Academy of Ophthalmology
http://www.aao.org

American Optometric Association
http://www.aoanet.org

Canadian Ophthalmological Society
http://www.eyesite.ca

See also: Acanthamoeba infection; Adenovirus infections; Airborne illness and disease; Bacterial infections; Children and infectious disease; Contagious diseases; Dacryocystitis; Eye infections; Inflammation; Keratitis; Ophthalmia neonatorum; Staphylococcal infections; Streptococcal infections; Trachoma; Viral infections.

Contagions. *See* Bacteria; Contagious diseases; Pathogens; Viruses.

Contagious diseases

CATEGORY: Epidemiology

DEFINITION

Contagious diseases are those diseases caused by pathogenic (disease-causing) agents, such as bacteria, viruses, and fungi, that infect the body. Contagious diseases, also called communicable diseases, are spread from person to person through direct contact or through contact with body fluids.

DISTINGUISHING FEATURES

Microorganisms are invisible and abundant residents of every habitat on Earth. Many have adapted to live inside the human body, and the vast majority reside there harmlessly or even with great benefit to the host. A small fraction of these microbes are pathogenic and can lead to infectious disease in humans. An even smaller number of pathogenic microbes can be transferred directly from one person to another, causing diseases that are termed "contagious."

Not all infectious diseases, however, are contagious. An example of an infectious but not contagious disease is malaria, which is caused by the protozoan *Plasmodium falciparum*, which is transferred from one person to another by the bite of a mosquito. Direct contact with the infected person or with that person's body fluids will not spread this disease. A notorious contagious infectious disease is influenza, which is caused by an orthomyxovirus that is easily spread from one person to another.

BIOLOGY OF PATHOGENIC ORGANISMS

There is great diversity among the types of microorganisms that are pathogenic. Contagious diseases are caused by viruses, bacteria, fungi, protozoa, and helminths. The specific biology of each organism determines what part of the body it will infect, what symptoms it will cause, how it will be spread from one person to another, and how it can be treated.

Viruses. Viruses are the smallest and simplest of all the pathogens that cause contagious diseases. They do not have cells and are not considered to be living organisms. Viruses are effectively designed containers, built to transport the genetic material they carry inside. They contain all the genetic information needed to re-create, so they have no materials or machinery for reproduction. After entering the body of a host animal, a virus reproduces by infecting a cell and taking over its reproductive machinery. New viral particles are assembled inside the cell and then released to the outside, where they can infect more cells.

Viruses cause a wide range of contagious diseases, many of which are serious or life-threatening. Treatment for viral infections is extremely limited or entirely unavailable. Because viruses exist inside human cells, it is difficult to destroy them without also killing the cells. Drugs that could potentially destroy a virus would be extremely toxic or fatal to the infected person. Antibiotics work only on bacteria, making the human immune system the most critical factor in recovery from viral infections.

Bacteria. Bacteria are living single-celled organisms

that are much more complex than viruses and about one hundred times larger. Bacteria are extremely significant to medicine, as they are responsible for large numbers of serious human illnesses. Bacteria are classified as prokaryotes because their cells have a simpler structure than those of plants and animals, which are eukaryotes. Despite their relatively simple structure, bacteria possess all the machinery necessary to grow and reproduce on their own. They are the smallest creatures on Earth that have this capacity. This feature sets them apart from viruses, which depend on host cells for reproduction. The small size and relatively simple structure of bacteria allows them to grow and reproduce rapidly.

A variety of antibiotics are available for the treatment of many bacterial diseases. These drugs target features of bacterial cells that are not present in eukaryotic cells. In this way, the drugs can kill the bacteria without damaging human cells. However, many bacteria have developed resistance to antibiotics. This worldwide problem limits the treatment options for a growing number of bacterial infections.

Fungi. Fungi are common eukaryotic microorganisms that only rarely cause disease in humans. Fungi have complex cells and a structure resembling those of plants. Unlike plants, fungi lack chlorophyll, so they cannot make their own sugars; they must live on nutrients found in their environment. Most take up residence on decaying plant matter and in soil. Fungi grow in two forms: molds and yeasts. Molds are quite common in nature. They are made of long filaments that branch and intertwine, creating the familiar mats that are often seen growing on bread and cheese. Yeasts are unicellular fungi that commonly live on fruits and flowers, thriving on the sugars provided there. Some are normal inhabitants of the human body.

Serious contagious diseases caused by fungi are quite rare in healthy persons. People who are seriously ill or have weak immune systems are more susceptible to fungal infections. Antifungal drugs are available and are effective against many fungal diseases.

Parasites. Parasites are eukaryotes that live on other living organisms for nutrition, without providing benefits to their hosts. Parasitic diseases are among the major causes of human suffering and death in the world. Contagious human parasites include protozoa and helminths. Protozoa are microscopic, unicellular eukaryotes, and as such are more complex than bacteria and have more in common with human cells. They are ten times larger than bacteria, and most can move or "swim." These organisms feed by taking in fluid from their surrounding environment, and they reproduce inside the body of the host. Helminths are multicellular macroscopic worms that find nutrients in body fluids and intestinal contents. Unlike protozoan parasites, most helminths must leave the host to lay eggs, which are the infective forms of the organism.

Drugs are available for the treatment of parasitic infections, but few of them are ideal. Similarities between human and parasite cells make it difficult to design drugs that can kill parasites without also being toxic to humans. Some drugs require long-term administration, which is not practical in many developing nations.

ROUTES OF TRANSMISSION

Pathogenic organisms vary in the way they spread from one host to another, a feature known as the route of transmission. For each pathogen, the route of transmission will determine where it enters and infects the body, how it spreads through a population, and how spread of the disease can be controlled. The routes of transmission for the agents of contagious diseases include airborne transmission, fecal-oral transmission, and direct transmission.

Airborne transmission. Airborne transmission occurs through the inhalation of infectious agents in aerosols that are released from an infected person. Aerosolized droplets are expelled by sneezing or coughing. The smallest of these droplets can remain suspended in air for a surprisingly long time (twenty minutes or longer). Inhaling the aerosol will introduce the pathogen into the respiratory tract. Different pathogens will infect different regions of the airways. Larger particles tend to settle from the air onto tissues sooner than do smaller particles, so the larger particles cause primarily upper respiratory infections. Smaller particles can infect the lower respiratory tract. Airborne pathogens can also be spread indirectly by contact with respiratory secretions that are on hands or inanimate objects. These organisms are then transferred to the airway through touching the nose, eyes, or mouth.

Organisms with airborne routes of transmission cause respiratory infections. The most common contagious infections worldwide are respiratory, because transmission through aerosols and contaminated

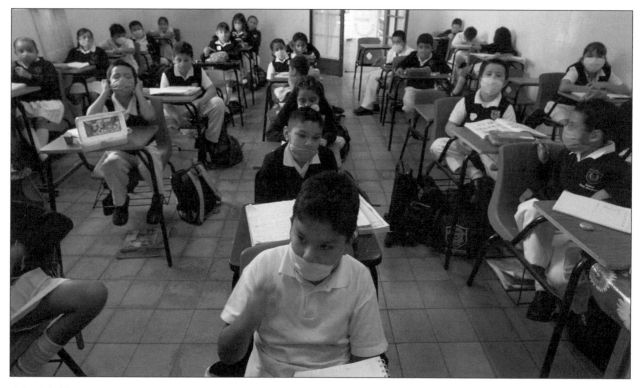

Schoolchildren in Mexico in 2009 wear protective masks to ward off the highly contagious H1N1 influenza, or swine flu. (AP/Wide World Photos)

objects occurs quite easily in normal daily activities. This mode of transmission is also known as casual contact. The majority of respiratory infections are caused by viruses. These include the common cold (rhinoviruses), influenza (orthomyxovirus), measles (paramyxovirus), and viral pneumonia (multiple virus types). Bacterial respiratory infections include tuberculosis (*Mycobacterium tuberculosis*), pneumonia (multiple species), strep throat (*Streptococcus pneumoniae*), and whooping cough (*Bordetella pertussis*). Some fungal diseases are respiratory. Most are caused by fungi that a healthy person's body can fight without consequence. The more common fungal respiratory infections include valley fever (*Coccidioides immitis*), histoplasmosis (*Histoplasma capsulatum*), and cryptococcosis (*Cryptococcus neoformans*).

Fecal-oral transmission. Fecal-oral transmission is a common route of spread of many bacterial, viral, and parasitic diseases. Organisms that are spread in this manner grow in the digestive tract, are present in feces, and usually cause diarrhea or vomiting. Infection occurs either by direct contact or through con-

sumption of food or water that has been contaminated with human feces. Food can become contaminated by a food handler who is ill, particularly if the handler's personal hygiene technique is inadequate. Raw shellfish, fruits, and vegetables that are washed in contaminated water can also spread disease. Waterborne pathogens are common in developing countries where sewage and drinking water are not treated. Natural disasters, such as earthquakes and floods, can breach water-treatment systems and cause outbreaks of waterborne illness.

Diarrheal diseases, which are the third leading cause of death in the world, are most often spread by fecal-oral transmission. Two of the most important are typhoid fever (*Salmonella typhi*) and cholera (*Vibrio cholerae*). These life-threatening bacterial illnesses are most often spread through contaminated water. Water purification methods have nearly eliminated these diseases in many countries, yet they remain a serious threat in many areas of the world. Outbreaks of intestinal illnesses, including those on cruise ships, are often caused by viruses (norovirus and rotavirus) that are spread through food by infected food handlers. Fecal contamination of food is the most common source of infection by the hepatitis A virus. Parasites can also be transmitted through food and water. *Cryptosporidium parvum, Entamoeba histolytica*, and *Giardia intestinalis* (also known as *G. lamblia*) are all protozoa that cause severe diarrhea. While rare in areas with good sanitation, these illnesses are still extremely common worldwide. It is estimated that 10 percent of the world's population and 2 to 3 percent of the U.S. population are infected with *E. histolytica*, which causes amebic dysentery.

Direct contact transmission. Some pathogens are so sensitive to the environment outside the human body that they cannot survive long enough to be transmitted by casual contact. These organisms must be transmitted from one person to another directly—through the exchange of body fluids during sexual contact, blood transfusion, birth, or breast-feeding. Bacterial infections that are transmitted through sexual contact only include syphilis (*Treponema pallidum*), gonorrhea (*Neisseria gonorrhoeae*), and chlamydia (*Chlamydia trachomatis*). A number of pathogenic viruses are transmitted through direct contact. These include human immunodeficiency virus (HIV); hepatitis virus B, C and D; and herpes simplex virus (HSV). Other pathogens are transmitted directly through contact with the skin, often entering through a wound or break in the skin. Staphylococcal infections (*Staphyloccocus aureus*) are transmitted in this manner. Antibiotic-resistant forms of staph infections are now common among athletes and are spread during contact sports and in locker rooms.

PREVENTION

Public sanitation programs have had a profound impact on the incidence of contagious diseases in developed countries. Public health measures to prevent the spread of waterborne and food-borne illnesses are generally quite effective. These measures include water purification and sewage treatment, waste removal, and enforcement of regulations to promote food safety during production and preparation.

A dramatic example of an effective public health program comes from data on typhoid fever in Philadelphia during the early twentieth century. In the ten years following the introduction of filtration and chlorination of the city's water, the number of cases of typhoid fever dropped steeply from nearly ten thousand cases each year to just more than one hundred cases. This result is a heartening reminder that the spread of contagious diseases can be controlled.

Vaccination is the most effective method of preventing a variety of contagious diseases. Recent innovations in molecular biology have enabled the development of new vaccines that provide coverage against more diseases. Despite the availability of a range of vaccines, many adults in developed countries are not effectively immunized. In some cases, this is because immunity from their childhood vaccines has faded or may not have been very effective to begin with. In other cases, adults may not be aware that new vaccines are available or that they need to be immunized against different organisms as they age. Vaccination rates for children and adults in developing countries are low because of financial barriers and a lack of infrastructure.

Certain measures for disease prevention are up to each person to adopt. Sexually transmitted diseases can be prevented by using condoms during intercourse. Handwashing is an effective way to avoid infection by organisms that are spread through respiratory and oral-fecal routes. One should wash his or her hands before and after handling food, after using the toilet or changing diapers, after sneezing or coughing, and before and after treating a wound. (Soap and warm water should be used to scrub hands for a minimum of twenty seconds. If water is not available, alcohol-based hand sanitizer is another good option.) One should often clean kitchen counter tops with soap and water. A disinfectant that destroys pathogenic organisms, such as 95 percent isopropyl alcohol, should be used occasionally in kitchens and bathrooms. One should avoid antibacterial soaps, however, because they are not more effective at killing bacteria than regular soap and can lead to the development of drug-resistant bacteria.

IMPACT

Contagious diseases have been intimately associated with human life throughout history. In fact, human history has been shaped by contagious diseases. These diseases continue to cause suffering, disability, and economic hardship for millions of people in both developed and developing nations. Every year, nearly one-quarter of all deaths worldwide (about 12 million) are caused by contagious diseases. Also, all nations face the financial burden of disease prevention and treatment. Widespread contagious illnesses can be so costly that they hamper the economic development and political stability of developing nations.

Kathryn Pierno, M.S.

FURTHER READING

Flint, S. J., et al. *Pathogenesis and Control. Vol. 2 in Principles of Virology.* 3d ed. Washington, D.C.: ASM Press, 2009. Discusses the general principles of infection by viruses, the mechanisms of infection and its spread in populations, immune responses, vaccination, and antiviral drugs.

Gilligan, Peter H., M. Lynn Smiley, and Daniel S. Shapiro. *Cases in Medical Microbiology and Infectious Diseases.* 3d ed. Washington, D.C.: ASM Press, 2003. The most common pathogens are presented by affected organ systems. Includes medical cases with descriptive examples of symptoms associated with infection by particular organisms.

Madigan, Michael T., and John M. Martinko. *Brock Biology of Microorganisms.* 12th ed. Upper Saddle River, N.J.: Pearson/Prentice Hall, 2010. A standard microbiology textbook for undergraduate college students, with detailed descriptions of cell structures and clear illustrations. Includes evolutionary perspectives and covers pathogenesis.

Percival, Steven L., et al. *Microbiology of Waterborne Diseases.* San Diego, Calif.: Academic Press/Elsevier, 2004. Major pathogenic waterborne microorganisms are described in terms of physiology, reproduction, clinical features and treatment of infection, and survival in the environment.

Ryan, Kenneth J., and C. George Ray. *Sherris Medical Microbiology: An Introduction to Infectious Diseases.* 5th ed. New York: McGraw-Hill Medical, 2010. Standard medical microbiology textbook covering pathogen biology, clinical presentation and diagnosis, treatment, and epidemiology.

Shannon, Joyce Brennfleck, ed. *Contagious Diseases Sourcebook.* Detroit: Omnigraphics, 2010. For general readers, this sourcebook provides information about the transmission and treatment of contagious diseases. Includes facts about prevention, self-care, and drug resistance.

Wilson, Michael. *Microbial Inhabitants of Humans: Their Ecology and Role in Health and Disease.* New York: Cambridge University Press, 2005. Biology and ecology of microorganisms indigenous to the human body. Describes environmental features of all organ systems in the human body and discusses microorganisms that reside in each.

WEB SITES OF INTEREST

Centers for Disease Control and Prevention
http://www.cdc.gov

National Institutes of Health
http://www.nlm.nih.gov

World Health Organization
http://www.who.int

See also: Airborne illness and disease; Bacteria: Classification and types; Bacterial infections; Bloodstream infections; Epidemiology; Fecal-oral route of transmission; Fungi: Classification and types; Hospitals and infectious disease; Immunization; Infection; Parasitic diseases; Protozoan diseases; Public health; Respiratory route of transmission; Rotavirus infection; Sexually transmitted diseases (STDs); Social effects of infectious disease; Superbacteria; Viral infections; Virulence; Viruses: Types.

Contaminated food. *See* Food-borne illness and disease.

Coronaviridae

CATEGORY: Pathogen
TRANSMISSION ROUTE: Direct contact, ingestion, inhalation

DEFINITION

The viral family Coronaviridae comprise RNA (ribonucleic acid) viruses that infect mammals and birds worldwide. The viruses pose potential pandemic challenges as several new strains emerge. Infection can range from mild to severe in humans, manifesting as respiratory tract illnesses, enteric infections in infants and, in rare cases, neurological syndromes.

NATURAL HABITAT AND FEATURES

The coronavirus, named for its "corona" or crown-shaped surface, is an enveloped, single-stranded, positive-sense RNA virus. It is the largest nonsegmented

Taxonomic Classification for Coronaviridae

Order: Nidovirales
Family: Coronaviridae
Subfamily: *Coronavirinae*
Genera:
Alphacoronavirus
Betacoronavirus
Gammacoronavirus
Subfamily: *Torovirinae*
Genera:
Bafinivirus
Coronavirus
Torovirus

RNA virus genome known, with a surface of 120 to 160 nanometers (nm) in diameter. Around the crown, viral spikes in the envelope glycoprotein bind to host surface glycoproteins to activate the virus.

Coronaviruses are divided into three antigenic groups. The first two include mammalian viruses such as HCoV-NL63, transmissible gastroenteritis virus, and bovine coronavirus. Group 3 includes avian coronaviruses. Studies indicate that there may be a fourth group that includes the SARS (severe acute respiratory syndrome) virus, which has distinct biologic and genomic features from both groups 1 and 2.

The most notorious coronavirus, SARS, has played a significant role in infectious diseases of the twenty-first century. The virus was discovered in February, 2003, by World Health Organization (WHO) physician Carlo Urbani. The original carrier of SARS was identified as a forty-eight-year old Vietnamese businessman who had traveled from the Guangdong Province of China, through Hong Kong to Hanoi, Vietnam. He died after spreading SARS to others throughout his journey. Urbani himself died from SARS in March of that year after monitoring the early progression of the disease. Within six weeks of the discovery of SARS, thousands of people had become infected throughout the world, causing panic and even disruption of national economies.

Fortunately, WHO staged an unprecedented rapid global response by issuing a worldwide global threat alert, travel advisories, and daily WHO updates that tracked the spread of SARS. Because of this aggressive public health approach, by June, the SARS epidemic had subsided. However, the virus has not disappeared, and WHO and other public health organizations continue to watch it closely.

PATHOGENICITY AND CLINICAL SIGNIFICANCE

SARS is a respiratory tract infection that damages the pneumocyte cells, causing alveolar damage and ultimately leading to adult respiratory distress syndrome. Diarrhea can be present; however, the intestinal tissue is not damaged. SARS manifests with a fever greater than 100.4° Fahrenheit, chills, malaise, dry cough, and chest infiltrates in the lower lobes. Tests used to diagnose SARS are a chest X ray or chest computed tomography scan and a complete blood count to measure white blood count, lymphocytes, and platelets.

SARS is a nosocomial illness, and health care workers are at high risk for the disease. Health care workers should wear protective masks and gowns and keep persons infected with SARS in isolation from healthy persons. Most infected persons, however, are not highly infectious outside conditions in which there is a high likelihood of other people handling their body fluids. For example, during the 2003 outbreak, infected persons had flown on several airliners without infecting other passengers. In contrast, certain other people appeared to be "super spreaders," a pattern often seen in other viral infections.

Another human respiratory epidemic, HCoV-NL63, was discovered in the Netherlands in 2004 and serves as another example of emerging coronaviruses. This virus infected mostly children and immunocompromised persons with mild upper respiratory symptoms and serious lower respiratory symptoms, including bronchiolitis and croup. HCoV-NL63 did not become epidemic, but it still exists as a potential threat.

DRUG SUSCEPTIBILITY

No vaccine exists for SARS. The epidemic is considered contained, but the likelihood of another SARS or SARS-like outbreak is high. Because of the high mutability of these viruses, the development of specific vaccines is unlikely.

Persons with SARS can be given antibiotics to treat associated bacterial infections. Antiviral medications may also be helpful. Persons with severe lung inflammation may need high doses of steroids, and those persons whose lungs have sustained damage may need mechanical ventilation for breathing support.

Lessons about vaccines can be learned by looking at work done with the transmissible gastroenteritis virus, a virus that is deadly to pigs. Studies have shown that vaccinating the sow confers passive immunity on the piglets, a strategy that can have implications for human coronavirus vaccine.

S. M. Willis, M.S., M.A.

FURTHER READING

Abdul-Rasool, Sahar, and Burtrum C. Fielding. "Understanding Human Coronavirus HCoV-NL63." *Open Virology Journal* 4 (2010): 76-84.

Peiris, M., et al., eds. *Severe Acute Respiratory Syndrome.* Malden, Mass.: Blackwell, 2005.

Saif, L. J., J. L. van Cott, and T. A. Brim. "Immunity to Transmissible Gastroenteritis Virus and Porcine Respiratory Coronavirus Infections in Swine." *Veterinary Immunology and Immunopathology* 43 (1994): 89-97.

Tambyah, P. A. "SARS: Responding to an Unknown Virus." *European Journal of Clinical Microbiology and Infectious Disease* 23 (2004): 589-595.

WEB SITES OF INTEREST

Centers for Disease Control and Prevention
http://www.cdc.gov/sars

Virus Pathogen Database and Analysis Resource
http://www.viprbrc.org/brc

World Health Organization
http://www.who.int/csr/resources/publications/sarsnewguidance

See also: Airborne illness and disease; Anthrax; Atypical pneumonia; Contagious diseases; Coronavirus infections; Epidemics and pandemics: History; Outbreaks; Pneumonia; Public health; Respiratory route of transmission; Respiratory syncytial virus infections; SARS; Viral infections; Viruses: Structure and life cycle; Viruses: Types; World Health Organization (WHO).

Coronavirus infections

CATEGORY: Diseases and conditions
ANATOMY OR SYSTEM AFFECTED: Gastrointestinal system, lungs, respiratory system
ALSO KNOWN AS: Common cold, SARS, viral bronchitis, viral pneumonia

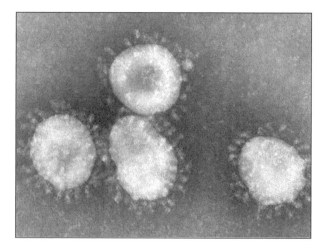

Coronavirus virions, or virus particles. (CDC)

DEFINITION

Exposure to the coronavirus results in a variety of infections, including approximately one-third of all cases of the common cold. The virus also may be responsible for viral bronchitis, pneumonia, and SARS (severe acute respiratory syndrome), especially in persons with weakened immune systems. The coronavirus is the largest positive-strand ribonucleic acid (RNA) virus; it is part of the Coronaviridae family.

CAUSES

Coronavirus is the underlying cause of a variety of illnesses that affect the respiratory system, the gastrointestinal system, and, in rare cases, the neurological system. Infections with the virus are often seasonal in nature, with more occurring in winter. Contact with contaminated droplets from sneezing and coughing and direct contact by touching contaminated objects, such as surfaces and tissues, may transmit the virus from person to person.

The virus may live six to nine hours, and the live virus has been found in the stool of people diagnosed with SARS. It is highly contagious, and reinfection may occur. The virus can affect humans, cattle, pigs, rodents, cats, dogs, and birds, but there is no evidence of animal and bird variations infecting humans.

RISK FACTORS

Risk factors for coronavirus infection are exposure to an infected person through kissing and sharing living spaces and contact with droplets or contaminated surfaces containing the virus. The severity of the infection increases if a person is immunocompromised (less able to fight infections because of a weakened immune system).

SYMPTOMS

Coronavirus infection that leads to the common cold comes with symptoms of fatigue, a scratchy throat, sneezing, nasal congestion, and a runny nose. Fever rarely occurs with a cold, except in children. A more serious infection, such as pneumonia or SARS, may be occurring if symptoms include fever, chills, muscle aches, an acute cough, a headache, dizziness, or diarrhea.

SCREENING AND DIAGNOSIS

A physical examination including listening to lung sounds, reviewing symptoms, chest X rays, and blood work may be used to determine if a person has a cold or has developed pneumonia or SARS. Blood work may include blood chemistries and a complete blood count to determine if white blood cell counts, lymphocytes, and platelets are low. Specific tests for SARS may be ordered too.

TREATMENT AND THERAPY

In the absence of fever, symptoms may be treated with over-the-counter medications, plenty of fluids, and rest. If symptoms worsen or if a fever develops, one should seek medical care. Antibiotics, antiviral medications, and high doses of steroids to decrease lung inflammation may be prescribed. In severe cases, the patient may need oxygen, breathing support with a respirator, and hospitalization.

PREVENTION AND OUTCOMES

The best prevention against coronavirus infection is to limit contact with infected persons. Hand hygiene, including handwashing or cleaning hands with an alcohol-based hand sanitizer, is an important part of prevention. Infected persons should cough or sneeze into tissue or into the arm to minimize droplets and airborne particles. Because coronavirus is contagious, one should not share food and drink, utensils, or personal supplies. Household areas, including door knobs, counter tops, and other surfaces, should be cleaned with disinfectant.

Patricia Stanfill Edens, R.N., Ph.D., FACHE

FURTHER READING

Eccles, Ronald, and Olaf Weber, eds. *Common Cold.* Boston: Birkhäuser, 2009.

Peiris, M., et al., eds. *Severe Acute Respiratory Syndrome.* Malden, Mass.: Blackwell, 2005.

Wagner, Edward K., and Martinez J. Hewlett. *Basic Virology.* 3d ed. Malden, Mass.: Blackwell Science, 2008.

WEB SITES OF INTEREST

American Lung Association
http://www.lungusa.org

American Public Health Association
http://www.apha.org

Centers for Disease Control and Prevention
http://www.cdc.gov

Clean Hands Coalition
http://www.cleanhandscoalition.org

See also: Airborne illness and disease; Bronchitis; Children and infectious disease; Contagious diseases; Coronaviridae; Pneumonia; Public health; Respiratory route of transmission; Respiratory syncytial virus infections; SARS; Schools and infectious disease; Sinusitis; Viral infections; Viral upper respiratory infections.

Corynebacterium

CATEGORY: Pathogen
TRANSMISSION ROUTE: Direct contact, ingestion, inhalation

DEFINITION

Corynebacterium is a gram-positive, non-spore-forming rod with a characteristic club-shaped appearance and worldwide distribution. *C. diphtheriae* is a major human pathogen.

NATURAL HABITAT AND FEATURES

Corynebacterium spp. are gram-positive, nonmotile, catalase-positive rods. Along with the *Mycobacteria* and *Nocardia*, they produce characteristic long-chain mycolic acids that can be used in their taxonomy. Their

Taxonomic Classification for *Corynebacterium*

Kingdom: Bacteria
Phylum: Actinobacteria
Class: Actinobacteria
Subclass: Actinobacteridae
Order: Actinomycetales
Suborder: Corynebacterineae
Family: Corynebacteriaceae
Genus: *Corynebacterium*
Species:
C. bovis
C. diphtheriae
C. glutamicum
C. jeikeium
C. pseudodiphtheriticum
C. pyogenes
C. striatum
C. ulcerans
C. xerosis

cent). The taxonomy of *Corynebacterium* is based on genomic deoxyribonucleic acid (DNA), 16-s ribonucleic acid (RNA), and cell wall lipids. A major taxonomic realignment was made in the 1990's. Some former *Corynebacterium* spp. have been moved to other related genera: *C. acnes* to *Propionobacterium acnes* and *C. hemolyticum* to *Arcanobacterium hemolyticum*. Other bacteria were added to *Corynebacterium*. For example, the JK bacterial group became *C. jeikeium*.

Many *Corynebacterium* spp. have industrial applications, producing complex organic nutritional factors and medically important compounds. They degrade hydrocarbons and age cheese. Arguably the most important of these species is *glutamicum*, which is the primary source of the food additive monosodium glutamate (MSG) and has been genetically engineered to produce human epiderman growth factor, among other applications. *Corynebacterium* spp. have a worldwide distribution, especially in temperate areas, and are found in soils and water and in and on animals and plants.

metabolism is varied, with both aerobic and facultatively anaerobic members of the genus. Those with anaerobic metabolism usually perform lactic acid fermentation. The bacteria are fastidious, and all strains require biotin and most require several other supplements. They are usually grown under an enriched carbon dioxide atmosphere and grow slowly, even on complex-enriched culture media.

The rods are pleiomorphic, some having club-shaped ends (the Greek word *koryne* means "club"), and often show incomplete separation during cell division. This has led some scientists to note their resemblance to Chinese characters. The incomplete separation is caused by a characteristic "snapping" cell division, which leads to their peculiar cell wall. The main wall constituent is commonly called mycolyl-AG-peptidoglycan and is made up of high-di-aminopimelic-acid peptidoglycans, arabinoglactans, and mycolic acid, all connected through disaccharide linkages. During cell division, the plasma membrane divides normally, but the cell wall may only partially separate, forming V- and other odd-shaped assemblages of two or more cells.

The genomes of three species have been sequenced and contain a single circular chromosome of about 2.5 million base pairs with a high G-C content (53.5 per-

PATHOGENICITY AND CLINICAL SIGNIFICANCE

Diphtheriae is the most important corynebacterial pathogen of humans and causes diphtheria. This disease is an upper respiratory infection with a characteristic pseudomembrane that covers parts of the pharynx and adjacent areas. *Diphtheriae* secretes diphtheria *Corynebacterium* toxin to epithelial cells at the site of infection, causing them to produce the fibrin-based pseudomembrane. The toxin can also be disseminated to many other areas of the body, leading to possible organ failure.

Only those strains with an integrated lysogenic phage that carries the gene for the diphtheria toxin are able to produce the toxin. The disease severity is often a consequence of the strain of *diphtheriae* that causes the infection, because different strains grow at different rates and produce different amounts of diphtheria toxin. The toxin regulatory gene (DtxR), located on the bacterial chromosome, also affects toxin levels. Iron serves as the corepressor of DtxR's product, so under normal iron concentrations, toxin production is greatly curtailed. Under iron starvation, toxin production is dramatically increased.

Diphtheriae also can cause cutaneous diphtheria, a skin infection, if it enters a break in the skin. In rare instances, it also can cause genital and eye infections.

Nonpathogenic *Corynebacterium* are often referred

to as diphtheroids, however, many of them can be opportunistic pathogens, especially in the elderly, the immune compromised, and those with prosthetic devices. *Bovis* and *ulcerans* have been isolated from skin ulcers, and *bovis* and *pyogenes* have caused systemic bacteremia. Corynebacteria that have been isolated from other infections include *xerosis, jeikeium, striatum,* and *pseudodiphtheriticum.* Many other diphtheroids, found as commensal organisms on healthy persons, might become pathogenic under the right circumstances.

DRUG SUSCEPTIBILITY

Treatment of diphtheria is two-pronged. Diphtheria antitoxin, produced in horses, is used to neutralize the toxin; antibiotics are used to kill the bacteria. The antibiotics of choice are penicillin and erythromycin, administered for fourteen days. Clindamicin, rifampin, and tetracycline can also be used. Antibiotic susceptibility of the diphtheroids varies, but penicillins, erythromycin, and rifampin are usually good choices. Penicillin resistance has been seen in some nontoxigenic *diphtheriae* strains.

Richard W. Cheney, Jr., Ph.D.

FURTHER READING

Burkovski, Andreas, ed. *Corynebacteria: Genomics and Molecular Biology.* Norfolk, England: Caister Academic Press, 2008. This book mainly focuses on C. glutamicim. Chapter 2, however, discusses the genomics of many Corynebacterium spp.

Guilfoile, Patrick G. *Deadly Diseases and Epidemics: Diphtheria.* New York: Chelsea House, 2009. This volume describes diphtheria in detail.

Krieg, Noel R., et al., eds. *Bergey's Manual of Systematic Bacteriology.* 2d ed. New York: Springer, 2010. Volume 5 of this multivolume work describes Corynebacterium and its relatives in detail.

Madigan, Michael T., and John M. Martinko. *Brock Biology of Microorganisms.* 12th ed. Upper Saddle River, N.J.: Pearson/Prentice Hall, 2010. This text outlines many common bacteria and describes their natural history, pathogenicity, and other characteristics.

WEB SITES OF INTEREST

Microbiology Information Portal
http://www.microbes.info

Todar's Online Textbook of Bacteriology
http://www.textbookofbacteriology.net

See also: Bacteria: Classification and types; Bacteriology; Diphtheria; DTaP vaccine; Microbiology; Pathogens.

Cowpox

CATEGORY: Diseases and conditions
ANATOMY OR SYSTEM AFFECTED: Skin

DEFINITION

Cowpox is an extremely rare zoonotic disease in humans, acquired from direct contact with an infected cow or other mammalian host. It is a skin disease that results in a rash and ulceration, but no long-term effects. Edward Jenner, observing that milkmaids who had had cowpox never were infected with smallpox, used biological material from a cowpox lesion as the basis of the first successful vaccination in 1796.

CAUSES

Cowpox is caused by infection with cowpox virus, a double-stranded deoxyribonucleic acid (DNA) virus of the Poxviridae family and related to variola virus, the agent of smallpox. Because the two viruses have similar antigenic sites, antibodies produced against the cowpox virus provide immunity to smallpox. In modern times, inoculation with the related vaccinia virus is used as the smallpox vaccination agent, providing cross-immunity to cowpox. Although found in cattle, from which it derives its name, the cowpox virus has many mammalian reservoirs, including wild rodents such as mice and voles, and cats. Pet cats are the most likely source of infections in humans. The virus also has been found in zoo animals, particularly feline species and elephants. Cowpox is found primarily in the United Kingdom and the former western states of the Soviet Union and adjacent areas of north and central Asia. Even at that, there are only a few cases reported each year worldwide. There have never been any reported cases in the United States.

RISK FACTORS

Infection can occur only through a break in the skin in direct contact with a cowpox lesion, especially

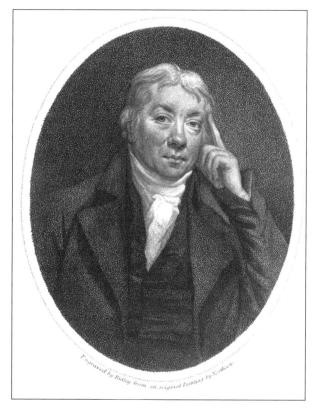

Edward Jenner. (Library of Congress)

from cats. Immune-compromised and eczematous persons are at higher risk of infection. Only one reported case of systemic involvement and death has been reported, and this occurred in an immune-compromised person.

SYMPTOMS

At the site of infection, which is usually the hands, the normal symptoms is a rash followed by a pustular blister that then ulcerates, scabs over, and leaves a scar. The rash and infection do not spread. Normally, only one lesion is found. Swollen nodes, slight fever, chills, loss of appetite, headache, and muscle aching may occur.

SCREENING AND DIAGNOSIS

Because cowpox is so rare, a physician will often misdiagnose the condition as bullous impetigo and treat it with antibiotics, which are ineffective. A patient history of contact with cats, and subsequent scratches, may help in diagnosis. Polymerase chain reaction

(PCR) analysis can be used to identify the virus, but this would normally not be done.

TREATMENT AND THERAPY

Generally, treatment is only supportive, as the disease is mild. Poxvirus infections can be treated with cidofovir or vaccinia immunoglobulin in immuno-compromised persons.

PREVENTION AND OUTCOMES

Because of its rarity, cowpox prevention techniques are not needed. If traveling in countries with endemic infections, one should avoid contact with cats.

Ralph R. Meyer, Ph.D.

FURTHER READING

Essbauer, Sandra, Martin Pfeffer, and Hermann Meyer. "Zoonotic Poxviruses." *Veterinary Microbiology* 140 (2010): 229-236.

Fenner, Frank. "Adventures with Poxviruses of Vertebrates." *FEMS Microbiology Reviews* 24 (2000): 123-133.

Knorr, Corinna W., et al. "Effects of Cidofovir Treatment on Cytokine Induction in Murine Models of Cowpox and Vaccinia Virus Infection." *Antiviral Research* 72 (2006): 125-133.

Rusnock, Andrea. "Catching Smallpox: The Early Spread of Smallpox Vaccination, 1798-1810." *Bulletin of the History of Medicine* 83 (2009): 17-36.

WEB SITES OF INTEREST

Centers for Disease Control and Prevention
http://www/cdc.gov

National Organization for Rare Disorders
http://www.rarediseases.org

See also: Chickenpox; Immunization; Monkeypox; Poxviridae; Poxvirus infections; Skin infections; Smallpox; Smallpox vaccine; Vaccines: History; Viral infections; Zoonotic diseases.

Coxsackie virus infections

CATEGORY: Diseases and conditions
ANATOMY OR SYSTEM AFFECTED: All
ALSO KNOWN AS: Hand, foot, and mouth disease

Definition

The coxsackie virus is a single-stranded ribonucleic acid (RNA) virus that belongs to the genus *Enterovirus*. The viruses are categorized as group A or B, with twenty-three and six types in each respective group. They cause common infections that are often mild; infrequently, they can be more severe. Rarely, they lead to death. Type B1 is the most common type in the United States, but type B4 has the highest risk for fatal complications.

Causes

Coxsackie viruses are spread by human contact, mainly through the fecal-oral route. Transmission by objects (fomites) contaminated with nasal and oral excretions is also possible. Improper handwashing often leads to the spreading of the disease. Some coxsackie viruses may be transmitted from a pregnant girl or woman to her fetus during pregnancy.

Risk Factors

Coxsackie virus infections may occur at any age but are most common during the first year of life and are most common among males. Newborns and immunocompromised persons have the greatest risk for more severe disease manifestations. The time of year with the greatest risk for getting the infections is the spring and fall seasons.

Symptoms

Most people with a coxsackie virus infection are asymptomatic or have an isolated fever. Both groups of coxsackie viruses may additionally cause rashes and upper respiratory tract infections. Group A viruses cause hand, foot, and mouth disease, cause mouth blisters and a rash on the hands and feet, and cause eye infections. Group B viruses infect the heart, pancreas, and liver and are more commonly associated with meningitis and inflammation of the muscles. Group B coxsackie virus infection has been found to be associated with insulin-dependent diabetes.

Screening and Diagnosis

It is possible to isolate coxsackie viruses from a rectal or oral swab in cell culture, although false-positive results are possible because the virus can remain in the system for up to two months following infection. Polymerase chain reaction (PCR) is a genetic technique that amplifies the virus for a faster result, but this test too lacks 100 percent accuracy.

Treatment and Therapy

Mildly affected persons do not require treatment as the infection independently resolves. No approved therapies exist for the treatment of coxsackie virus infections. Acetaminophen may be given for fever and nonsteroidal anti-inflammatory drugs for pain in mildly affected persons. If a more severe infection has been diagnosed, medical care is provided based on the specific symptoms. In persons with meningitis or a cardiac infection, experimental treatments have been attempted, but their overall effectiveness has yet to be proven.

Prevention and Outcomes

To reduce the chance of becoming infected with a coxsackie virus, one should avoid contact with infected persons and with contaminated items and should follow proper hygiene, including proper handwashing, techniques.

Janet Ober Berman, M.S., CGC

Further Reading

Richer, M. J., and M. S. Horwitz. "Coxsackievirus Infection as an Environmental Factor in the Etiology of Type 1 Diabetes." *Autoimmunity Reviews* 8 (2009): 611-615.

Rotbart, H. A., et al. "Clinical Significance of Enteroviruses in Serious Summer Febrile Illnesses of Children." *Pediatric Infectious Disease Journal* 18 (1999): 869-874.

Tebruegge, M., and N. Curtis. "Enterovirus Infections in Neonates." *Seminars in Fetal and Neonatal Medicine* 14 (2009): 222-227.

Web Site of Interest

Centers for Disease Control and Prevention
http://www/cdc.gov

See also: Children and infectious disease; Echovirus infections; Enterovirus infections; Fecal-oral route of transmission; Hospitals and infectious disease; Hygiene; Neonatal sepsis; Pregnancy and infectious disease; Viral infections.

Crab lice

CATEGORY: Diseases and conditions
ANATOMY OR SYSTEM AFFECTED: Genitalia, hair, skin
ALSO KNOWN AS: Pubic lice

DEFINITION

Crabs are tiny, barely visible parasites (*Pthirus pubis*) that live in the pubic area of humans and cause itching. (The word "lice" is plural, and the singular is "louse.") Pubic lice are commonly called crabs because they are shorter and rounder than head and body lice, making them resemble crabs. They are usually found in the pubic hair but can also be found in other body areas with short hair (such as eyelashes, eyebrows, armpits, and mustaches).

CAUSES

Crabs are spread by personal contact, usually during sexual activity. They also may be spread by sharing personal items, such as bedding, towels, and clothing; however, this form of transmission is less common.

RISK FACTORS

Risk factors for crab lice include sexual contact with people who have crabs and contact with contaminated items (fomites), such as bedding, towels, clothing, toilet seats, and furniture.

SYMPTOMS

Symptoms of crab lice include itchiness (from mild to severe), tiny blue-gray bumps called macula caerulea that are stuck to the skin, skin breaks, and possible bacterial infection (caused by scratching).

SCREENING AND DIAGNOSIS

A doctor will ask about symptoms and medical history and will perform a physical exam. He or she will examine the patient's pubic area for lice, lice eggs (called nits), and macula caerulea.

TREATMENT AND THERAPY

Treating crabs involves applying over-the-counter shampoo or cream rinse containing permethrin or pyrethrins. For resistant cases, the doctor may prescribe topical malathion (a highly effective medication approved only for persons older than six years of age) or lindane.

Lindane, a second-line treatment, is prescribed only to persons who are unable to take other medications or who have not responded to them. According to the U.S. Food and Drug Administration, lindane, rarely, can cause serious side effects, including seizure and death. Those especially susceptible are infants, the elderly, children and adults weighing under 110 pounds, and persons with other skin conditions. Lindane is a toxin and should not be overused. Infected persons are given small amounts (one to two ounces) of the shampoo or lotion and are instructed to apply a thin layer and to not reapply.

Treatment steps include the following: Wash the infested area and then towel dry.

Thoroughly saturate hair with lice medication. If using permethrin or pyrethrins, leave medication on for ten minutes; if using lindane, leave on for only four minutes. Thoroughly rinse off medication with water. Dry off with a clean towel.

Following treatment, most lice eggs will still be attached to hair shafts. The lice eggs can be removed with fingernails or tweezers. Following treatment, one should put on clean underwear and clothing. If lice is in the eyebrows, the eyebrows should be coated thoroughly with petroleum jelly.

To kill any lice and nits that may be left on clothing or bedding, one should wash all items used during the two to three days before treatment. Items should be washed in hot water (130° Fahrenheit) and dried using the hot cycle for a minimum of twenty minutes. Clothing that is not washable should be dry cleaned.

One should avoid sexual activity until partners have been treated. If necessary, the condition can be treated again in seven to ten days.

PREVENTION AND OUTCOMES

To reduce the chance of getting crabs or spreading crabs, one should limit sexual partners and watch for signs of crabs, such as itching in the genital area. At home, one should thoroughly wash and dry bedding, towels, and clothing, and vacuum carpets, rugs, and upholstered furniture. Any person who has had crabs should inform his or her sexual partner that he or she is at risk for crabs. Also, one should avoid sexual activity until all partners have been treated.

Jennifer Hellwig, M.S., RD;
reviewed by David L. Horn, M.D., FACP

FURTHER READING

American Academy of Dermatology. "Parasitic Infestations." Available at http://www.aad.org/education/students/parainfest.htm.

Berger, Stephen A., and John S. Marr. *Human Parasitic Diseases Sourcebook.* Sudbury, Mass.: Jones and Bartlett, 2006.

Centers for Disease Control and Prevention. "Pubic 'Crab' Lice." Available at http://www.cdc.gov/parasites/lice/pubic.

Despommier, Dickson D., et al. *Parasitic Diseases.* 5th ed. New York: Apple Tree, 2006.

Diaz, J. H. "Crab Lice (Pediculosis pubis)." In *Mandell, Douglas, and Bennett's Principles and Practice of Infectious Diseases,* edited by Gerald L. Mandell, John E. Bennett, and Raphael Dolin. 7th ed. New York: Churchill Livingstone/Elsevier, 2010.

Pickering, Larry K., et al., eds. *Red Book: 2009 Report of the Committee on Infectious Diseases.* 28th ed. Elk Grove Village, Ill.: American Academy of Pediatrics, 2009.

U.S. Food and Drug Administration. "Lindane Shampoo and Lindane Lotion." Available at http://www.fda.gov.

Weedon, David. *Skin Pathology.* 3d ed. New York: Churchill Livingstone/Elsevier, 2010.

Web Sites of Interest

American Academy of Dermatology
http://www.aad.org

American Congress of Obstetricians and Gynecologists
http://www.acog.org

Centers for Disease Control and Prevention
http://www.cdc.gov/parasites

See also: Body lice; Contagious diseases; Head lice; Jock itch; Parasitic diseases; Scabies; Sexually transmitted diseases (STDs); Skin infections; Skin infections.

Creutzfeldt-Jakob disease

CATEGORY: Diseases and conditions
ANATOMY OR SYSTEM AFFECTED: Brain, central nervous system, muscles, musculoskeletal system
ALSO KNOWN AS: Corticostriatospinal degeneration, new variant Creutzfeldt-Jakob disease, spastic pseudosclerosis, subacute spongiform encephalopathy

Definition

Creutzfeldt-Jakob disease (CJD) is a transmissible neurodegenerative disorder that was first described in the 1920's and later recognized as the most common human prion disease. It occurs worldwide, with an incidence rate of approximately one per one million people. The rare disease leads to dementia, mainly in middle-aged and elderly persons, and is invariably fatal. The late twentieth century saw the emergence of new variant CJD (nvCJD), which occurs in younger persons.

Causes

Prions, the putative transmitting agents, are proteinaceous pathogens. Unlike viruses, they do not contain detectable nucleic acid. They exhibit resistance to nucleic-acid-modifying agents such as heat and ultraviolet light but prove susceptible to treatments that denature protein.

The prion protein (PrP) is found in two isoforms. One is the normal cellular form (PrPC), a membrane-bound protein of unknown function, that is highly expressed in the brain. The second form (PrPSC), which is abnormally configured, is found in sheep scrapie and in other animal and human prion diseases. PrPSC appears not only inside the cell but also outside the cell, in abnormal protein deposits. PrPSC can bind to PrPC and convert it into PrPSC, thus triggering a self-perpetuating cycle. This conversion and the subsequent accumulation of PrPSC alter neuronal function and viability.

Most CJD cases (85 percent) occur sporadically (sCJD), probably through a spontaneous conformational change of PrPC into PrPSC or through an isolated, spontaneous gene mutation. Even though no environmental source is evident, sCJD might also result from contamination. Approximately 10 percent of cases have a genetic basis, with autosomal dominant inheritance linked to mutations in the prion protein gene (PRNP) on chromosome 20.

Infectious causes lead to disease variants and cases of iatrogenic origin (those resulting from medical procedures). The causal agents can be experimentally transmitted from animal to animal or from humans to other humans and animals. Brain tissue represents the most contagious material. It is assumed that prions reach the brain through the blood or by ascending through nerve fibers.

RISK FACTORS

Most CJD cases occur for unknown reasons. Genetic and infectious (acquired) disease types, however, are associated with specific factors.

Inheriting only one copy of the mutated gene, from one parent, is sufficient to develop the disease. The chance of passing the mutation to an offspring is 50 percent. In addition, genetic studies show that inheriting identical copies of certain PRNP variants may predispose a person to develop CJD if exposed to contaminated tissue.

Risk factors for acquired CJD include living in rural areas and eating raw meat or brains. The clearest relationship between CJD and animal product consumption characterizes nvCJD, which may result from eating meat infected with bovine spongiform encephalopathy (BSE), or mad cow disease.

A number of iatrogenic cases resulted from the use of pituitary extracts, corneal transplants, dural grafts, and contaminated electrodes. All forms of CJD, including sporadic disease, are also transmissible by transplanted organs. A number of persons with nvCJD had donated blood before their diagnoses; some of the recipients subsequently developed nvCJD.

It appears that CJD cannot be transmitted through casual respiratory or skin contact. Spouses and other household members of persons with CJD have the same risk of exhibiting the disease as the general population.

SYMPTOMS

After a long preclinical phase, sCJD becomes clinically manifest (on average in the sixth decade) and progresses rapidly to death within one year. Dementia with unusual behavior and ataxia (lack of coordination) constitute important initial manifestations. Other signs include myoclonus (muscle jerks), tremors, rigidity, difficulty speaking, seizures, and visual impairment.

Psychiatric symptoms, sensory disturbances, and ataxia characterize the onset of nvCJD. Eventually, most persons with the disease will suffer from dementia and involuntary movements. Patients are generally young, with a mean age at onset of twenty-eight years. The clinical course of this variant is slower and takes up to two years. Familial CJD has an earlier age

of onset and slower progression than does sCJD, but the outcome is also uniformly fatal.

SCREENING AND DIAGNOSIS

In typical cases, a clinical diagnosis is feasible based on dementia, myoclonus, and characteristic electroencephalograph (EEG) abnormalities. Other presentations may pose diagnostic difficulties and necessitate cerebrospinal fluid (CSF) testing for a brain marker protein known as 14-3-3. A definite diagnosis can be made only by analyzing brain tissue. Although rarely necessary, microscopic examination of brain biopsy samples can reveal neuronal loss and characteristic spongiosis (small "holes" in the brain's gray matter), hence the name spongiform encephalopathy. These changes occur anywhere in the central nervous system but predominate in the cortex and basal ganglia. Magnetic resonance imaging (MRI) shows increased signals, primarily in the basal ganglia. Also, genetic testing is available for familial cases.

TREATMENT AND THERAPY

Treatment is symptomatic. No successful therapeutic approach exists that can arrest or reverse the disorder. All forms of CJD end in death. Intense research efforts focus on pharmacological agents (such as polyanions, antimalarial derivatives, and amphotericin B), short peptide homologs to PrPC, and immunological therapies (such as anti-PrP antibodies).

PREVENTION AND OUTCOMES

The risk of contracting nvCJD is low. Successful policies aimed at preventing the transmission of BSE to humans have been implemented in several countries. High-risk bovine tissues are excluded from the animal and human food chains. The possibility, however, remains of secondary CJD transmission from human to human through blood and blood products, organs and tissues, and contaminated surgical instruments and medical devices. The potential for new iatrogenic cases has declined because of the use of recombinant growth hormone, synthetic or decontaminated dura mater, and disposable medical instruments.

There is no test for nvCJD in the donor population. The concern for donor transmission had prompted the deferral of blood donations from persons considered high risk. Reporting the diagnosis and any suspected case of nvCJD became imperative. During the clinically silent period, biological material from the affected person is potentially infectious. This warrants a complete investigation of the person's history of blood or other tissue donation.

One should exercise caution in surgical settings and pathology laboratories that manipulate brain-derived biological material. It is important to eliminate exposure to CSF, blood, or tissue, especially of open sores or conjunctiva.

Prions resist routine antiseptic practices. Special safety measures become necessary when handling infected material. One should use disposable instruments for spinal tap, brain biopsy, or histological processing. If this is not possible, special autoclaving procedures and chemical agents (for example, household bleach and detergents) help inactivate the prions.

Mihaela Avramut, M.D., Ph.D.

Further Reading

Bosque, Patrick J., and Kenneth L. Tyler. "Prions and Prion Diseases of the Central Nervous System (Transmissible Neurodegenerative Diseases)." In *Mandell, Douglas, and Bennett's Principles and Practice of Infectious Diseases,* edited by Gerald L. Mandell, John F. Bennett, and Raphael Dolin. 7th ed. New York: Churchill Livingstone/Elsevier, 2010. This chapter describes both human and animals forms of prion diseases and their modes of transmission.

Bradley, Walter G., et al. *Neurology in Clinical Practice.* 5th ed. Philadelphia: Butterworth-Heinemann, 2007. Includes basic information on prion diseases with continually updated online references.

Brown, David R., ed. *Neurodegeneration and Prion Disease.* New York: Springer, 2005. A textbook on the neurological effects of prion diseases.

Jubelt, Burk. "Prion Diseases." In *Merritt's Neurology,* edited by Lewis P. Rowland. 11th ed. Philadelphia: Lippincott Williams & Wilkins, 2005. Includes a well-written chapter on prion diseases.

Korth, Carsten, and Peter J. Peters. "Emerging Pharmacotherapies for Creutzfeldt-Jakob Disease." *Archives of Neurology* 63 (2006): 497-501. Reviews the main disease features of CJD and the most promising experimental therapies.

Nolte, John. *Human Brain: An Introduction to Its Functional Anatomy.* 6th ed. Philadelphia: Mosby/Elsevier, 2009. An introductory textbook on the anatomy of the human brain.

Prusiner, Stanley B. "The Prion Diseases." *Scientific American* 272, no. 1 (January, 1995): 48-57.

_____, ed. *Prion Biology and Diseases.* 2d ed. Cold Spring Harbor, N.Y.: Cold Spring Harbor Laboratory Press, 2004. Two important sources on prion diseases.

Web Sites of Interest

Creutzfeldt-Jakob Disease Foundation
http://www.cjdfoundation.org

Dana.org
http://www.dana.org

Genetic and Rare Diseases Information Center
http://rarediseases.info.nih.gov/gard

National Institute of Allergy and Infectious Diseases
http://www.niaid.nih.gov/topics/prion

National Institute of Neurological Disorders and Stroke, Transmissible Spongiform Encephalopathies Information Page
http://www.ninds.nih.gov/disorders/tse

See also: Encephalitis; Fatal familial insomnia; Foodborne illness and disease; Gerstmann-Sträussler-Scheinker syndrome; Guillain-Barré syndrome; Iatrogenic infections; Kuru; Prion diseases; Prions; Progressive multifocal leukoencephalopathy; Subacute sclerosing panencephalitis; Variant Creutzfeldt-Jakob disease.

Croup

CATEGORY: Diseases and conditions
ANATOMY OR SYSTEM AFFECTED: Larynx, lungs, respiratory system, throat, tissue
ALSO KNOWN AS: Laryngotracheobronchitis

Definition

Croup is inflammation or infection of the larynx (voice box) and trachea (windpipe). The inflammation causes tissue in the respiratory tract to swell, making it difficult for air to reach the lungs. Croup occurs in young children. As children grow older, their air passages widen, so swelling that is severe enough to block breathing is less likely in older children.

CAUSES

Causes of croup include viral infections such as parainfluenza, paramyxovirus, influenza virus type A, respiratory syncytial virus, adenovirus, rhinovirus, enterovirus, coxsackie virus, enteric cytopathogenic human orphan virus, reovirus, and measles virus.

Tests for specific viruses are rarely performed, so the actual cause of croup is usually not known. Conditions that resemble croup can also be caused by bacterial infections, allergies, and softening of cartilage in the larynx.

RISK FACTORS

Risk factors include attending day care, having a personal or family history of croup, and having frequent upper respiratory infections. Children ages three years and younger are at greatest risk, and there is a greater risk of developing croup in the colder months of October through March.

SYMPTOMS

Symptoms are usually preceded by an upper respiratory infection. Croup symptoms come on suddenly, often at night and include cough spasms; cough that sounds like a barking seal; hoarseness; fever; harsh, high-pitched breath sounds, especially when crying or upset; trouble breathing; and poor appetite and fluid intake.

More serious symptoms of croup that require immediate medical attention include a bluish color of the nails and lips or around the mouth. Other serious symptoms are decreased alertness, restlessness or agitation (possibly from a dangerous lack of oxygen); struggling for each breath; harsh, high-pitched breathing sounds, even at rest; trouble swallowing; drooling; and an inability to speak because of troubled breathing.

SCREENING AND DIAGNOSIS

A doctor will ask about the child's symptoms and medical history and will perform a physical exam. Tests may include blood tests, to check for signs of infection; neck X rays, to look for changes associated with croup; laryngoscopy (in which a thin tube is inserted into the mouth to look at throat tissue); and a culture of mucus from the trachea, to test for infection.

TREATMENT AND THERAPY

Treatment aims to keep the airway open while the infection resolves on its own in five to seven days. Severe symptoms usually resolve in three to four days. Treatments include self-care and humidification. One should try to keep the child calm and quiet. Crying can make the symptoms worse.

Moist air will help to keep the airways open. One should take the child into a bathroom, close the door, and run hot water in the shower, which will fill the room with moisture, and do so for fifteen to twenty minutes. (One should never leave a child unattended with hot water running or with a tub of water nearby.) The bathroom steam treatments can be repeated as needed. A warm- or cold-water humidifier in the child's bedroom is also helpful. If the moist-air treatments do not help breathing or the child's condition is getting worse, one should seek medical care immediately.

Another treatment is medication. The doctor may prescribe steroids to reduce swelling in the airways; this treatment has been shown to benefit croup and may keep a child from becoming sick enough to need hospitalization. Breathing treatments with a medicine called racemic epinephrine may provide temporary help until steroid medications (usually dexamethasone) start to work. Because most croup is caused by a viral infection, antibiotics are not usually given unless there is an accompanying problem, such as an ear infection or pneumonia.

A child with serious croup may be hospitalized and placed in a plastic croup tent, in which cool, moist air is delivered. Medications may be given to treat inflammation and respiratory distress. If the child continues to get worse, a breathing tube may be inserted in his or her throat to help keep the airway open. Fluids can be given through a vein if necessary. The child's oxygen level and heart rhythm are monitored. In severe cases, a surgical procedure called a tracheotomy can be performed to keep the airway open.

PREVENTION AND OUTCOMES

Croup usually occurs in response to an upper respiratory infection. Minimizing exposure to viruses that cause colds and flu may help prevent croup. Yearly influenza immunization can prevent those cases of croup caused by influenza A. Influenza immunization is strongly recommended for all children between the ages of six months and five years.

Debra Wood, R.N.;
reviewed by Christine Colpitts, M.A., CRT

FURTHER READING

American Academy of Pediatrics. "What Is Croup and How Is it Treated?" Available at http://www.aap.org/publiced/br_croup.htm.

Andreoli, Thomas E., et al., eds. *Andreoli and Carpenter's Cecil Essentials of Medicine.* 8th ed. Philadelphia: Saunders/Elsevier, 2010.

Behrman, Richard E., Robert M. Kliegman, and Hal B. Jenson, eds. *Nelson Textbook of Pediatrics.* 18th ed. Philadelphia: Saunders/Elsevier, 2007.

Dambro, Mark R., et al., eds. *Griffith's Five-Minute Clinical Consult.* 14th ed. Philadelphia: Lippincott Williams & Wilkins, 2006.

Mandell, Gerald L., John E. Bennett, and Raphael Dolin, eds. *Mandell, Douglas, and Bennett's Principles and Practice of Infectious Diseases.* 7th ed. New York: Churchill Livingstone/Elsevier, 2010.

Mason, Robert J., et al., eds. *Murray and Nadel's Textbook of Respiratory Medicine.* 5th ed. Philadelphia: Saunders/Elsevier, 2010.

Rakel, Robert E., Edward T. Bope, and Rick D. Kellerman, eds. *Conn's Current Therapy 2011.* Philadelphia: Saunders/Elsevier, 2010.

WEB SITES OF INTEREST

American Academy of Family Physicians
http://familydoctor.org

American Academy of Pediatrics
http://www.healthychildren.org

American Lung Association
http://www.lungusa.org

Canadian Lung Association
http://www.lung.ca

KidsHealth
http://www.kidshealth.org

See also: Airborne illness and disease; Allergic bronchopulmonary aspergillosis; Aspergillus; Atypical pneumonia; Bronchiolitis; Bronchitis; Children and infectious disease; Common cold; Influenza; Laryngitis; Measles; Paramyxoviridae; Pleurisy; Pneumonia; Schools and infectious disease; Strep throat; Tuberculosis (TB); Viral infections; Viral upper respiratory infections; Whooping cough.

Cryptococcosis

CATEGORY: Diseases and conditions
ANATOMY OR SYSTEM AFFECTED: All

DEFINITION

Cryptococcosis is a serious fungal infection most frequently acquired in tropical and subtropical areas of the world. People with compromised immune function, such as those with human immunodeficiency virus (HIV) infection and acquired immunodeficiency syndrome (AIDS), are often affected.

CAUSES

Cryptococcosis can be caused by either of two types of fungi—*Cryptococcus neoformans* or *C. gattii*–which are found in soil and bird droppings and in and around tropical trees. Because the fungi enter the body through inhalation of airborne fungal spores, the most common site of infection is the lungs. However, cryptococcosis can develop in any part of the body, including skin, eyes, central nervous system, and bones.

RISK FACTORS

Risk factors for cryptococcosis include exposure to areas with a high concentration of bird droppings and to soil or trees contaminated with *C. neoformans* or *C. gattii*, in combination with low immunity caused by previous infection, the use of corticosteroids, or chronic disease. People with AIDS are particularly susceptible to cryptococcosis, especially persons with low levels of a particular type of white blood cell, CD4+ T cells. Persons with AIDS who receive ongoing treatment with antiretroviral medications are afforded some protection.

SYMPTOMS

When the lungs are affected, symptoms include fever, cough, shortness of breath, and coughing up blood (hemoptysis). If the central nervous system becomes involved, symptoms of meningitis occur, these include stiff neck, headache, vomiting, and seizures. Skin infection may appear as a rash, swollen area, or blister. Cryptococcosis involving the eyes may cause eye pain and vision loss.

SCREENING AND DIAGNOSIS

A complete physical exam will reveal impaired immunity in combination with symptoms that lend suspicion for cryptococcosis. To confirm the diagnosis, the patient may receive a chest X ray; routine laboratory testing and culture of skin lesions, blood, urine, or sputum; and a lumbar puncture, which involves aspiration of cerebrospinal fluid for analysis.

TREATMENT AND THERAPY

Cryptococcosis is treated with oral or intravenous antifungal medication, such as amphotericin B and flucanozole, for a minimum of fourteen days. In many patients, symptoms are mild and resolve quickly once treated on an outpatient basis, but persons with AIDS typically have more severe symptoms, require hospitalization, and often experience a recurrence of infection.

PREVENTION AND OUTCOMES

Avoiding infested tropical and subtropical areas is key to preventing cryptococcosis. Persons with AIDS should be made aware that they may be infected with cryptococcosis more than once because of their suppressed immune systems, but that treatment with antiretroviral medications can increase CD4+ T cell counts and reduce the risk of being infected.

Carita Caple, M.S.H.S., R.N.

FURTHER READING

Bennet, John E. "Cryptococcosis." In *Harrison's Principles of Internal Medicine,* edited by Joan Butterton. 17th ed. New York: McGraw-Hill, 2008.

Bellissimo-Rodrigues, Fernando, et al. "Cutaneous Cryptococcosis Due to Cryptococcus gattii in a Patient on Chronic Corticotherapy." *Revista da Sociedade Brasileira de Medicina Tropical* 43 (2010): 211-212.

Dromer, Françoise, et al. "Major Role for Amphotericin B-Flucytosine Combination in Severe Cryptococcosis." *PLoS One* 3 (2008): e2870.

Jong, Elaine C., and Russell McMullen, eds. *Travel and Tropical Medicine Manual.* 4th ed. Philadelphia: Saunders/Elsevier, 2008.

Murray, Patrick R., Ken S. Rosenthal, and Michael A. Pfaller. *Medical Microbiology.* 6th ed. Philadelphia: Mosby/Elsevier, 2009.

Sarosi, George A., and Scott F. Davies, eds. *Fungal Diseases of the Lung.* 3d ed. Philadelphia: Lippincott Williams & Wilkins, 2000.

Webster, John, and Roland Weber. *Introduction to Fungi.* New York: Cambridge University Press, 2007.

WEB SITES OF INTEREST

AIDS.gov
http://www.aids.gov

American Lung Association
http://www.lungusa.org

Centers for Disease Control and Prevention, National Center for Zoonotic, Vector-Borne, and Enteric Diseases
http://www.cdc.gov/nczved/divisions/dfbmd/diseases/cryptococcus

See also: AIDS; Antifungal drugs: Types; Aspergillosis; Birds and infectious disease; Chromoblastomycosis; Coccidioides; Coccidiosis; Cryptococcus; Fecal-oral route of transmission; Fungal infections; Fungi: Classification and types; Histoplasmosis; HIV; Mycetoma; Paracoccidioidomycosis; Pneumocystis pneumonia; Respiratory route of transmission; Soilborne illness and disease; Stachybotrys; Tropical medicine.

Cryptococcus

CATEGORY: Pathogen
TRANSMISSION ROUTE: Inhalation

DEFINITION

Cryptococcus is a type of fungus that can be found worldwide in soil and in areas on and around trees. *Cryptococcus* causes cryptococcosis, an invasive mycosis in humans.

NATURAL HABITAT AND FEATURES

A *Cryptococcus* infection, or cryptococcosis, is typically caused by contaminated soil. *Neoformans* and *gattii* are the only two forms of cryptococcosis that are transmitted to humans. *Neoformans* is the most common species found in the United States and comes from the aged feces of wild birds, such as pigeons. The feces become dry and, once disrupted, produce spores that are released into the air.

Gattii, which is typically found in tropical and subtropical climates, has also been identified in Canada and the United States. *Gattii* is not associated with bird feces; rather, it is associated with the bark, leaves, and plant debris of eucalyptus trees and gum trees.

```
┌─────────────────────────────────────────┐
│        Taxonomic Classification          │
│           for Cryptococcus               │
│                                          │
│  Kingdom: Fungi                          │
│  Phylum: Basidiomycota                   │
│  Class: Tremellomycetes                  │
│  Order: Tremellales                      │
│  Family: Tremellaceae                    │
│  Genus: Cryptococcus Vuill. Filobasidiella│
│  Species:                                │
│    C. neoformans                         │
│    C. gattii                             │
│    C. laurenti                           │
│    C. albidus                            │
└─────────────────────────────────────────┘
```

Cryptococcus cells are round or oval shaped and are surrounded by a polysaccharide capsule comprising mannose, xylose, and glucuronic acid. During sexual reproduction of the *Cryptococcus* cell, two fungal cells fuse and develop threadlike extensions called hyphae. *Neoformans* and *gattii* are considered to be two distinct species. Each species has five serotypes based on the antigenic specificity of the capsular polysaccharide. *Neoformans* includes serotypes A, D, and AD. *Gattii* includes serotypes B and C. Serotype A causes most cryptococcal infections in immunocompromised persons.

C. *neoformans* is an encapsulated yeast that grows at 98° Fahrenheit (37° Celsius). Its identification is based on its microscopic appearance: smooth, convex, and yellow or tan colonies on solid media at 68° to 98° F (20° to 37° C).

PATHOGENICITY AND CLINICAL SIGNIFICANCE

Cryptococcal infection response mainly depends on the infected person's immune status before infection and on the involved sites. Responses include harmless colonization of the airway and asymptomatic infections to meningitis and disseminated disease. This organism's primary transmission is respiratory, but not directly from human to human. C. *neoformans* can also develop in nonhuman animals.

Once the fungal elements have been inhaled, the yeast spores deposit themselves in the pulmonary alveoli. They must survive the neutral to alkaline pH (acidity) and physiologic concentrations of carbon dioxide before they can be phagocytized by alveolar macrophages. Both *neoformans* and *gattii*, once inhaled,

may cause pneumonia-like symptoms, including shortness of breath, cough, chest pain, and fever. A chest X ray may reveal focal or diffuse infiltrates and a nodule or mass.

The mode of entry for *Cryptococcus* is through the lungs; however, the central nervous system is the main site of clinical involvement. Cryptococcal meningitis and meningoencephalitis are the most common and most serious forms of cryptococcal disease affecting the central nervous system. These forms can be fatal if not treated appropriately; death can occur from two weeks to years following the onset of symptoms. Headache, altered mental status, confusion, lethargy, obtundation (decreased alertness), seizures, and coma are the most common symptoms. Other organ involvement sites for infection are the skin, prostate, bones, eyes, heart (as myocarditis), liver (as hepatitis), and adrenals.

Neoformans typically infects immunocompromised persons, yet it has also infected persons who are not immunocompromised. At high risk of developing cryptoccus are persons who have human immunodeficiency virus infection and other immunocompromised persons, including those undergoing organ transplantation and persons receiving corticosteroid treatment. The incubation period for *neoformans* is unknown.

Gattii rarely infects immunocompromised persons; it usually infects persons with healthy immune systems. Persons infected with this type of *Cryptococcus* may begin to exhibit symptoms two to fourteen months following exposure. Persons infected with *gattii* respond much slower to treatment than those infected with *neoformans*, thereby increasing the risk of developing significant central nervous system sequela.

Cryptococcal-encapsulated yeast cells can be visualized using an India ink preparation on cerebral spinal fluid. In addition, blood, urine, tissue, and sputum can also be examined microscopically for the presence of *Cryptococcus*. A rapid cryptococcal antigen test also can be done using blood or cerebral spinal fluid. To definitively determine the infection type, the organism must be cultured, which requires special testing at state health-department laboratories or at the Centers for Disease Control and Prevention. Computed tomography scans and magnetic resonance imaging studies may help in distinguishing cryptococcal infections from other symptomology.

DRUG SUSCEPTIBILITY

Meningeal and other serious cryptococcal infections can have a rapid onset of symptoms, so the administration of the appropriate antibiotic "cocktail" is critical. Amphotericin B, in combination with oral flucytosine or fluconazole, is first-line drug therapy for cryptococcosis. This combination penetrates the blood-brain barrier more effectively. Amphotericin B has a rapid onset of action, leading to faster clinical improvement. For persons with renal impairment, liposomal amphotericin B is used (this type of amphotericin has sparing renal-function properties). Ketoconazole or itraconazole should not be used in the initial treatment of cryptococcosis because they do not adequately penetrate the blood-brain barrier.

Cryptococcosis includes varying degrees of treatment regimens following initial drug therapy. These regimens depend on immune system involvement. An immunocompromised person with an human immunodeficiency virus (HIV) infection will begin initial aggressive treatment with the therapeutic goal of controlling the acute cryptococcal infection, followed by lifelong suppression therapy. The therapeutic goal for persons with cryptococcosis but who are not HIV-positive is permanent cure, with no chronic suppressive therapy.

When systemic therapy becomes refractory, intrathecal or intraventricular amphotericin B may be required. Successful therapy is considered only after cerebral spinal fluid cultures are negative and the infected person has had significant clinical improvement.

Stephanie McCallum Blake, M.S.N.

FURTHER READING

"Cryptococcus neoformans Infections." *In Red Book: 2009 Report of the Committee on Infectious Diseases*, edited by Larry K. Pickering et al. 28th ed. Elk Grove Village, Ill.: American Academy of Pediatrics, 2009. The bible on infections of children and the official source for American Academy of Pediatrics policy.

King, John W., and Meredith L. DeWitt. "Cryptococcosis." Available at http://emedicine.medscape.com/article/215354-overview. Discusses background, differential diagnosis, workup, treatment, medications, and follow-up.

Sarosi, George A., and Scott F. Davies, eds. *Fungal Diseases of the Lung*. 3d ed. Philadelphia: Lippincott Williams & Wilkins, 2000. This resource covers a wide range of topics, including cryptococcosis, blastomycosis, coccidioidomycosis, and sporotrichosis.

Thomas, Nancy J., D. Bruce Hunter, and Carter T. Atkinson, eds. *Infectious Diseases of Wild Birds*. Ames, Iowa: Blackwell, 2007. A detailed description of the health risks to birds, other animals, and humans from avian-related infectious diseases.

Webster, John, and Roland Weber. *Introduction to Fungi*. New York: Cambridge University Press, 2007. An introductory text on all types of fungi, including Cryptococcus.

WEB SITES OF INTEREST

AIDSgov
http://www.aids.gov

American Lung Association
http://www.lungusa.org

Centers for Disease Control and Prevention
http://www.cdc.gov/nczved/divisions/dfbmd/diseases/cryptococcus

See also: AIDS; Antifungal drugs: Types; Aspergillosis; Birds and infectious disease; Coccidiosis; Cryptococcosis; Fecal-oral route of transmission; Fungi: Classification and types; Histoplasmosis; HIV; Paracoccidioidomycosis; Respiratory route of transmission; Soilborne illness and disease.

Cryptosporidiosis

CATEGORY: Diseases and conditions
ANATOMY OR SYSTEM AFFECTED: Gastrointestinal system, intestines
ALSO KNOWN AS: Crypto

DEFINITION

Cryptosporidiosis is an infection of the intestine that can cause severe diarrhea. Most healthy adults recover from this infection within a few weeks, but it can be life-threatening for young children, the elderly, and very sick people.

CAUSES

Cryptosporidiosis is caused by the parasite *Cryptosporidium parvum*. These protozoa live in the intestines of infected people and animals. They can also contaminate objects and surfaces that people touch. They may also be in soil where food is grown. The parasite can also be found in recreational waters where people swim.

The infection is caused by swallowing the parasite. When the parasite enters the intestine, it comes out of its shell. It will multiply and may cause an infection. Eventually, it is passed from the body through a bowel movement.

Sources of cryptosporidiosis include contact with diapers or clothing that are contaminated with the infection; contact with animal feces by touching animals, cleaning cages, or visiting barns; and sexual activity that involves contact with feces. Another source of crypto is eating food grown in, or contaminated by, infected soil; drinking unpasteurized milk or other dairy products; drinking apple juice; and eating food that was handled by an infected person or a person who has washed his or her hands in contaminated water.

Another source of infection is water. One can be infected by accidentally swallowing water from contaminated recreational sites, such as lakes, oceans, bays, streams, rivers, hot tubs, swimming pools, and water parks; and by drinking water or using ice that is contaminated.

RISK FACTORS

People who are at increased risk for cryptosporidiosis include young children, especially if they are in day care; day-care staff or those who work in other group settings; people whose immune system is weakened by cancer, human immunodeficiency virus (HIV) infection, acquired immunodeficiency syndrome (AIDS), or an organ transplant; people who engage in oral-anal sex; and international travelers, backpackers, hikers, and campers.

SYMPTOMS

Symptoms usually begin about one week after infection, but some people will not have any symptoms. Symptoms consist mainly of watery diarrhea; stomach cramps; upset stomach, vomiting; slight fever; weakness; weight loss; and dehydration. The symptoms may come and go before the infected person feels better.

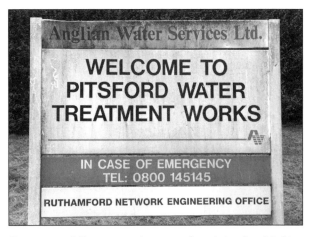

Cryptosporidium *parasites were found in the drinking water of the British town of Pitsford in 2008. The local water treatment facility issued a warning to the community of about 250,000 people.* (AP/Wide World Photos)

SCREENING AND DIAGNOSIS

A doctor will take one or more stool samples, which will be sent to a laboratory to be examined.

TREATMENT AND THERAPY

People with healthy immune systems usually recover without needing treatment. Recovery can take several weeks. The infected person with severe diarrhea may be given IV fluids and antidiarrheal drugs. Nitazoxanide is approved to treat the diarrhea associated with cryptosporidiosis in healthy people.

People with a weakened immune system (such as those living with AIDS) have a greater risk of getting this infection. They are also likely to have a more severe and longer infection. Also, they might become permanently infected.

PREVENTION AND OUTCOMES

There are several important measures one can take to lower the risk of getting cryptosporidiosis. These measures include good hygiene, such as washing one's hands after using the toilet, after changing a diaper, before handling or eating food, after contact with animals or soil, and after contact with infected people. Other measures are boiling water and avoiding swallowing water when swimming, washing vegetables that will be eaten raw, drinking only pasteurized milk and juice, and using precautions during sexual activity.

If infected with cryptosporidiosis, one should take measures to avoid spreading the parasite to others; these measures include frequent handwashing, avoiding swimming in recreational waters, and taking precautions during sexual activity.

Julie J. Martin, M.S.;
reviewed by David L. Horn, M.D., FACP

FURTHER READING

Centers for Disease Control and Prevention. "Cryptosporidiosis." Available at http://www.cdc.gov/parasites/crypto.

Despommier, Dickson D., et al. *Parasitic Diseases.* 5th ed. New York: Apple Tree, 2006.

Kapadia, Cyrus R., James M. Crawford, and Caroline Taylor. *An Atlas of Gastroenterology: A Guide to Diagnosis and Differential Diagnosis.* Boca Raton, Fla.: Pantheon, 2003.

Porter, Robert S., et al., eds. *The Merck Manual Home Health Handbook.* 3d ed. Whitehouse Station, N.J.: Merck Research Laboratories, 2009.

Roberts, Larry S., and John Janovy, Jr. *Gerald D. Schmidt and Larry S. Roberts' Foundations of Parasitology.* 8th ed. Boston: McGraw-Hill, 2009.

WEB SITES OF INTEREST

Centers for Disease Control and Prevention
http://www.cdc.gov/parasites

Clean Hands Coalition
http://www.cleanhandscoalition.org

National Center for Emerging and Zoonotic Infectious Diseases
http://www.cdc.gov/ncezid

Public Health Agency of Canada
http://www.phac-aspc.gc.ca

See also: Amebic dysentery; Antiparasitic drugs: Types; Diagnosis of protozoan diseases; Enteritis; Fecal-oral route of transmission; Food-borne illness and disease; Giardia; Giardiasis; Intestinal and stomach infections; Norovirus infection; Parasitic diseases; Peritonitis; Prevention of protozoan diseases; Protozoa: Classification and types; Protozoan diseases; Sexually transmitted diseases (STDs); Soilborne illness and disease; Treatment of protozoan diseases; Waterborne illness and disease.

Cysticercosis

CATEGORY: Diseases and conditions
ANATOMY OR SYSTEM AFFECTED: All

DEFINITION

Cysticercosis is an infectious disease caused by the parasite *Taenia solium*, which is a pork tapeworm. This parasite invades the central nervous system and causes cysts to form in various parts of the body, including the eyes, muscles, brain, and nervous system. Cysticercosis is a major cause of epileptic seizures, especially in the developing world. Although the prognosis is usually good, cysticercosis can lead to serious consequences, including blindness, brain damage, and heart failure.

CAUSES

Cysticercosis is caused by ingestion of *T. solium* eggs, which are found in foods that have been contaminated or cooked improperly. Once consumed, the eggs hatch and their embryos penetrate the intestinal wall and enter the bloodstream.

RISK FACTORS

Risk factors for cysticercosis include eating meats, vegetables, or fruits that are contaminated with *T. solium*. Such contamination can occur if foods are not washed or cooked properly.

SYMPTOMS

In many cases, cysticercosis does not produce symptoms. If the parasite invades muscle tissue, lumps may be visible beneath the skin. If the eyes are involved, symptoms may include blurred vision and detachment or swelling of the retina. If the disease invades the nervous system, it is often accompanied by seizures, headaches, brain swelling, and problems with balance.

SCREENING AND DIAGNOSIS

Establishing the diagnosis of cysticercosis can be challenging and requires various tests. Blood tests can be used to detect antibodies to *T. solium*. Imaging studies such as X rays, computed tomography, ultrasonography, and magnetic resonance imaging can aid in visualizing the cysts. Biopsies can be performed on infected tissue. Electroencephalographs are useful if seizures are present. A spinal tap (lumbar puncture) may be appropriate for some persons.

TREATMENT AND THERAPY

Consultation with an infectious disease specialist is highly recommended. Treatment should be tailored to each patient, based on multiple factors, including the symptoms, the stage of cyst development, and the site and quantity of cysts. Treatment may involve corticosteroids, anticonvulsant medications, and antiparasitic agents. Although antiparasitic agents are effective for expelling parasites, they may produce a reactive localized inflammation. Multiple courses of treatment may be needed to fully eliminate the cysts. If seizures are present, referral to a neurologist is helpful for determining appropriate therapy. In some cases, surgery or shunting may be needed.

PREVENTION AND OUTCOMES

Public education is extremely important for preventing cysticercosis. One should properly handle and cook food; fruits and vegetables should be washed thoroughly. One should not consume raw or undercooked pork. The risk of person-to-person transmission can be reduced by exercising good personal hygiene, including frequent handwashing. No vaccine against *T. solium* infection is available.

Lynda A. Seminara, B.A.

FURTHER READING

Garcia, H. H., et al. "Taenia solium Cysticercosis." *The Lancet* 16 (2003): 547-556.

Icon Group. *Cysticercosis: Webster's Timeline History, 1909-2007.* San Diego, Calif.: Author, 2009.

Penrith, M. L. "Cysticercosis Working Group in Eastern and Southern Africa." *Journal of the South African Veterinary Association* 80 (2009): 206-207.

Roberts, Larry S., and John Janovy, Jr. *Gerald D. Schmidt and Larry S. Roberts' Foundations of Parasitology.* 8th ed. Boston: McGraw-Hill, 2009.

Singh, Gagandeep, and Sudesh Prabhakar. "Taenia solium." *Cysticercosis: From Basic to Clinical Science.* Cambridge, Mass.: CAB International North America, 2002.

World Health Organization. "Taeniasis/Cysticercosis." Available at http://www.who.int/zoonoses/diseases/taeniasis.

WEB SITES OF INTEREST

National Center for Emerging and Zoonotic Infectious Diseases
http://www.cdc.gov/ncezid

U.S. Department of Agriculture, Food Safety Information Center
http://foodsafety.nal.usda.gov

World Health Organization
http://www.who.int/zoonoses/diseases/taeniasis

See also: Food-borne illness and disease; Parasites: Classification and types; Parasitic diseases; Pigs and infectious disease; Taeniasis; Tapeworms; Worm infections; Zoonotic diseases.

Cytomegalovirus infection

CATEGORY: Diseases and conditions
ANATOMY OR SYSTEM AFFECTED: All

DEFINITION

Cytomegalovirus (CMV) infection is a common viral infection. It can cause swollen lymph glands, fever, and fatigue. Most people with CMV do not show symptoms of infection and are not aware they have it. CMV infection rarely causes health problems except for people with compromised immune systems and for fetuses.

CAUSES

A herpesvirus causes CMV. The disease is passed by an exchange of body fluids with an infected person. A person can be exposed through kissing, sexual intercourse, breast-feeding, and changing the diaper of an infected infant. The virus is found in saliva, tears, blood, urine, semen, stool, vaginal fluids, and breast milk.

RISK FACTORS

This virus is common throughout the United States. Everyone is considered at risk for CMV. However, people with the highest risk of acquiring this virus include children and child-care providers in day care and preschool, because of their frequent exposure to body fluids that carry the infection; people with suppressed or impaired immune systems; transplant recipients; persons with cancer undergoing chemotherapy; and persons with human immunodeficiency virus (HIV) infection or acquired immunodeficiency syndrome (AIDS). Fetuses are at high risk too. Exposure in utero can result in congenital CMV (congenital means born with the condition). About 1 percent of babies born in the United States are born with congenital CMV.

SYMPTOMS

The virus often remains inactive in the body, and there are often no symptoms. Sometimes, the virus is activated. Reactivation of the virus can happen if a person's immune system becomes impaired. This can happen because of medication or illness. In this case symptoms can occur.

The symptoms are like those of mononucleosis, another herpesvirus infection, and include swollen lymph glands, sore throat, fever, and fatigue. People with suppressed or impaired immune systems can also develop pneumonia, colitis (inflammation of the large intestines), retinitis (an eye infection that can cause blindness), and chronic liver disease.

Babies born with congenital CMV infection often have hearing loss, deafness, blindness, mental retardation, developmental problems, and chronic liver disease. Infants who get a CMV infection after birth rarely have any symptoms or complications.

SCREENING AND DIAGNOSIS

CMV infection is not often diagnosed because the virus rarely produces symptoms. If CMV is suspected, it can be diagnosed through a blood test to detect CMV antibodies (disease-fighting proteins in the blood) and a laboratory test of fluid samples. Not all laboratories are equipped to perform this test, however. Other tests include amniocentesis, for pregnant women, to check for signs of infection in the fetus, and a biopsy of any affected organ.

TREATMENT AND THERAPY

Most people will not need specific therapy for CMV infection. Once a person has this virus, he or she has it for life. No vaccine exists to prevent the spread of this disease. For people undergoing organ transplants, people living with AIDS, and other persons with immunosuppression, specific antiviral drugs may be used, such as ganciclovir and valganciclovir.

PREVENTION AND OUTCOMES

There is no definitive way to prevent CMV. One should, however, wash hands frequently, dispose of di-

apers properly, and avoid intimate contact with people known to have a CMV infection.

Vonne Sieve, M.A.; reviewed by David L. Horn, M.D., FACP

FURTHER READING

Martin, Richard J., Avroy A. Fanaroff, and Michele C. Walsh, eds. *Fanaroff and Martin's Neonatal-Perinatal Medicine: Diseases of the Fetus and Infant.* 2 vols. 8th ed. Philadelphia: Mosby/Elsevier, 2006.

The Merck Manuals, Online Medical Library. "Cytomegalovirus Infection (Cytomegalic Inclusion Disease)." Available at http://www.merck.com/mmhe.

Roizman, Bernard, Richard J. Whitley, and Carlos Lopez, eds. *The Human Herpesviruses.* New York: Raven Press, 1993.

Scheld, W. Michael, Richard J. Whitley, and Christina M. Marra, eds. *Infections of the Central Nervous System.* 3d ed. Philadelphia: Lippincott Williams & Wilkins, 2004.

Wagner, Edward K., and Martinez J. Hewlett. *Basic Virology.* 3d ed. Malden, Mass.: Blackwell Science, 2008.

WEB SITES OF INTEREST

American Pregnancy Association
http://www.americanpregnancy.org

Centers for Disease Control and Prevention
http://www.cdc.gov

HerpesGuide.ca
http://www.herpesguide.ca

National Institutes of Health
http://www.nih.gov

Public Health Agency of Canada
http://www.phac-aspc.gc.ca

See also: Breast milk and infectious disease; Childbirth and infectious disease; Cytomegalovirus vaccine; Herpes simplex infection; Herpesviridae; Herpesvirus infections; Lymphadenitis; Mononucleosis; Neonatal sepsis; Pregnancy and infectious disease; Reinfection; Saliva and infectious disease; Sexually transmitted diseases (STDs); Viral infections.

Cytomegalovirus vaccine

CATEGORY: Prevention

DEFINITION

No vaccine exists for cytomegalovirus (CMV) infection, the most common congenital infection in the United States. Severely affected newborns may have hearing loss, vision loss, mental retardation, cerebral palsy, seizures, and liver disease. CMV is also frequently acquired in immunocompromised persons, such as those with human immunodeficiency virus (HIV) infection or cancer and those who have had organ transplants. Persons with compromised immune systems are consequently at risk for developing additional life-threatening infections.

CMV is primarily spread by contact with young children who excrete the virus. Earlier attempts to prevent CMV transmission by increased hygienic practices, such as handwashing and avoiding handling of children, proved unsuccessful, and antiviral medications have low efficacy. Therefore, in 1999 the Institute of Medicine listed CMV vaccine development as its top new vaccine priority for the twenty-first century.

POTENTIAL CMV VACCINES

Pregnant women without a history of CMV infection and who have close contact with young children are at greatest risk of contracting the virus and transmitting it to a fetus. Therefore, the primary goal of the CMV vaccine would be to give at-risk women immunity to the virus before giving birth. Several potential vaccine candidates, including the Towne and MF59 vaccines, are in clinical trials. Antibodies from the Towne vaccine were detected eighty-four months after administration, demonstrating long-term established immunity. Additionally, the MF59 vaccine showed 50 percent efficacy for preventing disease transmission; there was one case of congenital CMV reported after vaccination.

Immunocompromised persons are at risk of reactivating an old infection. The Towne vaccine protected kidney transplant patients from developing symptoms, although it did not prevent the acquisition of CMV. Another vaccine, TransVax, boosted immunity and reduced reactivation of the virus in immunocompromised persons. While promising, these vaccines all require further research.

DEVELOPMENT CHALLENGES

All vaccines have been shown to be safe, but studies are limited by difficulty in recruiting study subjects because of a lack of public awareness of CMV, by the need for a large sample size, and by the need for long-term follow-up. Additionally, many women enrolled in vaccine trials have increased their handwashing frequency and have decreased exposure to young children, making it difficult to determine if the vaccine, or the change in behavior, is determining outcome. Also, debate remains about what population should be targeted for vaccine administration.

IMPACT

Approximately eight thousand newborns annually have severe medical and neurological concerns related to congenital CMV infection, translating into a yearly national health care cost of $1.86 billion. An effective CMV vaccine not only would decrease the rate of infection but also would reduce the economic burden for treating the related diseases. Despite ongoing research efforts from the Centers for Disease Control and Prevention, the U.S. Food and Drug Administration, and National Institutes of Health, no approved CMV vaccine is available.

Janet Ober Berman, M.S., CGC

FURTHER READING

Adler, Stuart, et al. "Recent Advances in the Prevention and Treatment of Congenital Cytomegalovirus Infections." *Seminars in Perinatology* 31 (2007): 10-18.

Arvin, Ann, et al. "Vaccine Development to Prevent Cytomegalovirus Disease: Report from the National Vaccine Advisory Committee." *Vaccines* 39 (2004): 233-239.

Dekker, Cornelia, and Ann Arvin. "One Step Closer to a CMV Vaccine." *New England Journal of Medicine* 360 (2009): 1250-1252.

Martin, Richard J., Avroy A. Fanaroff, and Michele C. Walsh, eds. *Fanaroff and Martin's Neonatal-Perinatal Medicine: Diseases of the Fetus and Infant.* 2 vols. 8th ed. Philadelphia: Mosby/Elsevier, 2006.

WEB SITES OF INTEREST

Center for the Evaluation of Risks to Human Reproduction
http://cerhr.niehs.nih.gov

March of Dimes
http://www.modimes.org

Pediatric Infectious Diseases Society
http://www.pids.org

Women's Health Matters
http://www.womenshealthmatters.ca

See also: Breast milk and infectious disease; Childbirth and infectious disease; Children and infectious disease; Cytomegalovirus infection; Herpesviridae; Herpesvirus infections; HIV; Neonatal sepsis; Pregnancy and infectious disease; Vaccines: Experimental; Vaccines: Types; Viral infections; Women and infectious disease.

D

Dacryocystitis

CATEGORY: Diseases and conditions
ANATOMY OR SYSTEM AFFECTED: Eyes, nose, vision
ALSO KNOWN AS: Blocked tear duct, dacryostenosis

DEFINITION

Dacryocystitis is infection of the lacrimal sac, which is located on the side of the nose near the inner corner of the eye. The lacrimal sac drains tears from the eye into the tear ducts leading into the nose. Dacryocystitis is sometimes a congenital condition, which means it is present at birth. The condition affects as many as one-third of all newborn babies.

CAUSES

Dacryocystitis is typically caused by a blocked tear duct. When tears are unable to drain, they accumulate in the tear duct system, leading to the growth of bacteria, which leads to the infection.

RISK FACTORS

The risk from untreated dacryocystitis is bacterial infection, which could cause a number of problems, including fever and infection elsewhere in the body. The condition occurs most often in infants.

SYMPTOMS

Dacryocystitis can cause excessive tearing or watering of the eye when the infant is not crying; reddening of the side of the nose near the inner corner of the eye; tenderness of the side of the nose near the inner corner of the eye; swelling or a bump on the side of the nose; fever; mucus or pus in the corner of the eye; and crusty eyelids or eyelashes after sleep.

SCREENING AND DIAGNOSIS

A doctor will ask about symptoms and medical history and will perform a physical exam. Tests may include a culture of the fluid from the lacrimal sac. The fluid is examined to determine the type of bacteria present and to determine which antibiotics may help. The physical examination includes looking at the eye and the lacrimal system.

TREATMENT AND THERAPY

Treatment options for dacryocystitis include eye drops, oral antibiotics, and antibiotic ointments to kill the bacteria and clear up the infection. For severe infections, persons may be admitted to a hospital to receive antibiotics intravenously. Treatment for the infection does not treat the usual underlying cause of the infection: the blocked tear duct. To treat the blocked tear duct, the tear duct system may need to be massaged (once the infection has healed) to help remove the obstruction. If the obstruction cannot be removed, surgery may be required to prevent recurring dacryocystitis.

PREVENTION AND OUTCOMES

There are no known ways to prevent dacryocystitis except for attempting to open a blocked tear duct system.

Diana Kohnle; reviewed by Kari Kassir, M.D.

FURTHER READING

Cohen, Adam, Michael Mercandetti, and Brian Brazzo, eds. *The Lacrimal System: Diagnosis, Management, and Surgery.* New York: Springer, 2006.

Miller, Stephen J. H. *Parsons' Diseases of the Eye.* 19th ed. New York: Elsevier, 2002.

National Library of Medicine. "Blocked Tear Duct." Available at http://www.nlm.nih.gov/medlineplus/ency/article/001016.htm.

Nemours Foundation. "Tear Duct Obstruction and Surgery." Available at http://www.kidshealth.org.

Sutton, Amy L., ed. *Eye Care Sourcebook: Basic Consumer Health Information About Eye Care and Eye Disorders.* 3d ed. Detroit: Omnigraphics, 2008.

Van Haeringen, N. J. "Aging and the Lacrimal System" *British Journal of Ophthalmology* 81 (1997): 824-826.

WEB SITES OF INTEREST

American Academy of Ophthalmology
http://www.aao.org

KidsHealth
http://www.kidshealth.org

Penn State Hershey Children's Hospital
http://www.pennstatehershey.org/web/childrens

Public Health Agency of Canada
http://www.phac-aspc.gc.ca

See also: Bacterial infections; Cellulitis; Children and infectious disease; Conjunctivitis; Eye infections; Hordeola; Keratitis; Nasopharyngeal infections; Ophthalmia neonatorum.

Dandruff

CATEGORY: Diseases and conditions
ANATOMY OR SYSTEM AFFECTED: Hair, scalp, skin
ALSO KNOWN AS: Pityriasis simplex capillitii, scurf, seborrheic dermatitis

DEFINITION

Dandruff is the excessive scaling of dead cells on the scalp that produces itching and white or yellow flakes. Though not a serious condition, dandruff can be a nuisance and an embarrassment to the person with the condition.

CAUSES

Infrequent hair washing can result in an oily scalp and in the flaking of dead scalp cells. Dry skin on the head may cause itching, which produces small dry flakes. Persons with eczema or psoriasis can experience dandruff. Irritation from hair products can cause contact dermatitis, with itching and flaking. Seborrheic dermatitis occurs with irritated oily skin and results in white flaking wherever there is hair and in excess oil such as on the scalp, the eyebrows, or the groin area. A fungus called *Malassezia*, or *Pityrosporum ovale*, sometimes results in an itchy head and flaking. Newborns and infants experience a form of dandruff called cradle cap that usually resolves on its own.

RISK FACTORS

All persons are at risk for dandruff, but certain factors are associated with getting dandruff. Young and middle age persons tend to have more dandruff than older adults. Males exhibit more dandruff than females, possibly because of hormones and oil-producing glands in the scalp. An oily scalp provides a fertile breeding ground for fungi, resulting in dandruff. A diet that lacks zinc and B complex vitamins may put a person at risk for dandruff. Certain conditions, such as Parkinson's disease, can predispose a person to dandruff. Other factors, including a stressful lifestyle, chronic disease, or lowered immunity, can increase the chance of dandruff.

SYMPTOMS

Dandruff manifests with excessive flaking of dead cells and itching of the scalp. Flakes vary in size, texture, and color based on the causative factor. Dandruff flakes can be observed on the shoulders of dark clothes, on hair, and on the scalp.

SCREENING AND DIAGNOSIS

Dandruff rarely requires the attention of a physician. It is diagnosed by physical examination of the hair and scalp for white or yellow flakes and itching.

TREATMENT AND THERAPY

Dandruff can be controlled by different therapies based on the cause and extent of the problem. Frequent washing with a mild shampoo or with tea-tree oil may control dandruff caused by an oily scalp. Some cases require an antibacterial or antifungal shampoo that contains ketoconazole, zinc pyrithione, salicylic acid, selenium, or tar. However, if the scalp becomes red and swollen, a physician may provide a prescription-strength shampoo or a topical steroid lotion.

PREVENTION AND OUTCOMES

The key to preventing dandruff is to address the cause. One should keep the scalp clean with frequent hair washing; use a special shampoo for dandruff and leave it on the scalp for three to five minutes to assist with cleansing; and avoid chemical treatments of the hair, including permanents, hair color, and hair products that contain chemicals such as hair spray. Dandruff may present less in the summer when the head is exposed to sunlight. Basic good health with proper diet and stress management can help prevent this condition.

Marylane Wade Koch, M.S.N., R.N.

FURTHER READING

Khalsa, Karta. "Brush Off Dandruff." *Better Nutrition* 70, no. 4 (April, 2008): 34, 36.

Weedon, David. *Skin Pathology.* 3d ed. New York: Churchill Livingstone/Elsevier, 2010.

Wolff, Klaus, and Richard Allen Johnson. *Fitzpatrick's Color Atlas and Synopsis of Clinical Dermatology.* 6th ed. New York: McGraw-Hill Medical, 2009.

WEB SITE OF INTEREST

American Academy of Dermatology
http://www.aad.org

See also: Dermatomycosis; *Malassezia; Piedraia;* Pityriasis rosea; Skin infections; Tinea capitis.

DDT

CATEGORY: Prevention
ALSO KNOWN AS: Dichloro-diphenyl-trichloroethane

DEFINITION

DDT is a persistent, lipophilic, broad-spectrum, organochlorine pesticide used to control insects and thereby reduce insect-borne illness and disease. Paul Müller was awarded the Nobel Prize in Physiology or Medicine in 1948 for his discovery of the insecticidal properties of DDT.

The pesticide was used extensively during World War II to prevent and ameliorate typhus and malaria epidemics, saving hundreds of thousands of lives. DDT was used in the United States, Europe, Africa, India, and other regions to wipe out malaria and other diseases. Insect resistance to the pesticide and its effects on wildlife led to the ban of DDT in the United States and many other countries in 1972.

For decades, DDT has been used for imminent epidemics only. In 2006, the World Health Organization reassessed the risks versus the benefits of DDT use and deemed indoor residual spraying of homes to be one of the major mechanisms to control malaria, which affected 500 million people and

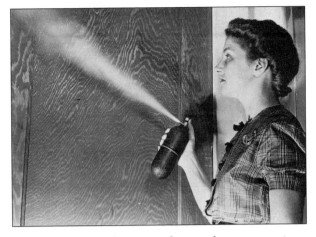

In this mid-twentieth century photograph, a woman sprays toxic DDT with an aerosol can, hoping to kill flies in her home. (AP/Wide World Photos)

killed more than 1 million people worldwide in 2006 alone.

INSECT CONTROL

DDT acts on sodium channels and mainly affects the peripheral nervous system, causing paralysis in insects. It kills the insects within hours or days. Because DDT is not water soluble, it remains effective for months or years after application. In powder form, it is used to control lice; it was used during a typhus epidemic during World War II in Naples, Italy, that was controlled within a few weeks. DDT is most often used in liquid form for spray application.

HEALTH CONCERNS

Studies conducted on volunteers and reports of applicators and chemical manufacturing workers in the 1940's showed that DDT can have neurologic effects and can cause cardiac and liver damage, birth disorders and defects, and chromatid aberrations. It is also an environmental estrogen, so it leads to a range of developmental issues in animals and humans. DDT remains in the human body for years after exposure and accumulates in fatty tissue.

ENVIRONMENTAL ISSUES

DDT has had far-reaching consequences for the natural environment. The pesticide, for example, thins the egg shells of birds, which has led to the near extinction of some bird species. DDT is toxic to fish and to some beneficial insects. In a process called biomagnification, the pesticide becomes more concentrated in creatures as they exist higher and higher along the food chain.

IMPACT

DDT was considered a miracle pesticide in the 1940's and 1950's, and it has saved millions of lives since its introduction. It played a significant part (not a positive one) in the development of the environmental movement and helped lead to an awareness of the biomagnification of other toxic chemicals. Although DDT continues to be controversial, its renewed but limited use has had a powerful positive effect on the lives of millions of people, especially in sub-Saharan Africa.

Dawn M. Bielawski, Ph.D.

FURTHER READING

Centers for Disease Control and Prevention. *Fourth National Report on Human Exposure to Environmental Chemicals* (2009). Available at http://www.cdc.gov/exposurereport.

Davies, T. G. E., et al. "DDT, Pyrethrins, Pyerethroids, and Insect Sodium Channels." *IUBMB Life* 59 (2007): 151-162.

Enayati, A., and J. Hemingway "Malaria Management: Past, Present, and Future." *Annual Review of Entomology* 55 (2010): 569-591.

Klaassen, Curtis D., ed. *Casarett and Doull's Toxicology: The Basic Science of Poisons.* 7th ed. New York: McGraw-Hill, 2008.

National Pesticide Information Center. "DDT (Technical Fact Sheet)." Available at http://npic.orst.edu/factsheets/ddttech.pdf.

Roy, Jonathan R., Sanjoy Chakraborty, and Tandra R. Chakraborty. "Estrogen-Like Endocrine Disrupting Chemicals Affecting Puberty in Humans: A Review." *Medical Science Monitor* 15 (2007): RA137-145.

Solomon, Gina, Oladele A. Ogunseitan, and Jan Kirsch. *Pesticides and Human Health: A Resource for Health Care Professionals.* San Francisco: Physicians for Social Responsibility, 2000.

Van den Berg, Henk. "Global Status of DDT and Its Alternatives for Use in Vector Control to Prevent Disease." *Environmental Health Perspectives* 117 (2009): 1656-1663.

WEB SITES OF INTEREST

Centers for Disease Control and Prevention, Agency for Toxic Substances and Disease Registry
http://www.atsdr.cdc.gov

Centers for Disease Control and Prevention, Division of Vector Borne Infectious Diseases
http://www.cdc.gov/ncidod/dvbid

National Pesticide Information Center
http://npic.orst.edu

World Health Organization: Pesticide Evaluation Scheme
http://www.who.int/whopes

See also: Biochemical tests; Chemical germicides; Developing countries and infectious disease; Epidemics and pandemics: Causes and management; Disease eradication campaigns; Insect-borne illness and disease; Insecticides and topical repellants; Malaria; Mosquitoes and infectious disease; Prevention of viral infections; Sleeping nets; Tropical medicine; Typhus; Vectors and vector control; World Health Organization (WHO).

Dead tissue. *See* Gangrene.

Decontamination

CATEGORY: Treatment
ALSO KNOWN AS: Disinfection

DEFINITION

Decontamination is the process of eliminating or inactivating unsafe materials and substances on a person or object. This process involves physical, chemical, or thermal means, depending on the contaminant, and it should be performed quickly and thoroughly. Substances removed or destroyed by decontamination include poisons, radioactivity, and microbial pathogens (bacteria, viruses, and parasites). Decontamination renders objects safe for use and handling and keeps persons from spreading contaminants.

Situations Requiring Decontamination

The most common use of decontamination is the inactivation of microbial pathogens on medical and dental instruments and equipment to prevent disease transmission between patients and to prevent infection of health care personnel. Another common use of decontamination is the removal of dirt, vegetation, and animal matter from utensils and preparation surfaces in the cooking and serving of meals to prevent the transmission of food-borne illnesses.

Examples of poisons and chemicals that require decontamination include the spray of a skunk, noxious pesticides, and the toxins of poison ivy and poison sumac. Other contaminants include the hazardous chemicals that may be released in transportation accidents and laboratory mishaps.

Radiation spills require prompt decontamination. Often, persons who participate in the clean-up efforts inadvertently spread the radiation on their shoes and clothing. Thus, one should confine the area and screen all affected persons before they can be allowed to leave the area.

Procedures

Decontamination may be performed by physical, chemical, or thermal means or by combinations of these methods. Medical and dental instruments are autoclaved, that is, they are subjected to high heat and pressure for an adequate period of time to kill the pathogens. Utensils placed in a dishwasher are effectively cleaned by the heat of the water and the chemicals in the detergent. Hands and other skin surfaces are disinfected by the use of a soaps and the mechanical action of scrubbing. Surfaces and equipment are decontaminated with disinfectant sprays.

Impact

Decontamination became a special public concern when the human immunodeficiency virus (HIV) was discovered to be a contagious blood-borne pathogen that leads to acquired immunodeficiency syndrome, an incurable disease. Standards of infection control known as universal precautions were devised to prevent cross-contamination among infected persons and to prevent occupational exposure by health care workers. Human blood and body fluids are assumed, since the discovery of HIV especially, to be contaminated and treated accordingly. These practices include the use of personal protective equipment, the handling and disposal of sharps, and the decontamination of equipment and surfaces.

Bethany Thivierge, M.P.H.

Further Reading

Manivannan, Gurusamy, ed. *Disinfection and Decontamination: Principles, Applications, and Related Issues.* New York: CRC Press, 2007.

National Institutes of Health. Division of Occupational Health and Safety. "Medical Aspects of Chemical and Biological Warfare: Decontamination and Sterilization." Available at http://dohs.ors.od.nih.gov/decontamination.htm.

Rutala, William A., David J. Weber, and the Healthcare Infection Control Practices Advisory Committee. *Guideline for Disinfection and Sterilization in Healthcare Facilities, 2008.* Atlanta: Centers for Disease Control and Prevention, 2008.

Web Sites of Interest

American Public Health Association
http://www.apha.org

Centers for Disease Control and Prevention
http://www.cdc.gov

See also: Bacteria: Classification and types; Biological weapons; Chemical germicides; Disease eradication campaigns; Disinfectants and sanitizers; Epidemiology; Hospitals and infectious disease; Hygiene; Iatrogenic infections; Infection; Outbreaks; Parasites: Classification and types; Pathogens; Prevention of bacterial infections; Prevention of fungal infections; Prevention of parasitic diseases; Prevention of viral infections; Public health; Viruses: Types; Water treatment; Waterborne illness and disease.

Dengue fever

Category: Diseases and conditions
Anatomy or system affected: All
Also known as: Break bone fever

Definition

Dengue fever is a flulike illness that is caused by a virus. The infection is passed to humans through the bite of a mosquito. Children and infants who are infected may have no symptoms or only a minor, flulike illness. Adults who become infected may develop a life-threatening illness.

CAUSES

There are four types of dengue viruses that can cause this illness. The viruses are carried by *Aedes* mosquitoes and enter the human bloodstream through the bite of an infected mosquito. The virus may then cause illness. The infection is not passed between humans.

RISK FACTORS

The main factor that increases a person's chance of developing dengue fever is travel to tropical or subtropical areas such as Africa, India, China, and Southeast Asia; and travel to the Middle East, the Caribbean, Central America, South America, Australia, and the central and south Pacific.

SYMPTOMS

A person experiencing any of the following symptoms should not assume he or she has dengue fever. These symptoms may be caused by other, less serious health conditions. Symptoms of dengue fever may include headaches, severe pain behind the eyes, fever, chills, red throat, nasal congestion, muscle pain, and bone pain. Skin symptoms include reddened skin, increased sensitivity of skin to touch, skin rash, and purple spots on the skin. Other symptoms include loss of appetite, nausea, vomiting, liver and spleen enlargement, hepatitis, bad taste in the mouth, minor bleeding from gums, nosebleeds, and blood in urine and stool. During recovery, a patient might have low energy, fatigue, and depression.

Severe complications are dengue hemorrhagic fever and dengue shock syndrome. Persons with these diseases may develop dangerously low blood pressure, a weak pulse, abdominal pain, sweatiness, pale or blue skin and lips, and uncontrolled bleeding (hemorrhaging) from the gums or the nose or from the urinary and gastrointestinal tracts.

SCREENING AND DIAGNOSIS

A doctor will ask about symptoms and medical history and will also ask about recent travel to tropical areas. The doctor may refer the patient to a specialist after performing a physical examination.

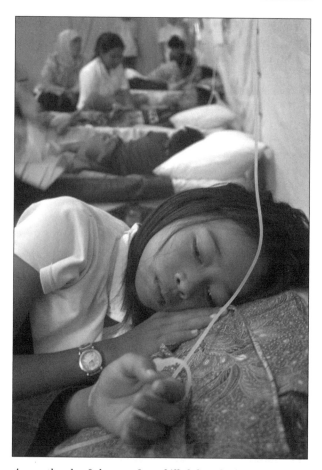

An outbreak of dengue fever killed hundreds and infected thousands in Indonesia in 2004. Tents were set up outside an overcrowded military hospital. (AP/Wide World Photos)

Tests to determine if a person has dengue fever include blood tests, antibody tests (to see if the body is producing substances that fight dengue fever viruses), and a reverse transcriptase polymerase chain reaction test, to determine the presence and quantity of virus in the bloodstream.

TREATMENT AND THERAPY

There are no medications available that can provide a cure. Treatment addresses the symptoms. It also attempts to avoid potential complications. Possible treatments include extra rest while recovering from the illness; adequate hydration (drinking increased amounts of beverages to help replace fluids, sugars, and salts lost during the illness; if unable to drink enough, the patient may need to receive IV fluids);

and medications to decrease fever and pain, such as acetaminophen (Tylenol). One should not use aspirin because it may increase the risk of bleeding.

PREVENTION AND OUTCOMES

To help reduce the chance of getting dengue fever, one should take the following steps when traveling in areas where dengue fever is common: Spend time in locations that are protected by good screens and are air conditioned; wear long-sleeved shirts and pants, and also wear socks and shoes; and use insect repellents (preferably those containing NN-diethyl metatoluamide, or DEET) on skin and clothing. Persons should either stay inside or take extra precautions during the times of day when mosquitoes are most likely to bite (early morning and late afternoon and early evening). Mosquitoes breed in standing water, so one should not leave standing water in buckets or other containers.

Rosalyn Carson-DeWitt, M.D.;
reviewed by David L. Horn, M.D., FACP

FURTHER READING

Centers for Disease Control and Prevention. "Dengue and Dengue Hemorrhagic Fever, Information for Health Care Practitioners." Available at http:/// www.cdc.gov.

Halstead, S. B. "More Dengue, More Questions." *Emerging Infectious Diseases* 11, no. 5 (May, 2005): 740-741.

Mandell, Gerald L., John E. Bennett, and Raphael Dolin, eds. *Mandell, Douglas, and Bennett's Principles and Practice of Infectious Diseases.* 7th ed. New York: Churchill Livingstone/Elsevier, 2010.

National Institute of Allergy and Infectious Diseases. "Dengue Fever." Available at http://www.niaid. nih.gov/factsheets/dengue.

WEB SITES OF INTEREST

American Society of Tropical Medicine and Hygiene
http://www.astmh.org

Centers for Disease Control and Prevention
http://www.cdc.gov

National Institute of Allergy and Infectious Diseases
http://www.niaid.nih.gov

Public Health Agency of Canada
http://www.phac-aspc.gc.ca

See also: Cholera; Developing countries and infectious disease; Eastern equine encephalitis; Encephalitis; Fever; Insect-borne illness and disease; Mosquito-borne viral encephalitis; Mosquitoes and infectious disease; Poliomyelitis; Sleeping nets; Tropical medicine; Viral infections; Viral meningitis; Waterborne illness and disease; West Nile virus; Yellow fever.

Deoxyribonucleic acid. *See* DNA.

Dermatomycosis

CATEGORY: Diseases and conditions
ANATOMY OR SYSTEM AFFECTED: Feet, genitalia, hair, head, nails, scalp, skin

DEFINITION

Dermatomycosis is a superficial fungal infection of the skin and its appendages (hair and nails) caused by dermatophytes, yeasts, and other fungi. The condition includes candidal (yeast) infections and skin disorders such as tinea barbae (ringworm of the beard), tinea capitis (ringworm of the scalp and hair), tinea corporis (ringworm of the body), tinea cruris (jock itch, or ringworm of the groin), tinea pedis (ringworm of the foot, or athlete's foot), and tinea unguium (ringworm of the nail).

CAUSES

Fungi are a large group of eukaryotic microorganisms that include molds and yeasts. Approximately four hundred species have been found to cause disease in humans, forty of which are common causes of skin disease. The genera of fungi that most commonly cause dermatomycosis are *Microsporum*, *Epidermophyton*, and *Trichophyton*. These species, which are also known as dermatophytes, colonize the outer layer of the skin and feed on keratinized material.

In addition to dermatophytes, yeasts such as *Candida albicans* are also common causes of dermatomycosis. *C. albicans* is part of the normal flora of the skin, vagina, and gastrointestinal tract. However, ill health, impaired immunity, and antibiotic treatment can disrupt the normal balance of bacterial flora and can trigger the yeast to multiply and cause disease.

RISK FACTORS

Dermatomycosis can occur in healthy persons. However, immunocompromised persons, such those with human immunodeficiency virus (HIV) infection or acquired immunodeficiency syndrome (AIDS), and those in poor health are at increased risk of severe, chronic, and recurrent dermatomycosis. Persons taking antibiotics may also be at increased risk.

SYMPTOMS

The signs and symptoms of dermatomycosis vary depending on the type and location of the infection. Most types cause symptoms of inflammation and itching.

Tinea barbae causes both mild superficial lesions that resemble tinea corporis and leads to severe lesions characterized by deep, pustular folliculitis. Tinea capitis causes scaly erythematous lesions and alopecia that can become severely inflamed; this leads to the formation of keloids and scarring with permanent alopecia. Tinea corporis causes lesions that vary from simple scaling, scaling with erythema, and vesicles to deep granulomata.

Tinea cruris causes lesions that are usually sharply demarcated and with a raised erythematous margin and thin dry epidermal scaling. Tinea pedis causes lesions that vary from mild, chronic, and scaling to acute, exfoliative, pustular, and bullous.

Tinea unguium can cause infection that is restricted to patches or pits on the surface of the nail or infection that is invasive and involves the lateral or distal edges of the nail. The infection then spreads beneath the nail plate.

SCREENING AND DIAGNOSIS

The diagnosis of dermatomycosis is made by the finding of characteristic hyphae or spores on microscopic analysis of skin, nail, and scalp scrapings. Cultures are also used to definitively identify the responsible species of fungus.

TREATMENT AND THERAPY

The treatment of dermatomycosis may include topical antifungal medications such as clotrimazole, butenafine, and miconazole, and systemic medications such as fluconazole, griseofulvin, terbinafine, and itra-

conizole. Antibiotics may also be necessary to treat secondary bacterial infections that occur as a result of scratching.

PREVENTION AND OUTCOMES

Dermatophytes are transmitted by direct contact with infected human or animal hosts or by direct or indirect contact with contaminated exfoliated skin or hair in the environment. Preventive measures, thus, include reducing or eliminating exposure to sources of disease transmission. In addition, one can help prevent dermatomycosis by keeping skin clean and dry, receiving immediate and concurrent treatment to prevent spreading, and taking prophylactic medicine to prevent recurrence.

Diep Koly, M.D.

FURTHER READING

Andrews, M. D., and M. Burns. "Common Tinea Infections in Children." *American Family Physician* 77 (2008): 1415-1420.

Berger, T. G. "Dermatologic Disorders." In *Current Medical Diagnosis and Treatment 2011*, edited by Stephen J. McPhee and Maxine A. Papadakis. 50th ed. New York: McGraw-Hill Medical, 2011.

National Library of Medicine. "Tinea Capitis." Available at http://www.nlm.nih.gov/medlineplus/ency/article/000878.htm.

Richardson, Malcolm D., and Elizabeth M. Johnson. *The Pocket Guide to Fungal Infection.* 2d ed. Malden, Mass.: Blackwell, 2006.

Wolff, Klaus, and Richard Allen Johnson. *Fitzpatrick's Color Atlas and Synopsis of Clinical Dermatology.* 6th ed. New York: McGraw-Hill Medical, 2009.

WEB SITES OF INTEREST

American Academy of Dermatology
http://www.aad.org

Canadian Dermatology Association
http://www.dermatology.ca

Microbiology and Immunology On-line: Mycology
http://pathmicro.med.sc.edu/book/mycol-sta.htm

See also: Antifungal drugs: Types; Athlete's foot; *Candida*; Chromoblastomycosis; Dermatophytosis; *Epidermophyton*; Fungal infections; Fungi: Classification and types; Jock itch; *Malassezia*; *Microsporum*; Mycoses; Onychomycosis; *Piedraia*; Ringworm; Scabies; Skin infections; Tinea capitis; Tinea corporis.

Dermatophytosis

CATEGORY: Diseases and conditions
ANATOMY OR SYSTEM AFFECTED: Feet, hair, head, nails, scalp, skin
ALSO KNOWN AS: Tinea

DEFINITION

Dermatophytosis is a superficial fungal infection of the skin, hair, and nails caused by dermatophytes. The condition is generally classified according to the location of the infection and is often referred to as tinea because of its resemblance to infections caused by parasitic worms that burrow beneath the skin.

CAUSES

Dermatophytes are fungi that can grow and colonize on keratinized, or nonliving, tissues of human and animal hosts. The genera of fungi that most commonly cause dermatophytosis are *Microsporum*, *Epidermophyton*, and *Trichophyton*. These fungi usually remain on the outer layer of the skin in healthy people and generate metabolic by-products that trigger an allergic and inflammatory response.

RISK FACTORS

Dermatophytosis can occur in healthy persons who come in direct or indirect contact with dermatophytes. Exposure to common transmission routes, such as shower stalls containing the species that causes athlete's foot, can increase the risk of infection. Preexisting injury to the skin, such as scars, burns, and excessive temperature and humidity, also can increase susceptibility to infection. Immunocompromised persons, such those with human immunodeficiency virus (HIV) infection or with acquired immunodeficiency syndrome (AIDS); persons with chronic disease; and persons who are sick or elderly are at increased risk of severe, subcutaneous, chronic, and recurrent dermatophytosis.

SYMPTOMS

The symptoms of dermatophytosis vary according to the type of fungus involved and the location of the infection. The different types of dermatophytosis include tinea barbae (ringworm of the beard), tinea capitis (blackdot ringworm, or ringworm of the scalp and hair), tinea corporis (ringworm of the body), tinea cruris (jock itch, or ringworm of the groin), tinea pedis (ringworm of the foot, or athlete's foot), tinea manuum (ringworm of the hands), and tinea unguium (ringworm of the nail). All cause inflammation that can be mild to severe, and many cause varying degrees of itchiness.

The common symptoms of athlete's foot, for example, include cracked, flaking, and peeling skin between the toes; red and sometimes blistering, oozing, or crusting skin; and itching, burning, or stinging sensations. Athlete's foot can also affect the toe nails, causing them to become discolored, thick, and crumbly.

SCREENING AND DIAGNOSIS

The diagnosis of dermatophytosis is made by the presence of fungi in skin, nail, and scalp scrapings seen under microscopy or by the isolation of fungi in culture. Information obtained during the patient history and physical examination, such as the appearance of the lesion, travel history, animal contacts, and race, are also helpful in diagnosing dermatophytosis.

TREATMENT AND THERAPY

The treatment of dermatophytosis varies according to the type of infection. Both topical and systemic antifungal agents are used. Antibiotics may also occasionally be necessary to treat secondary bacterial infections that occur as a result of scratching. In the case of tinea capitis, treatment often includes oral antifungal agents such as griseofulvin, terbinafine, and itraconazole, and a medicated shampoo to reduce the spread of infection.

PREVENTION AND OUTCOMES

Dermatophytosis can be transmitted by direct contact with infected people and animals and by indirect contact with organisms on exfoliated skin or hair found in the environment. Reducing or eliminating exposure to infected hosts and contaminated objects, such as combs, shoes, and locker room floors, can help prevent dermatophytosis. Prompt treatment can also help prevent the spread of the organisms to other parts of the body and to other people.

Diep Koly, M.D.

FURTHER READING

Berger, T. G. "Dermatologic Disorders." In *Current Medical Diagnosis and Treatment 2011*, edited by Stephen J. McPhee and Maxine A. Papadakis. 50th ed. New York: McGraw-Hill Medical, 2011.

Burns, Tony, et al., eds. *Rook's Textbook of Dermatology.* 8th ed. 4 vols. Hoboken, N.J.: Wiley-Blackwell, 2010.

Wolff, Klaus, and Richard Allen Johnson. *Fitzpatrick's Color Atlas and Synopsis of Clinical Dermatology.* 6th ed. New York: McGraw-Hill Medical, 2009.

WEB SITES OF INTEREST

American Academy of Dermatology
http://www.aad.org

Canadian Dermatology Association
http://www.dermatology.ca

Microbiology and Immunology On-line: Mycology
http://pathmicro.med.sc.edu/book/mycol-sta.htm

See also: Antifungal drugs: Types; Athlete's foot; *Candida*; Chromoblastomycosis; Dermatomycosis; *Epidermophyton*; Fungal infections; Fungi: Classification and types; Jock itch; *Malassezia*; *Microsporum*; Mycoses; Onychomycosis; *Piedraia*; Ringworm; Scabies; Skin infections; Tinea capitis; Tinea corporis; *Trichophyton*.

Developing countries and infectious disease

CATEGORY: Epidemiology

DEFINITION

Infectious diseases cause between 40 and 50 percent of all deaths in developing countries. For children younger than five years of age in these countries, infectious diseases cause almost 70 percent of deaths. Poverty, lack of education, inadequate or absent clean water and sanitation systems, crowded living conditions, unsafe sex, limited health care facilities, and lack of vaccines lead to the disproportionate burden of infectious diseases in the developing world. The chronic infectious disease-related disabilities suffered by adults in their prime working years leads to more poverty, continuing the cycle for the next generation.

In 2010, respiratory infections, including tuberculosis and pneumonias; diarrheal illnesses; malaria; and human immunodeficiency virus (HIV) contribute most to the infectious disease death toll in economically impoverished areas of the world; these and other infections, including the neglected tropical diseases, also contribute to substantial rates of chronic disease and disability.

MALARIA

Malaria is a parasitic disease transmitted by the bite of the female *Anopholes* mosquito, which is endemic to more than one hundred countries, including areas of Africa, Southeast Asia, Central America, South America, India, and parts of India and Oceania. Infection with any of the four species of *Plasmodium* causes fever, chills, and muscle aches, but the most dangerous kind of malaria, *falciparum* malaria, can cause serious disease in all ages. It results in significant mortality in children younger than five years of age.

The battle against malaria is fought on two fronts: with mosquito control and with effective antimalarial medication. In developing countries, there are many inherent difficulties with both methods. Mosquito control has historically been approached by widespread use of insecticides, including dichloro-diphenyl-trichloroethane (DDT). Because of worldwide bans on the use of DDT, other approaches have been taken, including very limited use of DDT.

The main mosquito-control tool in campaigns against malaria is the insecticide-treated bed net (ITN), which keeps mosquitoes away from people who are sleeping at night, the time when biting mosquitoes are most active. As of 2008, about 31 percent of African households in malarious areas had an ITN, and about 24 percent of children younger than the age of five slept under one. Several countries, including Rwanda, Tanzania, Eritrea, Sao Tome and Principe, Zambia, and Zanzibar, have achieved even higher ITN coverage, with a resultant 50 percent reduction in malaria cases and deaths in those areas. These significant improvements were aided by expanded international funding of malaria control programs to help meet the goal of the United Nations (U.N.) to decrease childhood mortality by two-thirds by 2015; this effort is part of the U.N. Millennium Development Goals program.

The other major goal of malaria control campaigns is the widespread availability and use of artemisinin drugs to treat malaria. Although older malaria drugs, such as quinine and chloroquine, are inexpensive and available in most developing countries, the malaria parasites have developed resistance to these drugs, rendering them ineffective in many areas of the world. Artemisinin drugs, though more expensive, are much more effective as long as they are used in combination with a second drug; otherwise, resistance will quickly develop. The use of these combination drugs is called artemisinin-based combined therapy (ACT). Because some signs of resistance to artemisinins have been reported in Southeast Asia, the World Health Organization is leading an initiative to carefully monitor malarious countries for the presence of artemisinin resistance and to contain it if found. International funding continues to go to agencies working on wider access to artemisinins.

HIV AND TUBERCULOSIS

More than thirty-three million people worldwide are infected with HIV, and a disproportionate number of them reside in developing countries. HIV is most prevalent in sub-Saharan Africa, and in that region, 75 percent of new infections are in teenage girls and in women. In Africa, HIV is transmitted nearly exclusively by heterosexual sex. Culturally and socially, females lack the ability to protect themselves from diseases transmitted by male sex partners or by rape, which is a widespread practice in some areas.

As more girls and women become infected, more newborns will become infected with maternally transmitted HIV. Transmission also occurs through breast milk, which is the only economical way to nourish infants in many impoverished areas. Decreasing the risk of mother-to-child HIV transmission is possible and requires only one dose of an antiretroviral drug during labor and one dose for the newborn to reduce risk by about 40 percent. More complicated and probably more effective regimes require girls and women to take multiple drugs during late pregnancy and until breast-feeding ends, but these practices have been difficult to implement in many areas. Maternal and paternal deaths from acquired immunodeficiency syndrome (AIDS), the advanced stage of HIV infection, have resulted in an enormous increase in the number of so-called AIDS orphans in many areas of Africa.

Outside Africa, growing areas of concern are in Asia, especially in Thailand, Cambodia, Myanmar, and Vietnam. Contributing to dramatically increased rates of HIV infection in these areas are the female sex-worker trade, a lack of condom use, stigmatization of HIV testing, and the transient population.

A surge in the number of new cases of tuberculosis (TB) has accompanied the HIV epidemic in both developed and undeveloped countries, but the latter are particularly unprepared to deal with increases in this serious disease. Some of these cases represent strains of TB that are resistant to many of the existing tuberculosis drugs. Asymptomatic TB infection is common in developing countries; when a healthy person inhales *Mycobacterium tuberculosis*, the body effectively walls off the infection in the lung, and the infected person does not become ill or contagious. As that person is infected with HIV, which gradually destroys the immune system, however, inactive TB becomes active, causing cough, fever, weight loss, and death if untreated. Coinfection with HIV and TB is a disabling, deadly combination.

Treatment of TB requires accurate diagnosis, which is often unavailable in undeveloped areas, and also requires long-term compliance with a daily medication regimen. Both factors contribute to the increase in new infections and incompletely treated infections. With the HIV epidemic in these areas, tuberculosis has become a priority in many disease-control programs.

International efforts to contain both the HIV epidemic and the upsurge in TB have focused on prevention, testing, and treatment. Prevention has focused on safer-sex practices and the empowering of girls and women to avoid sexually transmitted infection. HIV testing has increased but remains problematic because testing is stigmatized, and the stigma increases for persons whose test results are positive.

Progress has been made in the availability of antiretroviral drugs for HIV treatment, but 2008 data show that only 44 percent of those in need of these expensive drugs in sub-Saharan Africa received them and only 37 percent of those in need in Asia received them.

DIARRHEAL ILLNESS AND MEASLES

Diarrheal illness and its nearly inevitable complications of dehydration and malnutrition are large contributors to the disease burden in developing countries, particularly in children younger than age five years. While diarrhea is considered a minor, self-limiting illness in the developed world, in undeveloped countries, diarrhea kills more children each year than HIV, measles, and malaria combined. Diarrhea can be caused by many types of viruses, bacteria, and protozoa, but it is mostly a result of impure drinking water and fecal contamination of the living environment.

Even with access to decent sanitation and clean water, a child who does contract a diarrheal illness in a developing country is much less likely to have access to simple treatments that could save his or her life. One simple diarrhea treatment strategy that can save lives includes giving an ill child oral rehydration with a special salt solution (often referred to as ORS) and a zinc supplement, while continuing to feed the child to avoid malnutrition. WHO and other public health entities have also launched social marketing campaigns encouraging stigmatization of defecation in public (a significant problem in India, in particular) and encouraging handwashing with soap to avoid infection.

Immunization with rotavirus vaccine is another strategy that can decrease diarrhea in children, but this vaccine has yet to be included in immunization programs in developing countries. Better access to measles vaccine might also reduce the number of deaths from childhood diarrhea, as diarrhea is often a debilitating symptom of measles in very young children.

Measles is another childhood disease that affects children in undeveloped countries significantly more than it does in developed countries, primarily because, in developed countries, measles vaccination is routine at age twelve to fifteen months (with a booster at school entrance in most developed countries). Vaccination of young children in some areas of Africa and Asia has been limited.

The Measles Initiative, a consortium including the American Red Cross, the United Nations Foundation, the Centers for Disease Control and Prevention (CDC), United Nations Children's Fund (UNICEF), and WHO, had committed to reducing measles worldwide by 90 percent by 2010. Since 2001, the initiative has helped provide six hundred million doses of measles vaccine. As a result, measles cases decreased by 74 percent by 2008. The biggest impact has been in Africa, with an 89 percent reduction in measles deaths, and in the eastern Mediterranean region, which includes Afghanistan, Iran, Iraq, Pakistan, and Somalia.

For children not immunized and who are infected with measles, the disease can manifest as a mild respiratory infection, or it can be a serious illness. Serious complications of the infection include pneumonia, ear infection, blood abnormalities, and encephalitis (inflammation of the brain), which can cause permanent neurologic effects or death.

NEGLECTED TROPICAL DISEASES

Neglected tropical diseases (NTDs) infect billions of people worldwide, yet they are often unknown in developed countries. As a result, less funding has gone to NTDs for disease control or elimination programs. In the later decades of the twentieth century, the attention to NTDs increased somewhat. The NTDs contributing the largest burden of disease are lymphatic filariasis (elephantiasis), onchocerciasis (river blindness), schistosomiasis, soil-transmitted helminth (worm) infections, and trachoma.

Lymphatic filariasis (LF) is a disfiguring disease caused by thin, microscopic worms and is transmitted by mosquito bites. The tiny worms live in and damage the lymphatic system and, after long periods of time, can result in severe swelling of the arms, legs, breasts, and genitalia, leading to substantial disability. When chronically swollen areas become thickened and hardened, the resultant condition is referred to as elephantiasis. LF affects a minimum of one billion people in eighty-three countries, primarily in tropical and subtropical areas of India, Indonesia, Bangladesh, and Nigeria. LF can be treated with annual doses of inexpensive antiparasitic drugs, including albendazole and diethylcarbazine, which do not kill adult worms in the body but kill the immature worms that can transmit the disease person-to-person through mosquito bites and thereby interrupt the cycle of transmission.

Onchocerciasis, also known as river blindness, is transmitted from person to person by the bite of a black fly; the disease affects eighteen million people in thirty-five countries. The disease causes skin rashes with intense itching and eye damage that can result in blindness. An annual dose of the drug ivermectin can prevent the disease.

Schistosomiasis affects two hundred million people in seventy-four countries. It is caused by a parasite called a fluke, which lives in fresh-water snails and causes several different syndromes in humans; these syndromes can result in kidney, bladder, and liver disease, and death.

Soil-transmitted helminths (worms) cause malnutrition, vitamin deficiencies, anemia, and intestinal obstruction in more than one billion people world-wide, with many more persons at risk. It is easily treated by administration of mebendazole or albendazole twice yearly. Partners for Parasite Control, a WHO group, is working toward the goal of treating 75 percent of all at-risk children with these drugs.

Trachoma is a bacterial infection of the eye caused by *Chlamydia trachomatis*, which causes scarring of the lining of the upper eyelid and leads to blindness. It is spread from person to person by direct contact and affects more than eighty-four million people in fifty-five countries. The International Trachoma Initiative is dedicated to eradicating this disease by using a treatment and prevention strategy known as SAFE: surgery, antibiotics, face-washing hygiene, and environmental changes.

IMPACT

Infectious diseases in developing countries remain a huge global problem. Recognizing their responsibility to respond in a humanitarian way, many of the wealthy nations of the world are committed to finding solutions to these diseases. WHO, the Global Health Council, UNICEF, and other international organizations are working toward disease eradication, with polio and measles the most likely initial targets for eradication. National efforts, such as the U.S. President's Emergency Plan for AIDS Relief (PEPFAR), which was reauthorized in 2008, will continue to pump economic aid to programs that are researching ways to control HIV/AIDS, tuberculosis, malaria, and other diseases around the world.

Lindsey Marcellin, M.D., M.P.H.

FURTHER READING

Abdool, Karim S. S., et al. "HIV Infection and Tuberculosis in South Africa: An Urgent Need to Escalate the Public Health Response." *The Lancet* 374 (September 12, 2009): 921-933. Also available at http://www.ncbi.nlm.nih.gov/pmc/articles/pmc2803032. A study of the public health issues surrounding HIV infection and tuberculosis in South Africa.

Batterman S., et al. "Sustainable Control of Water-Related Infectious Diseases: A Review and Proposal for Interdisciplinary Health-Based Systems Research." *Environmental Health Perspectives* 117, no. 7 (July, 2009): 1023-1032. Also available at http://www.ncbi.nlm.nih.gov/pmc/articles/ PMC2717125. Focuses on the possibilities of controlling waterborne infectious diseases through effective interdisciplinary research.

Greenwood, Brian M., et al. "Malaria: Progress, Perils, and Prospects for Eradication." *Journal of Clinical Investigation* 118, no. 4 (2008): 1266-1276. Also available at http://www.ncbi.nlm.nih.gov/pmc/articles/pmc2276780. Examines the state of malaria and its eradication.

Packard, Randall M. *The Making of a Tropical Disease: A Short History of Malaria.* Baltimore: Johns Hopkins University Press, 2007. Discusses the many reasons that malaria continues to flourish in some parts of the world, despite being eradicated in others.

Plotkin, Stanley A., Walter A. Orenstein, and Paul A. Offit. *Vaccines.* 5th ed. Philadelphia: Saunders/Elsevier, 2008. An excellent description of the role of vaccines in the prevention of disease. Begins with a history of immunization practices. Each chapter deals with a specific disease and the role and history of vaccine production in disease prevention.

Santosham, Mathuram, et al. "Progress and Barriers for the Control of Diarrhoeal Disease." *The Lancet* 376 (July 3, 2010): 63-67. Argues for the revitalization of efforts to control diarrhea disease mortality rates worldwide.

WEB SITES OF INTEREST

Carter Center
http://www.cartercenter.org/health

Emerging and Reemerging Infectious Diseases Resource Center
http://www.medscape.com/resource/infections

Global Health Council
http://www.globalhealth.org/infectious_diseases

Malaria Foundation International
http://www.malaria.org

Partners for Parasite Control
http://www.who.int/wormcontrol

United Nations Development Programme
http://www.undp.org/mdg

See also: AIDS; Carriers; Cholera; Disease eradication campaigns; Emerging and reemerging infectious diseases; Epidemics and pandemics: Causes and management; Epidemics and pandemics: History; Epidemiology; Globalization and infectious disease; HIV; Hosts; Malaria; Mosquitoes and infectious disease; Outbreaks; Parasitic diseases; Public health; Sleeping nets; Social effects of infectious disease; Tropical medicine; Tuberculosis (TB); World Health Organization (WHO); Worm infections.

Diagnosis of bacterial infections

CATEGORY: Diagnosis

ALSO KNOWN AS: Bacteria identification, diagnostic testing

DEFINITION

Diagnosis is the process of identifying a disease by its symptoms and identifying the causes of disease. Bacterial diagnosis is the determination of disease caused by bacteria.

BACTERIA IN THE BODY

The human body is inhabited by hundreds of different species of bacteria that make up millions of individual bacteria in the body. Most of these microscopic organisms are harmless, and some are beneficial and help the body function at its best.

However, some bacteria, called pathogens, are harmful and cause illness. Pathogens enter the body usually through the respiratory system. Once inside the body, they multiply, resulting in a bacterial infection. Symptoms of bacterial infection vary according to the type of bacterium and according to where the infection forms. To treat symptoms, and cure the illness, health care providers need first to identify the cause of a disease; they can then diagnose the disease. Pathologists, doctors who specialize in diagnosing diseases, use a number of tests to arrive at a diagnosis of a bacterial infection.

COLLECTING SPECIMENS

The first steps in diagnostic testing for bacterial infection involve collecting samples, or specimens. Typical test specimens include fluids collected from a person's blood, throat, lungs, urine, or spine. Pathologists prescribe a four-step process for collecting specimens of suspected pathogens. This process includes the following:

Collect the right specimen. Doctors collect specimens for diagnostic testing based on the person's symptoms. For example, to test for lung or bronchial diseases such as pneumonia or bronchitis that are caused by bacteria, doctors need to collect secretions from the lungs, called sputum, that the person coughs up into a sterile cup.

Collect the specimen properly. Collecting a specimen from the throat, for example, requires the doctor or nurse to use a throat swab to collect tissue by inserting the swab deep enough into the throat to make the person gag.

Package and label the specimen correctly. Secure packaging prevents contamination of the specimen, and accurate labeling ensures appropriate testing.

Transport and store the specimen carefully. Controlled transport and storage prevent possible harmful bacteria from escaping and endangering public health.

TESTING PROTOCOLS

Medical professionals test for contagious, or communicable, diseases in a variety of settings. Portable assay machines allow doctors to perform quick, simple tests almost anywhere, including a person's home. Most tests, however, are done in clinic and hospital laboratories or in independent labs, known as clinical reference labs.

To ensure the highest standards for professionalism and safety, all labs must be certified and licensed by various medical, professional, and government organizations or boards. One of the main certifications is the Clinical Laboratory Improvement Amendments, administered by the Centers for Disease Control and Prevention, an agency of the U.S. Department of Health and Human Services.

Medical professionals who perform the tests must also be properly trained and certified. Pathologists and medical laboratory technologists, also known as technicians or clinical laboratory scientists, receive their specialized training from accredited medical education programs. They also are required to maintain their certification through continuing education and periodic recertification.

TYPES OF DIAGNOSTIC TESTS

Culturing is the standard method for testing the presence and type of bacteria in the lab. A technologist places the specimen on a special plate—called a cell culture plate, or, more often, a petri dish—that

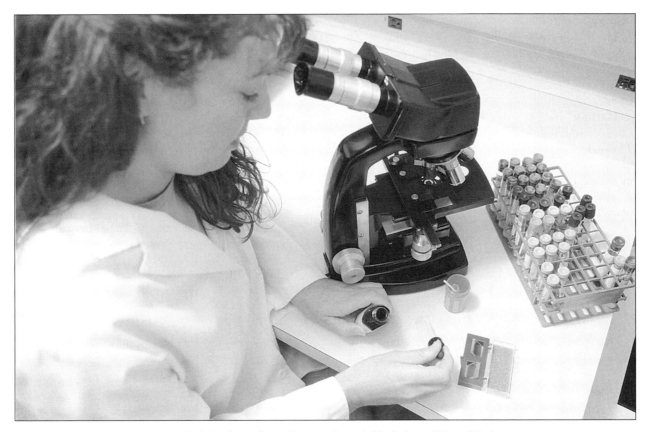

A laboratory technician examines biological samples to diagnose bacterial infections. (PhotoDisc)

has been treated with a special substance. This substance, called a culture medium, is a mixture of chemicals, including nutrients, that encourages the bacteria to multiply. If they do not multiply, that is, if no bacteria are present in the specimen, the technologist scores the test "negative." If they do multiply, the bacteria are then viewed under a microscope or analyzed through chemical testing for the type and numbers. Pathologists can identify specific bacteria based on certain characteristics, such as shape, staining (the color they turn after a certain chemical treatment), and whether they thrive with or without oxygen.

One of the first steps in testing is to determine if the infection is in fact caused by a bacterium. An infection caused by a virus, which is another type of disease-causing microorganism, does not respond to the same treatment as a bacterial infection. (Antibiotics kill or the stop the growth of bacteria but have no effect on viruses.) The problem for patients and doctors is that often the symptoms of both types of infec-

tions are similar. Bacterial cultures, and blood tests, help differentiate bacterial infections from viral infections.

The blood test, known as a complete blood count, or CBC, yields a count of white blood cells, red blood cells, and platelets in a patient's blood. The test can help determine the presence of a bacterial infection. A high white-blood-cell count indicates a bacterial infection.

Cultures help determine the type of bacterial infection. A blood culture shows if bacteria have entered the bloodstream and reveals such diseases as osteomyelitis (a bone infection) and sepsis (a serious, life-threatening blood infection). A throat culture checks only for *Streptococcus*, the pathogen that causes strep throat, rheumatic fever, and toxic shock syndrome. A sputum culture detects bacterial infections of the lungs or breathing passages and infections such as pneumonia, tuberculosis, and sinusitis. A urine culture is most commonly done to identify the cause of urinary tract infections. A spinal culture detects the origin of infections of the brain or nervous system, infections such as meningitis and brain abscess, a swelling of the brain.

IMPACT

Harmful bacteria that invade the human body cause many dangerous, debilitating, and fatal diseases. Through diagnostic testing for bacterial infections, medical professionals can pinpoint the specific species of bacteria and its numbers. Once pathologists identify the pathogen, doctors devise the proper treatment plans for their patients.

Wendell Anderson, B.A.

FURTHER READING

Beers, Mark H., et al. *The Merck Manual of Diagnosis and Therapy.* 18th ed. Whitehouse Station, N.J.: Merck Research Laboratories, 2006. Published since 1899, this classic work is well indexed and easy to use. Discussions are usually brief but thorough.

Cimolai, Nevio, ed. *Laboratory Diagnosis of Bacterial Infections.* New York: Marcel Dekker, 2001. A large, comprehensive desk reference covering the detection, epidemiology, and treatment of bacterial infections.

Professional Guide to Diseases. 9th ed. Philadelphia: Wolters Kluwer Health/Lippincott Williams & Wilkins, 2009. An encyclopedic guide to common diseases for health professionals. Includes descriptions, diagnoses, and treatments.

Richardson, Harold, and Fiona Smaill. "Medical Microbiology." *British Medical Journal* 317 (1998): 1060. A review of studies of diagnostic testing methods.

WEB SITES OF INTEREST

International Classification of Diseases
http://www.cdc.gov/nchs/icd/icd10cm.htm

Lab Tests Online
http://www.labtestsonline.org

See also: Acid-fastness; Bacteria: Classification and types; Bacteria: Structure and growth; Bacterial infections; Bacteriology; Biochemical tests; Epidemiology; Gram staining; Immunoassay; Microbiology; Microscopy; Pathogenicity; Polymerase chain reaction (PCR) method; Serology; Virulence.

Diagnosis of fungal infections

CATEGORY: Diagnosis

DEFINITION

The approach to the diagnosis of a fungal infection depends on the complexity of the infection and on the health status of the infected person. Noninvasive infections can usually be diagnosed based on a physical examination. Invasive or systemic infections require laboratory tests to confirm the diagnosis.

Key Terms: Fungal Infections

- *Filamentous fungus.* A threadlike fungus (mold)

- *Fungus.* A nonphotosynthetic, plantlike organism

- *Hyphae.* Thin tubes in fungi that secure food and grow, expanding the size of molds and yeasts

- *Mold.* A filamentous fungus that grows by branching and extending

- *Mycelium.* A collection of threadlike fungal strands (hyphae) making up the thallus, or nonreproductive portion, of a fungus

- *Mycology.* The study of fungi

- *Mycosis.* A disease of humans, plants, or animals caused by a fungus; the prefix myco- means "fungus"

- *Mycotoxin.* A poison released by fungi

- *Pleomorphic fungus.* A fungus whose morphology changes markedly from one phase of its life cycle to another, or according to changes in environmental conditions

- *Tinea.* A medical term for fungal skin diseases, such as ringworm and athlete's foot, caused by a variety of fungi

- *Yeast.* A unicellular fungus that grows by budding off smaller cells from the parent cell; yeasts belong to several different groups of fungi, and some fungi are capable of growing either as a yeast or as a filamentous fungus

---

NONINVASIVE INFECTIONS

Noninvasive infections include superficial and cutaneous infections. Superficial infections affect hair, nails, and the surface layer of the skin. Cutaneous infections affect living cells of the inner layers of the skin and mucous membranes. The location, appearance, and other distinctive signs and symptoms of an infection are used to obtain a diagnosis. Through diagnosis, one needs to distinguish between fungal infections (and similar infections caused by bacteria) and noninfectious inflammatory skin disorders, such as contact dermatitis and psoriasis. Some fungal infections, such as athlete's foot (tinea pedis) and jock itch (tinea cruris), are identified by where they occur. Common signs and symptoms of noninvasive fungal infections include characteristic itchy, red, scaly, and peeling areas of skin; brittle, thickened, or deformed nails (tinea unguium); brittle hair (tinea capitis); and vaginal itching and discharge (vaginal candidiasis).

The presence of pathogenic fungi is confirmed by studying a sample of infected matter under a light microscope. Typical samples, depending on the site of infection, are skin scrapings, nail or hair clippings, vaginal discharge, and sputum. Spores and yeasts that cause noninvasive infections are relatively large microorganisms that will be apparent on standard magnification. Staining enhances the image. A KOH preparation (a 10 percent potassium hydroxide solution) dissolves nonfungal components and distinguishes the rigid walls and other morphologic characteristics of fungi. A calcofluor white stain is more sensitive than a KOH prep. It binds to fungi and illuminates them under ultraviolet light. Both staining methods are easy to perform and provide rapid results. However, neither identifies specific fungi.

INVASIVE AND SYSTEMIC INFECTIONS

Invasive (subcutaneous) and systemic infections can cause a variety of symptoms, depending on the part of the body affected. Lung infections may cause flulike symptoms such as coughing, fever, muscle ache, headache, and rash. Blood infections (sepsis) may cause chills, fever, nausea, and rapid heartbeat. Central nervous system infections (meningitis) may cause severe, persistent headache, stiff neck, and sensitivity to light. Systemic infections may cause night sweating, chest pain, weight loss, and enlarged lymph nodes. These symptoms are nonspecific to fungal infections.

As for superficial infections, obtaining a fungal stain is usually the first step in confirming fungal involvement. Some invasive fungal pathogens (for ex-

ample, those that cause histoplasmosis) are too small or too few (for example, those that cause cryptococcosis) to be observed under light microscopy. For all invasive and systemic infections, it is essential to isolate the specific pathogen to confirm the diagnosis and to direct treatment.

To identify the specific pathogen, fungi obtained by sampling are grown in a culture media that inhibits bacterial growth while encouraging fungal growth. Depending on the location of the presenting symptoms, samples are taken from the blood, the lungs, a tissue biopsy, or cerebrospinal fluid. Care must be taken to avoid contamination. For example, when *Aspergillosis* species are suspected, it may be necessary to perform a biopsy of lung tissue, lung aspiration, or bronchoalveolar lavage to avoid contamination.

The most commonly used medium for culturing fungi is Sabouraud agar. Most bacteria associated with human infections do not grow or grow poorly in this medium. Because many fungi are slow-growing, it may take several weeks to obtain sufficient fungi to confirm a diagnosis.

As a follow-up to a culture, a susceptibility test can help in selecting the most effective antifungal or antifungals for addressing specific infections. Antigen or antibody testing of blood, cerebrospinal, or other body fluids may be ordered, especially if the infection is systemic or at risk of becoming so. Antigen testing detects proteins associated with a specific fungus for which a test has been developed. Effective antigen tests have been developed for the detection of the pathogens causing histoplasmosis and coccidioidomycosis. Antibody testing detects the immune response to specific fungi. Antibody testing is not effective for detecting aspergillosis, as healthy persons also have antibodies against *Aspergillus*.

An AFB (acid-fast bacillus) smear and culture may be ordered to rule out tuberculosis or infection caused by nontuberculous mycobacteria. If a fungal mass is suspected, an imaging scan, such as an X ray of the lungs, may be ordered.

IMPACT

In immunocompromised persons or in persons with an underlying disease, care must be taken to identify the specific pathogen or pathogens, even with noninvasive infections. Such care applies to all persons who present with an invasive or systemic infection. Knowing what fungal pathogen is causing the infection confirms the diagnosis and is instrumental in directing treatment.

Ernest Kohlmetz, M.A.

FURTHER READING

Chandrasekar, Pranatharthi. "Diagnostic Challenges and Recent Advances in the Early Management of Invasive Fungal Infections." *European Journal of Haematology* 84 (2009): 281-290.

Gladwin, Mark, and Bill Trattler. *Clinical Microbiology Made Ridiculously Simple.* 4th ed. Miami: MedMaster, 2007.

Richardson, Malcolm D., and Elizabeth M. Johnson. *The Pocket Guide to Fungal Infection.* 2d ed. Malden, Mass.: Blackwell, 2006.

Ryan, Kenneth J., and George Ray. *Sherris Medical Microbiology: An Introduction to Infectious Diseases.* 5th ed. New York: McGraw-Hill Medical, 2010.

Webster, John, and Roland Weber. *Introduction to Fungi.* New York: Cambridge University Press, 2007.

WEB SITES OF INTEREST

Centers for Disease Control and Prevention, Division of Foodborne, Bacterial, and Mycotic Diseases
http://www.cdc.gov/nczved/divisions/dfbmd

Lab Tests Online
http://www.labtestsonline.org

Microbiology and Immunology On-line: Mycology
http://pathmicro.med.sc.edu/book/mycol-sta.htm

Systematic Mycology and Microbiology Laboratory
http://www.ars.usda.gov

See also: Airborne illness and disease; Antifungal drugs: Mechanisms of action; Antifungal drugs: Types; Biochemical tests; Fungal infections; Fungi: Classification and types; Fungi: Structure and growth; Immune response to fungal infections; Microbiology; Microscopy; Pathogens; Treatment of fungal infections; Virulence.

Diagnosis of parasitic diseases

CATEGORY: Diagnosis

DEFINITION

Parasites, including helminths and ectoparasites, are organisms that depend on a host organism for their food source and survival. This relationship does not benefit the host and often leads to infection. Helminths of medical importance comprise roundworms, tapeworms, and flukes. Ectoparasites are arthropods that infest the skin of humans, from which they derive sustenance. The most significant ectoparasites are mites, lice, and fleas.

HELMINTHS

Diagnosis of parasitic infections begins with a clinical evaluation of symptoms presented by the affected person; epidemiology (such as the geographical region in which the person lives or has traveled, and his or her exposure to contaminated food and water) is considered too. Most helminths infect the intestinal tract, so detection and differentiation is usually accomplished by preparing smears of fecal samples and examining them under a microscope.

Microscopic examinations are unsatisfactory under conditions of low parasitic infection, if the person does not exhibit symptoms, or if the parasite cannot be identified. In these instances, serology tests are more sensitive and specific. These tests include enzyme-linked immunoabsorbent assay (ELISA), hemagglutination test, and immunoblot. Newer molecular methods use nucleic-acid-based technologies to diagnose parasitic infections. The polymerase chain reaction (PCR) is the primary technology used. The primary advantages of molecular methods are speed and sensitivity. Although much promising research has been done, the methods have not progressed to the stage of routine clinical use.

Roundworm (nematode) infections can be confined to the intestines, or they can invade other tissues, depending on the species. Pinworms (*Enterobius vermicularis*) commonly infect children in the United States. Diagnosis is accomplished by patting a sticky tape in the anal folds of the child and examining for ova.

Strongyloidiasis (*Strongyloides stercoralis*), or threadworm, infection occurs when feces contaminated with larva come in contact with and penetrate the skin. Examination of feces of infected persons for larva is a confirmed diagnosis. Larva migrans are diseases in which larva of various nematode parasites normally infecting dogs or cats migrate in human tissues as an unnatural host. Cutaneous larva migrans is caused by a hookworm that produces a winding, threadlike trail of inflammation in the epidermis. Discovery of larva in a skin biopsy confirms diagnosis. Visceral larva migrans is caused by ingestion of soil or food contaminated with *Toxocara* roundworm ova. The disease can be confirmed by liver biopsy or serologic tests. Larva migrans is usually self-limiting (it goes away on its own).

Trichinosis (*Trichinella spiralis*) is caused by eating inadequately cooked pork. Infection can cause a painful burrowing of larvae in muscle tissue. Larvae or cysts found in a muscle biopsy is a confirmed diagnosis. Large roundworm (*Ascaris lumbricoides*) infection may result after handling infected pets or soil and then not washing one's hands properly (or at all). Eggs can be found in the feces.

Tapeworms (cestodes) can infect the intestines or other parts of the body. Humans can be infected by consuming raw or undercooked meats from animals infected with beef (*Taenia saginata*), pork (*T. solium*), or fish (*Diphyllobothrium latum*) tapeworms. Tapeworms, which attach to the intestinal wall, contain a chain of segments (proglottids) that grow and mature. The segments break off and become part of the stool. Examining segments obtained from the stool allows differentiation between the three tapeworm species. Infection with *Echinococcus granulosis* tapeworm is largely limited to shepherds and their families, with dogs or other canines acting as intermediates. The infection can be diagnosed by the presence of cysts in the liver, which are detected by ultrasound scans or computerized tomography.

Flukes (trematodes) can be significant parasites in many world regions, but they are not common in the United States. Schistosomiasis is a major debilitating disease caused primarily by three species of *Schistosoma*. The parasite enters the skin of persons who drink or bathe in polluted water and migrates to the liver and other internal organs. Eggs are found in the stool or urine. Clonorchiasis is a liver fluke particularly significant in Asia. Eggs are found in the feces or the duodenal contents.

ECTOPARASITES

Scabies is caused by the itch mite *Sarcoptes scabiei*. The mite burrows in the external layer of skin (stratum corneum) to deposit its eggs. To diagnose scabies, a clinician takes scrapings of burrows and then examines them microscopically for the presence of mites or

their eggs. Burrows appear as dark wavy lines in the epidermis, but they can be difficult to find because they may be obscured by secondary lesions.

Lice infestations (pediculosis) feed on human blood and can be caused by three species. *Pediculus humanus capitis* affects the head, *P. h. corporis* affects the body, and *Phthirus pubis* affects the genital area. Diagnosis of head lice is confirmed by examining the scalp with a magnifying glass. Ova (nits) are found fixed to the hair shafts. Body lice are most readily found in clothing worn next to the skin. Pubic lice are difficult to find, but may be present as brown spots on the undergarments. *Tunga penetrans* (sand flea) is an important parasite of tropical regions.

Insects that cause bites and stings, such as bed bugs, mosquitoes, spiders, bees, ticks, and ants, do not invade the body and are, therefore, not considered here. Insects can, however, act as vectors that transmit protozoan parasites.

IMPACT

Parasitic infections are generally much less of a problem in the developed world than in tropical and subtropical areas. However, travelers to developing nations should be fully aware of the possibility of contracting a parasitic disease and should take the necessary precautions. The importation of foods from endemic regions represents a potential source of infection, particularly for produce that is eaten raw.

Many organizations around the world are involved in programs to reduce the incidence of parasitic infections in developing countries. These organizations are working in diagnostic research and applications.

David A. Olle, M.S.

FURTHER READING

Fritsche, Thomas, and Rangaraj Selvarangan. "Medical Parasitology." In *Henry's Clinical Diagnosis and Management by Laboratory Methods*, edited by Richard A. McPherson, Matthew R. Pincus, and John B. Henry. 22d ed. Philadelphia: Saunders/Elsevier, 2011. A detailed discussion of parasitic infections, with illustrations of parasites' life cycles and characteristics.

Garcia, Lynne Shore. *Diagnostic Medical Parasitology.* 5th ed. Washington, D.C.: ASM Press, 2007. A good reference source on the diagnostic aspects of parasitology.

Weller, P. F., and T. B. Nutman. "Intestinal Nematodes."

In *Harrison's Principles of Internal Medicine*, edited by Anthony Fauci et al. 17th ed. New York: McGraw-Hill, 2008. A good clinical reference on intestinal nematodes, including roundworms.

WEB SITES OF INTEREST

Centers for Disease Control and Prevention
http://www.cdc.gov/parasites

Microbiology and Immunology On-line: Parasitology
http://pathmicro.med.sc.edu/book/parasit-sta.htm

Neglected Tropical Diseases Coalition
http://www.neglectedtropicaldiseases.org

Partners for Parasite Control
http://www.who.int/wormcontrol

See also: Blood-borne illness and disease; Developing countries and infectious disease; Epidemiology; Fecal-oral route of transmission; Flukes; Food-borne illness and disease; Hosts; Intestinal and stomach infections; Oral transmission; Parasites: Classification and types; Parasitic diseases; Pinworms; Roundworms; Scabies; Tapeworms; Tropical medicine; Vectors and vector control; Waterborne illness and disease; Worm infections.

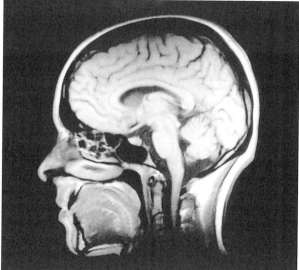

Diagnosis of prion diseases includes the use of magnetic resonance imaging, which provides detailed images of soft tissues, including those of the brain. (Digital Stock)

Diagnosis of prion diseases

CATEGORY: Diagnosis

DEFINITION

Prion diseases diseases are rare and fatal degenerative brain disorders caused by an abnormal version of a protein in the brain. This protein aggregates and forms visible "holes" that show a spongy appearance seen through a microscope; hence, the name "spongiform encephalopathies." Approximately 10 to 15 percent of prion diseases are genetically transmissible, whereas the remainder occur from unknown risk factors or are acquired through infection with prions.

The word "prion" was termed in 1982 by neurologist and biochemist Stanley B. Prusiner, who won the Nobel Prize in Physiology or Medicine in 1997. The term is derived from the words "protein" and "infectious."

TYPES

Prion diseases occur in both human and non-human animals. The most common human diseases are Creutzfeldt-Jakob disease (CJD), kuru, fatal familial insomnia, and Gerstmann-Sträussler-Scheinker syndrome. Animal prion diseases include bovine spongiform encephalopathy (mad cow disease), scrapie, chronic wasting disease, and transmissible mink encephalopathy. Human prion diseases are classified into three categories: sporadic, genetic, and acquired.

CJD, the most common of the human prion diseases, usually occurs spontaneously and most often in persons age fifty years and older. Other human prion diseases are genetic in nature and can be inherited. Acquired prion diseases include the variant form of CJD, which is caused by eating beef infected with a prion disease. Kuru is a human prion disease that was spread by ritualistic cannibalism among New Guineans until the 1950's.

SYMPTOMS

Symptoms of the various prion diseases vary, but generally include personality changes, psychiatric problems such as depression, lack of coordination, and an unsteady gait. Other symptoms include jerking or spontaneous movements called myoclonus, unusual sensations, insomnia, confusion, and memory problems. As disease progresses, patients may exhibit mental impairment and loss of speech or movements.

POSTMORTEM DIAGNOSIS

Because prion diseases tend to progress rapidly and may cause death within a few months of severe symptoms, many diagnoses may not be determined until postmortem examination. This exam is called a conformation-dependent immunoassay (CDI). CDI tests identify prions in human brain tissue by using highly specific antibodies that bind to all disease-causing prions in the brain. Immunohistochemistry testing measures the prion proteins that are resistant to an enzyme called protease. Protease-resistant prions are abnormal, usually infectious, and will cause a disease state. The presence of these prions in the brain leads to a diagnosis of a prion disease.

GENETIC TESTING

Another approach to diagnosing a subset of prion diseases is genetic testing. Only one gene is known to be associated with prion diseases. The gene, PRNP, encodes for a protein called prion protein, which is active in the brain and other tissues of the body. The exact function of PRNP is not known, but it is thought to be involved in the transport of charged copper ions into cells. This protein may also be involved in cell signaling, cell protection, and the formation of synapses, in which cell to cell communication occurs.

More than thirty mutations of the PRNP gene have been identified in people with prion diseases (mutations in this gene cause disease). Genetic tests have been established to identify the mutations known for prion diseases by sequence analysis of the entire coding region and by targeted mutation analysis. These test methods, however, will not detect all disease-causing mutations, so the absence of a PRNP mutation does not rule out the diagnosis of a prion disease.

CLINICAL FEATURES AND NEUROPATHOLOGIC FINDINGS

Prion disease should be considered when symptoms include dementia, neurologic signs, psychiatric problems, lack of coordination of movements, weakness, or seizures. The next step is to identify neuro-

pathologic characteristics of prion diseases. Such findings include spongiform degeneration and astrogliosis (an increase of the number of astrocytes as nearby neurons die), distributed diffusely throughout the cortex and deep nuclei of the brain. Amyloid plaques may also be present, in which antiprion protein antibodies will bind.

BRAIN IMAGING

Brain imaging through electroencephalogram (EEG) and examination of cerebrospinal fluid (CSF) may help support the diagnosis, but these alone are not enough to diagnose a prion disorder. These methods are often used to diagnose other disorders of the central nervous system and may not be reliable with genetic forms of prion diseases. However, EEG findings that show sharp periodic wave complexes, in which bursts of waves are seen every one-half to two seconds, may suggest a prion diagnosis. Prion diseases also show a characteristic magnetic resonance imaging (MRI) pattern, with diffusion weighted MRI, of mild to moderate generalized atrophy and hyperintensity of the basal ganglia. Patients with prion diseases often show a 10 percent increase in CSF protein concentration, which may be the result of the release of normal neuronal protein (14-3-3 protein) into the CSF as neurons die; however, this phenomenon is not specific to prion diseases.

IMPACT

Human prion diseases are rare. The worldwide incidence of genetic mutations and sporadic forms of disease is approximately one case per million humans. In the United States, there are approximately three hundred new human cases of prion diseases per year. About 10 percent of cases involve a genetic mutation.

The future for prion-disease diagnosis includes devising tools that will permit widespread screening for carriers of the infectious agent that causes the disease. This attempt at presymptomatic testing would signal who should receive treatment and, thus, would help prevent prions from spreading within the brain or from reaching the central nervous system that triggers disease.

Susan M. Zneimer, Ph.D., FACMG

FURTHER READING

Brown, David R., ed. *Neurodegeneration and Prion Disease.* New York: Springer, 2005.

Herbst, A., et al. "Prion Disease Diagnosis by Proteomic Profiling." *Journal of Proteome Research* 8 (2009): 1030-1036.

Mastrianni, James A. "Genetic Prion Diseases." *Gene Reviews* (March 27, 2003). National Center for Biotechnology Information. Available at http://www.ncbi.nlm.nih.gov/bookshelf.

Prusiner, Stanley B. "The Prion Diseases." *Scientific American* 272, no. 1 (January, 1995): 48-57.

_____, ed. *Prion Biology and Diseases.* 2d ed. Cold Spring Harbor, N.Y.: Cold Spring Harbor Laboratory Press, 2004.

Safar, J. R., et al. "Diagnosis of Human Prion Disease." *Proceedings of the National Academy of Science* 102 (2005): 3501-3506.

WEB SITES OF INTEREST

Creutzfeldt-Jakob Disease Foundation
http://www.cjdfoundation.org

Genetic and Rare Diseases Information Center
http://rarediseases.info.nih.gov/gard

National Institute of Allergy and Infectious Diseases
http://www.niaid.nih.gov/topics/prion

National Institute of Neurological Disorders and Stroke, Transmissible Spongiform Encephalopathies Information Page
http://www.ninds.nih.gov/disorders/tse

National Organization for Rare Disorders
http://www.rarediseases.org

See also: Creutzfeldt-Jakob disease; Encephalitis; Fatal familial insomnia; Gerstmann-Sträussler-Scheinker syndrome; Guillain-Barré syndrome; Kuru; Prion diseases; Prions; Sleeping sickness; Subacute sclerosing panencephalitis; Variant Creutzfeldt-Jakob disease.

Diagnosis of protozoan diseases

CATEGORY: Diagnosis

DEFINITION

Protozoa are members of an informal grouping of simple, usually unicellular, heterotrophic phyla that share similar characteristics. Some protozoa are pathogenic.

DIAGNOSTIC TOOLS

Diagnosis of protozoan infections begins with a clinical evaluation of symptoms presented by the affected person; epidemiology (such as the geographical region in which the person lives or has traveled, and his or her exposure to contaminated food and water) is considered too. Definitive diagnosis has traditionally been accomplished by microscopically detecting the protozoa or their eggs in stool, blood, or tissue samples.

Immunodiagnostic (serologic) tests can be valuable in those situations in which insufficient protozoa or eggs are available for detection. Similar to other infecting organisms, protozoa have unique proteins known as antigens on or in the organism. These antigens stimulate the body to produce specialized antibodies to react against the parasite. Serologic tests have been developed to detect either antigens or antibodies. These tests include the enzyme-linked immunoabsorbent assay (ELISA), hemagglutination, immunofluorescence, immunoblot, and rapid diagnostic tests.

Molecular methods use nucleic-acid-based technologies to diagnose protozoan infections. The polymerase chain reaction (PCR) is the primary technology used. The primary advantages of molecular methods are speed and sensitivity. Although much promising research has been done, the methods have not progressed to the stage of routine clinical use.

INTESTINAL PROTOZOANS

In the United States, the most common protozoan parasites that infect the intestinal tract include *Giardia lamblia* (giardiasis) and *Cryptosporidium parvum* (cryptosporidiosis). *Cyclospora cayetanensis*, which causes cyclosporiasis, is related to *Cryptosporidium*. Significant infectious intestinal protozoa worldwide include *Isospora belli* (isosporiasis), *Cyclospora* species, *Enterocytozoon bieneusi* (microsporidosis), and *Entamoeba histolytica* (amebiasis).

Diagnosis of intestinal protozoans is definitive with the microscopic detection of the organism in fecal contents and its differentiation from other species. Wet mounts from watery or loose stools that are prepared to detect the motile stage of the parasite (known as trophozoites) are particularly important to detect amebiasis. Permanent mounts prepared with various stains are used to detect the cyst, oocyst, or spore stages of protozoa species.

PROTOZOA INFECTING BLOOD AND TISSUE

Malaria is the most significant parasitic disease in humans. It is caused principally by four species of the genus *Plasmodium*. The disease is endemic to most tropical regions.

Malaria is transmitted by the bite of infected *Anopheles* mosquitoes. The asexual part of the malaria life cycle affects humans and is known as schizogony. The parasite first enters the liver and then the red blood cells.

For diagnosis, a clinician draws blood from the affected person; slides are then prepared for microscopic examination. Diagnosis is confirmed by the presence of parasitized erythrocytes. Newer tests known as rapid antigen detection tests have been applied in many laboratories to avoid misdiagnosis of malaria. This test involves applying a blood sample to a nitrocellulose strip containing antibodies. If positive, the resultant antigen-antibody can be visualized.

Babesiosis caused by *Babesia* species also infects red blood cells. *Babesia* resembles malarial parasites morphologically, so a differential diagnosis is necessary upon examining blood samples. This increasingly important parasite is found primarily in the northeastern United States and is spread by ticks. The initial symptoms of babesiosis are quite similar to bacterial Lyme disease, which also is contracted from ticks in the same geographical region.

Trichomoniasis, caused by *Trichomonas vaginalis*, is considered to be the most common parasitic infection in the United States. It is a sexually transmitted disease that affects the genitourinary tract. The usual diagnosis is to examine slides of vaginal secretion (women) or urethral secretion (men) under a dark field, phase-contrast, or ordinary light microscope. The parasite, if present, will exhibit rapid motility and flagella.

Toxoplasmosis, caused by *Toxoplasma gondii*, is also an important parasitic infection in the United States. Transmission usually takes place by oral ingestion of food or soil contaminated by the feces of infected cats. From the intestinal tract, the parasite invades a variety of tissues. This invasion stimulates a strong immune response from the host person and serves as a diagnostic tool.

Trypanosomiasiss consists of two separate diseases depending on the region where they occur. In South America, Chagas' disease is caused by *Trypanosoma cruzi*, while in Africa, African sleeping sickness is caused by *T. brucei*. Diagnosis depends upon identifying the organism. Blood samples are easy to obtain, but if the protozoan is not found under observation, the parasite can be concentrated by centrifugation before microscopic examination. The parasite is more concentrated in lymph node fluid, and *T. brucei* is found in cerebrospinal fluid during the latter stages of the disease.

Leishmaniasis is a collective term for the many diseases caused by species of the genus *Leishmania*. Visceral leishmaniasis (kala-azar) is caused by *L. donovani* and occurs over a wide geographical area. The parasite invades the blood and becomes established in spleen, liver, bone marrow, and lymph nodes. Diagnosis is established by finding the parasite in biopsies of those tissues or in cultures from those tissues or from blood. Cutaneous leishmaniasis (oriental sore) is caused many species, and results in skin lesions. The parasite can be found in aspirates, smears, or dermal scrapings of the ulcer. Mucosal leishmaniasis is caused by species of the *Viannia* subgenus. The parasite causes lesions in the nasal and pharyngeal mucosal lining. Diagnosis is made by examining biopsy material or culture of aspirated material from the lesion.

IMPACT

Protozoan infections are generally much less of a problem in the developed world than in tropical or subtropical areas. However, travelers to developing countries should be fully aware of the possibility of contracting parasitic diseases and should take the necessary precautions.

David A. Olle, M.S.

FURTHER READING

Fauci, Anthony, et al., eds. *Harrison's Principles of Internal Medicine*. 17th ed. New York: McGraw-Hill, 2008. A good clinical reference that also provides a summary table and extensive discussions of all significant protozoan diseases.

Fritsche, Thomas, and Rangaraj Selvarangan. "Medical Parasitology." In *Henry's Clinical Diagnosis and Management by Laboratory Methods*, edited by Richard A. McPherson, Matthew R. Pincus, and John B. Henry. 22d ed. Philadelphia: Saunders/Elsevier, 2011. A detailed discussion of parasitic infections, with illustrations of parasites' life cycles and characteristics.

McPhee, Stephen J., and Maxine A. Papadakis, eds. *Current Medical Diagnosis and Treatment 2011.* 50th ed. New York: McGraw-Hill, 2011. Chapter 35 of this classic reference text gives a complete review of the most common types of protozoan diseases.

Parker, Steve. *Protozoans, Algae, and other Protists.* Mankato, Minn.: Compass Point Books, 2009. Although written for middle-school students, this book provides good coverage for all general readers needing to understand the basics of protozoa.

WEB SITES OF INTEREST

Centers for Disease Control and Prevention
http://www.cdc.gov/parasites

Microbiology and Immunology On-line: Parasitology
http://pathmicro.med.sc.edu/book/parasit-sta.htm

See also: Developing countries and infectious disease; Immune response to protozoan diseases; Parasites: Classification and types; Parasitic diseases; Prevention of protozoan diseases; Protozoa: Classification and types; Protozoa: Structure and growth; Treatment of protozoan diseases; Tropical medicine.

Diagnosis of viral infections

CATEGORY: Diagnosis

DEFINITION

Viruses are intracellular parasitic organisms that infect the cells of other organisms. Viruses consist of nucleic acids surrounded by a protein coat known as a capsid. The clinical signs presented by a person during a suspected viral infection determine the samples collected for laboratory tests. Traditional tests such as serology and tissue culture, along with electron microscopy, remain the mainstays of viral diagnosis, but molecular methods have become more popular too.

SEROLOGY

Virus proteins are known as antigens when they elicit an immune response by the body. This immune

response leads to the body's formation of antibodies. Antibodies, also known as immunoglobulins, comprise five classes (IgM, IgG, IgA, IgD, and IgE), which are based on the structural characteristics and biological activity of the antigen. Serological tests detect virus antigens, measure serum antibody levels (titers), and relate these titers to the clinical state of the affected person.

All serological tests are based on the formation of an antigen-antibody complex. Typically, after infection, the IgM antibody is the first to appear, followed by a much larger rise in IgG antibodies; however, the dynamics of the antibody levels can vary greatly depending on many factors.

Standard or classical serological tests are those that have been in long-time use. The hemagglutination inhibition test determines the presence and quantity of virus antigen or antibody by the clumping of red blood cells. The single radial hemolysis technique determines the amount of virus antibody present in a serum sample by reacting it with red blood cells containing antigen and complement and by measuring the resultant circular zone of hemolysis. The complement fixation test measures the amount of antibody in serum or spinal fluid by the amount of complement consumed in the test medium.

The immunofluorescence test detects virus antigen that binds to a fluorescent-labeled antibody. In neutralization tests, virus and serum are mixed and inoculated into cell culture, eggs, or animals. The loss of resultant infectivity of the virus is called neutralization. The particle agglutination test involves coating the surface of latex particles with antigen (or antibody). A sample containing an antibody (or antigen) is added; resultant agglutination is a positive test.

Newer serological methods have been developed. In radioimmunoassay, either the antigen or the antibody is tagged with a radioactive molecule, and the radioactivity of the resultant complex is measured. In the enzyme-linked immunoabsorbent assay (ELISA), antibodies are attached to a solid support. A sample that contains virus is added; the antigen binds to the antibodies and an antibody-enzyme conjugate is added, which binds to the antigen. Finally, the substrate of the enzyme is added to form a colored complex. The reverse is also possible, starting with antigen bound to the solid support. The Western blot test can detect multiple antibodies directed against a single virus antigen.

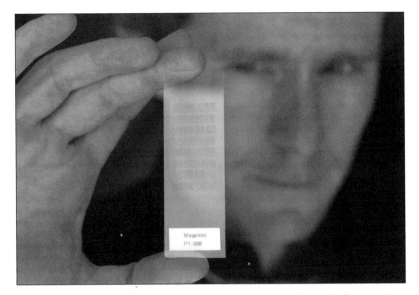

A researcher holds a slide containing a glass computer chip with the genetic sequence of every known virus. The slide is used to help determine the cause of suspected viral diseases. (AP/Wide World Photos)

MICROSCOPIC EXAMINATION

Electron microscopy (EM) has filled an essential, long-time role in virus diagnosis, helping to detect new and unusual disease outbreaks. EM requires the isolation of the virus for examination, which can require concentration of sample fluids. However, visualizing the pathogen can provide important preliminary identification clues that can help determine correct follow-up tests. Typically, a negative stain is prepared in which the virus appears clear or light colored against a darker background. Immunoaggregation, or the clumping of virus particles, is sometimes practiced to help visualize virus particles.

EM can be important for studying structural features, as it can help determine the function of various viral components. The findings can lead to the development of methods of treatment or of vaccines. Atomic force microscopy is now being used to improve the visualization of viruses.

Although viruses cannot be visualized by light microscopy, the procedure is used to examine cells or tissues for the effects of viral infections. The presence of inclusion bodies is an example.

TISSUE CULTURE

Growing virus in tissue culture is the traditional means to augment the quantity of virus for identifica-

tion. Three types of cell cultures are in use: primary cells from adult animals; semi-continuous cells from embryonic tissue; and continuous cells (immortalized tumor cell lines). The blood or tissue sample containing the suspected virus is inoculated into the cell culture, and the presence of growing virus is observed. The growing virus can kill the cells (cytopathic effect) or acquire the ability to stick to red blood cells (hemadsorption). Tissue culture is declining in importance because of the extended time required to obtain results, because of its low sensitivity, and because many viruses will not grow in cell culture.

MOLECULAR METHODS

Molecular methods are based on determining the genome, or genetic makeup, of the virus. Virus genomes are made up of nucleic acids, either deoxyribonucleic acid (DNA) or ribonucleic acid (RNA). Before testing, RNA must be converted to DNA by a process known as reverse transcriptase. To ensure sufficient amounts for detection, the small amounts of viral DNA present in a serum sample must then be amplified by the polymerase chain reaction (PCR) process. The development of what is called real-time PCR, which combines the rapid assay time of PCR amplification with an inbuilt detection system, is considered to be a major advance in virus disease diagnosis.

Another advance is the development of multiplex PCR, which can amplify several regions of DNA simultaneously. This technology can result in considerable savings in time and cost while facilitating the screening and identification of virus species. Another test, Western blotting, can measure antibody to several viral antigens simultaneously.

Finally, nanotechnology has entered the field of virus diagnostics. Its proponents claim that it can provide simple, rapid, and sensitive solutions. Semiconducting nanowires, magnetic nanoparticles, and fluorescent nanoparticles are finding applications in viral diagnoses.

IMPACT

The newer molecular methods are usually more sensitive and specific than tissue culture for virus diagnosis. However, traditional immunoassay methods, such as ELISA or immunofluorescence, may still have the advantages of speed, convenience, and ease of use, so they continue to be used for early diagnosis.

David A. Olle, M.S.

FURTHER READING

Croft, William J. *Under the Microscope: A Brief History of Microscopy.* Hackensack, N.J.: World Scientific, 2006. A straightforward history of microscopy.

Goldsmith, Cynthia, and Sara Miller. "Modern Uses of Electron Microscopy for Detection of Viruses." *Clinical Microbiology Reviews* 22, no. 4 (2009): 552-563. Describes the unique benefits of electron microscopy over other diagnostic methods.

Ratcliff, R., et al. "Molecular Diagnosis of Medical Viruses." *Current Issues in Molecular Biology* 9 (2007): 87-102. Excellent discussion of the latest diagnostic tools, focusing on PCR and other applications.

Wong, D. "Diagnostic Methods in Virology." Available at http://virology-online.com/general/tests.htm. Outlines all the important diagnostic tools, including microscopy, serology, tissue culture, and molecular methods.

WEB SITES OF INTEREST

International Classification of Diseases
http://www.cdc.gov/nchs/icd/icd10cm.htm

Lab Tests Online
http://www.labtestsonline.org

See also: Acid-fastness; Biochemical tests; Biostatistics; Diagnosis of bacterial infections; Gram staining; Immunoassay; Microbiology; Parasites: Classification and types; Pathogens; Polymerase chain reaction (PCR) method; Pulsed-field gel electrophoresis; Serology; Virology; Viruses: Structure and life cycle; Viruses: Types>

Dichloro-diphenyl-trichloroethane. *See* DDT.

Diphtheria, tetanus, and acellular pertussis vaccine. *See* DTaP vaccine.

Diphtheria

CATEGORY: Diseases and conditions
ANATOMY OR SYSTEM AFFECTED: Throat, tissue, tonsils, upper respiratory tract

DEFINITION

Diphtheria is a highly contagious and life-threatening infection caused by bacteria. The infection most commonly attacks the mucous membranes associated with the breathing system (the tonsils, throat, and nose) and can also infect the skin. In addition, some types of the bacterium can cause damage to the heart, nerves, kidneys, and brain.

The vaccine for diphtheria is safe and is effective at preventing the disease. A series of shots are given during childhood, then booster shots are required every ten years to keep the immunity strong. Before vaccines and medications were available to prevent and treat the disease, nearly one of every ten infected people died. Diphtheria was the leading cause of death among children.

Diphtheria is a medical emergency that requires immediate care from a doctor. Not everyone who gets diphtheria shows signs of illness, though they may be able to infect others. The sooner the infection is treated, the more favorable the outcome.

CAUSES

Diphtheria is caused by the bacterium *Corynebacterium diphtheriae*. The infection spreads from person to person through contact with droplets of moisture that are coughed or sneezed into the air and breathed in by a noninfected person, through contaminated personal items (fomites) such as tissues or drinking glasses that have been used by an infected person, and through skin that is infected with diphtheria.

RISK FACTORS

Risk factors include having never been immunized against diphtheria, not having had a booster dose in the past ten years, living in crowded or unsanitary conditions, having a compromised immune system, and being undernourished.

SYMPTOMS

Signs and symptoms of diphtheria usually begin two to five days after a person is infected. The most telltale sign of diphtheria is a gray covering on the back of the throat, which can detach and block the airway. If left untreated, the bacterium can produce a poison (toxin) that spreads through the body, causing damage to the heart, nerves, and kidneys. Symptoms include sore throat and painful swallowing, fever up to 103° Fahrenheit, swollen glands in the neck, difficulty breathing, difficulty swallowing, weakness, and a gray covering on the back of the throat.

SCREENING AND DIAGNOSIS

A doctor will ask about symptoms and medical history and will perform a physical exam. Diphtheria will be suspected if the throat and tonsils are covered with a gray membrane. Tests to confirm a diagnosis may include taking a sample of the gray membrane that coats the back of the throat and taking a sample of tissue from an infected area of skin.

TREATMENT AND THERAPY

If a doctor suspects diphtheria, the patient's treatment will start immediately, even before the lab results are returned. Treatment options include antitoxin, a substance injected into the body that neutralizes the diphtheria poison that is traveling in the body; antibiotics, a substance injected or given as a pill that kills the diphtheria bacteria in the body and heals the infection (also reduces the length of time a person is contagious); and isolation and bed rest. It takes much time, up to six weeks, to recover from diphtheria, especially if the heart is affected. Isolation may be necessary while a person is still contagious.

PREVENTION AND OUTCOMES

To help reduce the chance of getting diphtheria, persons should get immunized and stay up-to-date on future immunizations. If a person has been in contact with someone who has diphtheria, that person should be watched closely for symptoms and should work with a doctor to determine appropriate treatment, if necessary.

Julie J. Martin, M.S.;
reviewed by David L. Horn, M.D., FACP

FURTHER READING

Krieg, Noel R., et al., eds. *Bergey's Manual of Systematic Bacteriology.* Vol. 5. 2d ed. New York: Springer, 2010.
Pan American Health Organization. *Control of Diphtheria, Pertussis, Tetanus, "Haemophilus influenzae"*

Type B, and Hepatitis B Field Guide. Washington, D.C.: Author, 2005.
Parker, James N., and Philip M. Parker, eds. *The Official Patient's Sourcebook on Diphtheria.* San Diego, Calif.: Icon Health, 2002.

WEB SITES OF INTEREST

Caring for Kids
http://www.caringforkids.cps.ca

Centers for Disease Control and Prevention, National Immunization Program
http://www.cdc.gov/nip

National Institute of Allergy and Infectious Diseases
http://www.niaid.nih.gov

World Health Organization
http://www.who.int

See also: Airborne illness and disease; Bacterial infections; Bronchiolitis; Bronchitis; Children and infectious disease; Contagious diseases; *Corynebacterium*; Croup; DTaP vaccine; Epiglottitis; Mononucleosis; Pleurisy; Skin infections; Strep throat; Tuberculosis (TB); Vaccines: Types; Whooping cough.

Disease eradication campaigns

CATEGORY: Epidemiology

DEFINITION

True eradication of an infectious disease is rare; in fact, only one infectious disease, smallpox, has been completely eradicated. While many other infectious diseases have been controlled to various degrees, for a disease to be considered totally eradicated, that disease must no longer be occurring anywhere in the world and must no longer require control measures, such as vaccination. Elimination of a disease means that the disease is still occurring, but at a very low and predictable level. Control of a disease means that organized plans and programs are in place for decreasing the number of new cases.

VACCINES

Vaccines are considered the best tools for eventual

eradication of infectious diseases, but simply having a vaccine does not guarantee eradication or elimination of a disease. Vaccines to prevent some of the world's most burdensome diseases have been available for decades, but a lack of public health programs, infrastructure, money, and political resolve have kept these vaccines from being as successful as hoped for in eradicating polio, measles, and other diseases, particularly in developing countries. To address this problem, the World Health Organization (WHO) and its partner agencies began the Expanded Program on Immunization in 1974 to increase the formerly abysmal rate of childhood vaccination in developing countries.

A vaccine that requires only one dose to induce immunity is more likely to be successful in eradicating disease than is a vaccine, such as the hepatitis B vaccine, that requires multiple doses, because fewer people will receive a complete immunization series. Vaccines that can be given at convenient times, particularly on the same schedule as other vaccines, are also more likely to aid in disease eradication than are those requiring an additional trip to a clinic. Also, vaccines that do not need precisely controlled storage conditions are easier to use in undeveloped areas than are those that need to be kept frozen.

Other strategies are also important in the quest for disease eradication. Surveillance for new cases needs to be active and ongoing, at both local and global levels, so that small outbreaks can be controlled before they become large outbreaks. Sufficient stockpiles of drugs and vaccines must be available when needed.

Characteristics of the infectious agent and the disease itself can also impact the likelihood of eradication. For instance, a disease, such as smallpox, that becomes symptomatically obvious at the same time it becomes contagious will allow isolation of the infected person before he or she infects others. A virus, such as that which causes measles, can be contagious for days before symptoms appear, allowing the disease to spread to many contacts before the infection is recognized. Infectious agents that can live and reproduce in nonhuman animals or in insects will likely persist in those organisms even after elimination from humans, making them difficult to eradicate.

SMALLPOX

Smallpox, caused by the variola virus, was a deadly contagious disease that killed 20 to 60 percent of those infected. Records of smallpox epidemics go back thou-

sands of years, including records suggesting smallpox scars on the mummified body of the Egyptian pharaoh Ramses V, who died in 1157 B.C.E. The development of a vaccine in 1796, in which Edward Jenner used material from cowpox lesions to successfully inoculate against smallpox, led to a gradual decline in the disease. The last case of smallpox was seen in Somalia in 1977. The World Health Organization declared the disease eradicated in 1980.

ERADICABLE DISEASES

Dracunculiasis, also referred to as guinea worm disease, will likely be the first parasitic disease eradicated. This painful and debilitating disease is acquired by drinking stagnant water containing worm larvae. Once swallowed by a human, the larvae mature, multiply, and migrate throughout the body, eventually eroding through the skin. They must be carefully and slowly pulled from the skin during a period of a month. Guinea worm disease has decreased from about four million cases in twenty countries in the late 1980's to about three thousand cases in only four African countries in 2009. There is no drug that will cure the disease and no vaccination against it, so eradication efforts have concentrated on supplies of clean water and on educating people at risk about the need to filter drinking water.

Polio too is considered an eradicable disease. The last large-scale outbreaks of polio in the United States occurred in the 1950's, and routine childhood immunization for this disease began after the development of an injectable vaccine in the 1950's and an oral vaccine in the 1960's. By 2002, polio remained in only a few countries, including Afghanistan, India, Pakistan, Egypt, and Nigeria. However, the number of cases has begun to climb, in part because of the decrease in the number of immunized children and young adults in Nigeria, where concern about the vaccine's safety has derailed immunization efforts. Increased numbers of polio cases are now also being reported there and in countries bordering Nigeria.

IMPACT

The Carter Center's International Task Force for Disease Eradication considers several infectious diseases to be potentially eradicable in the future, but notes that there are impediments to success for each. Lymphatic filariasis eradication will require strengthening of health care systems in Africa. Eradication of measles could require development of a vaccine that can be given to infants before they are first exposed. The task force has categorized other infectious diseases as having the potential for elimination, but not for eradication, in limited geographical areas. These diseases include Chagas' disease, hepatitis B, malaria, rabies, and onchocerciasis (river blindness).

Lindsey Marcellin, M.D., M.P.H.

FURTHER READING

Delves, Peter J., et al. *Roitt's Essential Immunology.* 11th ed. Malden, Mass.: Blackwell, 2006.

Duclos, P., et al. "Global Immunization: Status, Progress, Challenges, and Future." *BMC International Health and Human Rights* 9, suppl. 1 (October 14, 2009): S2. Available at http://www.ncbi.nlm.nih.gov/pmc/articles/pmc2762311.

Fletcher, Robert H., and Suzanne W. Fletcher. *Clinical Epidemiology: The Essentials.* 4th ed. Baltimore: Lippincott Williams & Wilkins, 2005.

Henderson, D. A. *Smallpox: The Death of a Disease—The Inside Story of Eradicating a Worldwide Killer.* Amherst, N.Y.: Prometheus Books, 2009.

Morens, David M., Gregory K. Folkers, and Anthony S. Fauci. "The Challenge of Emerging and Reemerging Infectious Diseases." *Nature* 430 (July 8, 2004): 242-249.

Oshinsky, David M. *Polio: An American Story.* New York: Oxford University Press, 2006.

Plotkin, Stanley A., Walter A. Orenstein, and Paul A. Offit. *Vaccines.* 5th ed. Philadelphia: Saunders/Elsevier, 2008.

Rinaldi, Andrea. "Free, at Last! The Progress of New Disease Eradication Campaigns for Guinea Worm Disease and Polio, and the Prospect of Tackling Other Diseases." *EMBO Reports* 10 (2009): 215-221. Also available at http://www.ncbi.nlm.nih.gov/pmc/articles/pmc2658554.

Sherman, Irwin W. *The Power of Plagues.* Washington, D.C.: American Society for Microbiology Press, 2006.

World Health Organization. "Immunization Service Delivery and Accelerated Disease Control—Measles." Available at http://www.who.int/immunization_delivery/adc/measles/measles.

WEB SITES OF INTEREST

Carter Center
http://www.cartercenter.org/health

Centers for Disease Control and Prevention
http://www/cdc.gov

Emerging and Reemerging Infectious Disease Resource Center
http://www.medscape.com/resource/infections

Global Health Council
http://www.globalhealth.org

Global Polio Eradication Initiative
http://www.polioeradication.org

Guinea Worm Eradication Program
http://www.cartercenter.org/health/guinea_worm

World Health Organization
http://www.who.int

See also: Biosurveillance; Centers for Disease Control and Prevention (CDC); Cowpox; Developing countries and infectious disease; Dracunculiasis; Emerging and reemerging infectious diseases; Epidemics and pandemics: Causes and management; Epidemics and pandemic: History; Epidemiology; Globalization and infectious disease; Immunity; Koch's postulates; Outbreaks; Poliomyelitis; Public health; Smallpox; Smallpox vaccine; U.S. Army Medical Research Institute of Infectious Diseases; Vaccines: Types; World Health Organization (WHO).

Disinfectants and sanitizers

CATEGORY: Prevention

DEFINITION

Disinfectants and sanitizers are antimicrobials. A "disinfectant" destroys pathogens (disease-causing microorganisms, such as bacteria) but not spores and not all viruses. A "sanitizer" reduces the number of harmful microorganisms, or germs, so that they are not an infectious hazard. Disinfection and sanitization are effective only if a surface area is clean. "Clean" means that a surface has been cleared of soil, dust, organic matter (such as blood or stool), and microorganisms. Cleaning usually can remove large amounts of harmful microorganisms, but it usually does not kill them and does not disinfect or sanitize surfaces.

According to industry standards, a disinfectant must be capable of reducing the level of pathogenic bacteria by 99.999 percent during a time frame greater than five but less than ten minutes under conditions of the AOAC Use-Dilution Test. A disinfectant destroys all pathogens on a surface or object. Disinfectant products or processes can be ranked as low, medium, or high level. A sanitizer must reduce the level of harmful microorganisms by in a specific bacterial test population 99.999 percent (in a process known as a 5 log reduction) within thirty seconds under conditions of the AOAC Germicidal and Detergent Sanitizers Test (GDS).

One substance may work both as a sanitizer and a disinfectant. For example, an iodophor, when used at 25 ppm (parts per million of available iodine), is a sanitizer. However, that same product, when applied at 75 ppm, is a disinfectant. After using the sanitizer, which kills 99.999 percent of bacteria, five thousand bacteria per square foot would remain. These remaining microorganisms reproduce by splitting into two every fifteen minutes. The result is that those five thousand bacteria per square foot have now become 1 million bacteria per square foot within, for example, five hours.

The U.S. Environmental Protection Agency (EPA) is the governing body for antimicrobials. It places antimicrobials into four categories: sterilizers, disinfectants, sanitizers, and antiseptics and germicides. A sterilizer is equipment used in medical procedures. Cleaning professionals are concerned only with disinfectants and sanitizers, which are chemical antimicrobial agents, in contrast to physical antimicrobial agents, such as heat and radiation. Antiseptics and germicides are for use on living beings and are governed by the U.S. Food and Drug Administration (FDA). A sanitizer may be called an antiseptic when it is used on tissue. (Antiseptics are safe to use in this case because they do not have the same killing power as disinfectants.)

DEVELOPMENT OF SANITIZERS AND DISINFECTANTS

Infection control was pioneered by hospitals in the nineteenth century. Out of the filth, disease, and poverty of the early nineteenth century came sanitary reform. One of the more significant contributors to the health revolution was the technological, sociological, and environmental phenomenon now known as the sanitary era or the public health campaign. The goal of this campaign was to destroy all possible harmful microorganisms.

Health officials believed it was practical to allow a minimum of ten minutes of contact time with a sanitizer or disinfectant to accomplish this objective. As a result, most disinfectant tests were developed to ascertain whether any bacteria could survive exactly ten minutes of contact. When contact times that are significantly less than ten minutes are allowed, it becomes difficult to get a meaningful result from the Use-Dilution Test.

In food service and public-health related industries, interest in antimicrobials appeared much later than it did in hospitals. Conditions of use were different, so tests based on ten minutes of contact were not practical. In many cases even today, thirty seconds is about the maximum time one can realistically expect for contact in food and drink service (such as when a bartender washes a glass).

Because it is not realistic to expect complete kill in thirty seconds, the GDS test was developed to count microbes. (The Use-Dilution Test, in contrast, indicates the presence of bacteria but yields no counts.) Experts figured that it was possible to get, in thirty seconds, a 99.999 percent reduction in the amount of bacteria with the use of practical agents (such as detergents).

COMMON MECHANISM OF ACTION

A wide range of substances are used as disinfectants. These include alcohols, aldehydes, hydrogen peroxide, iodine, and potassium permanganate solution. Bromine and chlorine are the most common disinfectants and sanitizers for drinking and recreational waters.

The most widely used disinfectants and sanitizers are powerful oxidizers, which means that the atoms of these elements can accept electrons or hydrogens, or both. Hydrogen peroxide, bromine, and chlorine compounds oxidize the complex molecules present on the surface of bacteria, causing their cell walls and cell membranes to disrupt. The proteins on the surface become irreversibly damaged and start to stick together, forming clumps. This happens quickly: A strong solution of sodium hypochlorite ($NaOCl$, also known as household bleach) solution that is used to disinfect a toilet, for example, kills bacteria within seconds. The bacterial cell cannot respond to the damage quickly enough, and the whole cell simply splits open and dies.

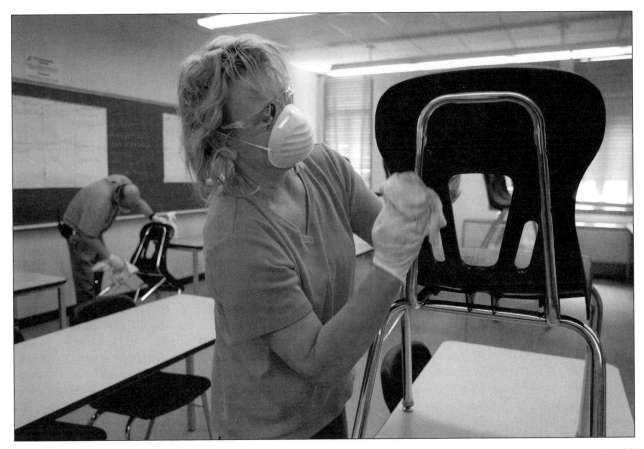

A Michigan high school staffer cleans classroom equipment with a disinfectant in 2009. The school district and local health department feared the transmission of H1N1 influenza, or swine flu. (AP/Wide World Photos)

Later research has shown that bacteria do have some capacity to resist an attack by bleach. Contact with hypochlorous acid was found to switch on a gene in some bacteria. This gene is part of the pathway that bugs use to cope with heat stress and the bleachlike substances that cells of the immune system produce to fight infection. If the concentration of bleach solution is low, bacteria with genes that resist this sort of cellular attack might survive.

IMPACT

It has been claimed that the major decline in mortality in the late nineteenth and early twentieth centuries resulted from innovations in environmental sanitation. About one century later, in 1997, *Life* magazine considered drinking water chlorination and filtration to be "probably the most significant public health advancement[s] of the millennium."

Today, modern hospital disinfectants must show efficacy in eliminating three primary organisms: *Staphylococcus aureus*, *Salmonella*, and *Pseudomonas aeruginosa*. However, hospital administrations generally require disinfectants with even more efficacy.

Many people in developed countries have grown to accept reduced rates of illness as the norm, and outbreaks that once would have been accepted as an unavoidable part of life are now considered crises of public health that require swift and decisive interventions. However, much of the developing world has yet to reap the benefits. According to World Health Organization (WHO) data, worldwide, two of every ten people live with no source of safe drinking water and four of every ten people lack access to a simple pit latrine.

There remains more work to be done. WHO has promoted as one of its Millennium Development

Goals the reduction by one-half, by the year 2015, of the proportion of people without sustainable access to safe drinking water and basic sanitation. Efficacious and inexpensive, chlorine disinfectants have been employed to help achieve this critical humanitarian goal.

Stephanie Eckenrode, B.A.

FURTHER READING

Block, Seymour S., ed. *Disinfection, Sterilization, and Preservation.* 5th ed. Philadelphia: Lippincott Williams & Wilkins, 2001. A comprehensive and practical reference on contemporary methods of disinfection, sterilization, and preservation and their medical, surgical, and public health applications.

Fraise, Adam P., Peter A. Lambert, and J.-Y. Maillard, eds. *Russell, Hugo, and Ayliffe's Principles and Practice of Disinfection, Preservation, and Sterilization.* Malden, Mass.: Wiley-Blackwell, 2004. A highly respected established text covering in detail many methods to prevent and eliminate microbial growth.

Novick, Lloyd F., Cynthia B. Morrow, and Glen P. Mays, eds. *Public Health Administration: Principles for Population-Based Management.* Sudbury, Mass.: Jones and Bartlett, 2008. The principles, practices, and skills essential to successful public health administration. Includes information on the Healthy People 2010 objectives and chapters on bioterrorism and emergency preparedness, public health systems research, and public health law.

WEB SITES OF INTEREST

Association for Professionals in Infection Control and Epidemiology
http://www.knowledgeisinfectious.org

Charity: Water
http://www.charitywater.org

Cleaning Industry Research Institute
http://www.ciriscience.org

UN-Water
http://www.unwater.org/discover.html

See also: Chemical germicides; Decontamination; Epidemiology; Hospitals and infectious disease; Hygiene; Iatrogenic infections; Infection; *Pseudomonas*; Public health; *Salmonella*; *Staphylococcus*; Water treatment; Waterborne illness and disease; Wound infections.

Disseminated intravascular coagulation

CATEGORY: Diseases and conditions
ANATOMY OR SYSTEM AFFECTED: Blood, circulatory system
ALSO KNOWN AS: Consumption coagulopathy, defibrination syndrome

DEFINITION

Disseminated intravascular coagulation, or DIC, is a serious disruption in the body's clotting mechanism. Normally, the body forms a blood clot in reaction to an injury. With DIC, the body overproduces many small blood clots throughout the body, depleting the body of clotting factors and platelets.

These small clots are dangerous and can interfere with the blood supply to organs, causing dysfunction and failure. Massive bleeding can occur because of the body's lack of clotting factor and platelets. DIC is life-threatening and must be treated promptly.

CAUSES

There are many causes of DIC. The disorder is usually caused by a release of chemicals into the bloodstream from one of the following conditions: asepticemia (a systemwide infection), especially with gram-negative bacteria; labor and delivery complications; eclampsia; amniotic fluid clots; retained placenta; certain cancers; extensive tissue injury; burns; head injury; reaction to blood transfusion; and shock. Less common causes include severe head trauma, prostate surgery complications, and venomous snake bites.

RISK FACTORS

Certain conditions increase the chance of developing DIC. When making a diagnosis, a doctor will look for a recent episode of bacteremia or septicemia, a recent injury or trauma, a recent surgery or anesthesia, labor and delivery complications, leukemia or widespread cancer, a recent reaction to a blood transfusion, and severe liver disease.

Key Terms: DIC

- *Acute DIC.* A disorder of the blood-clotting mechanism that develops within hours of an initial attack on an underlying body system

- *Chronic DIC.* A disorder of the blood-clotting mechanism that persists in a suppressed state until a coagulation disorder worsens

- *Coagulation.* The process of blood clot formation

- *Coagulation cascade.* The series of steps starting with the activation of the intrinsic or extrinsic pathways of coagulation and proceeding through the common pathway of coagulation leading to the formation of fibrin clots

- *Ecchymosis.* Bleeding into the skin, subcutaneous tissue, or mucous membranes, resulting in bruising

- *Hemostasis.* The stopping of blood flow through the blood vessels, usually as a result of blood clotting

- *Platelets.* Cells, found in the blood of all mammals, that are involved in the coagulation of blood and the contraction of blood clots

- *Thrombocytopenia.* A markedly decreased number of platelets in the blood

SYMPTOMS

Symptoms of DIC can vary in severity, depending on the cause and time of diagnosis. DIC is a life-threatening condition that must be treated promptly. Symptoms of DIC include bleeding, sometimes severe and from multiple locations in the body; bleeding from an unknown cause; gastrointestinal bleeding; blood clot formation causing fingers or toes to look blue; and sudden bruising.

SCREENING AND DIAGNOSIS

A doctor will make a diagnosis of DIC based on the patient's signs and symptoms and on results to certain blood tests. Like symptoms of DIC, blood levels will vary according to the severity of the DIC. The blood will be examined for abnormal levels of certain tests, including platelet count (usually reduced in DIC); fibrinogen (usually reduced in DIC); fibrin degradation products (usually elevated in DIC); prothrombin time (PT; usually prolonged in DIC); partial thromboplastin time (PTT; usually prolonged in DIC); thrombin test time (prolonged in DIC); and D-dimer test (high level in DIC).

TREATMENT AND THERAPY

Treatment of DIC depends on identifying and treating the underlying cause quickly. A doctor may give certain blood products or medications to treat the condition. Septicemia is usually treated with antibiotics. Treatment options include using fresh frozen plasma to replace low levels of coagulation factors caused by DIC. Platelets may also be given to restore low levels. Other treatments are the use of cryoprecipitates to correct low levels of fibrinogen and the use of heparin, a blood thinner. Doctors sometimes give heparin in combination with blood products to reduce blood clots. Persons with cancer whose DIC is difficult to control may receive heparin to control blood clots. Another medication, antithrombin III, is sometimes used to slow down clotting in certain patients.

PREVENTION AND OUTCOMES

To help reduce the chance of getting DIC, one should obtain prompt treatment for any of the conditions that can cause this disorder.

Patricia Griffin Kellicker, B.S.N.;
reviewed by Igor Puzanov, M.D.

FURTHER READING

Bick, Roger L. *Disorders of Thrombosis and Hemostasis: Clinical and Laboratory Practice.* 3d ed. Philadelphia: Lippincott Williams & Wilkins, 2002.

_____. "Disseminated Intravascular Coagulation: Objective Criteria for Diagnosis and Management." *Medical Clinics of North America* 78 (1994): 511-543.

Dahlback, Bjorn. "Blood Coagulation." *The Lancet* 355, no. 9215 (May 6, 2000): 1627-1632.

Karnik, L., and J. Murray. "Anticoagulation in the Trauma Patient." *Trauma* 7 (2005): 63-68.

Lichtman, Marshall A., et al., eds. *Williams Hematology.* 7th ed. New York: McGraw-Hill, 2006.

The Merck Manuals, Online Medical Library. "Bleeding and Clotting Disorders." Available at http://www.merck.com/mmhe.

_____. "Hemostasis and Coagulation Disorders." Available at http://www.merck.com/mmhe.

National Library of Medicine. "Disseminated Intravascular Coagulation (DIC)." Available at http://www.nlm.gov/medlineplus/ency/article/000573.htm.

Rodak, Bernadette, ed. *Hematology: Clinical Principles and Applications.* 3d ed. St. Louis, Mo.: Saunders/Elsevier, 2007.

Zucker-Franklin, D., et al. *Atlas of Blood Cells: Function and Pathology.* 3d ed. Philadelphia: Lea & Febiger, 2003.

WEB SITES OF INTEREST

National Heart, Lung, and Blood Institute
http://www.nhlbi.nih.gov

National Library of Medicine
http://www.nlm.gov

Public Health Agency of Canada
http://www.phac-aspc.gc.ca

See also: Bacterial infections; Behçet's syndrome; Bloodstream infections; Gangrene; Iatrogenic infections; Idiopathic thrombocytopenic purpura; Pregnancy and infectious disease; Sepsis; Wound infections.

Diverticulitis

CATEGORY: Diseases and conditions
ANATOMY OR SYSTEM AFFECTED: Colon, gastrointestinal system, intestines
ALSO KNOWN AS: Acute colonic diverticulitis, acute diverticulitis

DEFINITION

A pouch that forms in the wall of the large intestine is called a diverticulum. When the diverticulum becomes infected or inflamed, the condition is called diverticulitis.

CAUSES

It is not clear why the pouches form. Experts believe that a constant pressure is built up when food moves too slowly through the bowel. This pressure is thought to increase, push along the side walls, and then create pouches. Digested food or stool can become trapped in one of the pouches, leading to inflammation and infection.

Factors that may contribute to diverticulitis include a low-fiber diet. Fiber is critical because it softens stools and makes them pass through the bowel more easily. Other causes include increased pressure in the bowel from straining to pass a hard stool, defects in the colon wall, and chronic constipation.

Key Facts: Diverticulosis and Diverticulitis

- Diverticulosis occurs when small pouches called diverticula bulge outward through weak spots in the colon, or large intestine.

- Most people with diverticulosis never have any discomfort or symptoms.

- Diverticula form when pressure builds inside the colon wall, usually because of constipation.

- The most likely cause of diverticulosis is a low-fiber diet, which increases constipation and pressure inside the colon.

- For most people with diverticulosis, eating a high-fiber diet is the only treatment needed.

- Fiber intake can be increased by eating whole-grain breads and cereals; fruits such as apples and pears; vegetables such as peas, spinach, and squash; and starchy vegetables such as kidney and black beans.

- Diverticulitis occurs when the pouches become inflamed and cause pain and tenderness in the lower left side of the abdomen.

- Diverticulitis can lead to bleeding, infections, small tears called perforations, or blockages in the colon. These complications always require treatment to prevent them from progressing and causing serious illness.

- Severe cases of diverticulitis with acute pain and complications will likely require a hospital stay. When a person has complications or does not respond to medication, surgery may be necessary.

Source: National Digestive Diseases Information Clearinghouse

RISK FACTORS

Factors that increase the chance of getting diverticulitis include eating a low-fiber diet or a high meat or protein diet, previous episodes of diverticulitis, and chronic constipation. Also, persons age fifty and older are at higher risk.

SYMPTOMS

Symptoms can come on suddenly, and they vary depending on the degree of the infection. Symptoms include abdominal pain and tenderness, usually in the left lower abdomen; a swollen and hard abdomen; fever; chills; poor appetite; nausea; vomiting; diarrhea, constipation, or both; cramping; and rectal bleeding.

SCREENING AND DIAGNOSIS

A doctor will ask about symptoms and medical history and will perform physical and rectal exams. Finding the disease early is important to prevent the pouch from breaking and releasing stool into the abdomen. If this occurs, the patient will need emergency surgery. Tests may include an analysis of a stool sample to look for blood; blood tests to look for signs of infection, inflammation, and bleeding; X rays to look for a rupture; and a computed tomography (CT) scan or ultrasound to locate and determine the size of the inflamed pouch.

Once the inflammation subsides, other tests may be performed. These tests include a barium enema (injection of a dye into the rectum that makes the colon show up on an X ray so the doctor can see abnormal pouches in the colon); a flexible sigmoidoscopy (a thin, lighted camera is inserted into the rectum to examine the rectum and the lower colon); and a colonoscopy (a thin, lighted camera is inserted through the rectum and into the colon to examine the entire lining of the colon).

TREATMENT AND THERAPY

The goals of immediate treatment are to resolve the infection and inflammation, rest the bowel, and prevent complications. Treatment includes antibiotics and other drugs to fight the infection. Pain medications are given to decrease abdominal pain.

For mild inflammation, one should drink clear liquids for the first two to three days. More severe cases will require hospitalization so that fluids and antibiotics can be administered intravenously. To help with nausea and vomiting, a plastic tube may be inserted

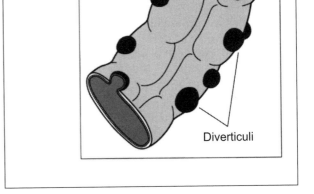

In diverticulitis, the outpouchings of the colon wall become inflamed.

through the patient's nose into his or her stomach. This will help decrease the vomiting and increase comfort.

Changes in diet can help prevent future attacks of diverticulitis. Diet changes include increasing the amount of fiber by eating more fruits, vegetables, and whole grains; supplementing one's diet with a fiber product, as recommended by a doctor; and avoiding laxatives, enemas, and narcotic medications that can lead to constipation.

Surgery to remove the section of the bowel with pouches may be recommended if the patient has had multiple attacks during a two-year period or if a pouch breaks and the contents spread into the abdominal cavity (which will require cleaning out). When surgery is done on an elective basis, a surgeon will remove part of the diseased bowel and hook the normal bowel together. Surgery also treats complications of diverticulitis, such as an abscess, which occurs if the infected pouch fills with pus; a blocked bowel (scar tissue that forms and blocks movement of stool through the intestine); or a fistula, which occurs if the infection spreads and colon tissue attaches to another organ, such as the bladder or the uterus/vagina.

During emergency surgery, the surgeon will remove the diseased bowel. Because of the serious infection, the two ends of the bowel will not be hooked together. The patient will most likely have a piece of bowel coming out to the abdomen (colostomy). After six to twelve weeks, the surgeon will hook the bowel back together.

PREVENTION AND OUTCOMES

The following recommendations may help prevent diverticulitis by improving the movement of stool through the bowel and decreasing constipation: eating a balanced, high-fiber diet with extra fruits, vegetables, and whole grains; drinking eight 8-ounce glasses of water every day; and exercising regularly.

Debra Wood, R.N.; reviewed by Daus Mahnke, M.D.

FURTHER READING

American Society of Colon and Rectal Surgeons. "Diverticular Disease." Available at http://www.fascrs.org/patients/conditions/diverticular_disease.

Feldman, Mark, Lawrence S. Friedman, and Lawrence J. Brandt, eds. *Sleisenger and Fordtran's Gastrointestinal and Liver Disease: Pathophysiology, Diagnosis, Management.* New ed. 2 vols. Philadelphia: Saunders/Elsevier, 2010.

Jacobs, D. O. "Clinical Practice: Diverticulitis." *New England Journal of Medicine* 357 (2007): 2057.

Kapadia, Cyrus R., James M. Crawford, and Caroline Taylor. *An Atlas of Gastroenterology: A Guide to Diagnosis and Differential Diagnosis.* Boca Raton, Fla.: Pantheon, 2003.

National Institute of Diabetes and Digestive and Kidney Diseases. "Diverticulosis and Diverticulitis." Available at http://digestive.niddk.nih.gov/ddiseases/pubs/diverticulosis.

Rakel, Robert E., Edward T. Bope, and Rick D. Kellerman, eds. *Conn's Current Therapy 2011.* Philadelphia: Saunders/Elsevier, 2010.

Strate, L. L., et al. "Nut, Corn, and Popcorn Consumption and the Incidence of Diverticular Disease." *Journal of the American Medical Association* 300 (2008): 907.

WEB SITES OF INTEREST

American College of Gastroenterology
http://www.acg.gi.org

American Dietetic Association
http://www.eatright.org

American Gastroenterological Association
http://www.gastro.org

American Society of Colon and Rectal Surgeons
http://www.fascrs.org

Dietitians of Canada
http://www.dietitians.ca

National Digestive Diseases Information Clearinghouse
http://digestive.niddk.nih.gov

See also: Duodenal ulcer; Enteritis; Gastritis; Infection; Inflammation; Intestinal and stomach infections; Norovirus infection; Peptic ulcer; Peritonitis; Viral gastroenteritis.

Dogs and infectious disease

CATEGORY: Transmission

DEFINITION

Dogs were the first animal species to become domesticated. Fossil evidence from fourteen thousand years ago shows that dogs lived among humans as a species physically distinct from their wolf ancestors. Genetic sequencing suggests dogs split from wolves as long as 100,000 years ago, perhaps because they began to live in close contact with humans. However, dogs remain close relatives to wolves; some scholars argue that dogs are simply a subspecies because dogs and wolves (and coyotes and dingoes) interbreed and produce fertile offspring. As canines, dogs belong to a group of social carnivores and scavengers. In practice, however, dogs, even feral dogs, are not effective

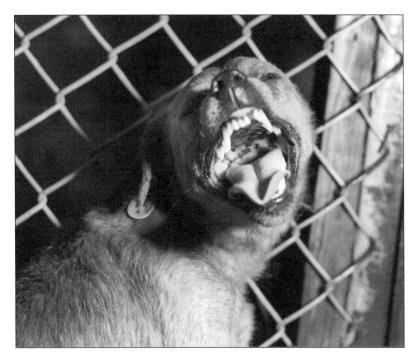

A dog shows the characteristic rabies signs of aggression and restlessness. (CDC)

hunters, depending instead on human provisioning and garbage.

Physically and behaviorally, dogs resemble juvenile wolves, a development called neotony. Juvenile features and behavior probably make them more appealing to humans and more amenable to human lifestyles.

NATURAL HISTORY AND RISK FACTORS

Dogs have adapted to the ecological niche of human society. They are so well adapted to humans that they understand human signals, such as pointing, gaze direction, and tapping, better than humans' closest primate relatives. These adaptations support and attest to the intimate nature of the human-dog bond. Although cultural norms and the role assigned to dogs vary, dogs worldwide still share homes, meals and sleeping spaces with humans. Given this, it is surprising that dogs do not form a great public health risk.

Globally, dogs remain the primary transmitters of rabies. They are the primary transmitters of *Echinococcus granulosus* and, along with cats and wild species, are sources of visceral and ocular larval migrans. Dogs can be one source of infection with *Leptospira*, and they reportedly occasionally transmit other bacterial and protozoan diseases.

RABIES

Recognition of the role dogs play in the transmission of rabies, a nearly 100 percent fatal form of encephalitis, is ancient. A four-thousand-year-old Eshnunna civil code sets fines for the owners of "mad-dogs"; that is, dogs with rabies. Early scholars described a venom, then called a virus, in the saliva of rabid dogs that they believed transmitted the disease. Rabies is actually a collection of viruses, with strains propagating best in a single mammalian species. There are dog strains, fox strains, raccoon strains, bat strains, and others; all can cause disease in any mammal. Although eradicated in developed nations, dog rabies has long been a major threat to humans.

Dog rabies became an epizootic and epidemic threat when humans began to live in cities and keep dogs as pets. Abandoned pets then became feral and depended on garbage to survive. Feeding at single sites brought dogs into close contact, allowing for efficient transmission of rabies.

Prevention of dog-rabies epizootics and human exposures can be achieved through the control of strays, licensing and leash laws, and vaccinations of susceptible dogs. These measures have eradicated dog strain rabies from the United States, Japan, and Europe.

CYSTIC *ECHINOCOCCUS*

Dogs are the natural host for the tapeworm *E. granulosus* and one of the natural hosts for *E. multicularis*. The worms mature in the dog's small intestines, shedding eggs that drop to the ground. Herbivores (especially sheep and goats, but also wild animals and bovines) ingest the eggs, and dogs are reinfected when they eat uncooked organ meats containing larval cysts. Humans can be infected if they ingest water or soil contaminated by dog feces or if they do not practice appropriate hygiene when handling dogs. The highest prevalence of infection with *E. granulosus* occurs in pastoral societies, particularly in sub-Saharan Africa.

Ingested eggs develop into larvae that migrate to organs such as the liver, lung, and brain, where they form cysts. Cysts may not cause disease unless they are large or if they rupture. Cystic *Echinococcus* is debilitating but rarely fatal. Prevention includes hygiene, keeping dogs from eating uncooked offal from abattoirs, and regular deworming of dogs.

E. multicularis is a similar tapeworm that uses wild canines, especially the red fox, as its definitive host. Dogs and cats also serve as hosts and can transmit the parasite to humans. *E. multicularis* most often causes alveolar echinococcosis when cysts develop in the host's lungs.

NEMATODE ZOONOSES

Dogs are natural hosts for a number of roundworms, including *Toxocara canis* and the Ancylostomatoidea, or hookworms. Humans have their own set of roundworm parasites, and often people assume dogs are a source; for the most part, dog roundworms do not develop into adult roundworms in humans.

T. canis larvae migrate in human tissues, most often in children, causing abdominal pain, respiratory signs, and allergy-like syndromes called visceral larval migrans. Occasionally, the larvae cause granulomatous lesions (ocular larval migrans) in the retinas of the eyes, which can limit vision and cause blindness. These diseases result from the ingestion of soil contaminated with *T. canis* eggs. Ancylostomatoidea roundworms comprise the group called hookworms and attach to the intestinal wall. These parasites cause anemia in both dogs and humans. Species of canine hookworms cannot mature in human organs and instead cause skin lesions and, rarely, enteritis.

BACTERIAL ZOONOSES

Dogs are one of many reservoir hosts for *Leptospira*, a spirochete bacteria. There are several pathogenic serovars of *Leptospira*, some of which can cause disease in humans and dogs. Rodents are the major reservoir. Infective bacteria are excreted with urine into standing water. *Leptospira* causes a flulike illness that can lead to liver and kidney failure.

Dogs have been the source of a variety of bacterial diseases in humans, including brucellosis, campylobacteriosis, salmonellosis, yersiniosis, and *Helicobacter* infections. Dogs may bring humans into contact with ticks and fleas, which can result in the transmission of vector-borne diseases such as Lyme disease, ehrlichiosis, and spotted fever group rickettsiosis. In addition,

dogbites can occasionally become infected, most commonly with *Staphylococcus, Streptococcus, Corynebacterium,* and *Bacteroides* spp.

PROTOZOAN ZOONOSES

Dogs are reservoir hosts for leishmaniasis. The disease, spread by sandflies, is caused by single-celled parasites. Skin lesions, disfigurement, and a rare, potentially fatal visceral syndrome called kala-azar may result.

IMPACT

Rabies kills about fifty-five thousand people every year around the world, and most of these infections are transmitted by dogs. The other diseases transmitted by dogs are not well documented and cause few fatalities. In developed nations, where dogs are controlled and receive veterinary care, public health concerns are limited. Indeed, there is evidence that owning a pet has salutary benefits, such as encouraging owners to exercise and helping to lower stress.

Cynthia L. Mills, D.V.M.

FURTHER READING

Krauss, Hartmut, et al. *Zoonoses: Infectious Diseases Transmissible from Animals to Humans.* 3d ed. Washington, D.C.: ASM Press, 2003. Explores the myriad infections introduced by human-animal contact.

Macpherson, Calum N. L., et al., eds. *Dogs, Zoonoses, and Public Health.* New York: CABI, 2000. A comprehensive survey of all potential zoonoses transmitted by dogs.

Morgan, Marina, and John Palmer. "Dog Bites." *British Medical Journal* 334 (2007): 413-417. A journal article on infections caused by dog bites.

Serpell, James, ed. *The Domestic Dog: Its Evolution, Behaviour, and Interactions with People.* 1995. Reprint. New York: Cambridge University Press, 2002. Explores the history and evolution of the domestic dog and its relationship with peoples around the world.

World Health Organization. "WHO Expert Consultation on Rabies: First Report." Technical Report Series 931. Geneva: Author, 2004. Experts' consensus with summaries of experience on controlling rabies. Emphasis on controlling dog populations and on mass vaccination administration.

See also: Bacteria: Classification and types; Bacterial infections; *Capnocytophaga* infections; Cat scratch fever; Cats and infectious disease; *Echinococcus*; Fecal-oral route of transmission; Parasitic diseases; Rabies; Rat-bite fever; Rodents and infectious disease; Roundworms; Saliva and infectious disease; Transmission routes; Worm infections; Wound infections; Zoonotic diseases.

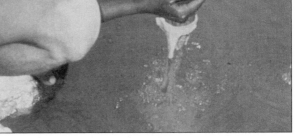

A child holds a strainer to filter water suspected of containing the parasitic worm Dracunculus. (CDC)

Dracunculiasis

CATEGORY: Diseases and conditions
ANATOMY OR SYSTEM AFFECTED: Gastrointestinal system, intestines, skin
ALSO KNOWN AS: Guinea worm disease

DEFINITION

Dracunculiasis, or guinea worm disease (GWD), is caused by the parasitic guinea worm, a long, thin worm that can grow inside humans. Dracunculiasis affects people living in certain parts of rural Africa who drink water contaminated by guinea worm larvae. GWD is one of the few diseases specifically mentioned in the Bible, where it is called *dracunculiasis medinensis*, or "fiery serpents." An adult female worm can reach up to three feet long.

CAUSES

People get dracunculiasis by drinking contaminated water infested with water fleas that have ingested the guinea worm larvae. The guinea worms, usually female, move through the body, and about one year later, protrude through the skin, usually on the lower leg or feet, causing immense pain. At the site of protrusion, there is a blister or an ulcer, and the worm can be seen emerging. Some people seek relief by placing the infected area in open water (such as a pond, lake, or river) that is used for drinking, which allows the female worms to release larvae into the water and repeat the process of infestation.

RISK FACTORS

This disease tends to affect people living in rural or poorer communities in certain countries in Africa, where water sources are scarce and where drinking water most often comes from open, and exposed, sources.

SYMPTOMS

Symptoms do not appear until about one year after a person has become infected with dracunculiasis. When the guinea worm prepares to emerge from the body, a person usually experiences intense pain and itching or burning, often followed by nausea, vomiting, and fever. A blister forms at the site of where the worm will emerge, leaving the person virtually incapacitated, sometimes for many months, as the worm is gently pulled from the body and removed.

SCREENING AND DIAGNOSIS

There is no screening for dracunculiasis. A person does not know he or she has the disease until the worm begins to exit the body, about one year after contaminated water has been ingested.

TREATMENT AND THERAPY

Once the worm emerges at the site of the blister, it is pulled out in a slow and painful process; the infection is then cleaned. The only treatment for the infection is to help alleviate symptoms once the worm emerges.

PREVENTION AND OUTCOMES

Preventive methods against dracunculiasis include using a cloth filter to remove water fleas from drinking water and to drink water from protected (closed) sources. Persons already infected with a dracunculiasis blister should not enter any water source that is used for drinking.

Although this disease was once widespread throughout Asia and Africa, public health experts and others are getting closer to eradicating the disease, aided by disease education and the use of chemicals to treat potentially unsafe drinking water.

Micki Pflug Mounce, B.A.

FURTHER READING

Berger, Stephen A., and John S. Marr. *Human Parasitic Diseases Sourcebook.* Sudbury, Mass.: Jones and Bartlett, 2006.

Centers for Disease Control and Prevention. "Progress Toward Global Eradication of Dracunculiasis, January, 2008-June, 2009." *Morbidity and Mortality Weekly Report* 58, no. 40 (2009): 1123-1125.

Muller, Ralph. *Worms and Human Disease.* 2d ed. New York: CABI, 2002.

Parker, James N., and Philip M. Parker, eds. *The Official Patient's Sourcebook on Dracunculiasis: A Revised and Updated Directory for the Internet Age.* San Diego, Calif.: Icon Health, 2002.

Roberts, Larry S., and John Janovy, Jr. *Gerald D. Schmidt and Larry S. Roberts' Foundations of Parasitology.* 8th ed. Boston: McGraw-Hill, 2009.

Weedon, David. *Skin Pathology.* 3d ed. New York: Churchill Livingstone/Elsevier, 2010.

WEB SITES OF INTEREST

American Society of Tropical Medicine and Hygiene
http://www.astmh.org

Carter Center, Guinea Worm Eradication Program
http://www.cartercenter.org/health/guinea_worm

Centers for Disease Control and Prevention
http://www.cdc.gov/parasites

See also: Ascariasis; Cholera; Developing countries and infectious disease; Flukes; Giardiasis; Hookworms; Infection; Intestinal and stomach infections; Parasitic diseases; Pinworms; Roundworms; Skin infections; Taeniasis; Tapeworms; Tinea corporis; Toxocariasis; Travelers' diarrhea; Trichinosis; Tropical medicine; Waterborne illness and disease; Whipworm infection; Worm infections.

Drug resistance

CATEGORY: Epidemiology
ALSO KNOWN AS: Antibiotic resistance, antimicrobial resistance, drug tolerance

DEFINITION

Drug resistance is the decreased ability of a medication to cure or reduce disease symptoms. Typically, drug resistance is caused by a pathogenic organisms' decreased susceptibility to a medication over time.

HISTORY

The discovery of medications that target disease-causing, pathogenic organisms was a great medical victory against infection. The most famous of these medications, often called antimicrobials, is bacteriologist Alexander Fleming's 1928 discovery that a specific kind of mold, *Penicillium notatum* (now called *P. chrysogenum*), kills many forms of disease-causing bacteria. However, this discovery was closely followed by the realization that bacteria can develop drug resistance. By the late 1940's, multiple strains of bacteria had been found to be resistant to antibiotics. These bacteria developed a variety of mechanisms to overcome the damaging effect of the antimicrobial medications.

Since the mid-twentieth century, the natural ability of pathogenic organisms to overcome biological barriers and the use, overuse, and misuse of antibiotics and related medications to treat human and animal illnesses have allowed disease-causing agents to become less and less affected by agents such as penicillin; thus, the related diseases are not as effectively treated. To complicate the issue, some organisms have developed a resistance to treatment with several, often unrelated, antimicrobial medications. This is particularly true in hospitals. It is estimated that more than 70 percent of the disease-causing bacteria found in hospitals are resistant to at least one of the standard antibiotics used to treat them.

CLASSIFICATION

Drug resistance occurs in a variety of disease-causing (pathogenic) organisms that are characterized by their ability to reproduce, thrive, and efficiently increase their numbers. The pathogens are bacteria, viruses, fungi, and parasites.

Bacteria. Bacteria are microorganisms characterized by the lack of a distinct nuclear membrane and a cell wall. Most bacteria are one-celled organisms and are found everywhere on Earth: in the soil, water, and air, and in and on the human body and the bodies of nonhuman animals. Although not all bacteria cause disease, strains of streptococci, *Escherichia coli, Haemophilus influenzae, Salmonella,* and staphylococci cause diseases such as the flu, strep throat, and food poisoning. Most bacterial infections are transmitted by direct contact with contaminated people or by indirect contact with contaminated objects. Although mild bacterial infections are usually effectively fought by the body's immune system, antibiotic medications such as penicillin, cephalosporin, tetracycline, aminoglycoside, and quinolones damage or prevent creation of bacterial cell walls, interrupt normal bacterial function, and disrupt their genetic code. All these medications assist the immune system in combating bacterial infections.

Viruses. Viruses are microscopic infectious organisms composed of a small piece of genetic information (deoxyribonucleic acid, or DNA, and ribonucleic acid, or RNA) and an external protein "body." Most viruses are disease-causing and can replicate only inside the cells of other organisms. Common viruses cause diseases such as influenza, chickenpox, and AIDS (acquired immunodeficiency syndrome). Most viral infections are transmitted by direct contact with contaminated people or by indirect contact with contaminated objects; however, some viral infections, such as human immunodeficiency virus (HIV), occur only by contact with specific bodily fluids (namely blood, semen, vaginal fluid, pre-ejaculate, and breast milk). Antiviral medications have been developed to inhibit infection by specific viruses. However, because of their rapid rate of reproduction, viruses have been able to adapt quickly and have become resistant to many antiviral medications.

Fungi. Fungi are organisms that include a variety of mushrooms, yeasts, and molds. They reproduce through spores and obtain food from breaking down organic matter. Some categories of fungi infect humans and cause disease. Several fungi cause common conditions such as yeast infection and athlete's foot. Other fungi species, such as *Aspergillus,* can cause significant health issues for persons who are chronically ill and immunocompromised, especially persons with cancer or immune or autoimmune disorders. Antifungal drugs are less effective than antibiotics or antiviral medications because most fungi are made of cells that are like human cells in design, with membranes enclosed in genetic material. As the number of persons susceptible to fungal infections and requiring treatment has increased, fungal drug resistance has increased as a significant clinical problem too. Fungi have been found that are resistant to an array of antifungal agents, such as the azoles, flucytosine, and amphotericin B.

Parasites. A parasite is an organism that takes its nourishment from another organism (a host) without providing any direct benefit to that host. There are numerous parasites that infect humans, including bacteria, fungi, viruses, lice, worms, fleas, amebas, and other small organisms. Like bacteria, viruses, and fungi, other parasitic organisms have developed resistances to drugs. For example, parasitic hookworms have developed a genetic resistance to the anthelmintics that are designed to kill or stun them sufficiently to expel them from the body.

CAUSAL MECHANISMS

Pathogenic organisms have an unparalleled ability to adapt to their environments and survive the attacks of antimicrobial medications. In many cases, natural selection is the key to pathogen success, as the few disease-causing organisms that are not killed by a medication have an advantage over susceptible organisms. The keys to adaptation in pathogenic organisms are their fast rate of reproduction and fast development and transmittal of new, beneficial traits to the next generation.

Frequently, an organism's advantageous feature is the result of a particular genetic change or mutation that codes for a feature that decreases a medication's effectiveness. Bacteria, parasites, and other disease-causing microbes sometimes undergo random mutations that spontaneously confer resistance. More frequently, one microbe will acquire survival-enhancing characteristics from another as they exchange genetic information through gene transfer systems. For example, one strain of pathogenic bacteria develops a mutation coding for a medication "pump" that sends the antibiotic tetracycline out of their systems before causing damage. Over time, this resistant bacteria strain will exchange genetic material with another set of bacteria and, in turn, provide them with the pump feature. These genetic changes are also transmitted to bacterial offspring. This innate ability of the organisms to transmit favorable mutations means that many have multiple defense mechanisms to combat antimicrobial medications. In the case of drug resistance, the microbes are simply using their natural approach to obstacles that decrease their primary functions, which are to reproduce, thrive, and spread quickly and efficiently.

Although the development of drug resistant genes is a natural process, specific human behaviors have accelerated the success of these pathogens. The first is excessive or inappropriate use of antibiotics and related antimicrobials. To provide some measure of comfort to ill patients, some physicians will prescribe an antibiotic for a viral infection or an antiviral for someone with an undefined illness. Additionally, to speed the time to wellness, a physician may prescribe stronger or broader spectrum medications when a targeted antibiotic would be sufficient. The exposed disease-causing organisms may develop resistance to medications that were not designed for optimum effectiveness against them and, over time, produce a strain of microbes with multiple resistances.

An additional increase in drug resistant organisms is related to human behavior in taking medications. Physicians optimize the use of medications based on the perceived strength of the disease-causing organism and the effectiveness of the medication. Often patients will begin taking the medication at the prescribed strength and dose, but than stop taking the medication when they feel symptoms decrease. In some instances, they will keep the remaining pills and use them without a physician's prescription to address a similar, future illness. A similar concern arises in lower income or uninsured patients, who may not be able to afford a full course of medication. This practice of undertreatment eliminates the drug-sensitive microbes while allowing more disease-causing organisms to survive and to adapt a drug resistance to the medication being used.

Another reason antimicrobial medications have accelerated drug resistance is the increased number of chronically ill and immunocompromised persons treated in hospitals and clinics. These critically ill persons acquire more frequent infections and require more frequent use of medications to treat them. Over time, the antimicrobials weed out the weaker microbe strains, leaving the strong, more virulent, and more resistant pathogens to cause infections. This, in turn, requires stronger medications for treatment, bringing about more adaptations to other drugs. Also, in a hospital setting, infection transmission from one person to another is increased because of proximity.

A final accelerant in the development of drug resistance is the overuse in livestock of antibiotics, antiparasitics, antifungals, and related medications. Scientists estimate that 70 percent of all antibiotics in the United States are put into the food and water of healthy livestock. The use of these medications is to control disease, improve metabolism, and stimulate the growth of microbes that produce vitamins and other related, useful, metabolic products. The overuse of these medications increases the number of drug resistant organisms in the livestock, the food derived from the livestock, and the environment surrounding the livestock's feeding area.

TREATMENT AND RESEARCH

Physicians, scientists, epidemiologists, and others in public health have been working to combat drug-resistant microbes through a multimodal approach. First, they have focused on infection prevention through lifestyle habits such as frequent handwashing and good hygiene to decrease the spread of drug resistant microbes. Hospitals and clinics have developed detailed policies and procedures on identifying affected persons, preventing disease spread, and the provision and use of protective gear such as gloves and alcohol-based hand rubs. Educational efforts focus on patients, physicians, and family members to decrease the incidence of disease.

When disease does occur, physicians are encouraged to use diagnostic techniques to identify the exact cause of illness and to prescribe the most targeted antimicrobial treatment. Appropriate diagnosis, as a result, would limit the use of broad spectrum medications. Also, physicians and patients should be counseled on the importance of taking all prescribed medication and of not keeping pills for later use.

When a particular disease-causing organism is resistant to all front-line antibiotics and related medications, physicians often use strong antimicrobial medications that have more side effects. In many cases, the overseeing physicians must then monitor subjects more closely to ensure that they take all their medication and return for follow-up care. A good example of this is the practice of tuberculosis (TB) clinics that monitor patient medication use closely, hoping to decrease the speed of development of drug resistant TB strains.

Although it has met with considerable resistance, the U.S. Food and Drug Administration and other North American organizations have been working with farmers and veterinarians to determine the best ways to reduce the use of antibiotics and related medications in livestock and food-producing animals.

Beyond medical and agricultural practices, scientists are working to determine the basic mechanisms of function, infection, genetics, and drug resistance in a variety of pathogenic organisms. This research is helping scientists develop ways to avoid triggering increased drug resistance and to circumnavigate identified organism defense mechanisms to restore the effectiveness of known medications. Much of this new information comes from scientists delving into an organism's genetic code to learn exactly what mutation causes a particular defense system. As an example, after determining that some bacteria resistant to tetracycline have developed a protein to shield their ribosomes, scientists found other forms of tetracycline that render the shield ineffective.

Scientists are also working on new medications based on knowledge of the structure and function of pathogenic organisms. Some of these antibiotics are naturally occurring and others are synthetic and were created in a laboratory. For example, researchers are working on the development of a medication against a strain of staphylococci bacteria that makes specific proteins that destroy the white blood cells of the immune system. The hope is that compounds formed in the lab will be different enough from those found in nature that it will take longer for disease-causing organisms to develop resistance. Whether used to work around current resistant organism defenses or to develop new drugs, increased knowledge about the pathogenic organisms is helping combat drug resistant strains of organisms.

IMPACT

Disease-causing organisms have developed multiple levels of drug resistance to many crucial antimicrobial medications. Drug resistant microbes that were once considered completely treatable can be life-threatening. A prime example of this is methicillin-resistant *Staphylococcus aureus* (MRSA), which is now common in hospitals and community settings.

A global health crisis also has emerged with drug resistant malaria and tuberculosis. The crisis began in countries without modern medication systems that have relied instead upon lower-cost traditional medications, such as chloroquine, to treat these frequent infections exclusively; however, the resistant strains of the microbes have spread across the world. This loss of effectiveness has led to increased death, suffering, and disability, and to higher health care costs. Physicians, scientists, public health workers, government agencies, and pharmaceutical companies are working to decrease the spread of drug resistant microbes through education, research, and better health care procedures.

Dawn Laney, M.S.

FURTHER READING

Arias, Cesar A., and Barbara E. Murray. "Antibiotic-Resistant Bugs in the Twenty-first Century: A Clinical Super-Challenge." *New England Journal of Medicine* 360 (2009): 439-443. Discusses the history and specific characteristics of antibiotic resistant bacteria.

Gorman, Christine. "Playing Chicken with Our Antibiotics." *Time,* January 21, 2002, pp. 98-99. Describes the ways in which overtreatment is creating dangerous drug resistant germs.

Mellon, Margaret, Charles Benbrook, and Karen L. Benbrook, "Hogging It: Estimates of Antimicrobial Abuse in Livestock." Cambridge, Mass.: Union of Concerned Scientists, 2001. This article provides information about the misuse of antibiotics in raising farm animals.

Nash, J. Madeleine. "The Future of Drugs: The Antibiotics Crisis." *Time*, January 15, 2001, pp. 90-93. Discusses antibiotic resistant medications and impending medical crises.

Nicolaou, K. C., and Christopher N. Boddy. "Behind Enemy Lines: A Close Look at the Inner Workings of Microbes in this Era of Escalating Antibiotic Resistance Is Offering New Strategies for Designing Drugs." *Scientific American*, May, 2001, p. 54. A detailed discussion about scientific exploration into microbe characteristics that will provide strategies for designing drugs in overcoming antibiotic resistance.

Rosenblatt-Farrell, Noah. "The Landscape of Antibiotic Resistance" *Environmental Health Perspectives* 117, no. 6 (2009): 244-250. A detailed article examining the issue of antibiotic resistance and the future of existing antibiotic therapies.

Science 321, no. 5887 (July 18, 2008). A special issue devoted to antibiotic resistance, highlighting some particularly difficult infections and discussing issues pertaining to the genetics of antibiotic resistance.

State of New Hampshire. Communicable Disease Control and Surveillance. "State of New Hampshire Recommendations for the Prevention and Control of Multi-Drug-Resistant Organisms (MDROs)." Available at http://www.dhhs.state.nh.us/dhhs/cdcs/library. Clearly describes a series of preventive measures being taken to reduce transmission of organisms resistant to multiple medications.

Walsh, Christopher. *Antibiotics: Actions, Origins, Resistance*. Washington, D.C.: ASM Press, 2003. Examines such topics as how antibiotics block specific proteins, how the molecular structure of drugs enables such activity, the development of bacterial resistance, and the molecular logic of antibiotic biosynthesis.

WEB SITES OF INTEREST

Centers for Disease Control and Prevention
http://www.cdc.gov/drugresistance

National Institute of Allergy and Infectious Diseases
http://www.niaid.nih.gov/topics/antimicrobialresistance

Todar's Online Textbook of Bacteriology
http://www.textbookofbacteriology.net

World Health Organization
http://www.who.int/drugresistance

See also: Alliance for the Prudent Use of Antibiotics; Alternative therapies; Antibiotic resistance; Antibiotics: Experimental; Antibiotics: Types; Antifungal drugs: Types; Antiparasitic drugs: Types; Antiviral drugs: Types; Bacterial infections; Home remedies; Hospitals and infectious disease; Iatrogenic infections; Infection; Microbiology; Over-the-counter (OTC) drugs; Parasitic diseases; Pathogens; Public health; Secondary infection; Virulence.

DTaP vaccine

CATEGORY: Prevention

ALSO KNOWN AS: Diphtheria, tetanus, and acellular pertussis vaccine

DEFINITION

The DTaP vaccine protects against three different bacterial illnesses. The first disease, diphtheria, is caused by the bacterium *Corynebacterium diphtheriae*. Infection with this bacterium causes a severe sore throat and difficulty breathing and swallowing. The second disease, tetanus, is caused by the bacterium *Clostridium tetani* and leads to what is commonly referred to as lockjaw. This disease causes intense muscle contractions and can interfere with breathing. The last disease, pertussis, or whooping cough, is caused by the bacterium *Bordetella pertussis*. This bacterium produces a severe persistent cough with a characteristic whooping sound on inspiration between coughing fits and can lead to respiratory failure.

MECHANISM OF ACTION

The vaccine incorporates the three toxins that are produced by the bacteria in their inactivated forms (known as toxoids). These toxoids are then administered, leading to an immune response without actually causing the disease, therefore providing protection from future illness.

HISTORY

Individual vaccines against diphtheria, tetanus, and pertussis were first developed in the late nineteenth and early twentieth centuries. The combination vaccine that incorporated all three was first licensed in 1948. The vaccine was further modified in 1991 in response to a high rate of side effects thought to be caused by the original whole-cell pertussis component. A new, acellular pertussis element was developed at that time and has resulted in a significant decrease in the side effect profile of the vaccine. The DTaP vaccine can be found as a component of combination vaccines such as Pediarix (with hepatitis B and inactivated poliovirus) and Pentacel (with *Haemophilus influenzae* type B and inactivated poliovirus).

ADMINISTRATION

Health experts recommended that children receive the DTaP vaccine at age two, four, six, and fifteen to eighteen months and again between the age of four and six years. Adolescents and adults should then receive one administration of the Tdap vaccine, which differs from the DTaP in that it contains less of the diphtheria and acellular pertussis components. After the Tdap, adults should receive the Td booster immunization against tetanus and diphtheria every ten years.

IMPACT

The impact of the DTaP vaccine on public health has been enormous. Diphtheria has been nearly eradicated in the United States, and the incidence of tetanus and pertussis has been greatly reduced. However, of the three diseases, pertussis continues to affect many adults and children in the United States, with morbidity and mortality rates rising among infants.

Jennifer Birkhauser, M.D.

FURTHER READING

Advisory Committee on Immunization Practices. "Recommended Adult Immunization Schedule: United States, 2010." *Annals of Internal Medicine* 152 (2010): 36-39.

Centers for Disease Control and Prevention. "Recommended Immunization Schedules for Persons Aged 0-18 Years—United States, 2008." *Morbidity and Mortality Weekly Report* 57 (2008): Q1-Q4. Also available at http://www.cdc.gov/mmwr/preview/mmwrhtml/mm5701a8.htm.

Harvey, Richard A., Pamela C. Champe, and Bruce D. Fisher. *Lippincott's Illustrated Reviews: Microbiology.* 2d ed. Lippincott Williams and Wilkins, 2006.

Loehr, Jamie. *The Vaccine Answer Book: Two Hundred Essential Answers to Help You Make the Right Decisions for Your Child.* Naperville, Ill.: Sourcebooks, 2010.

Pan American Health Organization. World Health Organization. *Control of Diphtheria, Pertussis, Tetanus, "Haemophilus influenzae" Type B, and Hepatitis B Field Guide.* Washington, D.C.: Author, 2005.

Playfair, J. H. L., and B. M. Chain. *Immunology at a Glance.* 9th ed. Hoboken, N.J.: Wiley-Blackwell, 2009.

Plotkin, Stanley A., Walter A. Orenstein, and Paul A. Offit. *Vaccines.* 5th ed. Philadelphia: Saunders/Elsevier, 2008.

WEB SITES OF INTEREST

Centers for Disease Control and Prevention
http://www.cdc.gov/vaccines/pubs/vis

Children's Hospital of Philadelphia, Vaccine Education-Center
http://www.chop.edu/service/vaccine-education-center

National Institutes of Health
http://www.nlm.nih.gov/medlineplus/ency/article/002021.htm

See also: Bacterial infections; *Bordetella*; Children and infectious disease; *Clostridium*; *Corynebacterium*; Diphtheria; Hib vaccine; Immunity; Immunization; Tetanus; Vaccines: Types; Whooping cough.

Duodenal ulcer

CATEGORY: Diseases and conditions
ANATOMY OR SYSTEM AFFECTED: Abdomen,digestive system, gastrointestinal system, intestines, stomach
ALSO KNOWN AS: Peptic ulcer, ulcer

DEFINITION

A duodenal ulcer is a peptic ulcer that is located in the duodenum, the upper part of the small intestine where it attaches to the stomach. The ulcer is a sore on the lining of the duodenum.

CAUSES

More than one-half of the cases of duodenal ulcer are caused by infection with a bacterium called *Helicobacter pylori* (*H. pylori*). Aspirin and ibuprofen are examples of nonsteroidal anti-inflammatory drugs (NSAIDs) that can also cause duodenal ulcers. Rarely, tumors that are benign (not cancerous) or malignant (cancerous) may cause ulcers. Eating spicy foods, stress, smoking, and drinking alcohol do not cause, but do often worsen the symptoms of, ulcers.

RISK FACTORS

Infection with *H. pylori* is common. Infections can develop in childhood without causing symptoms until later in life. Drinking contaminated water or eating contaminated food increases the risk of taking in the bacterium. Food that is not properly washed or cooked increases the chance of infection. Contact with the saliva, vomit, or feces of an infected person may also transfer the bacterium.

SYMPTOMS

Discomfort in the abdomen is the most common symptom, but some people have no symptoms or mild symptoms only. Discomfort may be a dull or burning pain (heartburn) that lasts a few minutes or hours when the stomach is empty, and episodes may continue for days or weeks. Discomfort may improve after eating or taking antacids. Weight loss, lack of appetite, burping, bloating, nausea, and vomiting are all common symptoms. If sharp, persistent, and severe pain or bloody vomit or bowel movements occur, one should consult a doctor immediately.

SCREENING AND DIAGNOSIS

A physician usually makes the diagnosis by taking a careful history of drugs used, especially prescription or over-the-counter NSAIDs, and by testing for *H. pylori*. A breath test or stool test are more accurate at finding *H. pylori* than are blood tests. If symptoms are severe, a thin, lighted tube with a camera on the end (endoscope) is threaded down the throat and through the stomach to the duodenum to look at the area (endoscopy). Radiology (X-ray) tests of the upper gastrointestinal tract may also be done.

TREATMENT AND THERAPY

The primary treatment for NSAID-related duodenal ulcers is stopping the drug and using medicines that reduce stomach acid to decrease pain and promote healing and coat the ulcer to protect it from stomach acid. For duodenal ulcers caused by *H. pylori*, antibiotic therapy for ten to fourteen days usually heals the ulcer. Different antibiotic regimens are used throughout the world because the *H. pylori* bacterium has become resistant to some antibiotics. This means that the drug is no longer effective in killing the bacterium. Medicines to reduce acid and coat the ulcer are also used. About four weeks after treatment, the person is tested again to see if the *H. pylori* bacterium is gone.

PREVENTION AND OUTCOMES

While it is not known how *H. pylori* spreads, the bacterium can be avoided with careful handwashing, especially after using the toilet and before eating, washing, and cooking food; drinking clean water; not sharing drinks and food with others; and using gloves when cleaning up vomit or bowel movements. Taking NSAIDs in recommended doses or only when needed may also prevent a duodenal ulcer.

Patricia Stanfill Edens, R.N., Ph.D., FACHE

FURTHER READING

Feldman, Mark, Lawrence S. Friedman, and Lawrence J. Brandt, eds. *Sleisenger and Fordtran's Gastrointestinal and Liver Disease: Pathophysiology, Diagnosis, Management.* New ed. 2 vols. Philadelphia: Saunders/Elsevier, 2010.

Kapadia, Cyrus R., James M. Crawford, and Caroline Taylor. *An Atlas of Gastroenterology: A Guide to Diagnosis and Differential Diagnosis.* Boca Raton, Fla.: Pantheon, 2003.

Kirschner, Barbara S., and Dennis D. Black. "The Gastrointestinal Tract." In *Nelson Essentials of Pediatrics*, edited by Karen J. Marcdante et al. 6th ed. Philadelphia: Saunders/Elsevier, 2011.

McColl, Kenneth E. L. "*Helicobacter pylori* Infection." *New England Journal of Medicine* 362 (2010): 1597-1604.

WEB SITES OF INTEREST

American College of Gastroenterology
http://www.acg.gi.org

Clean Hands Coalition
http://www.cleanhandscoalition.org

National Digestive Diseases Information Clearinghouse
http://digestive.niddk.nih.gov

See also: Amebic dysentery; Bacteria: Classification and types; Bacterial infections; Cancer and infectious disease; Food-borne illness and disease; Gastritis; Giardiasis; *Helicobacter*; *Helicobacter pylori* infection; Infectious colitis; Intestinal and stomach infections; Peptic ulcer.

E. coli infection. *See Escherichia coli* infection.

E

Eastern equine encephalitis

CATEGORY: Diseases and conditions
ANATOMY OR SYSTEM AFFECTED: Brain, central nervous
system

DEFINITION

Eastern equine encephalitis (EEE) is a virus affecting wild birds. It is carried by certain mosquitoes and is occasionally transmitted to horses and, rarely, to humans. EEE affects the brain and central nervous system.

Although EEE is more dangerous to horses than to humans (many people infected with the EEE virus do not have any apparent health problems), in some cases, people infected can become suddenly and seriously ill and may experience severe injury to the nervous system; death sometimes follows.

In areas where EEE is known to be present, one should take extra precaution to avoid mosquitoes and to protect against mosquito bites.

CAUSES

EEE, an arbovirus, is spread by infected invertebrate animals, mostly blood-sucking (hematophagous) insects. Arboviruses are usually spread by infected mosquitoes. Mosquitoes most often get the EEE virus by biting infected birds, and then spreading the virus to horses and other mammals, including humans.

RISK FACTORS

Because the only known way for humans to contract EEE is by being bitten by an infected mosquito, the risk factor most commonly associated with EEE is exposure to mosquito bites, or living near or visiting a wetland area or an area known to have incidents of EEE. People age fifteen years and younger and age fifty years and older seem to be more susceptible to the infection.

SYMPTOMS

If a person experiences any of the symptoms for EEE, he or she should not assume it is caused by EEE.

These symptoms may be caused by other, less serious health conditions. However, one should consult a doctor if any of the following symptoms are present: fatigue; fever; headache; nausea; restlessness or irritability; difficulty walking or unstableness; confusion, impaired judgment, or an altered mental state; or seizures.

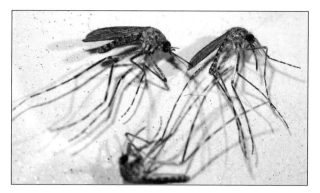

Dead cattail mosquitoes, which can transmit eastern equine encephalitis to humans, in containers for laboratory inspection. (AP/Wide World Photos)

SCREENING AND DIAGNOSIS

A doctor will ask about symptoms and medical history, will perform a physical exam, and may order the following tests: blood tests to check if the virus is present; a spinal tap to remove a small amount of spinal fluid to check for signs of infection; an electroencephalogram (EEG) to measure the brain's activity; a neurological exam to access reflexes, memory, and other brain function; a magnetic resonance imaging (MRI) scan (a scan that uses radio waves and a powerful magnet to produce detailed computer images); and a computed tomography (CT) scan (a detailed X-ray picture that identifies abnormalities of fine tissue structure).

TREATMENT AND THERAPY

There are no drug options to treat the EEE virus in humans, so medical treatment focuses on the symptoms of the infection. Such treatments may include antibiotics for secondary infections; anticonvulsants to treat seizures; a respirator to help with breathing; pain relievers to treat headache, fever, and body aches; corticosteroids to reduce swelling in the brain; and sedatives for restlessness or irritability.

PREVENTION AND OUTCOMES

To help reduce the chance of getting EEE, one should avoid areas of mosquito activity, if possible, and stay inside when mosquitoes are most active (at dawn and at dusk). When outside, one should wear insect repellent, long pants, and long-sleeved shirts to limit exposure to bites. To help limit mosquito populations in and around the home, one should eliminate the insects' breeding areas, such as standing water in ponds, bowls for pets, rain barrels, and other containers.

Diane Stresing;
reviewed by David L. Horn, M.D., FACP

FURTHER READING

Booss, John, Margaret Esiri, and Margaret M. Esin, eds. *Viral Encephalitis in Humans.* Washington, D.C.: ASM Press, 2003.

Centers for Disease Control and Prevention. "Eastern Equine Encephalitis Virus (EEEV)." Available at http://www.cdc.gov/easternequineencephalitis.

Marquardt, William C., ed. *Biology of Disease Vectors.* 2d ed. New York: Academic Press/Elsevier, 2005.

North Carolina Department of Health and Human Services. "Arboviruses: Eastern Equine Encephalitis." Available at http://www.epi.state.nc.us/epi/arbovirus/eee.html.

Stull, J. W., et al. "Eastern Equine Encephalitis—New Hampshire and Massachusetts, August-September 2005." *Journal of the American Medical Association* 296 (2006): 645-646. Available at http://jama.ama-assn.org/cgi/content/full/296/6/645.

WEB SITES OF INTEREST

Canadian Cooperative Wildlife Centre
http://www.ccwhc.ca

Centers for Disease Control and Prevention
http://www.cdc.gov/ncidod/dvbid

National Institute of Neurological Disorders and Stroke
http://www.ninds.nih.gov

U.S. Department of Agriculture, Animal and Plant Health Inspection Service
http://www.aphis.usda.gov/animal_health

See also: Arthropod-borne illness and disease; Avian influenza; Birds and infectious disease; Blood-borne illness and disease; Carriers; Cholera; Dengue fever; Encephalitis; Insect-borne illness and disease; Mosquito-borne viral encephalitis; Mosquitoes and infectious disease; Poliomyelitis; Psittacosis; Tropical medicine; Viral infections; Viral meningitis; West Nile virus; Yellow fever; Zoonotic diseases.

Ebola hemorrhagic fever

CATEGORY: Diseases and conditions
ANATOMY OR SYSTEM AFFECTED: Blood
ALSO KNOWN AS: Viral hemorrhagic fever

DEFINITION

Ebola hemorrhagic fever is a condition caused by the Ebola virus, leading to a serious disease that has an extremely high mortality rate. This condition is spread by contact with the body fluids of an infected person or animal, even after death, and can be spread in research laboratories from infected animals. The Ebola virus, which occurs naturally in Africa, damages the lining of blood vessels and interferes with blood clotting. Ebola hemorrhagic fever appears in sporadic outbreaks.

CAUSES

Ebola hemorrhagic fever is caused by a virus from the family Filoviridae and the genus *Ebolavirus*. There are five species of the virus: *Zaire, Sudan, Cote d'Ivoire, Bundibugyo,* and *Reston. Reston* and *Cote d'Ivoire* cause relatively mild symptoms and are usually not fatal. *Zaire, Sudan,* and *Bundibugyo* appear to be the cause of Ebola hemorrhagic fever. These species originate in the rain forests of Africa and reside in an unknown host. Less commonly, these species appear in the western Pacific in the Philippines. Although the reservoirs of the virus are unknown, scientists theorize the virus originates in animals, possibly bats.

RISK FACTORS

The main risk factor is direct contact with the body fluids of infected persons or animals. Other risk factors for Ebola hemorrhagic fever are living in or visiting areas where the Ebola virus is found, working in a laboratory where animal testing with the Ebola virus is being conducted, and caring for persons with Ebola virus infection.

SYMPTOMS

The incubation period for Ebola hemorrhagic fever ranges from two to twenty-one days after exposure. During this time, the infected person can have joint and muscle pain, low back pain, chills, a fever, diarrhea, a headache, malaise, nausea, vomiting, and a sore throat. The disease then rapidly progresses to symptoms of bleeding from the eyes, ears, nose, mouth, and rectum; internal bleeding; depression; conjunctivitis; swelling of the genitalia; skin pain; a body-wide rash; stomach pain; seizures; coma; and delirium. About 90 percent of persons who contract Ebola hemorrhagic fever will die from the condition.

SCREENING AND DIAGNOSIS

There is no routine screening for Ebola hemorrhagic fever. The isolated geographic areas in which the disease occurs affects diagnosis, which is often delayed because of a lack of medical care or because of inadequate medical care. Diagnosis is achieved through symptoms and blood tests, including complete blood count, blood electrolytes, blood coagulation tests, and identification of the virus or antibodies to the virus. If a person is infected, his or her blood cell counts will be low, electrolytes will be decreased, and blood coagulation rate will be decreased. Testing for the virus or its antibodies is performed using antigen-capture enzyme-linked immunosorbent assay or by polymerase chain reaction.

TREATMENT AND THERAPY

There is no cure for Ebola hemorrhagic fever. Existing antiviral medications do not seem to be effective against this virus. The treatment for Ebola hemorrhagic fever is intensive and supportive care. This care

---

In the News: Congolese Outbreak of Ebola

In December, 2002, reports that gorillas and chimpanzees were dying in remote forests within the northern region of the Republic of Congo alarmed Congolese authorities. The following month, word spread of a possible outbreak of Ebola virus in the country's Cuvette-Ouest district. At that point in time, twelve people had died of apparent hemorrhagic fever in the town of Kelle, and four more persons had died at Mbomo. The previous year, in the same area, a similar episode led to the deaths of forty-three people in the Republic of Congo and fifty-three residents of neighboring Gabon.

At the peak of the epidemic, most of the population of Kelle fled into the forest in an attempt to hide from the deadly virus. Volunteers from the Congolese Red Cross, clad in protective suits, cared for the sick and the elderly who were left behind. Few villagers believed that the epidemic was a natural disease brought about by eating infected primate meat: Rather, they suspected witchcraft. Four teachers, accused of causing the outbreak, were reportedly killed by a mob.

Medical teams from the World Health Organization (WHO), the Red Cross, and Médecins Sans Frontières/Doctors Without Borders set up makeshift hospital wards in the affected area. The U.S. Centers for Disease Control and Prevention (CDC) sent an expert epidemiologist. The European Commission's Humanitarian Aid Office appropriated 500,000 euros to support the relief work.

Aid workers began a public awareness campaign to halt the spread of the disease. WHO held meetings with local leaders to assure them they could limit the outbreak by avoiding primate meat and by not touching the bodies of those sick with the disease. People were urged to refrain from washing deceased family members, a ritual required by traditional burial practices.

By late April, the epidemic appeared to be under control, and people began to return to their homes. Fears that the returning villagers might start a new series of infections after eating the meat of dead gorillas while hiding in the forest proved unfounded. Out of 144 reported cases, the disease claimed 126 lives, a death rate approaching 90 percent.

Milton Berman, Ph.D.

---

includes intravenous fluids and blood transfusions; replacing electrolytes and blood coagulation factors; oxygen; maintaining blood pressure with medications; and treating complications, such as infections.

The types of treatments used are based on the symptoms and blood tests of the infected person. The transfusion of blood from Ebola fever survivors to persons with Ebola has been tried. Because the survivor blood has antibodies to the virus, experts believe this

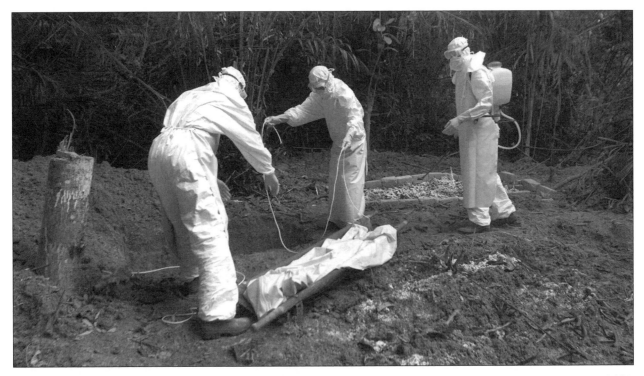

Health workers wear protective clothing and gear to bury a child who died from Ebola hemorrhagic fever in Gabon in 2001. (AP/Wide World Photos)

blood could assist the infected person in fighting the disease. There is limited data, however, on the effectiveness of this treatment.

PREVENTION AND OUTCOMES

The only way to prevent Ebola hemorrhagic fever is to avoid places where the virus is known to occur. This includes Africa, the Phillippines, and laboratories that perform animal testing with viruses. Because the reservoir of the Ebola virus is not known, there is no way to eliminate the virus. Caretakers of infected persons and workers in viral-testing animal laboratories should always wear personal protective clothing, such as a gown, gloves, goggles, and a facial mask.

Testing is underway to develop a vaccine against the Ebola virus. Most of the testing of this vaccine, however, has been performed on animals.

Education of persons living in areas where the Ebola virus resides can limit the spread of the disease. This education consists of teaching villagers to avoid unprotected contact with persons who have or had the disease, whether living or dead. It also includes teaching villagers to avoid unprotected contact with

dead animals in cases in which the cause of death is unknown.

Christine M. Carroll, R.N.

FURTHER READING

Centers for Disease Control and Prevention. "Ebola Hemorrhagic Fever Information Packet." Available at http://www.cdc.gov/ncidod/dvrd/spb/mnpages/dispages/ebola/qa.htm.

_____. "Outbreak Postings." Available at http://www.cdc.gov/ncidod/dvrd/spb/outbreaks.

Francesconi, Paolo, et al. "Ebola Hemorrhagic Fever Transmission." *Emerging Infectious Diseases* 9, no. 11 (2003).

Hewlitt, Barry S., and Bonnie L. Hewitt. *Ebola, Culture, and Politics: The Anthropology of an Emerging Disease.* Belmont, Calif.: Thomson Higher Education, 2008.

Knipe, David M., and Peter M. Howley, eds. *Fields' Virology.* 5th ed. Philadelphia: Wolters Kluwer Health/Lippincott Williams & Wilkins, 2007.

Peters, C. J., and J. W. LeDuc. "An Introduction to Ebola: The Virus and the Disease." *Journal of Infectious Diseases* 179, supp. 1 (1999): ix-xvi.

World Health Organization. "Ebola Heamorrhagic Fever." Available at http://www.who.int/media-centre/factsheets/fs103/en.

WEB SITES OF INTEREST

Centers for Disease Control and Prevention
http://www.cdc.gov

Emerging and Reemerging Infectious Diseases Resource Center
http://www.medscape.com/resource/infections

National Center for Emerging and Zoonotic Infectious Diseases
http://www.cdc.gov/ncezid

Public Health Agency of Canada
http://www.phac-aspc.gc.ca

World Health Organization
http://www.who.int

See also: Dengue fever; Developing countries and infectious disease; Emerging and reemerging infectious diseases; Fever; Filoviridae; Hemorrhagic fever viral infections; Marburg hemorrhagic fever; Plague; Primates and infectious disease; Tropical medicine; Viral infections; West Nile virus; Zoonotic diseases.

Echinocandin antifungals

CATEGORY: Treatment

DEFINITION

Echinocandin antifungal drugs inhibit the biosynthesis of a key component of many fungal cell walls called (1,3)beta-glucan. Because this compound does not exist in mammals, echinocandin antifungals inhibit the construction of a material that is critical for many fungal cells but does not directly target processes in human cells.

These drugs are active only against those fungi that possess appreciable quantities of (1,3)beta-glucan in their cell walls. Therefore, the antifungal spectrum of echinocandin antifungals is somewhat limited. Members of the fungal genera *Candida* and *Aspergillus* are the most susceptible to echinocandins. Pathogenic fungi such as *Cryptococcus, Trichosporon,* and members of Zygomycotina, however, are unaffected by these drugs. Likewise, echinocandin antifungals show only limited activity against fungi (such as *Fusarium, Scedosporium, Coccidioides, Blastomyces,* and *Histoplasma*) that cause systemic infections. Echinocandin antifungals are also effective against pneumonia caused by *Pneumocystis jiroveci* (formerly known as *P. carinii*).

The first echinocandin antifungal approved by the U.S. Food and Drug Administration (FDA) was caspofungin (Cancidas) in 2001. In 2005, the FDA approved micafungin (Mycamine) and in 2006 approved anidulafungin (Eraxis). These drugs are used to treat invasive *Candida* or *Aspergillus* infections, *Candida* infections of mucous membranes, and candidemia, an infection in which yeast colonizes the bloodstream. Micafungin is especially effective against infections with a specific species of *Candida* called *C. glabrata.*

Echinocandin antifungals must be given intravenously. In general, they are well tolerated, but they do cause some side effects. They all can cause headache, cough, and digestive problems. Additionally, caspofungin can cause chills and fever; micafungin can cause back pain, sleep disruptions, nosebleeds, loss of appetite, fatigue, and a sore mouth; and anidulafungin can cause pain and swelling at the injection site.

Persons at risk for systemic fungal infections, who typically require treatment with echinocandin antifungal drugs, include those who have cancer and those who have had a transplant. Also at risk are persons who are infected with the human immunodeficiency virus (HIV) and those who use steroid drugs, are malnourished, have uncontrolled diabetes mellitus, or have particular blood, bone marrow, or liver disorders. Echinocandin antifungals interact with some of the drugs given to transplant recipients that suppress the immune system. Caspofungin and micafungin, for example, can increase the blood levels of several antirejection drugs and produce toxic side effects.

Resistance can arise to echinocandin antifungals, as (1,3)beta-glucan is synthesized by an enzyme called (1,3)beta-glucan synthase, the active subunit of which is encoded by FKS genes. Specific mutations in FKS1 can lower the sensitivity of (1,3)beta-glucan synthase to echinocandin antifungals, and fungi that harbor such mutations show clinical resistance to these drugs.

Echinocandin antifungals can also work in combination with other antifungal drugs such as triazoles (fluconazole, posaconazole, voriconazole, itraconazole, and ketoconazole), and with polyenes, which are various preparations of amphotericin B, for particular fungal infections.

Michael A. Buratovich, Ph.D.

FURTHER READING

Bal, Abhijit M. "The Echinocandins: Three Useful Choices or Three Too Many?" *International Journal of Antimicrobial Agents* 35 (2010): 13-18.

Centers for Disease Control and Prevention. "Biofilms and Fungal Resistance." Available at http://www.cdc.gov/ncidod/eid/vol10no1/03-0119.htm.

Griffith, R. K. "Antifungal Drugs." In *Foye's Principles of Medicinal Chemistry*, edited by Thomas L. Lemke et al. 6th ed. Philadelphia: Lippincott Williams & Wilkins, 2008.

Murray, Patrick R., Ken S. Rosenthal, and Michael A. Pfaller. "Antifungal Agents." In *Medical Microbiology*. 6th ed. Philadelphia: Mosby/Elsevier, 2009.

Thompson, George R., Jose Cadena, and Thomas F. Patterson. "Overview of Antifungal Agents." *Clinics in Chest Medicine* 30, no. 2 (2009): 203-215.

Webster, John, and Weber, Roland. *Introduction to Fungi*. New York: Cambridge University Press, 2007.

WEB SITES OF INTEREST

Centers for Disease Control and Prevention, Division of Foodborne, Bacterial, and Mycotic Diseases
http://www.cdc.gov/nczved/divisions/dfbmd

DoctorFungus
http://www.doctorfungus.org

See also: Antifungal drugs: Mechanisms of action; Antifungal drugs: Types; Diagnosis of fungal infections; Fungal infections; Fungi: Classification and types; Imidazole antifungals; Immune response to fungal infections; Infection; Mycoses; Polyene antifungals; Prevention of fungal infections; Thiazole antifungals; Treatment of fungal infections; Triazole antifungals.

Echinococcus

CATEGORY: Pathogen
TRANSMISSION ROUTE: Ingestion

Taxonomic Classification for *Echinococcus*

Kingdom: Animalia
Phylum: Platyhelminthes
Class: Cestoda
Order: Cyclophyllidea
Family: Taeniidae
Genus: *Echinococcus*
Species:
E. granulosus
E. multicularis
E. vogeli
E. oligarthus

DEFINITION

Echinococcus species are tapeworms of carnivores that cause serious disease in humans and herbivores as intermediate hosts. This disease is known as echinococcosis.

NATURAL HABITAT AND FEATURES

Echinococcus species are cestodes (tapeworms) with complex life cycles requiring two mammalian hosts. Their definitive hosts (where sexual reproduction occurs) are carnivores, commonly dogs and foxes. In definitive hosts, the worms remain small, usually less than 6 millimeters in size, and consist of a head and three egg packets or proglottids. Proglottids pass with feces and contaminate the environment, where they are ingested by the intermediate species, typically herbivores and sometimes humans.

After ingestion by herbivores, *Echinococcus* species eggs develop into oncospheres that can penetrate intestinal epithelium. Once there, they pass into blood or lymph vessels and then travel passively to target organs, usually the liver or lung but occasionally the spleen, brain, heart, and kidneys. Once there, they form metacestodes, reproductive structures called hydatid cysts. These cysts grow to between 5 and 10 centimeters in size within one year and can persist and remain viable for years, growing, on occasion, so large they contain several liters of fluid. The cysts contain protoscoleces (called hydatid sand) and are ingested by carnivores, where they develop into adult *Echinococcus* cestodes.

PATHOGENICITY AND CLINICAL SIGNIFICANCE

The different species of *Echinococcus* cause different syndromes of disease in humans. *E. granulosus* causes the oldest known disease, cystic echinococcosis (CE). CE cysts are large, unilocular, and fluid-filled. Typically, CE occurs most commonly in humans living pastoral lives in contact with sheep, goats, and dogs. Signs of CE often take years to develop and include abdominal pain occurring when cysts have grown large enough to displace organs. Allergic signs and anaphylaxis can occur with cyst rupture. Treatment is usually a combination of chemotherapy and the surgical removal of cysts. CE is a disease of the Northern Hemisphere.

E. multicularis was recognized as a separate parasite in the nineteenth century that caused a syndrome known as alveolar echinococcosis (AE). *E. multicularis* is most often found in foxes and rodents. AE cysts differ from CE in that they are multilocular, solid, and frequently pulmonary. Signs are similar to CE, but pulmonary AE also causes coughing. AE is more likely to be fatal. Treatment of AE is usually a combination of chemotherapy and the surgical removal of cysts. AE is a disease of the Northern Hemisphere and of suburban regions where humans and wildlife are close.

E. vogeli and *E. oligarthus* cause polycystic echinococcosis (PE). PE cysts tend to be small. The disease is not well characterized because it has only recently been recognized; also, only a few cases have been described. Treatment is usually chemotherapy. PE occurs in Central America and South America.

DRUG SUSCEPTIBILITY

Albendazole, mebendazole, and praziquantal are drugs used to treat echinococcosis. High doses are used, and treatment may last for years or even be lifelong.

Cynthia L. Mills, D.V.M.

FURTHER READING

Deplazes, Peter, et al. "Wilderness in the City: The Urbanization of *Echinococcus multicularis*." *Trends in Parasitology* 20 (2004): 77-84.

Eckert, J., et al. *WHO/OIE Manual on Echinococcosis in Humans and Animals: A Public Health Problem of Global Concern.* Geneva: World Organization for Animal Health and World Health Organization, 2001.

Krauss, Hartmut, et al. *Zoonoses: Infectious Diseases Transmissible from Animals to Humans.* 3d ed. Washington, D.C.: ASM Press, 2003. Explores the myriad infections introduced by human-animal contact.

Zhang, Wenbao, et al. "Concepts in Immunology and Diagnosis of Hydatid Disease." *Clinical Microbiology Reviews* 16 (2003): 18-36.

WEB SITES OF INTEREST

American Veterinary Medicine Association
http://www.avma.org

National Center for Emerging and Zoonotic Infectious Diseases
http://www.cdc.gov/ncezid

See also: Dogs and infectious disease; Parasites: Classification and types; Parasitic diseases; Tapeworms; Worm infections; Zoonotic diseases.

Echovirus infections

CATEGORY: Diseases and conditions
ANATOMY OR SYSTEM AFFECTED: Respiratory system
ALSO KNOWN AS: Enteric cytopathic human orphan virus, nonpolio enterovirus

DEFINITION

Echoviruses are single-stranded ribonucleic acid (RNA) viruses that belong to the genus *Enterovirus.* Thirty-two types of echovirus have been identified. Echovirus infections are common infections that are often mild but may be more severe and life-threatening. Echoviruses are among the leading causes of hospital visits in febrile infants and young children.

CAUSES

Echoviruses are spread by human contact, mainly through the fecal-oral route but also during pregnancy or childbirth. Also, echoviruses are often spread in hospitals from staff to patients because of improper handwashing technique.

RISK FACTORS

Although any person can contract echovirus infection, persons of low socioeconomic status are most susceptible because of their often poor living conditions, which includes a higher incidence of eating contaminated food and using unsafe drinking water. Echovirus infections may occur at any age, but the younger the person, the higher the risk. There is a greater incidence too among males. The spring and fall seasons see the greatest risk for echovirus infections.

SYMPTOMS

Many persons with echovirus infection may be asymptomatic and require no follow-up or treatment. For infected persons, symptoms usually begin three to six days after initial infection with the virus. Most persons have a mild infection and may present with a fever, a rash, and mouth blisters. Infants may also present with pneumonia, upper respiratory infections, and lethargy. Newborns who have echovirus infection shortly after birth and persons who are immunocompromised have the greatest risk for more significant infections, including encephalitis, myocarditis, meningitis, and neonatal sepsis, all which could lead to death.

SCREENING AND DIAGNOSIS

It is possible to isolate echovirus from blood, cerebrospinal fluid, feces, and the throat in cell culture, although diagnostic results often take several days. Results from enterovirus polymerase chain reaction (EV-PCR) test is a genetic technique that amplifies the virus for a much quicker result; false-positive results are possible. The quicker turnaround time of one day favors the latter diagnostic testing option.

TREATMENT AND THERAPY

Mildly affected persons do not require treatment because the infection will self-resolve. No approved therapies exist for the treatment of echovirus infection. If a more severe type of echovirus infection has been diagnosed, medical care is provided based on the specific symptoms. Experimental treatments with an immunoglobulin and pleconaril have been attempted in persons who are immunocompromised; these treatments have shown some promise but have yet to be proven generally effective.

PREVENTION AND OUTCOMES

Regular, adequate hygiene, including handwashing, may reduce the spread of echovirus.

Janet Ober Berman, M.S., CGC

FURTHER READING

Abzug, M. J., M. J. Levin, and H. A. Rotbart. "Profile of Enterovirus Disease in the First Two Weeks of Life." *Pediatric Infectious Disease Journal* 10 (1993): 820-824.

Fauci, Anthony. "Enteroviruses and Reoviruses." In *Harrison's Principles of Internal Medicine*, edited by Joan Butterton. 17th ed. New York: McGraw-Hill, 2008.

Hawkes, Michael, and Wendy Vaudry. "Nonpolio Enterovirus Infection in the Neonate and Young Infant." *Paediatric Child Health* 7 (2005): 383-388.

Martin, Richard J., Avroy A. Fanaroff, and Michele C. Walsh, eds. *Fanaroff and Martin's Neonatal-Perinatal Medicine: Diseases of the Fetus and Infant.* 2 vols. 8th ed. Philadelphia: Mosby/Elsevier, 2006.

Modlin, J. F. "Perinatal Echovirus Infection: Insights from a Literature Review of Sixty-one Cases of Serious Infection and Sixteen Outbreaks in Nurseries." *Reviews of Infectious Diseases* 6 (1986): 918-926.

WEB SITES OF INTEREST

About Kids Health
http://www.aboutkidshealth.ca

American Academy of Family Physicians
http://familydoctor.org

American Academy of Pediatrics
http://www.healthychildren.org

See also: Childbirth and infectious disease; Children and infectious disease; Coxsackie virus infections; Encephalitis; Enterovirus infections; Fecal-oral route of transmission; Myocarditis; Pregnancy and infectious disease; Viral infections.

Ehrlichiosis

CATEGORY: Diseases and conditions
ANATOMY OR SYSTEM AFFECTED: All
ALSO KNOWN AS: Human granulocytic anaplasmosis, human granulocytic ehrlichiosis, human monocytic ehrlichiosis

DEFINITION

Ehrlichiosis is a rare infectious disease caused by a rickettsial bacteria. It is spread by tick bites and occurs in the United States in tick-infested areas. It can occur in humans and other mammals. There are two types of ehrlichiosis: human granulocytic ehrlichiosis (HGE) or anaplasmosis (HGA) and human monocytic ehrlichiosis (HME).

CAUSES

The bacteria that causes ehrlichiosis is from the genus *Ehrlichia* and the species *chaffeensis* and *ewingii*. *E. chaffeensis* causes HGE and *E. ewingii* causes HME. Nondomesticated animals are thought to be reservoirs of the bacteria. Ehrlichiosis is most commonly transmitted by the lone star tick, although it can be transmitted by the dog tick and the deer tick. A tick must be attached and feeding for a minimum of twenty-four hours to transmit this disease.

RISK FACTORS

The risk factors for ehrlichiosis are contact with an infected tick; living in or visiting an area with ticks; being outdoors in warm weather; and having a pet dog. Males are more at risk than are females. Ehrlichiosis usually occurs in the Northeast, Upper Midwest, Southeast, and south-central states and in California and Texas.

SYMPTOMS

The symptoms of ehrlichiosis develop within five to fourteen days of the tick bite. These symptoms include fever, headache, fatigue, muscle aches, nausea, vomiting, diarrhea, rash, chills, cough, joint pain, and confusion. The symptoms may be mild or severe. Severe or untreated cases of ehrlichiosis can lead to kidney failure, respiratory failure, heart failure, seizures, coma, and death.

SCREENING AND DIAGNOSIS

There is no routine screening for ehrlichiosis. Any person who is bitten by a tick should be tested for the disease. The diagnosis is based on the person's symptoms and on the results of blood tests. The tests used are complete blood counts, liver enzymes, antibody immunofluorescence assay, and a blood smear with the bacteria.

TREATMENT AND THERAPY

Ehrlichiosis is treated with antibiotics, such as tetracycline or doxycycline, which should be taken for seven to fourteen days. Tetracycline should not be taken by pregnant women (who instead should be prescribed the antibiotic rifampin). The tick should be removed as soon as possible from the body, using tweezers and wearing gloves. The tick's whole body and mouth parts should be extracted and then dropped into rubbing alcohol. One should carefully clean the bite with soap and water or with a hand antiseptic.

PREVENTION AND OUTCOMES

Ehrlichiosis is prevented by avoiding contact with ticks. Persons who plan to walk in wooded areas or in deep grass should take the following precautions: Wear insect repellant with DEET (NN-diethyl metatoluamide); wear long pants, light-colored clothing, closed shoes, and socks; tuck pants into socks; stay on trails; and, after hiking or walking, check clothes, body, and hair for ticks. One should also check pets for ticks.

Christine M. Carroll, R.N.

FURTHER READING

Bratton, R. L., and G. R. Corey. "Tick-Borne Disease." *American Family Physician* 71 (2005): 2323.

Dumler, J. S., et al. "Ehrlichioses in Humans: Epidemiology, Clinical Presentation, Diagnosis, and Treatment." *Clinical Infectious Diseases* 45, no. 15, suppl 1 (2007): S45-S51.

Dumler, Thomas, and J. A. Carlyon. "Current Management of Human Granulocytic Anaplasmosis, Human Monocytic Ehrlichiosis, and *Ehrlichia ewingii* Ehrlichiosis." *Expert Review of Anti-infective Therapy* 7, no. 6 (2009): 709-722.

Ganguly, S., and S. K. Mukhopadhayay. "Tick-Borne Ehrlichiosis Infection in Human Beings." *Journal of Vector Borne Diseases* 45, no. 4 (2008): 273-280.

WEB SITE OF INTEREST

Centers for Disease Control and Prevention
http://www.cdc.gov/ticks/diseases/ehrlichiosis

See also: Acariasis; Anaplasmosis; Arthropod-borne illness and disease; Bacterial infections; Blood-borne illness and disease; Colorado tick fever; Encephalitis; Hemorrhagic fever viral infections; Lyme disease; Mediterranean spotted fever; Mites and chiggers and infectious disease; *Rickettsia*; Rocky Mountain spotted fever; Ticks and infectious disease; Vectors and vector control.

Eikenella infections

CATEGORY: Diseases and conditions
ANATOMY OR SYSTEM AFFECTED: Genitalia, lungs, mouth, respiratory system, teeth

DEFINITION

Eikenella infection is caused by *E. corrodens*, a facultative, anaerobic, gram-negative rod that is part of the normal flora of the oral cavity, upper respiratory tract, and urogenital tract. This bacterium is an opportunistic pathogen. *E. corrodens* has been implicated in many types of infections, including juvenile periodontal disease, head and neck infections, pneumonia, intra-abdominal infections, cellulitis, and endocarditis.

CAUSES

Poor oral hygiene will allow *E. corrodens* to build up in plaque and damage the surrounding gum tissue, leading to gingivitis or abscesses (or both). A weakened immune system may allow infections to spread to the middle ear and sinuses then reach into the spinal fluid and cause meningitis. Dental extractions provide access to the bloodstream by *E. corrodens*, which can then infect damaged heart valves. Saliva from a human bite transfers this organism into the wound, where an infection may develop and lead to cellulitis. Virulence factors target macrophage activity and allow the organism to attach to epithelial cells. The cell wall of *E. corrodens* also has endotoxin activity.

RISK FACTORS

The following factors increase the chance of developing an *Eikenella* infection: poor oral hygiene; the presence of an underlying disease such as diabetes, rheumatoid arthritis, leukemia, and lung cancer; a compromised immune system; intravenous drug use; and preexisting heart valve damage.

SYMPTOMS

Symptoms are not specific and depend on the site of infection. Infected persons may have a fever and a heart murmur and feel malaise.

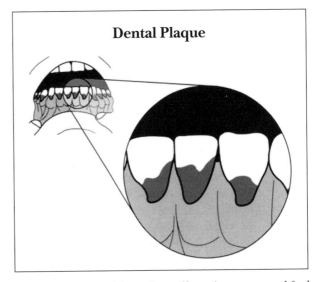

Dental Plaque

Dental plaque, which is made up of bacteria, mucus, and food debris, can lead to periodontal disease, a common result of infection with Eikenella corrodens.

SCREENING AND DIAGNOSIS

A doctor will suspect *Eikenella* infection if the patient has a history of recent dental work, has had a recent urologic procedure, has a history of intravenous drug abuse, or has wounds caused by a human bite. Diagnosis is made by isolating the organism from the infected site. *E. corrodens* is a fastidious organism (and a member of the slow-growing HACEK bacterial group) that requires agar for growth, supplemented with hemin and an atmosphere of 5 to 10 percent carbon dioxide. Colonies have a characteristic bleach-like odor, and most strains pit the agar.

TREATMENT AND THERAPY

Surgical drainage is required if an abscess is present. In severe hand infections, debridement may be needed. Because of the emergence of beta-lactamase-producing strains of *E. corrodens*, the antibiotics recommended for treatment of most infections are ampicillin/sulbactam or amoxicillin/clavulanate, unless susceptibility testing is performed. For treatment of endocarditis, effective drugs are ceftriaxone, cefotaxime, and cefepime.

PREVENTION AND OUTCOMES

To help prevent *Eikenella* infections, one should practice good dental hygiene, have routine dental check ups, take prophylactic antibiotics before dental work (patients with underlying diseases), and properly identify and treat underlying diseases.

Carol Ann Suda, B.S., MT(ASCP)SM

FURTHER READING

Engelkirk, Paul G., and Janet Duben-Engelkirk. *Laboratory Diagnosis of Infectious Diseases: Essentials of Diagnostic Microbiology*. Baltimore: Lippincott Williams & Wilkins 2008.

Garrity, G. M. *Bergy's Manual of Systematic Bacteriology*. 2d ed. New York: Springer, 2005.

Langlais, Robert P., and Craig S. Miller. *Color Atlas of Common Oral Diseases*. 4th ed. Philadelphia: Lippincott Williams & Wilkins, 2009.

Preus, Hans R., and Lars Laurell. *Periodontal Diseases: A Manual of Diagnosis, Treatment, and Maintenance*. Chicago: Quintessence, 2003.

Winn, W. C., et al. *Koneman's Color Atlas and Textbook of Diagnostic Microbiology*. 6th ed. Baltimore: Lippincott Williams & Wilkins, 2006.

WEB SITES OF INTEREST

American Dental Association
http://www.ada.org

Centers for Disease Control and Prevention
http://www.cdc.gov

See also: Abscesses; Antibiotics: Types; Bacteria: Classification and types; Bacterial infections; Bacterial meningitis; Bloodstream infections; Cellulitis; Endocarditis; Gingivitis; Mouth infections; Opportunistic infections; Saliva and infectious disease; Sepsis; Thrush; Tooth abscess; Vincent's angina.

Elderly persons. *See* Aging and infectious disease.

Elephantiasis

CATEGORY: Diseases and conditions
ANATOMY OR SYSTEM AFFECTED: Lymphatic system, skin, tissue
ALSO KNOWN AS: Lymphatic filariasis

DEFINITION

Elephantiasis is a rare and chronic medical condition characterized by extreme enlargement of an area of the body, most often the arms, legs, trunk, and external genitalia. ("Elephantitis" is a commonly used misnomer.) The disorder involves significant thickening of the skin and its underlying tissues. The skin can become infected and gangrenous. Elephantiasis, which is also known as lymphatic filariasis, is most common in Africa and other tropical regions.

CAUSES

Elephantiasis occurs as a consequence of obstructed lymph flow. Often responsible for this obstruction are threadlike parasitic roundworms (filaria), such as *Brugia malayi*, *B. timori*, and *Wuchereria bancrofti*, which harbor detrimental bacteria. These worms are introduced into the body by various types of mosquitoes. The adult worms live in the lymphatic system, where they cause obstruction, inflammation, and fibrosis (the formation of excess fibrous connective tissue). In turn, this results in thickening and enlargement of the skin. This type of elephantiasis is known as true elephantiasis.

Nonfilarial elephantiasis (which is not caused by parasites) is believed to be caused by continued exposure of barefooted populations to the soil in which they dwell—particularly red clay soils that have a high content of alkali metals (which is common in African regions). Small chemical particles enter the skin through the feet. These particles eventually end up in lymphatic tissue, where they generate harmful effects. This type of elephantiasis is common in Ethiopia.

RISK FACTORS

Exposure to mosquitoes is a common risk factor for elephantiasis, as is walking barefoot on soils rich in alkali metals. Lymphedema or any damage or obstruction to the lymphatic vessels also are risk factors. People who live in areas where elephantiasis is most common have the greatest risk for contracting the disease.

SYMPTOMS

Elephantiasis involves severe swelling, most commonly of the limbs, trunk, and genitalia. Skin-related symptoms include abnormal thickening, ulceration, brawny skin tone, excess fibrotic skin tissue, and pebble-like appearance. Lymphatic symptoms include blocked lymph ducts and impaired lymphatic

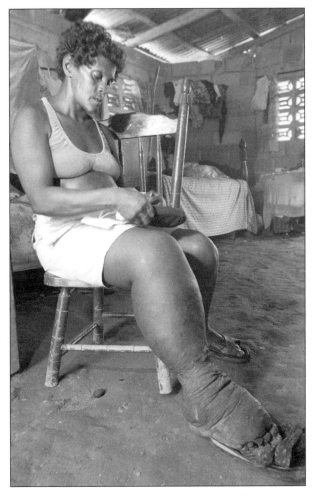

A woman in the Dominican Republic with disabling elephantiasis, which severely affects her leg and foot. (AP/Wide World Photos)

drainage. Fever, chills, headache, and general malaise also may be present. Symptoms develop slowly and may not occur until many years after the initial infection.

SCREENING AND DIAGNOSIS

Elephantiasis can be diagnosed by identifying the parasitic worm or worms by a finger-prick blood test. Physical examination to detect the common symptoms is also helpful for establishing the diagnosis, as is the infected person's medical history. Other useful screening tests include magnetic resonance imaging, computed tomography, Doppler ultrasonography, and radionucleotide imaging of the lymphatic system.

TREATMENT AND THERAPY

The treatment of elephantiasis varies according to geographic region and the availability of particular medications. The use of combination agents is a common strategy to eradicate the parasitic worms. In sub-Saharan Africa, a typical combination regimen is albendazole with ivermectin, anthelmintic medicines that kill parasites. In some cases, just a single dose of ivermectin can arrest the parasitic activity. Diethylcarbamazine (also an anthelmintic agent) often kills adult worms or impairs their ability to reproduce. Chemotherapy also can attack the adult worms. The antibiotic doxycycline kills bacteria that live inside the worms, leading to the death of the worms.

Rigorous daily cleaning of the affected areas can minimize the symptoms of elephantiasis. Light exercise can help to move excess lymphatic fluid from the limbs. Elevating the legs will improve circulation. The use of massage techniques and compression garments can aid in reducing inflammation. Surgical treatment can be helpful for scrotal elephantiasis, but it is generally not effective for elephantiasis of the limbs.

PREVENTION AND OUTCOMES

Worldwide efforts are in place to eliminate lymphatic filariasis by 2020, and results have been promising. Effective medications are being supplied to areas that have a high prevalence of the disease. International awareness of the causes and treatments is crucial for achieving this goal and includes emphasis on the importance of personal hygiene. Controlling the mosquito population is another key to reducing the incidence of elephantiasis. Precautions should be taken to prevent mosquito bites.

Lynda A. Seminara, B.A.

FURTHER READING

Dandapat, C. M., S. K. Mohapatro, and S. S. Mohanty. "Filarial Lymphoedema and Elephantiasis of a Lower Limb." *British Journal of Surgery* 73 (1986): 451-453.

Icon Group. *Elephantiasis: Webster's Timeline History, 1573-2007.* San Diego, Calif.: Author, 2010.

Lu, S., et al. "Localized Lymphedema (Elephantiasis): A Case Series and Review of the Literature." *Journal of Cutaneous Pathology* 36 (2009): 1-20.

Parker, James N., and Philip P. Parker, eds. *Elephantiasis: A Medical Dictionary, Bibliography, and Annotated*

Research Guide to Internet References. San Diego, Calif.: Icon Group, 2004.

Ryan, T. J. "Elephantiasis, Elastin, and Chronic Wound Healing: Nineteenth Century and Contemporary Viewpoints Relevant to Hypotheses Concerning Lymphedema, Leprosy, Erysipelas, and Psoriasis." *Lymphology* 42 (2009): 19-25.

Sisto, K., and A. Khachemoune. "Elephantiasis Nostras Verrucosa." *American Journal of Clinical Dermatology* 9 (2008): 141-146.

Tekola, F., et al. "Development and Testing of a De Novo Clinical Staging System for Podoconiosis (Endemic Non-Filarial Elephantiasis)." *Tropical Medicine and International Health* 13 (2008): 1277-1283.

WEB SITES OF INTEREST

Global Health Council
http://www.globalhealth.org/infectious_diseases

Neglected Tropical Diseases Coalition
http://www.neglectedtropicaldiseases.org

Partners for Parasite Control
http://www.who.int/wormcontrol

See also: Arthropod-borne illness and disease; Blastomycosis; Chromoblastomycosis; Developing countries and infectious disease; Filariasis; Inflammation; Leprosy; Parasites: Classification and types; Parasitic diseases; Ringworm; Roundworms; Skin infections; Soilborne illness and disease; Tropical medicine; Worm infections.

Emerging and reemerging infectious diseases

CATEGORY: Epidemiology

DEFINITION

First introduced by Nobel laureate Joshua Lederberg, the phrase "emerging infectious diseases" applies to those infectious diseases that newly appear in a populace, have been in existence for some time but are rapidly increasing in incidence or geographic range, or appear as new drug-resistant strains of viruses, bacteria, fungi, or parasitic species. Most emerging diseases are zoonotic in origin and are disseminated through a range of vectors, from insects such as mosquitoes to nonhuman primates.

While new infectious diseases continue to emerge, many of the old plagues remain, often appearing in more virulent and drug-resistant forms. While many outbreaks inexplicably appear, often there are specific identifiable ecological factors, such as climate change; agricultural development, such as land clearing; or demographic changes that may place people at increased risk through exposure to unfamiliar microbes or their natural zoonotic hosts.

Still another major challenge to the global health community is the growing drug resistance, particularly to antibiotics, of certain diseases. These diseases include tuberculosis (TB), typhoid, malaria, and sexually transmitted diseases such as HIV (human immunodeficiency virus) infection. There has been a renewed commitment to vaccine research to prevent and treat these infections and other preventable infectious diseases.

Often to blame for emerging diseases are megacities, with their increased urban crowding, general lack of potable water, and ability, through its populations, to rapidly spread contagious diseases around the world through air travel. Mostly, these are global problems and are viewed as global infectious disease threats.

BACKGROUND

Throughout history, populations have been afflicted by major outbreaks of emerging infectious diseases. These disease include the bubonic plague (also known as the Black Death), caused by the bacterium *Yersinia pestis* and spread by fleas that feed on rats. The plague emerged in the fourteenth century and decimated populations in Europe and Asia.

Even more deadly than *Y. pestis*, however, was the variola virus, the etiologic agent responsible for smallpox, which evolved from poxviruses in cattle and emerged into human populations thousands of years ago; from the fourteenth to sixteenth centuries, Spanish conquistadors vanquished Central America by causing a smallpox epidemic through introduction of the smallpox virus into indigenous populations, thereby disabling their armies. More than four hundred years later, in 1980, the World Health Organization (WHO) declared that smallpox had been eradicated worldwide. In 2003, however, the United States entered into war with Iraq, and U.S. president George W. Bush decreed that members of the U.S. Armed Forces be vaccinated against smallpox in anticipation of a biological attack. This order came on the heels of several acts of bioterrorism in 2001 in the United States, wherein anthrax infection caused by *Bacillus anthracis* emerged in Florida and New York.

The United States was also at war (World War I) in 1918 when the influenza pandemic of that year killed up to fifty million persons, more than the war itself. In 2010, emerging viral scourges include H1N1 influenza, or swine flu, which exhibited drug-resistant strains, and HIV, which was isolated in 1981 and continues to mutate in persons with HIV infection and AIDS (acquired immunodeficiency syndrome), mandating the need for new therapies and combinations. Emerging bacterial scourges include methicillin-resistant *Staphylococcus* A (MRSA), multi-drug resistant tuberculosis (MDR-TB), and extensively multi-drug resistant TB (XMDR-TB). In addition, malaria, a parasitic disease, has demonstrated resistant strains of its most lethal specie, *Plasmodium falciparum*.

EMERGING VIRUSES

Swine flu is a zoonotic disease resulting from a mix of swine, avian, and human flu viruses. Between 2006 and 2009, investigators in China isolated H1N1, H1N2, and H3N2 from pigs, observing a novel reassortment between contemporary swine and avian influenza viruses and hypothesizing that swine may serve as hosts for genetic reassortment between humans and avian panzoonotic viruses.

H1N1 first emerged in the Northern Hemisphere in Mexico, where the index case was isolated. Following the regular flu season of April, 2009, H1N1 appeared in the United States; during the 2008-2009 flu season, influenza A (H1), A (H3), and B viruses had cocirculated. In mid-April, the Centers for Disease Control and Prevention (CDC) documented the first two cases of novel influenza A pandemic (H1N1) in the United States. Beginning in September, the CDC had antigenically characterized flu viruses; one seasonal influenza A (H1N1), three influenza A (H3N2), four influenza B, and 412 influenza A (H1N1) 2009 viruses, the latter spread rapidly in the Northern Hemisphere and producing unprecedented morbidity and mortality in infants, young children, and

pregnant women. Most cases were found in persons age sixty and younger; only 1 percent of those age sixty-five years and older and 50 percent of those age twenty-five to forty-nine years were infected. Usually, the flu causes the greatest morbidity and mortality in those age sixty-five years and older. H1N1 infected about twenty-two million people in the United States and killed almost four thousand persons between April and October, 2009.

EMERGING RETROVIRIDAE

HIV/AIDS is of zoonotic origin and was first observed in nonhuman primates who came in close contact with hunters and with persons clearing land in the African plains. Since the time that HIV, the virus that causes AIDS, was isolated in the early 1980's, the virus has continued to emerge in new populations and new geographic locations and has continued to morph into new strains and variants, becoming resistant to available antiretroviral therapies (ART); new drugs and combinations of old and new therapies must be produced to help keep alive the more than 1.3 million persons in North America living with HIV and AIDS in 2008.

Although HIV infection is now treated as a chronic disease in many developed countries, developing nations continue to struggle to facilitate prevention programs and to obtain enough drugs to treat all those infected with the virus. The world awaits the first cure and vaccine to prevent the dreaded disease. Moreover, despite the advent of highly active antiretroviral therapy (HAART) in 1996, a range of comorbidities continues to affect those living with HIV and AIDS. These comorbidities include liver disease (hepatitis B and C), non-Hodgkin's lymphoma, neurological illnesses, malignancy, malnutrition, and increased susceptibility to TB and MDR-TB. In addition, socioeconomic factors such as poverty, unemployment, stigmatization, drug and alcohol addiction, and undocumented immigration status are often by-products of those infected with the disease.

In 2010, the CDC presented one of the first large-scale studies to demonstrate a strong association between poverty and HIV infection; poverty was shown to be a powerful driver of the AIDS pandemic. Of note, the study was conducted by surveying nine thousand heterosexual persons living in cities of the United States, a population not considered to be of high risk of contracting HIV infection. The results of the study

Global Emerging and Reemerging Infectious Diseases

AIDS
Campylobacteriosis
Chagas' disease
Cholera
Coccidioidomycosis
Creutzfeldt-Jakob disease
Cryptococcosis
Cryptosporidiosis
Cyclosporiasis
Cysticercosis
Dengue fever
Diphtheria
Drug-resistant infections
Ebola hemorrhagic fever
Escherichia coli infection
Group B streptococcal infection
Hantavirus pulmonary syndrome
Hendra virus infection
Hepatitis C

Histoplasmosis
HIV infection
Influenza
Lassa fever
Legionnaires' disease
Leptospirosis
Listeriosis
Lyme disease
Malaria
Marburg hemorrhagic fever
Measles
Meningitis
Methicillin-resistant *Staphylococcus
aureus*
Monkeypox
Nipah virus infection
Norovirus infection
Plague
Polio

Pontiac fever
Rabies
Rift Valley fever
Rotavirus infection
Salmonellosis
SARS
Shigellosis
Smallpox
Trypanosomiasis
Tuberculosis
Tularemia
Vancomycin-intermediate/resistant
Staphylococcus aureus
Variant Creutzfeldt-Jakob disease
West Nile virus infection
Whooping cough
Yellow fever

revealed a 2.1 percent incidence of HIV infection, twice the expected number.

Also, in 2010, U.S. president Barack Obama announced the implementation of a new strategy to prevent HIV infection and to better serve those living with HIV/AIDS. The president declared his commitment to continue the fight against HIV and AIDS in the United States and across the globe with an emphasis on prevention, and he allocated $30 million in funding in addition to an earlier pledge, in 2009, of $45 million over five years; the new strategy will focus on gay and bisexual men, on blacks and other persons of color, and on substance abusers. Program goals include reducing new HIV infections by 25 percent and increasing the number of those who know their HIV status from 79 to 90 percent.

EMERGING MYCOBACTERIAL DISEASES

The emergence and spread of *Mycobacterium tuberculosis* strains that are resistant to multiple drugs represent an emerging threat for global control of both TB and HIV; TB often coinfects patients with HIV and AIDS, whose weakened immune systems are more vulnerable to bacterial infections, especially TB, MDR-TB, and XMR-TB. WHO estimates that almost one-half million cases of MDR-TB emerged in 2006;

MDR-TB is defined as resistance to a minimum of the anti-TB drugs, isoniazid and rifampin, and in certain regions of the world, prevalence of MDR-TB may be greater than 20 percent. Although HIV may or may not be directly associated with the risk of developing MDR-TB, nosocomial outbreaks of MDR-TB in persons with HIV/AIDS have been noted. HIV/AIDS has also been linked to an increased risk for rifampin-monoresistant TB.

In addition, new cases of XMR-TB that are defined as MDR-TB resistant to a fluoroquinolone and to a (minimum of one) second-line injectable anti-TB agent, have been reported in forty-five countries and on all continents. Treatment of MDR-TB is complex and may result in the use of less effective and more toxic drugs that require treatment over longer periods of time, thereby threatening success; this is a serious problem for developing countries, especially countries (such as those in sub-Saharan Africa) with a high prevalence of HIV-1 infection. MDR-TB and XMR-TB also are of concern in developed countries because of mass immigration and global travel; even long-term visitors appear to significantly contribute to the burden of TB among foreign-born persons in the United States.

EMERGING PARASITIC DISEASES

Malaria continues to wreak havoc across the developing world. According to WHO, the disease killed 881,000 persons in 2008, 89 percent of whom were African; 88 percent of these persons were younger than age five years.

Malaria is spread through mosquito bites. While significant progress in malaria control has been made in some of the highly endemic nations, such as Zambia, Zanzibar, and Rwanda, where control relies on a combination of interventions that include the use of insecticides and sleeping nets, the number of patients treated for malaria with a confirmed diagnosis of malaria remains low in Africa. This can lead to the inappropriate administration of antimalarial medications, a practice that could foster the spread of resistance.

Of note, parasite resistance to almost all commonly used antimalarials has been observed in the most lethal parasite species, *P. falciparum*, presenting a huge barrier to successful disease management. Although artemisinin-based combination therapy (ACT) has made a significant contribution to malaria control by reducing transmission, its administration to infants and small children may be especially problematic. As such, educating health workers and entire communities about malaria prevention, diagnosis, and treatment remains vital to effective case management and to the forestalling of the emergence of resistance to both ACT and insecticides used in vector control.

GLOBAL IMPACT

The impact of emerging infectious diseases on global health is far reaching; new and reemerging infectious diseases that were once unknown or thought to have disappeared have reappeared, and diseases that were once treatable have become resistant to drug therapies that once worked. In addition, socioeconomic determinants and environmental factors have been shown to play a significant role in morbidity and mortality from emerging infectious diseases, which remain the world's leading cause of death (killing 34 percent of persons who succumb each year across the globe, 9 percent of whom are children). HIV/AIDS, malaria, and TB are the three leading threats to global health and are becoming more difficult to treat because of resistance to drug therapies and, in the case of malaria, resistance to insecticides.

Most prevalent in developing countries, TB and malaria are further retarding economic and social development. Malaria kills almost one million persons each year, and it can decrease a country's gross domestic product by 1.3 percent; for example, malaria costs African countries more than $12 billion per year. TB kills more than 1.7 million persons per year, costing affected countries more than $3.1 billion in 2008 (up from $2.3 billion in 2007). MDR-TB should be given high priority in global public health and biomedical research, and Greater efforts should be made to furnish appropriate resources to economically disadvantaged areas for fighting MDR-TB and preventing XMR-TB.

HIV/AIDS kills 2 million persons each year, and though the number of persons who contracted HIV infection declined from 3.2 million in 2001 to 2.7 million in 2008, there are 33.4 million persons living with HIV and AIDS worldwide; they are able to survive because of antiretroviral therapy (ART) and preventive measures. Sub-Saharan Africa is the global epicenter of the AIDS pandemic, with 71 percent of cases. According to the journal *Health Affairs*, if the pandemic continues unabated, more than 1 million persons will become infected each year through 2031, the fiftieth anniversary of the beginning of the HIV/AIDS pandemic, at a total cost of $722 billion.

Many other infectious diseases of zoonotic origin have emerged at considerable cost to human and animal life, with attendant economic losses when livestock are removed from the food chain: Emerging zoonotic infectious diseases, including bovine spongiform encephalitis (BSE, or mad cow disease) and avian influenza (or bird flu), cost an estimated $120 billion worldwide from 1995 to 2008.

Another zoonotic disease emerged in 2009 and soon became a pandemic. According to WHO, as of November, 2009, there were more than 40,600 cumulative confirmed and probable cases of H1N1 influenza and 7,826 deaths worldwide, though this may be an underestimate because the statistics are based on just 20 percent of the countries and communities that were able to provide confirmed laboratory data. In 2010, the Global Influenza Surveillance Network (GISN) reported that H1N1 continued to circulate in Malaysia, Singapore, India, Bangladesh, Bhutan, Chile, and Uruguay. During the height of the pandemic, many countries culled swine, resulting in economic hardship and adding to the losses incurred by human morbidity, mortality, and other related expenses.

Environmental factors such as climate change have influenced the emergence of disease, as was demonstrated with the appearance of vector-borne West Nile virus infection, which is endemic to the Near East and Africa. West Nile was observed in the Western Hemisphere for the first time in the northeastern United States in 1999, and it continues to return each summer to the same region as mosquitoes return to feed on the viral reservoir of infected birds; in July, 2010, the New York City Department of Health and Mental Hygiene issued an alert for the virus, which can sicken and kill humans. From 2004 through 2007, hospitalization costs for waterborne pathogens such as Legionnaires' disease (caused by a bacterium), cryptosporidiosis (caused by a fungus), and giardiasis (caused by a protozoan) were $154 million to $539 million.

Despite the foregoing statistics, there is growing worldwide recognition that science and public policy based on historical experience, international law, and ethics must intersect more effectively if the global community is to conquer the multitude of problems resulting from new and reemerging infectious diseases.

Cynthia F. Racer, M.P.H., M.A.

FURTHER READING

Drexler, Madeline. *Emerging Epidemics: The Menace of New Infections.* New York: Penguin Books, 2010. A comprehensive book that includes the history of a range of emerging diseases, including H1N1 and West Nile virus infection.

Fischback, M. A., and C. T. Walsh. "Antibiotics for Emerging Pathogens." *Science* 325, no. 5944 (August 28, 2009): 1089-1093. Discusses options for developing new antibiotics to circumvent existing bacterial resistance mechanisms.

Garrett, Laurie. *Betrayal of Trust: The Collapse of Global Public Health.* New York: Hyperion Books, 2001. Focuses on biopreparedness, bioterrorism, and public health preparedness.

Giles-Vernick, Tamara, and Susan Craddock, eds. *Influenza and Public Health: Learning from Past Pandemics.* London: Earthscan, 2010. Discusses lessons learned from past flu pandemics about transmission patterns and successful (and not so successful) interventions.

Hill, Stuart. *Emerging Infectious Diseases.* San Francisco: Benjamin Cummings, 2005. Includes historical data and updates on emerging diseases of the twenty-first century.

Leslie, T., et al. "Epidemic of *Plasmodium falciparum* Malaria Involving Substandard Antimalarial Drugs, Pakistan, 2003." *Emerging Infectious Diseases* 15 (2009): 1753-1759. Describes the role of substandard treatment of malaria in the formation of resistant malarial strains.

MacPherson, D. W., et al. "Population Mobility, Globalization, and Antimicrobial Drug Resistance." *Emerging Infectious Diseases* 15 (2009): 1727-1732. A timely assessment of the root causes of drug resistance.

Strickland, Thomas, et al., eds. *Hunter's Tropical Medicine and Emerging Infectious Diseases.* 8th ed. Philadelphia: W. B. Saunders, 2000. This is a classic textbook written by internationally known experts in the field. Although it uses some technical words, most readers should find the text understandable.

WEB SITES OF INTEREST

Centers for Disease Control and Prevention
http://www/cdc.gov

Emerging and Reemerging Infectious Diseases Resource Center
http://www.medscape.com/resource/infections

National Center for Emerging and Zoonotic Infectious Diseases
http://www.cdc.gov/ncezid

World Health Organization
http://www.who.int

See also: AIDS; Antibiotics: Experimental; Antibiotics: Types; Antiviral drugs: Types; Bacterial infections; Biosurveillance; Centers for Disease Control and Prevention (CDC); Developing countries and infectious disease; Disease eradication campaigns; Emerging Infections Network; Endemic infections; Epidemics and pandemics: History; Epidemiology; Globalization and infectious disease; HIV; Hospitals and infectious disease; Immunity; Immunization; Insecticides and topical repellants; Malaria; *Mycobacterium*; Outbreaks; Pathogenicity; Plague; Primates and infectious disease; Public health; Retroviral infections; Retroviridae;

Tropical medicine; Tuberculosis (TB); Typhoid fever; U.S. Army Medical Research Institute of Infectious Diseases; Vaccines: Types; Viral infections; World Health Organization (WHO); *Yersinia*.

Emerging Infections Network

CATEGORY: Epidemiology

DEFINITION

The Emerging Infections Network (EIN) is a group of physicians who specialize in the diagnosis and treatment of infectious diseases. These infectious disease physicians serve on the front-line in the detection of new and unusual cases of illness caused by microorganisms encountered in routine care. The member physicians are regularly queried on specific infectious diseases of interest and provide a source of data on infections. They work closely with their local and state health departments and with the Centers for Disease Control and Prevention (CDC). As such, they may also participate in outbreak investigations conducted by public health agencies or in studies through the identification of persons with an infectious disease of interest. Physicians in the network also share information among other members about diagnosis and treatment options. More than eleven hundred physicians are in the network, most of them in North America.

HISTORY

In 1995, the CDC and the Infectious Diseases Society of America (IDSA) entered into a cooperative agreement whereby the CDC would provide grant money to the ISDA to investigate the feasibility of developing a network of practicing infectious disease physicians. The network was to provide timely information on cases of microbial illness. A pilot study was conducted in the spring of 1996. Recruited for participation were 169 physicians from IDSA regional and state chapters. Physicians in urban (64 percent), suburban (26 percent), and rural (10 percent) settings participated in four initial surveys of infectious diseases, with a mean response rate of 85 percent. Most surveys took only two minutes to complete and were returned in two to three days. The pilot study was deemed a success, and all ISDA members were invited to participate in the network.

ACTIVITIES

Network physicians today are surveyed on a topic of interest approximately every eight weeks. Members also voluntarily report individual clinical findings that may lead to future surveys. In the case of a possible infectious disease outbreak, members are prepared to respond to questionnaires concerning individual patient cases within twenty-four hours. Members also share information with one another and with public health officers through the Internet.

IMPACT

Infectious diseases cross geographic borders. Reminders of this fact are the emergence of the H1N1 (swine flu) virus in 2009 and of SARS (severe acute respiratory syndrome) in 2002, among many other pandemics. Health surveillance organizations such as EIN played critical roles in preparing for the fallout from the diseases.

Economic globalization, climate change, unchecked population growth, and increasing gaps between the rich and the poor, all contribute to the increased likelihood that previously unrecognized infectious diseases will emerge. The sooner such diseases are recognized as threats to public health, the sooner resources can be mobilized to combat their spread and limit their impact. EIN members are integral to this mobilization.

Linda J Miwa, M.P.H.

FURTHER READING

Abraham, Thomas. *Twenty-first Century Plague: The Story of SARS*. Baltimore: Johns Hopkins University Press, 2007.

Drexler, Madeline. *Emerging Epidemics: The Menace of New Infections*. New York: Penguin Books, 2009.

Lashley, Felissa R., and Jerry D. Durham, eds. *Emerging Infectious Diseases*. 2d ed. New York: Springer, 2007.

Morens, David M., Gregory K. Folkers, and Anthony S. Fauci. "The Challenge of Emerging and Re-emerging Infectious Diseases." *Nature* 430 (July 8, 2004): 242-249.

WEB SITES OF INTEREST

Centers for Disease Control and Prevention: Emerging Infections Programs
http://www.cdc.gov/ncpdcid/deiss/eip

Emerging Infections Network
http://ein.idsociety.org

Infectious Diseases Society of America
http://www.idsociety.org

*National Center for Emerging and Zoonotic Infectious
    Diseases*
http://www.cdc.gov/ncezid

World Health Organization
http://www.who.int

See also: Biostatistics; Biosurveillance; Centers for Disease Control and Prevention (CDC); Disease eradication campaigns; Emerging and reemerging infectious diseases; Endemic infections; Epidemics and pandemics: Causes and management; Epidemiology; Globalization and infectious disease; Infectious disease specialists; Infectious Diseases Society of America; Outbreaks; Public health; World Health Organization (WHO).

Empyema

CATEGORY: Diseases and conditions
ANATOMY OR SYSTEM AFFECTED: Chest, lungs, skin
ALSO KNOWN AS: Empyema of the gallbladder, pelvic empyema, purulent or suppurative pleurisy, purulent pericarditis, subdural empyema, thoracic empyema

DEFINITION

Empyema is the collection of pus (a liquid that forms from leukocytes, cellular debris, and protein) in a natural body cavity. Empyema should not be confused with an abscess, which develops its own cavity. Empyema is most common in the pleural cavity, the space between the inside of the chest wall and the lung. Empyema may also occur in other body cavities, such as the pelvis, abdomen, subdural space, gallbladder, and the pericardial sac surrounding the heart.

CAUSES

Empyema is caused by an infection that leads to the development of pus in a body cavity or space. The amount of pus in such an infection can be as much as one pint (16 ounces), putting pressure on the adjacent body part or organ. A variety of bacteria, such as *Staphylococcus aureus*, *Streptococcus pneumoniae*, and *Haemophilus influenzae*, may cause empyema.

RISK FACTORS

Bacterial infection is the primary risk factor for empyema. Lung abscess, chest surgery, and injury or trauma to the chest are also risk factors for pleural empyema. Cholecystitis with contaminated bile is a risk factor for empyema of the gallbladder. People with chronic diseases may be more likely to develop empyema. Cancer may also contribute to empyema development.

SYMPTOMS

Symptoms will vary based on the location of the empyema. Fever is almost always present. Sweating, especially at night, often occurs. Sharp or shooting pains, undesired weight loss, headache, and a general poor feeling may occur. For empyema in the pleural space or chest cavity, shortness of breath and difficulty breathing are usually evident. For empyema in the pelvic cavity, foul smelling pus is present. A rigid or very tight abdomen may be noted.

SCREENING AND DIAGNOSIS

Screening and diagnosis are based on symptoms and careful evaluation of the physical condition of the infected person and his or her complaints. Decreased breath sounds (heard through a stethoscope) are often noted if pleural empyema is present. Taking a sample of pus from the pleural space by using a needle or plastic catheter (thoracentesis) is sometimes done to look for the causative bacteria. The doctor also will investigate any complaints of pain. Radiology tests, including X rays and computed tomography (CT) scans, are often used.

TREATMENT AND THERAPY

The primary goals of therapy are to cure the infection and to drain the pus if possible. Antibiotics are prescribed and may be given intravenously (in a vein), which requires hospitalization. If pleural empyema is the diagnosis, a chest tube inserted into the pleural cavity may be used to drain the pus from the body. In rare cases, a procedure to peel away part of the lining of the lung may be done so that the lung can inflate.

In empyema of the gallbladder, surgery to remove the gallbladder may be indicated. Other surgeries may be necessary, depending on the site of the empyema.

PREVENTION AND OUTCOMES

One can help prevent the development of empyema by treating infections promptly and using antibiotics appropriately.

Patricia Stanfill Edens, R.N., Ph.D., FACHE

FURTHER READING

Celli, B. R. "Diseases of the Diaphragm, Chest Wall, Pleura, and the Mediastinum." In *Cecil Medicine*, edited by Lee Goldman and Dennis Arthur Ausiello. 23d ed. Philadelphia: Saunders/Elsevier, 2008.

Levitzky, Michael G. *Pulmonary Physiology*. 7th ed. New York: McGraw-Hill Medical, 2007.

Madigan, Michael T., and John M. Martinko. *Brock Biology of Microorganisms*. 12th ed. Upper Saddle River, N.J.: Pearson/Prentice Hall, 2010.

Reed, James C. *Chest Radiology: Plain Film Patterns and Differential Diagnoses*. 5th ed. Philadelphia: Mosby, 2003.

Weedon, David. *Skin Pathology*. 3d ed. New York: Churchill Livingstone/Elsevier, 2010.

WEB SITES OF INTEREST

American Lung Association
http://www.lungusa.org

Canadian Lung Association
http://www.lung.ca

National Heart, Lung, and Blood Institute
http://www.nhlbi.nih.gov

See also: Abscesses; Bacterial infections; Cancer and infectious disease; Cholecystitis; Iatrogenic infections; Infection; Pleurisy; Skin infections; Wound infections.

Encephalitis

CATEGORY: Diseases and conditions
ANATOMY OR SYSTEM AFFECTED: Brain, central nervous system

DEFINITION

Encephalitis is inflammation of the brain. The inflammation may involve the whole brain or parts of the brain only.

CAUSES

Viral infection of the central nervous system can be asymptomatic, present with mild symptoms, or cause meningitis or encephalitis, or both. Most cases of encephalitis are caused by a viral infection. Encephalitis may be sporadic or epidemic. In the United States, the most common cause of sporadic encephalitis is the herpes simplex virus. Epidemic encephalitis is usually mosquito-borne or tickborne, which may be dependant on the geography and season. The most common viruses that cause encephalitis include West Nile, chickenpox, herpes simplex, poliovirus, Epstein-Barr virus, measles, mumps, rotavirus, influenza, rabies, and enterovirus.

RISK FACTORS

Risk factors for encephalitis include living, working, or playing in an area where mosquito-borne viruses are common; not being immunized against diseases such as measles, mumps, chickenpox, or polio; having cancer; taking immunosuppressive medicines after organ transplant; and having acquired immunodeficiency syndrome. Newborns of women who have genital herpes are at risk for herpes simplex encephalitis.

SYMPTOMS

The symptoms may range from mild, such as fever and headache, to severe, such as seizures, loss of consciousness, and permanent neurological damage; death also may occur. Symptoms include fever, weakness, severe fatigue, headache, sensitivity to light, stiff neck and back, vomiting, changes in consciousness, muscle aches, rash, personality changes, confusion, irritability, seizures, partial or complete paralysis, progressive drowsiness, yawning, trouble walking, trouble speaking, and trouble swallowing.

SCREENING AND DIAGNOSIS

A doctor will ask about symptoms and medical history and will do a physical exam. Tests may include blood tests to look for signs of infection; a spinal tap to test spinal fluid for signs of infection; computed tomography (CT) and magnetic resonance imaging (MRI) scans of the head, to look for abnormal areas

Common Brain Disorders

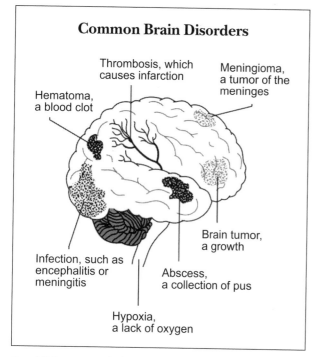

Thrombosis, which causes infarction

Meningioma, a tumor of the meninges

Hematoma, a blood clot

Infection, such as encephalitis or meningitis

Brain tumor, a growth

Abscess, a collection of pus

Hypoxia, a lack of oxygen

In addition to encephalitis, a number of diseases and disorders can affect the brain.

of enhancement, hemorrhage, or edema in the brain; an electroencephalogram (EEG) to look for abnormal electrical activity in the brain; and a brain biopsy (removal of a small sample of brain tissue to test for signs of infection).

TREATMENT AND THERAPY

Treatment is mostly supportive. It may include antiviral drugs (such as intravenous acyclovir for herpes simplex encephalitis) to potentially help shorten the duration of the illness; steroid medicines to decrease brain swelling; diuretics (such as mannitol) to decrease elevated intracranial pressure; intubation with hyperventilation to decrease elevated intracranial pressure and to maintain respiration and ventilation; and anticonvulsant medicines to prevent or treat (or both) seizures.

PREVENTION AND OUTCOMES

Vaccination against preventable viral illnesses is the best way to avoid encephalitis. Another preventive measure is avoiding areas with mosquitoes and ticks.

Rosalyn Carson-DeWitt, M.D.;
reviewed by Rimas Lukas, M.D.

FURTHER READING

Andreoli, Thomas E., et al., eds. *Andreoli and Carpenter's Cecil Essentials of Medicine.* 8th ed. Philadelphia: Saunders/Elsevier, 2010.

Booss, John, Margaret Esiri, and Margaret M. Esin, eds. *Viral Encephalitis in Humans.* Washington, D.C.: ASM Press, 2003.

EBSCO Publishing. *DynaMed: Herpes Simplex Encephalitis.* Available through http://www.ebscohost.com/dynamed.

Mandell, Gerald L., John E. Bennett, and Raphael Dolin, eds. *Mandell, Douglas, and Bennett's Principles and Practice of Infectious Diseases.* 7th ed. New York: Churchill Livingstone/Elsevier, 2010.

Marx, John A., et al., eds. *Rosen's Emergency Medicine: Concepts and Clinical Practice.* 7th ed. Philadelphia: Mosby/Elsevier, 2010.

National Institute of Neurological Disorders and Stroke. "Meningitis and Encephalitis Fact Sheet." Available at http://www.ninds.nih.gov.

Rakel, Robert E., Edward T. Bope, and Rick D. Kellerman, eds. *Conn's Current Therapy 2011.* Philadelphia: Saunders/Elsevier, 2010.

Woolsey, Thomas A., Joseph Hanaway, and Mokhtar Gado. *Brain Atlas: A Visual Guide to the Human Central Nervous System.* 3d ed. Hoboken, N.J.: Wiley, 2008.

WEB SITES OF INTEREST

Canadian Neurological Sciences Federation
http://www.ccns.org

Encephalitis Society
http://www.encephalitis.info

National Institute of Neurological Disorders and Stroke
http://www.ninds.nih.gov

See also: Acanthamoeba infection; Bacterial meningitis; Eastern equine encephalitis; Encephalitis vaccine; Enterovirus infections; Epstein-Barr virus infection; Herpes simplex infection; Herpesviridae; Herpesvirus infections; Inflammation; Insect-borne illness and disease; Japanese encephalitis; Mosquito-borne viral encephalitis; Mosquitoes and infectious disease; Poliomyelitis; Progressive multifocal leukoencephalopathy; Rotavirus infection; Sleeping sickness; Subacute sclerosing panencephalitis; Ticks and infectious disease; Viral infections; Viral meningitis; West Nile virus.

Encephalitis vaccine

CATEGORY: Prevention
ALSO KNOWN AS: Japanese encephalitis vaccine

DEFINITION

The encephalitis vaccine is used to prevent infection with Japanese encephalitis (JE), which is caused by a virus that affects the brain and can sometimes result in death. The virus, found primarily in Asia, is transmitted through infected mosquitoes.

HISTORY AND DEVELOPMENT

There are two types of JE vaccine licensed for use in the United States, JE-VAX and Ixiaro. JE-VAX, derived from mouse brains, was licensed for use in adult and pediatric (age one year and older) travelers in 1992. However, production of JE-VAX was discontinued in 2006, and stockpiles are expected to be depleted shortly. Ixiaro, a second-generation vaccine approved in 2009, is manufactured using cell culture technology. Research in the United States and Europe showed that Ixiaro produced sufficient levels of antibodies to protect against JE.

RECOMMENDATIONS

The Centers for Disease Control and Prevention (CDC) recommends vaccination against JE for people traveling to Asia who will spend one month or more in areas where JE occurs, who plan to visit rural areas or engage in outdoor activities, who expect to travel in areas of JE outbreak, and who are unsure of their exact plans while travelling. Laboratory workers who may be exposed to the JE virus should also be vaccinated.

Pregnant women are advised to avoid the vaccine, as are persons with a history of a severe allergic reaction to a previous dose of the JE vaccine or any other vaccine or vaccine component. Travelers who plan to return from Asia within thirty days and who will stay in major urban areas should consult a doctor before travel, because in these cases, the vaccine may not be recommended.

ADMINISTRATION

Ixiaro is given to people seventeen years of age and older in two separate doses, twenty-eight days apart. The second dose should be given a minimum of one week before travel. The need for and timing of Ixiaro booster shots is not yet known.

SIDE EFFECTS

The risk of Ixiaro causing serious harm or death is extremely small. Data on Ixiaro are limited thus far; severe reactions to Ixiaro are very rare, and other reported symptoms, including headache, muscle aches, pain, and tenderness, redness, or swelling at the injection site, are mild.

IMPACT

The impact of JE vaccination is expected to be significant, especially in countries where the disease is more prevalent. The vaccines will prevent illness, disability, and death. JE infection rates have fallen in Thailand and Japan as a result of vaccination.

Katherine Hauswirth, M.S.N., R.N.

FURTHER READING

Booss, John, Margaret Esiri, and Margaret M. Esin, eds. *Viral Encephalitis in Humans*. Washington, D.C.: ASM Press, 2003.

Centers for Disease Control and Prevention. "Japanese Encephalitis." In *CDC Health Information for International Travel 2010*. Available at http://wwwnc.cdc.gov/travel/content/yellowbook/home-2010.aspx.

Plotkin, Stanley A., Walter A. Orenstein, and Paul A. Offit. *Vaccines*. 5th ed. Philadelphia: Saunders/Elsevier, 2008.

United Nations International Children's Emergency Fund (UNICEF). "Vaccine Is Key to Preventing Outbreaks of Japanese Encephalitis." Available at http://www.unicef.org/infobycountry/india_28555.html.

WEB SITES OF INTEREST

Centers for Disease Control and Prevention
http://www.cdc.gov/vaccines

Encephalitis Society
http://www.encephalitis.info

Vaccine Research Center
http://www.niaid.nih.gov/about/organization/vrc

World Health Organization
http://www.who.int/immunization

See also: Arthropod-borne illness and disease; Bacterial meningitis; Eastern equine encephalitis; Encephalitis; Encephalitis vaccine; Insect-borne illness and disease; Japanese encephalitis; Mosquito-borne viral encephalitis; Vaccines: Types; Viral infections.

Endemic infections

CATEGORY: Epidemiology
ALSO KNOWN AS: Native diseases, regional diseases

DEFINITION

Endemic infections are diseases that are constant, that vary in numbers and severity, and that are localized to a particular region or population. Endemic infections, or diseases, are caused by any of the pathogens that plague humans: bacteria, viruses, fungi, and parasites. Most endemic diseases are contagious, or communicable. Health conditions too can be described as endemic, and they include those conditions that lead to disease, such as obesity, poor maternal nutrition, and impure drinking water, within a particular area or community.

The World Health Organization's list of some of the most common, and deadly, infectious diseases throughout the world include many that are endemic, particularly in developing countries where sanitation is poor. This list of diseases includes cholera, a bacterial infection spread mostly through contaminated drinking water (endemic to Russia, sub-Saharan Africa, and the Indian subcontinent); Japanese encephalitis, a viral infection spread by mosquitoes that live in rice paddies (endemic to parts of rural East Asia); malaria, which is widespread in tropical and subtropical climates, but is endemic to sub-Saharan Africa, where 90 percent of the world's cases of malaria are found; onchocerciasis, or river blindness (which is endemic to Africa), is caused by a parasitic worm than can live for years in the human body; and schistosomiasis, a parasitic infection that can damage the kidneys and is caused by a worm that swims freely in contaminated water (endemic to many developing countries).

LOCAL FACTORS

The local climate, or even microclimate, plays a major role in certain diseases endemic to a specific region, especially diseases that are spread by indigenous insects. For example, Chagas' disease, the leading cause of heart disease in Central America and South America, is spread by the triatomine bug, or kissing bug (*Triatoma pallidipennis*), that is found in tropical regions. This insect carries a parasite in its feces that infects humans who come in contact with the feces. This parasite can cause chronic heart problems and death.

Some diseases, ear infections in children, for example, are endemic to colder climates. Ear infections are not communicable. They develop when the eustachian tube (the air passage into the middle ear) becomes clogged and inflamed, usually as a secondary infection of the common cold, which is the endemic, ubiquitous scourge of cold climates.

POPULATIONS

The term "endemic" pertains to population groups, not individual persons. Persons who are perpetually ill suffer from a chronic condition, not an endemic condition. An endemic infection is entrenched and sustained within a population (but is not necessarily exclusive to that population). For a contagious disease such as chickenpox to be sustained or endemic, each member of the population who becomes infected must transmit, or pass along, the infection to a minimum of one other person, on average, in the group. Members of these population groups share certain characteristics (such as age, gender, and genetic heritage) and are affected by the same external influences (such as poverty, social stressors, and climate) that make them susceptible to certain pathogens.

CLASSIFICATIONS

"Endemic" is one of three broad categories used to describe the spread of infection. "Epidemic" and "pandemic" are the other two categories. Because these three words are related, they are often confused. The common root "demic" comes from the Greek *demos*, meaning "people."

Endemic infections. Endemic (*en* in Greek means "in") infections are always present at various levels of dissemination in a region or population and remain so without outside inputs. For example, meningococcal diseases, most notably meningitis, are endemic to Canada.

Epidemic infections. Epidemic (*epi* in Greek means "on" or "upon") infections are sudden, severe outbreaks in a region or population. They eventually become extinct. However, the number of infections and the aftermath of the outbreak can remain significant for a long time. For example, polio was an epidemic in the United States in the early 1950's.

Pandemic infections. Pandemic (*pan* in Greek means "all") infections are epidemics that are geographically widespread across a region or even the entire planet. An example is the Spanish flu pandemic of 1918.

Endemic infections are further classified in a number of ways. One distinction is between "holoendemic" and "hyperendemic" diseases.

Holoendemic diseases are those diseases that affect almost all the inhabitants of a particular area but are more prevalent in children than in adults (and usually more severe), because of the acquired immunity. For example, children under the age of five years account for 75 percent of the deaths from malaria in sub-Saharan Africa. Hyperendemic diseases are those diseases that affect nearly everyone in a given population, but the prevalence is more or less equal across all age groups. The common cold during cold season is an example of a hyperendemic disease.

A specific endemic infection can be quantified, or counted. One measure is "prevalence," the number of cases of a certain disease in a specified region or population at a given time. The prevalence can be low or high, and it can vary, but the disease remains; it is always in the region or within the group.

IMPACT

The socioeconomic impact of endemic infections on various regions and human populations is impossible to calculate. One ongoing debate is whether to focus resources on control or eradication. The rise in globalization in the twenty-first century has had an enormous effect on endemic infections.

Biological invasions are widespread. Travelers and transported goods carry insects and other living organisms all around the world. These invasions not only introduce new diseases but also increase the frequency and severity of local endemic diseases. Biologists have found that often the introduced species serve as suitable hosts for local endemic disease agents (such as bacteria and parasites). The introduced hosts help maintain the endemic status of the disease, making that disease increasingly difficult for local health organizations to control or eradicate.

Wendell Anderson, B.A.

FURTHER READING

Elliott, Charles W. "Prioritizing Endemic Diseases." *U.S. Army Medical Department Journal,* January-March, 2005. Presents ideas for using available resources to fight local endemic diseases affecting U.S. military personnel abroad.

May, Robert M., and Roy M. Anderson. "Endemic Infections in Growing Populations." *Mathematical Biosciences* 77 (1985): 141-156. A mathematical model for projecting the growth of endemic infections in growing populations.

Timmreck, Thomas C., ed. *An Introduction to Epidemiology.* 3d ed. Sudbury, Mass.: Jones and Bartlett, 2002. A basic guide to the topic for undergraduate students that includes the study of disease distribution in humans.

WEB SITES OF INTEREST

Disease Ecology Research Group
http://155.198.140.40/medicine/divisions/publichealth/ide/research_groups/diseco

Emerging Infections Network
http://ein.idsociety.org

Global Health Council
http://www.globalhealth.org/infectious_diseases

Infectious Diseases Society of America
http://www.idsociety.org

World Health Organization
http://www.who.int

See also: Biosurveillance; Centers for Disease Control and Prevention (CDC); Developing countries and infectious disease; Disease eradication campaigns; Emerging and reemerging infectious diseases; Emerging Infections Network; Epidemics and pandemics: Causes and management; Epidemiology; Globalization and infectious disease; Hospitals and infectious disease; Outbreaks; Public health; Tropical medicine; U.S. Army Medical Research Institute of Infectious Diseases; World Health Organization (WHO).

Endocarditis

CATEGORY: Diseases and conditions
ANATOMY OR SYSTEM AFFECTED: Blood, cardiovascular system, heart, tissue
ALSO KNOWN AS: Acute infective endocarditis, infective endocarditis

DEFINITION

Endocarditis is an inflammation of the endocardium, the lining of the interior surfaces of the heart. Endocarditis results from an endocardial injury, leading to the formation of a vegetation on the surface of the heart, often on a valve. The endothelial injury is most often the result of a preexisting heart condition, but it can be secondary to medical device implantation. The immune system's response to this injury is the formation of a blood clot, a thrombus, primarily composed of fibrin and platelets. Initially sterile, the thrombus is open for attack from microorganisms in the bloodstream.

CAUSES

Although there are many possible causes of endocarditis, including fungi, bacteria are the most common causes. The Duke criteria highlights the microorganisms most likely to be responsible for endocarditis and includes both gram-positive organisms and gram-negative organisms; gram-positive organisms are more common. Typical microorganisms include community acquired enterococci, *Staphylococcus aureus*, *Streptococcus bovis*, viridans streptococci, and the HACEK group (*Haemophilus* spp., *Actinobacillus actinomycetecomitants*, *Cardiobacterium hominis*, *Eikenella* spp., and *Kingella kingae*).

These microorganisms are able to enter the bloodstream from a trauma to a body surface. Body surfaces that are densely colonized and most likely to provide an avenue for bacteria to enter the bloodstream include the oral cavity, gastrointestinal tract, and genitourinary system.

RISK FACTORS

Risk factors for endocarditis include congenital heart abnormalities, intravenous drug use, and the implantation of prosthetic heart valves. Right-sided endocarditis is more likely to develop in persons who are drug users. In the past, it was commonly assumed that invasive procedures into highly colonized areas

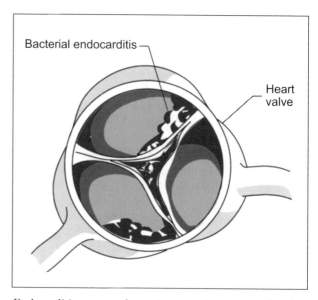

Endocarditis occurs when microorganisms, most often bacteria, cause inflammatory lesions on the lining of the interior surfaces of the heart.

also increased a person's risk for developing endocarditis, although the latest evidence does not support this theory. Preexisting structural abnormalities exist in about 75 percent of people who go on to develop endocarditis, and valvular conditions consist of a large percentage of these abnormalities. Other potential risk factors include a history of endocarditis and hemodialysis, diabetes, kidney disease, and human immunodeficiency virus infection.

SYMPTOMS

Most persons with endocarditis will present with nonspecific symptoms that include fever, fatigue, and malaise. A previously undetected heart murmur, a change in a preexisting heart murmur, and neurological impairment also may be present. Janeway lesions, Osler's nodes, and Roth spots are more specific for endocarditis; however, they are not always present. Janeway lesions are nonpainful red lesions found on the palms and soles; Osler's nodes are painful nodules found on the fingers and toes; and Roth spots are retinal hemorrhages that have a white center.

SCREENING AND DIAGNOSIS

Diagnosis of endocarditis is based on the Duke criteria, consisting of major and minor criteria. Major criteria include microbiologic evidence from blood samples (the number of positive samples depends on the organism) and positive echocardiogram findings. A minimum of three blood samples should be collected, preferably over the course of a few days; however, these samples can be collected within the span of an hour. The minor criteria include predisposition to infective endocarditis (such as previous endocarditis, injection drug use, prosthetic heart valve, or cardiac lesion causing turbulent blood flow), fever greater than 100.4° Fahrenheit (38° Celsius), a vascular phenomenon, an immunologic phenomenon, and a microbiologic finding not meeting major criteria.

TREATMENT AND THERAPY

Antibiotics are the mainstay of therapy for endocarditis. Surgery may be required for more severe cases. Therapy should be initiated with intravenous antibiotics, often at high doses, because of the hard-to-reach nature of the vegetation. Therapy should be continued for two to six weeks or longer, depending on the infected person's response. Antibiotics should be initiated as soon as feasible, depending on cultures.

In cases of complicated or severe endocarditis, empirical therapy may be initiated and targeted at *S. aureus* and enterococci. A recommended regimen for empiric therapy is a combination of vancomycin and gentamicin. Treatment regimens are as follows:

Enterococci. Ampicillin in combination with an aminoglycoside (gentamicin). In persons unable to take penicillin or penicillin-resistant isolates, vancomycin in combination with an aminoglycoside is recommended.

S. aureus. Semisynthetic penicillin or a first-generation cephalosporin is the first-line recommendation. Some studies support the addition of gentamicin or rifampin with either a semisynthetic penicillin or a first-generation cephalosporin for the first few days of therapy. In persons unable to take penicillin or penicillin-resistant isolates, vancomycin is recommended.

S. epidermis. Vancomycin with rifampin is recommended. An aminoglycoside may be added for two weeks.

Gram-negative microorganisms. A third-generation cephalosporin with an aminoglycoside is recommended; a broad-spectrum penicillin is a second option.

PREVENTION AND OUTCOMES

Perioperative prophylactic antibiotics are recommended for specific cardiovascular procedures, including surgery to insert a prosthetic heart valve and intravascular or intracardiac materials. The American Heart Association does not recommend the use of prophylactic antibiotics in persons who undergo either gastrointestinal or genitourinary surgical procedures. Historically, prophylactic antibiotics were given to a majority of persons undergoing even minimally invasive dental procedures, however, updated guidelines recommend prophylaxis only in persons with specific preexisting conditions.

Allison C. Bennett, Pharm.D.

FURTHER READING

Baddour, Larry, et al. "Infective Endocarditis Diagnosis, Antimicrobial Therapy, and Management of Complications." *Circulation* 111 (2005): e394-e433. Detailed guidelines directed at health care professionals. Includes information on drugs and dosing.

McDonald, Jay. "Acute Infective Endocarditis" *Infectious Disease Clinics of North America* 23 (2009): 643-664. Summary of the disease state, including coverage of the Duke criteria. Does not provide detailed information of treatment and dosing but covers demographics, epidemiology, mortality, and general topics.

Rakel, Robert E., Edward T. Bope, and Rick D. Kellerman, eds. *Conn's Current Therapy 2011.* Philadelphia: Saunders/Elsevier, 2010. Section 5, "The Cardiovascular System—Infective Endocarditis," provides good coverage of prophylaxis and background on the disease state.

WEB SITES OF INTEREST

American Heart Association
http://www.heart.org

National Heart, Lung, and Blood Institute
http://www.nhlbi.nih.gov

See also: Bacterial endocarditis; Behçet's syndrome; Bloodstream infections; Disseminated intravascular coagulation; Inflammation; Myocarditis; Pericarditis.

Endometritis

CATEGORY: Diseases and conditions
ANATOMY OR SYSTEM AFFECTED: Reproductive system, uterus
ALSO KNOWN AS: Endomyometritis

DEFINITION

Endometritis is an irritation or inflammation of the endometrium, the inner lining of the uterus, that sometimes extends into the myometrium and parametrial tissues. Pathologically, endometritis is classified as acute or chronic. Acute endometritis is distinguished by the presence of neutrophils in the endometrial glands and chronic endometritis is characterized by variable numbers of plasma cells and lymphocytes within the endometrial stroma.

CAUSES

Endometritis is a microbial infection that can be caused by normal vaginal bacteria and by chlamydia, gonorrhea, chronic pelvic inflammatory disease, or tuberculosis. In most cases, it is initiated by an ascending infection from organisms found in the normal vaginal flora. Infection may be produced by compromised abortions, complicated deliveries, miscarriages, medical exam instrumentation, and retention of placental fragments.

RISK FACTORS

The risk for endometritis increases after miscarriage or childbirth, particularly after a long labor or a cesarean section. Medical procedures that involve entering the uterus through the cervix such as hysteroscopy and placement of an intrauterine device increase the risk of developing endometritis. After vaginal delivery, incidence is between 1 and 3 percent, whereas for cesarean delivery, incidence ranges from 13 to 90 percent.

SYMPTOMS

The most common symptoms associated with endometritis are lower abdominal pain, fever, and increased vaginal discharge or bleeding. There may be yellow, foul-smelling vaginal discharge. Discomfort with bowel movement and constipation may also occur. Menstruation can be excessive after acute endometritis, but the excessive bleeding can usually be resolved after two weeks of antibiotic treatment. Patients suffering from chronic endometritis may have an underlying cancer of the cervix or endometrium.

SCREENING AND DIAGNOSIS

Physical and pelvic exams will be performed by a health care provider. The lower abdomen, uterus, and cervix may be tender. Cervical discharge and decreased bowel sounds may be present. Cultures may be taken from the cervix to test for microbial infectious agents. Other tests performed often include an endometrial biopsy, laparoscopy, white blood count, and microscopic examination of any vaginal discharge.

TREATMENT AND THERAPY

Broad-spectrum antibiotics are used to treat and prevent complications of endometritis. Treatments sometimes involve plenty of rest and administering fluids through a vein. For complicated cases of endometritis, hospitalization may be necessary.

PREVENTION AND OUTCOMES

The risk of endometritis can be reduced by employing careful, sterile techniques during the delivery of a baby, during an abortion, or during any gynecological procedures. Safer sex practices reduce the risk of endometritis caused by sexually transmitted infections.

Alvin K. Benson, Ph.D.

FURTHER READING

Beers, Mark H., et al., eds. *The Merck Manual of Diagnosis and Therapy*. 18th ed. Whitehouse Station, N.J.: Merck Research Laboratories, 2006.

Berek, Jonathan S., ed. *Berek and Novak's Gynecology*. 14th ed. Philadelphia: Lippincott Williams & Wilkins, 2007.

Dallenbach-Hellweg, Gisela, Dietmar Schmidt, and Friederike Dallenbach. *Atlas of Endometrial Histopathology*. 3d ed. New York: Springer, 2010.

Icon Health. *Endometritis: A Medical Dictionary, Bibliography, and Annotated Research Guide to Internet References*. San Diego, Calif.: Author, 2003.

Katz, V. I., et al., eds. *Comprehensive Gynecology*. 5th ed. Philadelphia: Mosby/Elsevier, 2007.

Wilson, Walter, and Merle Sande. *Current Diagnosis and Treatment in Infectious Diseases*. New York: McGraw-Hill Medical, 2001.

American Congress of Obstetricians and Gynecologists
http://www.acog.org

National Women's Health Information Center
http://www.womenshealth.gov

Women's Health Matters
http://www.womenshealthmatters.ca

See also: Bacterial vaginosis; Cervical cancer; Childbirth and infectious disease; Chlamydia; Gonorrhea; Iatrogenic infections; Inflammation; Pelvic inflammatory disease; Pregnancy and infectious disease; Tuberculosis (TB); Urinary tract infections; Vaginal yeast infection; Women and infectious disease.

Enteritis

CATEGORY: Diseases and conditions
ANATOMY OR SYSTEM AFFECTED: Digestive system, gastrointestinal system, intestines
ALSO KNOWN AS: Bacterial enteritis, food poisoning

DEFINITION
Enteritis is inflammation of the small intestine often caused by bacterial infection.

CAUSES
Enteritis is often caused by consuming food or water contaminated with bacteria or viruses, which can migrate to the small intestine and cause swelling and inflammation. Common organisms that may cause enteritis include *Escherichia coli, Salmonella, Shigella,* and *Staphylococcus aureus.* Enteritis is also caused by food poisoning, by some autoimmune diseases (such as Crohn's disease), by damage from radiation treatment, and by drugs such as ibuprofen and cocaine.

RISK FACTORS
Exposure to unclean or improperly handled food and water, travel in areas with poor water quality and questionable food hygiene, and contact with a person with diarrhea are risk factors for enteritis. Another risk factor is eating foods with mayonnaise or dairy products that have been unrefrigerated for long periods, such as at picnics or during parties. Autoimmune diseases may also contribute to the development of enteritis. Receiving radiation treatment to the abdomen can result in complications in the intestine, including enteritis.

SYMPTOMS
Symptoms of enteritis occur from hours to a few days after infection and include gas, diarrhea, pain or cramping in the abdomen, poor appetite, and rarely, vomiting. Bloody diarrhea and fever may indicate infection with *E. coli* bacteria. Severe diarrhea may cause dehydration, in which the body loses too much fluid. Babies and children with diarrhea may become dehydrated quickly. Severe dehydration may be life-threatening.

SCREENING AND DIAGNOSIS
There is no screening test for enteritis. Diagnosis is made based on a stool culture to identify bacteria, but this test does not always identify the specific causative organism. Because diarrhea is a common symptom in several diseases, the physician will ask questions about recent travel, exposure to others with diarrhea, and any diseases or treatments that may be present in the infected person. Diagnosis also includes a physical examination.

TREATMENT AND THERAPY
Symptoms usually disappear without treatment. Antidiarrheal medicines are not recommended because they may slow the bacteria's movement from the intestine. If dehydration occurs, electrolyte solutions may be recommended to replenish the fluids in the body. Consuming small amounts of liquid frequently will decrease the risk of dehydration. Persons taking diuretics, or water pills, are usually asked to stop the medication. In rare cases with children and the elderly, intravenous fluids, or fluids given through a vein, may be indicated; this may also require hospitalization. Avoiding dairy products is recommended because they can make the diarrhea worse. One should consult a doctor if the diarrhea persists, if a fever is present, or if the person becomes dehydrated.

PREVENTION AND OUTCOMES
Careful handwashing, especially after using a toilet; safe food handling; and drinking only clean water are helpful in preventing enteritis. Other preventive

measures include keeping cold foods cold and hot foods hot, carefully washing utensils and cutting boards after food preparation, and cooking food to recommended temperatures. When traveling, one should drink bottled water or use purification tablets and should ensure that food is cooked properly. One should not eat raw foods, such as salads, that are washed using the local water supply, and should avoid drinking from streams and rivers without first boiling the water.

Patricia Stanfill Edens, R.N., Ph.D., FACHE

FURTHER READING

Feldman, Mark, Lawrence S. Friedman, and Lawrence J. Brandt, eds. *Sleisenger and Fordtran's Gastrointestinal and Liver Disease: Pathophysiology, Diagnosis, Management.* New ed. 2 vols. Philadelphia: Saunders/Elsevier, 2010.

"Infectious Diarrheal Diseases and Bacterial Food Poisoning." In *Harrison's Principles of Internal Medicine*, edited by Joan Butterton. 17th ed. New York: McGraw-Hill, 2008.

Johnson, Leonard R., ed. *Gastrointestinal Physiology.* 7th ed. Philadelphia: Mosby/Elsevier, 2007.

Kirschner, Barbara S., and Dennis D. Black. "The Gastrointestinal Tract." In *Nelson Essentials of Pediatrics*, edited by Karen J. Marcdante et al. 6th ed. Philadelphia: Saunders/Elsevier, 2011.

WEB SITES OF INTEREST

American College of Gastroenterology
http://www.acg.gi.org

American Society of Tropical Medicine and Hygiene
http://www.astmh.org

Crohn's and Colitis Foundation of America
http://www.ccfa.org

National Digestive Diseases Information Clearinghouse
http://digestive.niddk.nih.gov

U.S. Department of Agriculture, Food Safety Information Center
http://foodsafety.nal.usda.gov

See also: *Campylobacter; Clostridium difficile* infection; Cryptosporidiosis; Diverticulitis; *Escherichia coli* infection; Food-borne illness and disease; Giardiasis; Inflammation; Intestinal and stomach infections; Norovirus infection; Peptic ulcer; Peritonitis; Salmonellosis; Shigellosis; Travelers' diarrhea; Tropical medicine; Typhoid fever; Viral gastroenteritis; Waterborne illness and disease; Worm infections.

Enterobacter

CATEGORY: Pathogen
TRANSMISSION ROUTE: Variable

DEFINITION

Enterobacter are gram-negative, aerobic, motile bacilli found in soil, water, and the human intestinal tract. *Enterobacter* is an opportunistic pathogen responsible for various infections.

**Taxonomic Classification
for *Enterobacter***

Kingdom: Bacteria
Phylum: Proteobacteria
Class: Gamma Proteobacteria
Order: Enterobacteriales
Family: Enterobactriaceae
Genus: *Enterobacter*
Species:
E. aerogenes
E. amnigenus
E. agglomerans
E. asburiae
E. cancerogenous
E. cloacae
E. cowanii
E. dissolvens
E. gergoviae
E. hormaechei
E. intermedium
E. kobei
E. ludwigii
E. nimipressuralis
E. pyrinus
E. sakazakii
E. taylorae

NATURAL HABITAT AND FEATURES

Enterobacter is a gram-negative bacillus that belongs to the family Enterobacteriaceae, which includes *Klebsiella*, *Escherichia*, *Citrobacter*, and *Serratia*. *Enterobacter* bacteremia exhibits symptoms similar to other gram-negative bacilli.

Not all *Enterobacter* species cause diseases in humans, but those that have the most encounters in humans include *aerogenes*, *agglomerans*, *cloacae*, and *sakazakii*. Various species can be found in water, plants, plant materials, insects, and dairy products and in human and nonhuman animal feces. *Cloacae* has been used in the biological control of plant diseases and in the control of insects on mulberry leaves.

Enterobacter species are rod-shaped bacteria that can be identified by large lactose-fermenting colonies of gram-negative rods that are either raised or mucoid. These mucoid colonies appear pink to purple because of lactose fermentation. *Enterobacter* strains are mainly fimbriate and slime-forming.

Species of *Enterobacter* can be differentiated by their ability to ferment particular sugars and by their possession of arginine dihydrolase, lysine, and ornithine decarboxylase. Most *Enterobacter* species grow well at 86° to 98.6° Fahrenheit (30° to 37° Celsius), using eosin methylene blue (EMB) agar. MacConkey agar, when used, will give a red stain to the growing colonies.

Aerogenes and *cloacae* can be differentiated by tests for lysine decarboxylase and arginine dihydrolase. *Sakazakii* can be differentiated from *cloacae* by its ability to ferment D-sorbitol and by its yellowish pigment on culture medium.

PATHOGENICITY AND CLINICAL SIGNIFICANCE

Gram-negative pathogens possess endotoxins, giving them pathogenetic properties. *Enterobacter* species are pathogenic; the most common species are *cloacae* and *aerogenes*. These types of bacteremia can cause opportunistic infections in immunocompromised persons. Rarely will *Enterobacter* become problematic in a healthy person. The urinary and respiratory tracts are the most common sites of infection.

Acquisition of *Enterobacter* infections can be by either endogenous or exogenous sources. Most nosocomial (hospital acquired) *Enterobacter* infections cannot be traced to a single common exogenous source. Endogenous sources of nosocomial *Enterobacter* infections typically arise from a previously colonized site, such as the skin, gastrointestinal tract, or urinary

tract. A person can be colonized with more than one *Enterobacter* species at any given time.

Nosocomial acquisition of *Enterobacter* is more common than community acquired *Enterobacter*. These infections are acquired from prolonged hospitalization, especially in intensive care units, and from poor handwashing technique, invasive procedures, mechanical ventilation (which causes ventilator-associated pneumonia), the use of hyperalimentation with dextrose, the use of indwelling catheters (such as intravenous catheters), and from prior use of antimicrobial agents.

Incubation times for *Enterobacter* are variable. Symptoms can appear from as early as two hours to three weeks, with the majority of symptoms occurring between two hours and two days.

Enterobacter bacteremia associated with skin and soft tissue infections, burn and surgical wound infections, intra-abdominal infections, endocarditis, septic arthritis, osteomyelitis, meningitis, and bloodstream infections further complicate an already ubiquitous pathogen. Morbidity and mortality rates with *Enterobacter* are significant. The most critical factor in helping to determine the risk of mortality in persons with *Enterobacter* bacteremia is the severity of the underlying disease. Additional factors include other aspects of treatment and the microorganism's virulence or resistance. *E. cloacae* has the highest mortality rate of all *Enterobacter* infections.

DRUG SUSCEPTIBILITY

Pharmacotherapy goals in the treatment of *Enterobacter* infection are to reduce morbidity, eradicate infection, and to prevent complications. Prior use of antimicrobial agents is the single most frequently cited risk factor in the development of *Enterobacter* resistance. Initial drugs of choice include aminoglucosides, carbapenems, fluoroquinolones, and fourth generation cephalosporins. Susceptibility testing is essential because some *Enterobacter* infections are resistant to the initial drugs of choice, making the choice of appropriate antimicrobial agents more complicated.

Carbapenems (imipenem and meropenum) continue to be the most effective drugs of choice against *cloacae*, *aerogenes*, and other *Enterobacter* species. First and second generation cephalosporins are virtually ineffective against *Enterobacter*. Third generation cephalosporins, which show good in vitro activity, appear, however, to increase the risk of developing drug resistance. Piperacillin/tazobactam (Zosyn) has been shown to lower *Enterobacter* bacteremia mortality rates.

Enterobacter species contain subpopulations of organisms that produce low levels of beta-lactamase. The subpopulation of these beta-lactamase producing organisms will predominate once exposed to broad spectrum cephalosporins. Thus an *Enterobacter* infection that initially appears sensitive to cephalosporins may eventually become resistant during therapy.

Antimicrobial drug resistance occurs as a result of the production of inactivating enzyme, alteration of the drug's target, and alteration in the ability of the drug to enter and or accumulate in the cell. Detection of resistance can be identified as soon as twenty-four hours after initiation and up to two to three weeks into therapy.

Bacterial resistance to antibiotics continues to be a significant threat. Multiple *Enterobacter* strains are already resistant to many antibiotics. Infectious disease specialists are instrumental in determining appropriate antibiotic treatment. Handwashing remains the single most helpful method in preventing the spread of *Enterobacter* infections.

Stephanie McCallum Blake, M.S.N.

FURTHER READING

Farmer, J. J., et al. "Enterobacteriaceae: Introduction and Identification." In *Manual of Clinical Microbiology*, edited by Patrick R. Murray et al. 9th ed. Washington, D.C.: ASM Press, 2007.

Frasier, Susan L., and Michael Arnett. "*Enterobacter* Infections." eMedicine. Discusses background, differential diagnosis, workup, treatment, medications and follow-up with *Enterobacter* infections.

Marcos, Miguel, et al. "Effect of Antimicrobial Therapy on Mortality in 377 Episodes of *Enterobacter* spp. Bacteremia." *Journal of Antimicrobial Chemotherapy* 62 (2008): 397-408.

Sanders, W. E., and C. C. Sanders. "*Enterobacter* spp: A Pathogen Poised to Flourish at the Turn of the Century." *Clinical Microbiology Reviews* 10 (1997): 220-241.

Tortora, Gerard J., Berdell R. Funke, and Christine L. Case. "Antimicrobial Drugs." In *Microbiology: An Introduction*. 10th ed. San Francisco: Benjamin Cummings, 2010.

WEB SITES OF INTEREST

Clean Hands Coalition
http://www.cleanhandscoalition.org

Todar's Online Textbook of Bacteriology
http://www.textbookofbacteriology.net

See also: Antibiotic resistance; Antibiotics: Types; Bacteria: Classification and types; Bacterial infections; Cephalosporin antibiotics; *Escherichia*; *Salmonella*; *Yersinia*.

Enterobiasis

CATEGORY: Diseases and conditions
ANATOMY OR SYSTEM AFFECTED: Gastrointestinal system, genitalia, intestines, skin
ALSO KNOWN AS: Pinworm infection, pinworms

DEFINITION

Enterobiasis is a parasitic infection of the large intestines by pinworms (*Enterobius vermicularis*), which are small white roundworms, or nematodes. Enterobiasis is most endemic to children. Pinworm infection is globally distributed with a higher prevalence in cool and temperate climates. It is the most common parasitic worm infection found in the United States.

CAUSES

Infection is possible from direct hand-to-mouth transmission when fingers come into contact with eggs either from scratching or from touching clothing containing live eggs; from exposure to contaminated objects, such as clothing, linens, or toys; from inhalation of airborne eggs; and from retroinfection, when the eggs hatch on the perianal skin and the larvae travel up the colon.

Once ingested, the eggs will take one to two months to reach sexual maturation. Males typically die after reproduction and females usually die after laying eggs. The intense itching in the perianal and perineal area of the skin occurs during the females' nighttime migration through the anus to deposit eggs. A person is considered infected as long as a female worm is depositing eggs.

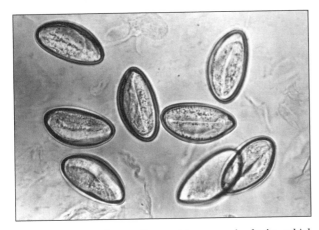

Eggs of the roundworm Enterobius vermicularis, *which causes enterobiasis.* (CDC)

RISK FACTORS

Scratching because of the itching tends to cause reinfection from hand-mouth transmission. Intense itching may also lead to bacterial skin infections from scratching. In severe cases, enterobiasis may cause appendicitis or intestinal blockage. Rarer complications include urinary tract infections and vulvovaginitis.

SYMPTOMS

The hallmark symptom of enterobiasis is the nighttime itching around the perianal and perineal area. Itching is caused by the migration of the female worm to deposit eggs. The itching often results in sleep disturbance and in some cases may lead to severe skin infections from scratching. Other symptoms that may be seen, especially in children, include nervousness, abdominal pain, vomiting, weight loss, and enuresis. It is not uncommon, however, for enterobiasis to be asymptomatic.

SCREENING AND DIAGNOSIS

Diagnosis is made by microscopic identification of the thick-shelled, ovoid eggs. Cellulose tape is used to collect samples of eggs by pressing the tape against the perineal area. The tape preparation is then used to prepare a slide to view under a microscope. Worms may also be visible. The collection of eggs with the tape may need to be taken over several consecutive days. Eggs are not typically observed in the stools.

TREATMENT AND THERAPY

The treatment of choice is chemotherapy with al-bendazole or mebendazole given in a single dose and repeated in two weeks. Pyrantel pamoate (available without a prescription) and piperazine may also be used. To avoid reinfection, one should seek counseling to discuss personal hygiene and environmental sanitation. Family members should also be treated, and the living environment should be decontaminated by washing bed linens and clothing.

PREVENTION AND OUTCOMES

The best method of preventing enterobiasis is good personal hygiene that includes daily bathing and frequent handwashing. Using well-laundered (in hot water) clothing and bed linens can also help to reduce and prevent reinfection. Sunlight and ultraviolet lamps will destroy eggs, and dry heat is useful in sterilizing metal toys. Eggs are not killed by swimming pool chlorine, however. Health experts believe that total prevention is unrealistic.

Susan E. Thomas, M.L.S.

FURTHER READING

Centers for Disease Control and Prevention. "Pinworm Infection (Enterobiasis)." Available at http://www.cdc.gov/ncidod/dpd/parasites/pinworm.

Despommier, Dickson D., et al. *Parasitic Diseases.* 5th ed. New York: Apple Tree, 2006.

"*Enterobius vermicularis.*" In *Human Parasitology*, edited by Burton J. Bogitsh, Clint E. Carter, and Thomas N. Oeltmann. 3d ed. Boston: Academic Press/Elsevier, 2005.

"Intestinal Nematodes." In *Diagnostic Medical Parasitology*, edited by Lynne Shore Garcia. 5th ed. Washington, D.C.: ASM Press, 2007.

Kucik, Corry Jeb, et al. "Common Intestinal Parasites." *American Family Physician* 69 (2004): 1161-1168.

Rett, Doug. "*Enterobius vermicularis.*" University of Michigan, Museum of Zoology. Available at http://animaldiversity.ummz.umich.edu/site/index.html.

Shorey, Harsha, Beverley-Ann Biggs, and Peter Traynor. "Nematodes." In *Manual of Clinical Microbiology*, edited by Patrick R. Murray et al. 9th ed. Washington, D.C.: ASM Press, 2007.

WEB SITES OF INTEREST

American Gastroenterological Association
http://www.gastro.org

Canadian Association of Gastroenterology
http://www.cag-acg.org

Centers for Disease Control and Prevention: Division of Parasitic Diseases
http://www.cdc.gov/ncidod/dpd

See also: Amebic dysentery; Anal abscess; Ascariasis; Children and infectious disease; Cryptosporidiosis; Dracunculiasis; Hookworms; Intestinal and stomach infections; Oral transmission; Parasitic diseases; Pilonidal cyst; Pinworms; Roundworms; Skin infections; Toxocariasis; Trichinosis; Whipworm infection; Worm infections.

Enterococcus

CATEGORY: Pathogen
TRANSMISSION ROUTE: Blood, direct contact

DEFINITION

Enterococcus is a bacterium that is normally found in the human intestinal tract. The bacterium can cause a number of infections in humans.

**Taxonomic Classification
for *Enterococcus***

Kingdom: Bacteria
Phylum: Firmicutes
Order: Lactobacillales
Family: Enterococcaceae
Genus: *Enterococcus*
Species:
E. faecalis
E. faecium

NATURAL HABITAT AND FEATURES

Enterococci are part of the normal bacterial flora of the human intestine. They are also found naturally in the intestines of nonhuman animals and of birds. Although most commonly found in the bowel, enterococci can also be present in the vagina, skin, and upper respiratory tract. In the environment, enterococci can be found in surface water, plants, and soil.

Although there are seventeen species of enterococci, the most common species found in humans are *faecalis* and *faecium*. Other species known to cause infection in humans include *avium, casseliflavus, durans, gallinarum, mundtii,* and *raffinosus*. Enterococci are gram-positive anaerobic cocci that grow in short chains. Under a microscope, enterococci appear spherical. They are extremely hardy and can grow and survive under a variety of conditions. They can survive in temperatures ranging from 50° to 113° Fahrenheit (10° to 45° Celsius), under aerobic or anaerobic conditions, under hypotonic or hypertonic conditions, and in acidic or alkaline environments. Unlike most microorganisms, they can grow in 6.5 percent sodium chloride and in concentrated bile salts.

PATHOGENICITY AND CLINICAL SIGNIFICANCE

There are a number of infections that are caused by enterococci. Common infections include those of wounds, the urinary tract, the heart valve (endocarditis), the bloodstream (bacteremia), and the intra-abdomen and pelvis, and infection and inflammation of the protective membranes of the brain (meningitis).

Many enterococcal infections are spread by colonized persons (people whose normal intestinal flora has spread to the urinary tract, the abdomen, or other parts of the body without causing disease). There are certain factors that may put a person at risk for enterococcus colonization. Colonization risk factors include the following: prolonged hospitalization, admission to an intensive care unit, receiving a transplant, having a compromised immune system, undergoing a lengthy course of antibiotics, having renal insufficiency, and providing patient care in a health care setting.

The majority of enterococcal infections are nosocomial (hospital acquired) infections, many of which are spread from colonized patients to other patients by health care workers. Enterococci can live on surfaces for several weeks, so infection can easily be spread through contact with contaminated items (fomites) such as bed rails, door knobs, faucets, and sinks. Inadequate handwashing technique also contributes to the spread of *Enterococcus*.

The most common type of nosocomial infection is urinary tract infection (UTI), although *Enterococcus* is not the only bacterium known to cause nosocomial UTI. Most nosocomial UTIs are the result of inadequate handwashing, the inappropriate use of urinary catheters, and the mismanagement of indwelling urinary catheters.

Another common nosocomial enterococcal infection is bacteremia, which is frequently associated with the use of central venous catheters. Serious catheter-related bloodstream infections can develop quickly because central venous catheters are placed in major veins. Nosocomial bacteremia is usually a result of inadequate handwashing, lack of appropriate barrier precautions during insertion, poor choice of placement site, improper cleaning of the insertion site, and a lack of patient education about site care at home.

Drug Susceptibility

Enterococcal infections can be difficult to treat because *Enterococcus* has not only an intrinsic resistance to antibiotics but also an acquired resistance. Before beginning treatment for an enterococcal infection, isolated organisms should be tested for resistance to beta-lactam antibiotics (such as penicillin and cephalosporin), glycopeptides (vancolycin and tycoplanin), aminoglycosides (gentamycin and streptomycin), macrolides (erythromycin and tetracycline), and quinolones (ofloxacin and ciprofloxacin).

Most enterococcal infections are treated using a combination of antibiotics: one (such as ampicillin or vancomycin) that attacks the cell wall and an aminoglycoside, which inhibits protein synthesis. In the past several years, enterococci have become resistant to vancomycin, making it increasingly difficult to treat enterococcal infections. There are some newer antibiotics that have been found to be effective against vancomycin-resistant enterococci (VRE). These antibiotics include quinupristin/dalfopristin, linezolid, daptomycin, and tigecycline. However, incidences of resistance to these newer antibiotics also have been reported. As with other types of enterococcal infection, treatment of VRE requires laboratory testing for resistance to determine what antibiotics will be effective as treatment.

Julie Henry, R.N., M.P.A.

Further Reading

Barie, Philip S., and Steven M. Opal. "Infectious Complications Following Surgery and Trauma: Bloodstream Infection." In *Cohen and Powderly Infectious Diseases*, edited by Jonathan Cohen, Steven M. Opal, and William G. Powderly. 3d ed. Philadelphia: Mosby/Elsevier, 2010. Addresses the risk of opportunistic infection, especially bloodstream infection, following surgery or injury.

Durack, David T., and Michael H. Crawford, eds. *Infective Endocarditis*. Philadelphia: W. B. Saunders, 2003. A text on all aspects of endocarditis, which is caused by bacteria, including *Enterococcus*.

EBSCO Publishing. *DynaMed: Vancomycin-Resistant Enterococci (VRE) Infection*. Available through http://www.ebscohost.com/dynamed.

Fraser, Susan, and Julie Lim. "Enterococcal Infection." Available at http://emedicine.medscape.com/article/216993-overview. A good discussion of enterococcal infections, including frequency, pathophysiology, history, diagnosis, treatment, prevention, and drug susceptibility.

Johns Hopkins Hospital and Johns Hopkins Health System. "Vancomycin Resistant Enterococci (VRE)." Available at http://www.hopkinsmedicine.org/heic/ID/vre. An overview of vancomycin-resistant enterococci that includes information about the organism, epidemiology, disease description, diagnosis, treatment, and infection prevention and control.

The Nurse's Role in Infection Prevention and Control. Oakbrook Terrace, Ill.: Joint Commission Resources, 2010. A book for health care workers and health care organization administrators that discusses methods for preventing and controlling the spread of infection in the health care setting.

Web Sites of Interest

Centers for Disease Control and Prevention
http://www.cdc.gov

Todar's Online Textbook of Bacteriology
http://www.textbookofbacteriology.net

See also: Acute cystitis; Antibiotics: Types; Bacterial endocarditis; Bacterial infections; Bacterial meningitis; Drug resistance; Endocarditis; Hospitals and infectious disease; Iatrogenic infections; Pathogens; Urinary tract infections; Vancomycin-resistant enterococci infection; Wound infections.

Enterovirus infections

CATEGORY: Diseases and conditions
ANATOMY OR SYSTEM AFFECTED: All
ALSO KNOWN AS: Enteroviral sepsis syndrome

DEFINITION

Enterovirus is a single-stranded RNA (ribonucleic acid) virus that belongs to the family Picornaviridae. The *Enterovirus* genus contains echoviruses, coxsackie A and B viruses, polioviruses, and the numbered enteroviruses. Enteroviruses are among the most common viruses causing disease symptoms in humans, although poliovirus has been eliminated in the United States. Approximately ten to fifteen million (nonpolio) enterovirus infections occur annually.

CAUSES

Enteroviruses are most commonly transmitted by the fecal-oral route or by the respiratory route. They also may be acquired during pregnancy through the placenta or during labor. Also, enteroviruses often are spread in hospitals because of improper handwashing or through contaminated equipment.

RISK FACTORS

Newborns, children, and immunocompromised persons are at greatest risk. Enterovirus infections may occur at any age, but the younger the person the greater the risk. Additional risk factors include prematurity, lower socioeconomic status, and poor sanitary living conditions. The majority of infections occur during the summer and fall seasons.

SYMPTOMS

Symptoms depend upon the type of enterovirus diagnosed. Common symptoms include a flulike fever, upper respiratory tract infection, and lethargy. Symptoms also include irritability, poor feeding, and a rash. More severe symptoms are inflammation of the liver (hepatitis), pancreas (pancreatitis), heart (myocarditis), and brain (encephalitis); these infections place a person at an increased risk for long-term complications, such as liver dysfunction, neurological deficits, and mortality (although these complications are rare). Enteroviruses may also predispose a person to diabetes.

SCREENING AND DIAGNOSIS

Testing is performed by sampling through a throat or rectal swab or stool sample, or through cerebrospinal fluid. The diagnosis is confirmed by isolating the virus in cell culture. Reverse transcriptase-polymerase chain reaction (RT-PCR) is also becoming a popular genetic technique, with the benefit of a shorter turnaround time. Prenatal diagnostic tests, such as amniocentesis, may be available for specific types of enteroviruses.

TREATMENT AND THERAPY

The majority of infected persons have mild symptoms that do not require treatment because the infection independently resolves within one week. Medical care is provided based on specific symptoms. Antiviral treatments, such as pleconaril, and immunoglobulin administration have shown benefit in some studies.

PREVENTION AND OUTCOMES

Poliovirus infections are very rare because of national immunization programs; the last reported case in the United States, related to the virus and not the vaccine, was in 1979. The spread of enteroviruses may be reduced through universal hygiene practices, including handwashing and avoiding contact with contaminated items.

Janet Ober Berman, M.S., CGC

FURTHER READING

Elfving, Maria, et al. "Maternal Enterovirus Infection During Pregnancy as a Risk Factor in Offspring Diagnosed with Type I Diabetes Between Fifteen and Thirty Years of Age." *Experimental Diabetes Research* 2008 (2008): 1-6.

Strauss, James, and Ellen Strauss. *Viruses and Human Disease.* 2d ed. Boston: Academic Press/Elsevier, 2008.

Tebruegge, Marc, and Nigel Curtis. "Enterovirus Infections in Neonates." *Seminars in Fetal and Neonatal Medicine* 14 (2009): 222-227.

Zaoutis, Theoklis, and Joel D. Klein. "Enterovirus Infections." *Pediatrics in Review* 19 (1998): 183-191.

WEB SITES OF INTEREST

American Academy of Family Physicians
http://familydoctor.org

American Academy of Pediatrics
http://www.healthychildren.org

Centers for Disease Control and Prevention
http://www.cdc.gov

See also: Antiviral drugs: Types; Childbirth and infectious disease; Children and infectious disease; Coxsackie virus infections; Echovirus infections; Encephalitis; Fecal-oral route of transmission; Hospitals and infectious disease; Iatrogenic infections; Picornaviridae; Picornavirus infections; Poliomyelitis; Pregnancy and infectious disease; Respiratory route of transmission; Viral infections; Viral meningitis.

Epidemic Intelligence Service

CATEGORY: Epidemiology

DEFINITION

The Epidemic Intelligence Service (EIS) is a U.S. government program that trains scientific professionals as public health investigators. The EIS is part of the Centers for Disease Control and Prevention (CDC).

CREATION AND PURPOSE

Cold War concerns regarding the potential of biological warfare motivated government scientists, including epidemiology expert Alexander Langmuir, to prepare effective medical defenses against epidemics infecting large populations. After World War II, Langmuir became chief epidemiologist at the Communicable Disease Center (now called the Centers for Disease Control and Prevention) in Atlanta. He emphasized surveillance techniques to evaluate the occurrence and distribution of diseases affecting groups. Seeking to train more epidemiologists to work for the CDC to document outbreaks, study pathogens, and reduce bioterrorism risks, Langmuir and colleagues created EIS in 1951.

Langmuir presented his goal for EIS in a March, 1952, article in the *American Journal of Public Health*, stressing the need for epidemiologists who can quickly respond to infectious disease crises. He reported that the initial EIS recruits began training in Atlanta in July, 1951, before conducting field work for the re-

mainder of a two-year commitment to EIS. Langmuir stated that EIS officers provided an essential epidemiological resource if the United States faced a biological attack. In peacetime, EIS personnel would aid in the comprehension of how infectious diseases are transmitted and how they can be prevented and controlled.

SELECTION AND TRAINING

EIS retained its basic structure into the early twenty-first century, adapting to incorporate scientific and medical developments and address evolving infectious diseases concerns. Initially, EIS sought applicants who were physicians. By the late twentieth century, EIS recognized the importance of an interdisciplinary approach to its work, encouraging applicants with expertise in pharmacology, biostatistics, nutritional sciences, and other fields that complement public health work. EIS expects applicants to have earned professional degrees in their specialties and to have secured relevant licenses. Because EIS investigations often occur in other countries, administrators consider qualified applicants from countries outside the United States who can gain a security clearance to access restricted information and laboratory materials.

Approximately seventy to ninety people are selected annually to join EIS. Several weeks of course work begin in Atlanta every year in July, in a program often compared with a hospital residency. Each EIS officer receives a position with health departments or CDC centers, such as the National Center for Emerging and Zoonotic Infectious Diseases, which focus on specific concerns. EIS officers perform various professional tasks, including writing scientific reports for the CDC's *Morbidity and Mortality Weekly Report* and attending the annual EIS conference, which is held each April.

EIS also offers a number of medical and veterinary medicine students the chance to participate in EIS epidemiology investigations for one to two months before they graduate from medical school. Some of those students are later selected for the main EIS program.

DISEASE RESPONSE

EIS officers respond to disease emergencies by traveling to infected areas, including disaster zones, immediately after learning of outbreaks. They collect specimens, interview patients, analyze causes and

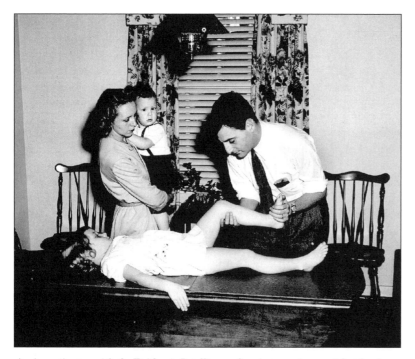

An investigator with the Epidemic Intelligence Service examines a girl at her home for signs of poliomyelitis, circa 1952. (CDC)

transmission of diseases, and immunize vulnerable or high-risk populations. EIS also sends representatives to areas affected by unidentified (and emerging) diseases.

Early EIS investigations frequently involved the diseases of histoplasmosis, rabies, and norovirus infection. EIS officers have also assisted in controlling diphtheria epidemics, in developing therapeutic oral hydration to treat cholera, and in identifying pathogens associated with Legionnaires' disease and acquired immune deficiency syndrome. They determined that West Nile virus is transmitted to humans by mosquitoes. EIS personnel also developed methods to counter lethal microbes, including Lassa, Ebola virus, and hantavirus. They have investigated SARS, H1N1 influenza, and the proliferation of antibiotic-resistant microbes that spread infectious diseases.

EIS officers were dispatched to New York City and Washington, D.C., after the September 11, 2001, terrorist attacks to survey sites around Ground Zero and the Pentagon for signs of biological warfare. EIS officers also investigated the distribution of anthrax spores through the U.S. mail. EIS officers now participate in bioterrorism exercises as part of their training to prepare as first responders in biological attacks.

IMPACT

By the early twenty-first century, the EIS had investigated more than ten thousand cases on six continents. A significant public health success attributed to EIS personnel includes eradicating smallpox.

Approximately three-fourths of the estimated three thousand EIS graduates have pursued public health work after they completed their EIS service, extending the reach and influence of EIS. As of 2010, almost one-half of state epidemiologists and forty percent of state health officials have received EIS training. Four EIS alumni have served as directors of the CDC. Former EIS officers also have been leaders in organizations such as the Infectious Diseases Society of America, the National Foundation for Infectious Diseases, and the World Health Organization.

EIS representatives have assisted other countries in establishing epidemiological services such as the Field Epidemiology Training Program (FETP) and the Field Epidemiology and Laboratory Training Program (FELTP). By 2010, FETP and FELTP had been established in twenty-nine countries, many in Asia and Africa. EIS alumni also helped create the European Programme for Intervention Epidemiology Training, a program that serves countries of the European Union.

Elizabeth D. Schafer, Ph.D.

FURTHER READING

Altman, Lawrence K. "An Elite Team of Sleuths, Saving Lives in Obscurity." *The New York Times*, April 6, 2010, D-5. An EIS alumnus comments on Langmuir's sometimes controversial actions as EIS director, actions such as not releasing complete information regarding flawed polio vaccines and controlling publicity concerning infectious diseases.

Koo, Denise, and Stephen B. Thacker. "In Snow's Footsteps: Commentary on Shoe-Leather and Applied Epidemiology." *American Journal of Epidemiology* 172, no. 6 (2010): 736-739. Distinguishes between applied and academic epidemiology, providing a table outlining differences in personnel, training, benefits, and other areas.

Koplan, Jeffrey P., and Stephen B. Thacker. "Fifty Years of Epidemiology at the Centers for Disease Control and Prevention: Significant and Consequential." *American Journal of Epidemiology* 154, no. 11 (2001): 982-984. A CDC director and an epidemiology program office leader identify U.S. and international public health precedents that inspired Langmuir, stressing how EIS constantly adjusts to improve its services.

McKenna, Maryn. *Beating Back the Devil: On the Front Lines with the Disease Detectives of the Epidemic Intelligence Service.* New York: Free Press, 2004. Atlanta-based journalist focuses on experiences of EIS officers from 2002 through 2003, preparing for bioterrorism and combating epidemics during wartime.

Pendergrast, Mark. *Inside the Outbreaks: The Elite Medical Detectives of the Epidemic Intelligence Service.* Boston: Houghton Mifflin Harcourt, 2010. Comprehensive chronological discussion of EIS, from the time of its founding into the early twenty-first century. Incorporates information from interviews with EIS and CDC personnel and from primary sources.

WEB SITES OF INTEREST

African Field Epidemiology Network
http://www.afenet.net

Epidemic Intelligence Service
http://www.cdc.gov/eis

European Programme for Intervention Epidemiology Training
http://www.epiet.org

Field Epidemiology Training Program
http://www.cdc.gov/globalhealth/fetp

Training Programs in Epidemiology and Public Health Interventions Network
http://www.tephinet.org

See also: Biosurveillance; Bioterrorism; Centers for Disease Control and Prevention (CDC); Developing countries and infectious disease; Disease eradication campaigns; Emerging and reemerging infectious diseases; Emerging Infections Network; Endemic infections; Epidemics and pandemics: Causes and management; Epidemiology; Infectious disease specialists; Koch's postulates; National Institute of Allergy and Infectious Diseases; National Institutes of Health; Outbreaks; Public health; Social effects of infectious disease; U.S. Army Medical Research Institute of Infectious Diseases; World Health Organization (WHO).

Epidemics and pandemics: Causes and management

CATEGORY: Epidemiology; Epidemics and pandemics: Causes and management

DEFINITIONS

An epidemic is a contagious, infectious, or viral disease affecting a disproportionate number of persons in a community, region, or population at the same time. A pandemic is a contagious, infectious, or viral disease occurring over a large geographical area or affecting a high proportion of a certain population.

Although both the terms "epidemic" and "pandemic" refer to a disease spreading through a population, a pandemic usually indicates either a larger geographical area or a higher number of people affected, or sometimes both. For example, a disease, such as influenza, may occur in a limited geographical area in many more people than would be expected. However, if the disease never spreads widely (perhaps only a few other cases appear nationwide), this situation would be an epidemic. However, if the disease spreads into a larger geographical area, for example, nationwide, with many more people contracting the disease than would be expected, this episode would then be termed a pandemic.

Another use of the term "pandemic" occurs when the disease affects an inordinate amount of people in a localized population. For example, in some areas of Africa, nearly 100 percent of the population is infected with the human immunodeficiency virus (HIV), making the situation a pandemic. Generally, a pandemic starts as an epidemic that, because of poor management, negligence, or ignorance, spreads into a larger area or affects a larger percentage of a population.

The application of the words "epidemic" and "pandemic" also depends on what is expected or what has been experienced in the past. For example, the common cold is a virus that is experienced worldwide; however, it is expected and it is known, from experience, that many people contract the virus that leads to the common cold. Even though the cold is a widespread illness, it is not a pandemic, or even an epidemic. However, hantavirus infection, being very rare and neither expected nor experienced by many, becomes epidemic when a few people do become infected.

The words "epidemic" and "pandemic" are often used in connection with a disease or condition, such as diabetes or obesity, that is not infectious. In their true scientific senses, epidemic and pandemic refer only to conditions that are contagious or transmittable from one person to another.

CAUSES

Disease epidemics have been recorded since at least the time of the pharaohs in ancient Egypt, and there are biblical references to plagues and diseases that spread rapidly and decimated human populations. Some of the most striking examples of past epidemics include the Black Death, or bubonic plague, which spread through Europe in the fourteenth century; the smallpox epidemic that affected Native Americans at first contact with Europeans in the New World; and the Spanish flu, a form of influenza that spread around the world in 1918, killing millions of people in just eighteen months.

Epidemics can be spread by many different means, including by an infectious carrier, contamination, mutation of an infectious agent, human behavior, and environmental change.

Infectious carrier. Sometimes animals carry disease that can spread rapidly through a population. For example, the bubonic plague, which killed an estimated 1 of every 4 people in Europe and 1 of every 2 people in Venice alone in 1347-1348, is thought to have been spread by rats carrying fleas infected with the disease. These fleas easily made the transition from being carried by rats to being carried by people, and through their bites, the fleas spread this disease. Other examples of vectors (organisms that carry disease) are the

ticks that carry Lyme disease.

It is also possible for a person to be a vector, to carry a disease without becoming or being infected. These carriers can infect others unknowingly. For example, in the early twentieth century case of Mary Mallon (also known as Typhoid Mary), who worked as a cook, Mallon infected more than forty people with typhoid fever. She was immune to typhoid, even though she carried the disease.

Contamination. Contamination of water or food can also be a source of epidemics, such as cholera, which is transmitted through contaminated water. Strange cases of outbreaks can be tied to contamination. For example, an outbreak of cases involving *Salmonella* bacteria in Minnesota in 1994 was traced back to a particular brand of ice cream. However, *Salmonella* can be found only in poultry and eggs. Because the ice cream contained neither, the outbreak was puzzling. Further investigation revealed that the ice cream was created with a mix that had been carried by trucks that had previously carried unpasteurized eggs. Another factor was inadequate cleaning, which had contaminated the ice cream mix.

Mutation of an infectious agent. Even when the infectious agent is known, as are the *Plasmodium* microbes that cause malaria, an agent's ability to quickly mutate to survive can foil attempts to prevent the spread of disease. These microbes reproduce so rapidly and change genetic material so often that it is difficult for malarial medicine to keep up with the changes. Another problem that continues the spread of malaria is that involving the mosquitos that carry the disease; they too can quickly mutate and thus survive the application of pesticides, making it difficult to control the population of the infected vectors.

Human behavior. Social and political issues also affect how disease is spread. For example, even though many studies have shown that the best way to prevent the spreading of disease is frequent handwashing, other studies show that people do not always comply with handwashing recommendations. Another example is the refusal by some parents to vaccinate their children against diseases, even though the benefits of vaccination far outweigh the risks. Also, sexual contact can transmit infectious diseases; some people refuse to practice safer sex, even though doing so has been proven to reduce sexually transmitted infections. Lack of education and access to medications are other issues that allow disease to spread.

Another factor in the spread of disease is the introduction of new diseases by nonindigenous populations. Early Native Americans had contact with settling Europeans, who had gained immunity to but still carried infectious agents, causing Native Americans, who had never been exposed to the smallpox virus and thus had no opportunity to develop immunity to it, to contract severe and oftentimes fatal infections from their first exposure. This type of disease transmission still occurs today. With more people traveling the globe, diseases are spread more quickly among populations; for example, severe acute respiratory syndrome (SARS) spread rapidly throughout the world in early 2003 because of the high number of international travelers who were infected.

Political issues also interfere with disease control. U.S. president Woodrow Wilson was roundly criticized for his policies during the influenza outbreak of 1918. Even though many people were dying from influenza, he refused to move resources focused on fighting in World War I to fighting the disease, thus possibly contributing to the spread of the disease and to many more deaths.

Environmental change. A short-term or long-term change in environmental conditions can contribute to the spread of a disease. An example of environmental change contributing to an epidemic is that of the hantavirus. This virus mysteriously appeared in Native Americans in the American Southwest in 1993, infecting three healthy people and rapidly killing them. The virus then spread through the population.

Through a series of investigations, epidemiologists discovered that after years of drought, a snowy winter and wet spring had led to an increase in pinion nuts in the area, which, in turn, led to an increase in mice that ate these nuts. The hantavirus can be carried in the feces and urine of these mice. Infection occurred when people cleaned up the mouse droppings, inhaled the virus that was in the contaminated dust, and then passed the virus to other humans. Because of the change in weather, the mice, who had always been in the area, increased in numbers. This led to greater contact with the human population.

Environmental change contributed to the spread of disease among the people of the Lyme, Connecticut, area. People began building homes farther into the woods, which led to more contact with deer that were native to the area. These deer carried ticks that, in turn, carried the bacterium *Borrelia burgdorferi.*

When the ticks began to leave their deer hosts and to infect humans with this bacterium, humans contracted what came to be called Lyme disease.

MANAGEMENT

Seventeenth century Dutch scientist Antoni van Leeuwenhoek first looked into his microscope and saw "little animals," thus inspiring scientists such as Robert Koch and Louis Pasteur to study and understand that microbes can cause diseases that can be transmitted from one person to another. Scientists still work at creating antibacterials, antivirals, and vaccines that will prevent people from getting or spreading disease.

However, even with all the medications that are available, there are other hurdles to overcome in managing diseases. Often, medications are too expensive, or, as in cases of war or other civil disruptions, medications do not get to those who need them. Also, a decline in sanitary conditions can lead to outbreaks of disease. Vaccination programs can fail to reach a critical mass of people to keep infectious diseases under control.

Public health agencies also have a role to play in managing disease. John Snow had been credited with the first public health action in managing the spread of disease after he investigated the London cholera outbreak in 1854. Cholera was raging through the city, and many still believed that disease was caused by bad air or humours. Snow, however, plotted the cholera outbreak by using a map to pinpoint the cases of the disease. He noticed that many of the people with the disease were getting water from the Thames River through a pump; the river, at the time, was severely polluted with human waste. Even though he made his findings public, some people refused to believe that the polluted water was causing their illnesses. The Reverend Harry Whitehead found Snow's evidence compelling and worked with Snow to convince city officials to remove the handle of the pump, rendering it unusable. This public health intervention led to a rapid decline in the cases of cholera in the area and to an overhaul and general cleanup of London water sources.

These types of outbreaks still occur, and public health officials resort to seemingly drastic measures to try to control the spread of disease. For example, during a cryptosporidium outbreak in 2007, public health officials in Utah intervened to ensure public safety by asking that children younger than age five years, persons wearing a diaper, and persons with diarrhea avoid using public swimming pools. Even after the outbreak subsided, small children were required to wear a swim diaper and plastic pants to help curb the disease.

IMPACT

Epidemics have raged through populations since the beginning of human existence, and the future will be no different. The ability of infectious agents to propagate and mutate far outstrips the human immune system's ability to adapt to and fight contagious diseases. However, fear and ignorance of how disease is transmitted have a huge societal and economic impact. For example, misunderstandings of how a particular disease is transmitted led to fear of touching persons with AIDS at the beginning of that pandemic. More recently, misunderstandings of how the H1N1 virus is transmitted led to the slaughter of pigs in certain countries. Neither of these actions impacted the infection rates of these diseases.

The keys to preventing epidemics and pandemics include understanding how a particular disease is transmitted and spread through a population; using public health pathways to provide and act upon scientifically proven information, both in controlling a disease and preventing it in the first place; and educating the public on good health practices, both socially and physically.

Marianne M. Madsen, M.S.

FURTHER READING

Baker, Robert. *Epidemic: The Past, Present, and Future of the Diseases that Made Us.* London: Vision, 2008. Discussion of human susceptibility to epidemic diseases. Includes information on how diseases have changed the human population around the world.

Barry, John M. *The Great Influenza: The Story of the Deadliest Pandemic in History.* New York: Penguin Books, 2005. A study of how biology met politics (the continuation of World War I at all costs) with deadly results for an overwhelming number of people in the United States.

DeSalle, Rob, ed. *Epidemic! The World of Infectious Disease.* New York: New Press, 2000. A companion to the American Museum of Natural History's exhibition on epidemics, methods of infection, pathogens, and means of transmission. Contains essays by experts, profiles of scientists, and case studies.

Giles-Vernick, Tamara, and Susan Craddock, eds. *Influenza and Public Health: Learning from Past Pandemics.* London: Earthscan, 2010. Discusses lessons learned from past flu pandemics about transmission patterns and successful (and not so successful) interventions.

Herring, Ann, and Alan C. Swedlund. *Plagues and Epidemics: Infected Spaces Past and Present.* New York: Berg, 2010. Addresses the growing realization that epidemics and pandemics are global problems that will remain a part of human life. Perspectives are from the sciences and from the social sciences, such as history and anthropology.

Johnson, Steven. *The Ghost Map: The Story of London's Most Terrifying Epidemic, and How It Changed Science, Cities, and the Modern World.* New York: Riverhead Books, 2007. A detailed view of London's cholera epidemic of 1854, with a focus on the Reverend Harry Whitehead and John Snow and the pioneering use of scientific methods to track the disease's origins.

McKenna, Maryn. *Beating Back the Devil: On the Front Lines with the Disease Detectives of the Epidemic Intelligence Service.* New York: Free Press, 2008. Explores the work of the Epidemic Intelligence Service, a division of the Centers for Disease Control and Prevention, with chapters devoted to different epidemic diseases.

Moore, Peter. *Little Book of Pandemics.* New York: Harper, 2008. Discusses major diseases with future pandemic possibilities, including those involving the Ebola virus and SARS. Includes maps of disease activity, statistics on infection and death rates, and drawings showing where the disease affects the human body.

Pendergrast, Mark. *Inside the Outbreaks: The Elite Medical Detectives of the Epidemic Intelligence Service.* Boston: Houghton Mifflin Harcourt, 2010. Case histories of disease told by Epidemic Intelligence Service officers and Centers for Disease Control and Prevention staff.

WEB SITES OF INTEREST

Centers for Disease Control and Prevention
http://www.cdc.gov

World Health Organization: Global Alert and Response
http://www.who.int/csr

See also: AIDS; Bacterial infections; Contagious diseases; Disease eradication campaigns; Emerging and reemerging infectious diseases; Endemic infections; Epidemics and pandemics: History; Epidemiology; Globalization and infectious disease; H1N1 influenza; HIV; Infectious disease specialists; Influenza; Koch's postulates; Mutation of pathogens; Outbreaks; Plague; Public health; SARS; Smallpox; Viral infections.

Epidemics and pandemics: History

CATEGORY: Epidemiology

DEFINITION

Although the definitions of the terms "epidemic" and "pandemic" remain inexact, authorities mostly agree that the difference between the two words is subtle and hinges on the geographical scale of the disease and the number of populations afflicted. Generally, an epidemic is a frequent, severe, and widespread outbreak of a specific disease, whereas a pandemic is a recurring epidemic that affects a very large area of the world.

EPIDEMICS BEFORE THE SEVENTEENTH CENTURY

Civilization's earliest written records periodically include accounts of devastating epidemics of unknown origin, epidemics that killed huge numbers of people and left behind disruption and despair. In 430 B.C.E., the city of Athens, Greece, was faced with a four-year epidemic known as the plague of Athens that appeared during the Peloponnesian War and reduced the Athenian population by 30 to 35 percent. Greek historian Thucydides, afflicted by a then-unknown disease, described its effects upon people, suggesting that it was not bubonic plague but, more likely, smallpox. Thought to have originated in Africa, smallpox was unknown to Athenians; consequently, Athens was likely a virgin-soil area.

Although by the fifth century B.C.E. in ancient Rome, malaria was endemic to certain low lying areas, reaching epidemic proportions during late summer and fall, no evidence suggests how it affected the population. However, a series of epidemics swept through the Roman Empire, one of the most deadly being the plague of the Antonines, which struck Rome in 166 C.E. and lasted about fifteen years. The famous Greco-Roman physician Galen, who lived during this time, recorded descriptions of those stricken that imply the disease was smallpox. Estimates of this disaster (from nineteenth and early twentieth century writings) insist that one-half the Roman Empire population died, but later research suggests a loss of 10 percent of the population.

In the eighth century, smallpox epidemics ravaged Japan, and attacks of leprosy (Hansen's disease) in Europe between 1000 and about 1350 led to the construction of institutions for isolating lepers. Thought by medieval Christians to be divine punishment for sin, and by physicians to reflect an imbalance in the four humours (blood, phlegm, yellow bile, and black bile) that are believed to inhabit the body, ideas about leprosy were influenced by medieval attitudes. People of the time believed that epidemics resulted from God's anger, especially the deadly epidemic known as French disease, or syphilis, which was spread through Europe by soldiers. Pustules appeared on infected bodies, which soon seemed to rot. Response to this disease included the first prepared and marketed remedy: mercuric ointment.

The encroachment of French disease into virgin-soil areas of Europe also was similar to the vast sixteenth century American epidemics originating with Spanish explorers and slaves who unwittingly spread microorganisms among the indigenous peoples (who had no previous exposure). Spreading from the Caribbean region to Mexico, in about 1520, smallpox took a huge toll on the Aztecs, on the peoples of Panama, and on the Incas in South America, therefore reducing the indigenous resistance to the Spanish conquerors. The later part of the century saw renewed outbreaks of smallpox, measles, and typhus.

EPIDEMICS: SEVENTEENTH TO TWENTY-FIRST CENTURIES

Few methods of disease exposure were more effective than war, particularly the Thirty Years' War, which involved vast numbers of people in a large area of central Europe. Most battles raged through the Germanic areas, with many areas losing one-half their populations between 1618 and 1648. This century's battles

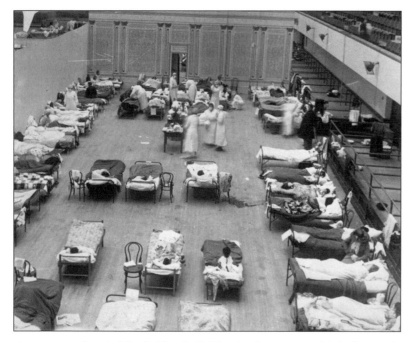

A temporary hospital in Oakland, California, for persons with influenza in 1918. The pandemic of 1918-1919 killed an estimated fifty million people worldwide. (Courtesy, Oakland Public library)

illustrated the interaction between war and epidemic disease that characterized armies in centuries to come. Wars carried diseases of influenza, typhus, and plague, yet, war's chaos prevented any response to the diseases.

Also in the seventeenth century, a sequence of disasters, including famines, floods, and epidemics that may have involved several different diseases (such as typhus, typhoid fever, malaria, dysentery, and bubonic and pneumatic plague), ravaged China between 1635 and 1644. Much conjecture pertains to the political implications of the losses of populations in certain areas and to whether the crop failures associated with disasters contributed to dietary deficiencies in a population more likely to succumb to disease.

In its devastation of huge areas of the world, smallpox attacked Iceland between 1707 and 1709, claiming the lives of one-quarter of the population. In 1721, Boston fell victim to a smallpox epidemic, leading to controversy between religion and science with regard to inoculation. The argument concerning inoculation continued during the eighteenth century smallpox rampage through European cities, with chil-

dren being the most susceptible to the disease.

A severe late-eighteenth century epidemic of yellow fever thwarted the efforts of British soldiers trying to take over Saint Domingue (now Haiti) and ultimately facilitated the island's bid for independence by its former slaves. Another yellow fever epidemic farther north afflicted Philadelphia and was possibly caused by fleeing Haitian refugees. As the capital of the new United States, Philadelphia's wresting with a deadly epidemic led to limitless political speculation. In 1853, yellow fever struck New Orleans, a site of frequent outbreaks, with its worst epidemic, leading to one-half of the recorded deaths in that city in 1853.

In 1916, the United States sustained the world's first major poliomyelitis epidemic, in the environs of New York City, striking mostly young children. Twenty-seven thousand Americans were afflicted by poliomyelitis and six thousand died from the disease. This epidemic initiated hysteria about poliomyelitis, whose numbers rose drastically between 1945 and 1955, and then declined spectacularly. In the 1980's, the number of diagnosed AIDS (acquired immunodeficiency syndrome) cases in the United States reached more than 160,000, soon declining significantly. Tuberculosis, sometimes connected with AIDS, is one of the most prevalent diseases in the world, as is malaria, whose death toll in the twentieth century varies between one and two million cases, most of these in Africa.

PANDEMICS: PLAGUE AND CHOLERA

The first plague pandemic began spreading from obscure origins in 540 B.C.E., moving through the Roman Empire into Asia in waves of disease for two hundred years. Although modern estimates of mortality vary widely, descriptions of those afflicted verify that the disease was bubonic plague. Thought to be sent by a vengeful God, the plague prompted changes in populations hitherto discussed only speculatively; however, recent archaeological discoveries have suggested more indirect answers.

The second plague pandemic began with the Black Death that originated in 1346 in southern Russia and spread, following trade routes, to the most densely populated areas in Europe, destroying more than one-third of its population by 1353. As the Black Death began to wane, other random but widespread outbreaks occurred in the next four hundred years, targeting Italian cities in the 1630's, London in 1665, Marseilles in 1721-1722, and Moscow in 1771; it remained in northern Africa until 1844. Before the second plague pandemic was extinguished in Asia, another disease site took hold in China that would expand into the third plague pandemic. This third plague pandemic continued in Asia and then into Africa and the United States in the twentieth century. An estimated thirteen million people perished in the third plague pandemic, with most deaths between 1894 and 1912.

All seven cholera pandemics that afflicted vast areas of the world began in Bengal, India, in the Ganges River delta, where cholera had long been endemic. The first pandemic began in Calcutta in 1817 and spread into Thailand, the Philippines, Asia, Japan, the Persian Gulf, Syria, and Persia; by 1823, it had spread to the Russian Empire. The second cholera pandemic spread from Bengal in 1827 into Russia and continued westward to, for the first time, Europe and North America in 1832. Americans were suspicious of the immigrant poor, while many Parisians believed the cholera pandemic was an elitist plot to rid Paris of the poor. In 1839, the third cholera pandemic began in paths that moved from Bengal to other parts of the world, some of which had never seen cholera. The disease reappeared in Europe and North America, spreading widely into areas of the Caribbean and South America, where a shocking number of deaths occurred in Brazil and in Latin America. These deaths initiated inquiries about the connection between cholera and race.

The fourth cholera pandemic, beginning in 1863, traveled around the world and convinced many that cholera moved with "human traffic." The fifth pandemic, beginning in 1881, extended across the Mediterranean to Italy, France, and Spain, then across the world to Argentina, Japan, and the Philippines. During this pandemic, Robert Koch, a German microbiologist, discovered a germ that is primarily in water (and in some food) and was responsible for cholera; but, as doubts and uncertainties reigned, positive response to his findings was slow in coming. The sixth cholera pandemic (1899) made less progress because of the growing insistence upon clean water supplies; and, the seventh cholera pandemic (1961), attacking Europe, Africa, Latin and Central America, and Mexico, left cholera endemic to some parts of the world.

PANDEMICS: INFLUENZA AND AIDS

In 1781-1782, a massive pandemic of influenza spread from Russia into Europe and afflicted an estimated three-fourths of the population of Europe. Despite its high morbidity rate (the number of ill persons), the mortality rate was relatively low, as the disease proved fatal mostly to the elderly. A second influenza pandemic (1889-1890), also beginning in Russia, extended worldwide by way of steamship and railroad travel. Morbidity was uncommonly high, calculated to be between one-third and one-half the world's population. Historian David Patterson has estimated that this pandemic killed between 270,000 and 360,000 people in Europe.

The third influenza pandemic (1918-1919) became the most extensive disease event in recorded history, with an estimated death toll of fifty million people. The pandemic traveled in three waves. The first one began in March of 1918 in Fort Riley, Kansas, and, following U.S. troops to battle in World War I, appeared in western Europe in April. It then moved to China, India, Australia, and Southeast Asia. The second wave of the influenza pandemic, experiencing a resurgence in France and crossing the Atlantic, entered Boston in October of 1918 and moved westward to the Pacific Coast. Mortality rates in the United States were estimated at 5.2 per 1,000 persons. Another surge of the second wave progressed from France, to the Mediterranean areas, and to Scandinavia, Great Britain, Germany, eastern Europe, and Russia. The second wave, far more lethal than the first, was especially harsh for young adults between the ages of eighteen and thirty-five years. Also, the populations in Asia, Africa, and India were at greater risk of death, suffering disastrous mortality rates that were twelve times greater than those of Europe and North America. The pandemic's third wave was milder than the second, raising the number of cases moderately as the disease was in decline.

After becoming known in the United States in 1981, AIDS began to spread worldwide within ten years, and by the end of the century, more than 25 million people had died in the pandemic. The region most affected by AIDS was Africa, with Zimbabwe, Zambia, and Malawi exceeding 500 cases per 100,000 persons. The number of persons in South Africa who are infected with the human immunodeficiency virus (HIV) reached 5.3 million by 2004. Since 2003, Asia has posted higher numbers of new infections than those of Africa, and India's 5.1 million HIV cases comes near to South Africa's total. In many African states, life expectancy has fallen below age forty years, as the disease strikes age groups between fifteen and forty-five years, and has increased the death rate of orphaned children. Also, the economic aspects are dire because the targeted age group is the most productive group of the African population.

IMPACT

Knowledge of major epidemics and pandemics from the beginning of recorded history provides insight into the beliefs and mind-sets peculiar to times that were unable to combat catastrophic diseases. With the gradual realization that epidemics demand responses from the medical community, world societies began to understand the need for clean water, antibiotics, vaccines, and quarantines. This knowledge also raises serious questions about the future of epidemics and pandemics from the standpoint of population shifts and growth, primarily in dense urban populations in warm climates, and about mass migration and the aging or younger populations who are especially at risk. Other serious considerations include the cost of public health measures, the effect of certain political imperatives, and the possibilities that those without money would be disregarded.

Mary Hurd, M.A.

FURTHER READING

Barry, John M. *The Great Influenza: The Story of the Deadliest Pandemic in History.* New York: Penguin Books, 2005. Riveting account of the influenza epidemic of 1918-1919, including Barry's indictment of the U.S. government's dishonesty in minimizing the dangers of the disease to keep the primary focus of the United States on World War I.

Behrman, Greg. *The Invisible People: How the U.S. Has Slept Through the Global AIDS Pandemic, the Greatest Humanitarian Catastrophe of Our Time.* New York: Free Press, 2004. Addresses the effect of the AIDS pandemic on social and economic conditions both in the United States and in other regions of the world.

Hays, Jo N. *Epidemics and Pandemics: Their Impacts on Human History.* Santa Barbara, Calif.: ABC-CLIO, 2005. A chronology of significant epidemics and pandemics throughout recorded history that includes backgrounds and unresolved issues.

Herring, Ann, and Alan C. Swedlund. *Plagues and Epidemics: Infected Spaces Past and Present.* New York: Berg, 2010. Addresses the growing realization that epidemics and pandemics are global problems that will remain a part of human life. Perspectives are from the sciences and from the social sciences, such as history and anthropology.

Oldstone, Michael B. A. *Viruses, Plagues, and History: Past, Present, and Future.* New York: Oxford University Press, 2010. This excellent book provides a detailed and fascinating account of historical epidemics and pandemics, including HIV/AIDS and West Nile virus. Each chapter deals with the history of an individual disease, its epidemiology, treatments, and the effect of the disease on human history.

Pendergrast, Mark. *Inside the Outbreaks: The Elite Medical Detectives of the Epidemic Intelligence Service.* Boston: Houghton Mifflin Harcourt, 2010. The story of the Epidemic Intelligence Service, founded in Atlanta in 1951 under the auspices of the Centers for Disease Control and Prevention to train disease "detectives" to address global epidemics.

Sherman, Irwin W. *Twelve Diseases That Changed Our World.* Washington, D.C.: ASM Press, 2007. A brief chronicle of one dozen diseases, not all of which infect humans but which greatly influenced human history. The author does provide useful sources in the chapter notes.

Shilts, Randy. *And The Band Played On: Politics, People, and the AIDS Epidemic.* Rev. ed. New York: St. Martin's Griffin, 2007. Detailed account of the first five years of the AIDS epidemic in the United States. Shilts is critical of the medical and scientific responses and the Ronald Reagan administration's dishonesty about the disease with the U.S. Congress.

Stine, Gerald J. *AIDS Update 2010.* New York: McGraw-Hill Higher Education, 2010. A thorough examination of the AIDS pandemic as it affected world populations in 2009-2010.

Trifonov, Vladimir, Hossein Khiabanian, and Raul

Rabadan. "Geographic Dependence, Surveillance, and Origins of the 2009 Influenza A (H1N1) Virus." *New England Journal of Medicine* 361 (2009): 115-119. This journal article discusses the various genetic origins of the 2009 H1N1 influenza virus.

Tucker, Jonathan B. *Scourge. The Once and Future Threat of Smallpox.* New York: Atlantic Monthly Press, 2001. A detailed account of the history of smallpox, the eradication of the disease from the earth, and the controversy surrounding whether or not the remaining smallpox stocks should be destroyed. The potential of smallpox as a biological weapon is also addressed.

WEB SITES OF INTEREST

AIDSgov
http://www.aids.gov

Centers for Disease Control and Prevention
http://www.cdc.gov

Emerging and Reemerging Infectious Diseases Resource Center
http://www.medscape.com/resource/infections

World Health Organization
http://www.who.int

See also: AIDS; Contagious diseases; Disease eradication campaigns; Emerging and reemerging infectious diseases; Endemic infections; Epidemics and pandemics: Causes and management; Epidemiology; Globalization and infectious disease; HIV; Infectious disease specialists; Influenza; Leprosy; Measles; Outbreaks; Plague; Public health; Quarantine; Smallpox; Typhus; Viral infections.

Epidemiology

CATEGORY: Epidemiology

DEFINITION

Epidemiology is the branch of medicine in which practitioners study the occurrence, causes, distribution, prevention, and control of diseases, illnesses, and injuries.

Epidemiologists follow and study disease distribu-

> **Key Terms: Epidemiology**
>
> - *Case-control study.* An epidemiological study that starts with identification of a group of cases with the disease of interest and a control group of persons without the disease; the association between risk factors and the disease is examined by comparing the two groups with regard to how frequently the risk factors are present in each group
>
> - *Cohort study.* An epidemiological study in which groups are identified by the status of exposure to risk factors of the disease of interest; the occurrences of the disease are observed during a follow-up and compared between different groups
>
> - *Cross-sectional study.* An epidemiological study that describes disease distribution or frequency by person, place, and time to identify a population at risk
>
> - *Epidemiological triangle model.* A model used to explain the interrelationship between agent, host, and environment, the three essential factors in the development of disease
>
> - *Population at risk.* A group of people who have an increased risk for a particular disease
>
> - *Public health.* The effort to protect, promote, and restore human health through programs that emphasize the prevention of diseases
>
> - *Risk factor.* An aspect of behaviors, lifestyle, environmental exposure, or heredity that is known to be associated with a particular disease

tion in particular groups rather than focus on one person and his or her disease. They study both epidemic (an outbreak that is above and beyond what is expected) and endemic (common and prevalent) diseases. The idea behind the epidemiological study of disease is that, most often, disease does not spread randomly; personal, social, and environmental characteristics affect the disease, its pattern of spreading, and who is likely to become infected.

Using field investigations, laboratory studies, and statistical and mathematical analyses, epidemiologists use data on a disease to identify the cause of the disease, determine who is at risk for the disease, ascertain where the disease is likely to occur, track how it changes over time, take measures to prevent or arrest the spread of the disease, and plan new types of public health services and interventions to control or eliminate the disease. They use sophisticated computer programming, mathematical modeling, and statistical analysis to determine how many cases of the disease could be avoided by preventive measures and uncover where the disease is likely to spread.

TYPES

There are two basic types of epidemiological practice that focus on different aspects of disease and its spread. Descriptive epidemiology examines a certain population, such as those of a particular age, gender, ethnic group, or occupation, to determine how this group as a whole is affected by a disorder and whether the disease is associated with certain risk factors. Public records (such as death certificates, school or police records, or population censuses) or specially designed tools (such as disease registries and surveys) are used to study the mortality rate (number of deaths in an at-risk population), incidence (number of new cases per year), and prevalence (number of currently existing cases) of a disease. Descriptive epidemiologists also follow changes in the disease or its infection or mortality rate over time in these particular groups, help predict the disease's spread to other groups with similar risk factors, and provide information for analytic epidemiologists, who develop and execute studies.

Analytic epidemiology focuses on further studies to test the findings from case studies, surveys, or laboratory observations. These studies help determine what specific factors increase or decrease the risk and spread of disease and attempt to quantify these risks. The studies may be observational, in which only a subject's behavior is observed (no attempt is made to change the behavior), or experimental, in which the epidemiologist looks at two groups, one with no change in behavior (a control group) and another group (an experimental group) whose members are asked to change their behavior to determine if that behavior has an effect on contracting or spreading the disease in question.

A cohort study is another type of analytical study in which epidemiologists analyze a defined population whose members are known or suspected to have risk factors at various levels for a particular condition. Epidemiologists then record the death and infection rates among these group members to see which of these people are truly at increased risk for the disease and to determine what factors seem to protect them

from or to help them avoid the disease. These types of studies must include many people who are usually studied over time. These studies, therefore, are expensive and labor intensive.

An example of a cohort study is the Framingham study, in which residents of Framingham, Massachusetts, have been the subjects of studies regarding heart disease risk factors since 1948, and have lent their name to an identified group of risk factors called the Framingham factors. Another cohort study is the Nurses' Health Study. Begun in 1976 and expanded in 1989, 238,000 nurses participate in this epidemiological study to determine what risk factors lead to particular diseases and to discover what social and behavioral factors lead to better health. The National Children's Study is a nationwide epidemiological study that, over time, will enroll 100,000 children to study the affect of environmental, biological, genetic, and psychosocial factors on humans from before a person's birth through the age of twenty-one years. The study seeks to determine which of these factors affect the health and well-being of children.

HISTORY

The history of epidemiology began informally with the curiosity about and the observation of the transmission of contagious diseases. At the beginning of human history, plagues and diseases appeared to have no logic. These tragedies were thought to be the wrath of gods, the doings of evil spirits, or emanations from the body itself. In ancient times, however, humans began to question how disease was transmitted. Around 400 B.C.E., Hippocrates described epidemics and listed some social, behavioral, and environmental factors that he thought may be associated with certain types of disease. Although ancient thinkers and healers did not fully understand the role of microorganisms in the transmission of disease, the concept of contagious disease was being formed. By the early sixteenth century, Fracastorius had identified what is now commonly known: that disease can be spread through recognizable paths, such as direct contact, through the air, or even by contacting contaminated objects.

One of the first public health studies was performed by John Snow, who tracked the transmission of cholera during a London epidemic by creating a map showing all cases of the disease. His map led him to realize that many of the sick were getting water from the same source, a pump close to the Thames River, which at that time was extremely polluted. Even though Snow showed others his findings, including people who lived in the area and who were likely to get the disease from the contaminated water from the pump, the pump was still used by people who did not want to travel far to get water. Snow, and others who believed his work, convinced London officials to remove the handle from the pump, making it unusable and forcing people to get water elsewhere. The spread of the disease was reduced considerably.

This type of mapping has been used throughout the history of epidemiological study to show the spread of other diseases, such as tuberculosis and measles. Careful scrutiny of disease maps can lead to connections that may not otherwise be seen. For example, a lethal type of pneumonia struck a far-flung group of men, seemingly randomly, in 1976. The Epidemic Intelligence Service (EIS) officers of the U.S. Centers for Disease Control and Prevention, through careful mapping and meticulous tracking of the men's behaviors before they became ill, discovered that the men had attended a conference of the American Legion in Philadelphia and had returned home before falling ill. Because of the painstaking work of the EIS, the source of the disease was discovered to be a bacterium that had spread through a heating and air conditioning system.

Past epidemiological studies have also focused on the link between chronic diseases and activities that seemingly have no connection. For example, one early study showed that there was some type of statistically significant link between those who worked as chimney sweeps and those who developed cancer of the scrotum. Another early study, dietary experiments with sailors, showed that those who ate fresh fruit on a voyage were statistically less likely to get scurvy than those who refused to eat fresh fruit. Modern epidemiology has shown how certain factors lead to chronic diseases too. These disease factors include smoking (linked to heart disease and cancer) and certain sexual practices, which are linked to human immunodeficiency virus (HIV) infection and acquired immunodeficiency syndrome (AIDS). Epidemiologists also study the effects of treatments or preventive measures on disease spread. For example, they found that mammography reduces mortality from breast cancer and that a reduction in cholesterol intake can reduce the risk of heart disease.

Epidemiologists use statistical modeling each year to determine what types of influenza are likely to be spread throughout a population. This helps public health officials determine who should be vaccinated and which types of vaccine the flu shot should contain for that year. In the case of outbreaks of diseases such as the seasonal flu, mathematical modeling can help determine public health actions, such as where and when schools should be closed to prevent the flu from spreading.

The rise of supercomputers, which can perform even more complicated statistical analyses, and the development of even more complex methodological approaches, have led to increased relevancy and applicability of epidemiological findings. Molecular biology has added an even more interesting dimension, the use of deoxyribonucleic acid (DNA) typing and biomarkers, to disease tracking and monitoring, which allows epidemiologists to trace the passage of a particular strain of infectious agent. This work is called molecular epidemiology. For example, it is now possible to track the exact strain of gonorrhea from person to person as it is transmitted through direct contact and to conclude with a great deal of certainty what persons have the same strain and thus are likely to have contracted it through the same source. Also, through the genetic identification of the particular strain of tuberculosis that an infected person has, it can be proven that the infected person transmitted the strain to others through coughing in a crowded place.

Genetic epidemiology raises questions at a new level. Moral issues arise when molecular genetics intersects with public, occupational, and environmental health issues. For example, should someone with a genetic disposition toward lung cancer be allowed to work in industries known to raise the risk of lung cancer? If this person knowingly chooses to do so, should he or she be made to cover any and all expenses associated with the costs of any lung cancer treatment?

IMPACT

Epidemiologists use studies to identify personal, environmental, and social factors that increase the risk of disease. The study of epidemiology leads to improvements in disease prevention and determines what vaccines and other public health measures will minimize the spread of disease. These scientists provide facts that lead to risk assessments and provide impetus to change public health policies. By educating the public with evidence-based specifics about disease, they help prevent the spread of disease.

Evidence-based medicine is the practice of medicine statistically based on the best patient outcomes determined by close attention to the nature and quality of evidence on which clinical decisions are made. Epidemiologists help provide this evidence and use best practices in making decisions about public health.

Epidemiology involves many different types of doctors and scientists who work together to identify, control, and prevent disease and put these findings into practice in the public health sector. Epidemiologists come from fields such as biomedical informatics, biostatistics, chemistry, computer programming, genetics, immunology, microbiology, and statistics. They work in and influence many fields, including agricultural science, population and family studies, social and behavioral sciences, and wildlife biology, engineering, law enforcement, and town planning.

The connection between disease and infection makes it necessary for epidemiologists to have a broad knowledge of microorganisms and how they spread. This knowledge of microorganisms includes how they can be used for biological attack, especially an attack on a civilian population, and includes methods such as DNA analysis of biological weapons. This analysis could help determine where an infectious agent originated and how it might spread.

Marianne M. Madsen, M.S.

Further Reading

Dworkin, Mark S., ed. *Outbreak Investigations Around the World: Case Studies in Infectious Disease Field Epidemiology.* Sudbury, Mass.: Jones and Bartlett, 2010. Includes the introductory chapter "How an Outbreak Is Investigated" and several case studies of infectious disease outbreaks worldwide, as told by investigators who tracked disease origins.

Fletcher, Robert H., and Suzanne W. Fletcher. *Clinical Epidemiology: The Essentials.* 4th ed. Baltimore: Lippincott Williams & Wilkins, 2005. Provides students and clinicians with the basic principles and concepts of clinical epidemiology. Discusses system development of outcomes assessment and the application of this knowledge to improve patient care. Includes illustrations and examples.

Friis, Robert, and Thomas Sellers. *Epidemiology for Public Health Practice.* Sudbury, Mass.: Jones and Bartlett, 2008. Includes comprehensive coverage of major topics, such as study designs, terminology, and quantitative analysis.

Gerstman, B. Burt. *Epidemiology Kept Simple: An Introduction to Classic and Modern Epidemiology.* 2d ed. Hoboken, N.J.: Wiley-Liss, 2003. An introduction to major areas of epidemiology. Includes the chapters "Epidemiology Past and Present" and "Causal Concepts."

Gordis, Leon. *Epidemiology.* Philadelphia: Saunders/ Elsevier, 2008. A readable textbook that includes many examples and illustrations of epidemiological practice.

Merrill, Ray M. *Introduction to Epidemiology.* Sudbury, Mass.: Jones and Bartlett, 2010. Includes tables, figures, case studies, and examples. Designed for those with limited training in the biomedical sciences and in statistics.

Rothman, Kenneth J. *Epidemiology: An Introduction.* New York: Oxford University Press, 2002. Discusses causal thinking, causal inference, confounding factors, chance, and interactions.

Rothman, Kenneth J., Sander Greenland, and Timothy Lash. *Modern Epidemiology.* Philadelphia: Lippincott Williams & Wilkins, 2008. Covers conceptual development and role of epidemiology in public health issues. Includes discussion of a broad range of concepts, such as basic measures of disease frequency, Bayesian analysis, and hierarchical regression, and discusses specific research areas, such as infectious disease and genetic, molecular, and clinical epidemiology.

Susser, Mervyn, and Zena Stein. *Eras in Epidemiology: The Evolution of Ideas.* New York: Oxford University Press, 2009. Shows the evolution of epidemiology from the early concepts of magic and humours through observational methods and systematic counts through the dawn of national public health systems.

Szklo, Moyses, and F. Javier Nieto. *Epidemiology: Beyond the Basics.* 2d ed. Sudbury, Mass.: Jones and Bartlett, 2007. A detailed discussion of key epidemiological principles, such as study design and research association. Includes examples and exercises with discussion of Rothman's causality model, sensitivity analysis, and meta-analysis.

WEB SITES OF INTEREST

American Public Health Association
http://www.apha.org

Association for Professionals in Infection Control and Epidemiology
http://www.knowledgeisinfectious.org

Centers for Disease Control and Prevention
http://www.cdc.gov

Pan American Health Organization
http://new.paho.org

Society for Healthcare Epidemiology of America
http://www.shea-online.org

World Health Organization
http://www.who.int

See also: Bacterial infections; Centers for Disease Control and Prevention (CDC); Contagious diseases; Disease eradication campaigns; Emerging and re-emerging infectious diseases; Endemic infections; Epidemics and pandemics: Causes and management; Epidemics and pandemics: History; Globalization and infectious disease; Infectious disease specialists; Koch's postulates; National Institutes of Health; Outbreaks; Plague; Public health; Quarantine; Viral infections.

Epidermophyton

CATEGORY: Pathogen
TRANSMISSION ROUTE: Direct contact

DEFINITION

Epidermophyton is a genus of filamentous fungi (molds). One species, *floccosum*, is a primary cause of human infections of the outer layer of the skin and the beds of the nails.

NATURAL HABITAT AND FEATURES

Both species of *Epidermophyton* are distributed worldwide. *Floccosum* is anthropohilic, meaning its natural habitat is the human body. *Stockdaleae* is geophilic, meaning its natural habitat is the soil. *Floccosum*, but not *stockdaleae*, causes human infection.

Taxonomic Classification for *Epidermophyton*

Kingdom: Fungi
Phylum: Ascomycota
Class: Onygenales
Family: Arthrodermataceae
Genus: *Epidermophyton*
Species:
E. floccosum
E. stockdaleae

Transmission of infection can be by direct human-to-human contact, from objects that came into direct contact with infected persons or from self-inoculation. Human-to-human transmission occurs most frequently within families or among children in day care or school settings. Infected inanimate objects (fomites) that can contribute to transmission include wet floors in gyms or locker rooms, shared towels, and contaminated tools in barber shops and hair and nail salons. Self-inoculation occurs when a person first touches an infected area of the body, then touches a noninfected, vulnerable area elsewhere on the body.

Colonies of *Epidermophyton* incubated on Sabouraud's dextrose agar at 77° to 86° Fahrenheit (25-30° Celsius) mature within seven to fourteen days. From the front, the colonies appear greenish-brown or khaki. The suedelike surface is raised and folded in the center and is otherwise flat, with a submerged fringe of growth at the outermost edges. From the reverse, the colonies usually are deep yellowish-brown.

Microscopic examination of colonies of *Epidermophyton* reveals septate, hyaline hyphae (partitioned and transparent tubelike filaments). Smooth, thin-walled, fusiform (spindle-shaped) macroconidia (large multicelled spores) are seen singly or in clusters growing directly from hyphae. The macroconidia of *floccosum* are shorter than those of *stockdaleae*. Microconidia (small one-celled spores) are typically not observed in *Epidermophyton* species. This absence differentiates *Epidermophyton* from *Microsporum* and *Trichophyton*, the two other genera of fungi responsible for dermatophytosis (infections of the outer layer of the skin, nails, and hair). In older lab cultures, chlamydoconidia (round thick-walled spores) and arthroconidia (jointed spores) are observed.

PATHOGENICITY AND CLINICAL SIGNIFICANCE

Floccosum, along with species of *Microsporum* and *Trichophyton*, is among the most common causes of superficial fungal infections of the skin and nails in otherwise healthy persons. Unlike *Microsporum* and *Trichophyton* species, however, it is not implicated in causing infections of the hair. *Floccosum* is highly adapted to the nonliving outer layer of the skin (the stratum corneum) and to nail beds.

Infection develops when fungi penetrate minor lesions, such as paper cuts and blisters, of the surface layer of the skin. The infection spreads sideways, with sharp, advancing margins. It remains limited to the nonliving outer layer of skin because *floccosum* cannot penetrate living tissue. *Floccosum* is a common cause of tinea corporis (ringworm of the body), tinea cruris or jock itch (ringworm of the groin), tinea manuum (ringworm of the hands), tinea pedis (athlete's foot), and tinea unguium or onychomycosis (ringworm of the nail). All the infections caused by *floccosum* are found worldwide, although tinea corporis is more common in tropical and subtropical regions.

Many infections caused by *floccosum* are asymptomatic and, even when symptomatic, are self-limiting and resolve spontaneously. Such infections do not require medical treatment. For most persons who require treatment, a topical agent (cream, ointment, or solution) is sufficient. Some infections, especially in immunocompromised persons, may require more aggressive treatment with oral agents alone or in combination with topical agents.

DRUG SUSCEPTIBILITY

Susceptibility methods for testing agents used to treat dermatophytosis caused by *floccosum* in infected persons (in vivo) have not been standardized. Limited testing and comparisons have shown that specific newer agents have lower minimum inhibitory concentrations (MICs) than do earlier agents, such as griseofulvin, amphotericin B, and fluconazole (formerly the drugs of choice). These newer agents also carry a lower risk of side effects.

Fluconazole, the first azole, has been replaced by newer, broad-spectrum azoles with much lower MICs. These include clotrimazole, econazole, imidazole, miconazole, and sulconazole, all of which are available as topical agents. Along with topical formulations of the allylamine drugs naftifine and terbinafine, these are the drugs of choice in otherwise healthy persons with infections caused by *floccosum*.

For persons with spreading, persistent, or recurring infections, oral drugs may be required in addition to or in place of topical agents. Oral terbinafine, which has an especially low MIC, is the drug of choice in these cases. Oral formulations of azoles, including itraconazole, ketoconazole, and voriconazole, may also be used. All these drugs are more effective and convenient than griseofulvin and do not have the risks associated with the use of griseofulvin. However, griseofulvin may be required for treating extensive infections of the nail beds.

Ernest Kohlmetz, M.A.

FURTHER READING

Richardson, Malcolm D., and David W. Warnock. *Fungal Infection: Diagnosis and Management*. New ed. Malden, Mass.: Wiley-Blackwell, 2010. Chapter 4 on dermatophytosis contains substantial information about *Epidermophyton*.

Ryan, Kenneth J., and C. George Ray, eds. *Sherris Medical Microbiology: An Introduction to Infectious Diseases*. 5th ed. New York: McGraw-Hill, 2010. A first text in microbiology for students in medicine and medical science, with a focus on infectious diseases. Chapter 44 covers dermatophytes, including *Epidermophyton*.

White, Gary M., and Neil H. Cox. *Diseases of the Skin: A Color Atlas and Text*. 2d ed. Philadelphia: Mosby/Elsevier, 2006. Chapter 26 provides an overview of fungal infections. Chapter 29 covers disorders of the nails. Includes full-color illustrations.

WEB SITES OF INTEREST

Centers for Disease Control and Prevention, Division of Foodborne, Bacterial, and Mycotic Diseases
http://www.cdc.gov/nczved/divisions/dfbmd

Microbiology and Immunology On-line: Mycology
http://pathmicro.med.sc.edu/book/mycol-sta.htm

See also: Antifungal drugs: Types; Athlete's foot; Chromoblastomycosis; Dermatomycosis; Dermatophytosis; Diagnosis of fungal infections; Fungi: Classification and types; Jock itch; *Malassezia*; *Microsporum*; Mold infections; Mycoses; Onychomycosis; Ringworm; Skin infections; *Trichophyton*.

Epididymitis

CATEGORY: Diseases and conditions
ANATOMY OR SYSTEM AFFECTED: Genitalia, reproductive system, skin
ALSO KNOWN AS: Epididymo-orchitis

DEFINITION

Acute epididymitis is an inflammation of the epididymis. This is a structure shaped like a tube that surrounds and attaches to each testicle. The epididymis helps transport and store sperm cells.

Chronic epididymitis causes pain and inflammation in the epididymis. There is often no swelling of the scrotum. Symptoms can last six weeks or more, but this type is less common.

CAUSES

Epididymitis is most often caused by bacterial infections such as those of the urinary tract, by sexually transmitted diseases (STDs) such as chlamydia and gonorrhea, by infection of the urethra (urethritis), by infection of the prostate (prostatitis), and by tuberculosis. Other causes include injury, viral infections such as mumps, genital abnormalities, treatment with the heart rhythm drug amiodarone (cordarone), and chemotherapy to treat bladder cancer.

RISK FACTORS

Risk factors for epididymitis include infection of the genitourinary tract (bladder, kidney, prostate, or testicle), narrowing of the urethra, use of a urethral catheter, infrequent emptying of the bladder, recent surgery or instrumentation of the genitourinary tract (especially prostate removal), birth disorders of the genitourinary tract, unprotected sex, and disease that affects the immune system. Most at risk are boys and men ages fifteen to thirty years and men older than age sixty years.

SYMPTOMS

Symptoms usually develop within a day and include pain in the testes; sudden redness or swelling of the scrotum; hardness, a lump, or soreness (or all three) in the affected testicle; tenderness in the nonaffected testicle; groin pain; chills; fever; inflammation of the urethra; pain during intercourse or ejaculation; pain or burning, or both, during urination; increased pain while having a bowel movement; lower abdominal discomfort; discharge from the penis; and blood in the semen.

SCREENING AND DIAGNOSIS

A doctor will ask about symptoms and medical history and will perform a physical exam. Tests may include a urinalysis to check for a high white blood cell (WBC) count and the presence of bacteria; a urine culture to identify the type of bacteria present; a culture of discharge from the penis; a blood test to measure the white blood cell count (WBC); and an ultrasound (a test that uses sound waves to examine the scrotum).

TREATMENT AND THERAPY

Treatment is essential to prevent the infection from worsening. Treatment may include bed rest. The patient should stay in bed to keep the testicles from moving and to promote healing. Bed rest might be necessary until the swelling subsides. Another treatment is antibiotics, prescribed for bacterial infections. If the patient has an STD, his partners will also need treatment. Another treatment is oral anti-inflammatory medication, which includes drugs such as ibuprofen, to help reduce swelling.

The patient may need to wear an athletic supporter for several weeks. Taking baths can ease the pain and help relieve swelling. One should not have sex until treatment is completed. Finally, surgery may be needed in severe cases that return.

PREVENTION AND OUTCOMES

To help decrease the risk of developing epididymitis, one should practice safer sex. One can protect against STDs by using condoms. Finally, one should empty one's bladder when feeling the need to do so.

Michelle Badash, M.S.;
reviewed by Adrienne Carmack, M.D.

FURTHER READING

Centers for Disease Control and Prevention. "Sexually Transmitted Diseases Treatment Guidelines 2010." Available at http://www.cdc.gov/std/treatment/2010.

Lunenfeld, Bruno, and Louis Gooren, eds. *Textbook of Men's Health.* Boca Raton, Fla.: Parthenon, 2007.

National Institutes of Health. "Men's Health." Available at http://health.nih.gov/category/menshealth.

Schrier, Robert W., ed. *Diseases of the Kidney and Urinary*

Tract. 8th ed. Philadelphia: Wolters Kluwer Health/ Lippincott Williams & Wilkins, 2007.

Simon, Harvey B. *The Harvard Medical School Guide to Men's Health.* New York: Free Press, 2004.

WEB SITES OF INTEREST

Canadian Health Network
http://www.canadian-health-network.ca

National Institute of Diabetes and Digestive and Kidney Diseases
http://www.niddk.nih.gov

National Kidney Foundation
http://www.kidney.org

UrologyHealth.org
http://www.urologyhealth.org

See also: Bacterial infections; Chlamydia; *Chlamydia*; Gonorrhea; Inflammation; Men and infectious disease; Mumps; Prostatitis; Sexually transmitted diseases (STDs); Urethritis; Urinary tract infections.

Epiglottitis

CATEGORY: Diseases and conditions
ANATOMY OR SYSTEM AFFECTED: Lungs, pharynx, respiratory system, throat, tissue

DEFINITION

Epiglottitis is the severe swelling of the epiglottis, a flaplike, cartilage structure located in the throat. During swallowing, the epiglottis folds over the trachea (windpipe) and vocal cords to prevent food and liquids from entering the lungs. Swelling can quickly seal off a person's airway, making it difficult to breathe.

Epiglottitis is rare and requires immediate medical attention, as it can quickly turn deadly. Persons who believe they have epiglottitis should seek emergency care.

CAUSES

Factors that can cause epiglottitis include bacteria, viruses, and fungi. Bacteria include *Haemophilus influenzae* type B (Hib), which is the most common cause

(in adults) and the cause of the most deadly type of epiglottitis (but it is not the same germ that causes the flu); *Streptococcus pneumoniae* (also the cause of meningitis); *Streptococcus* A, B, and C (also the cause of strep throat and blood infections); *Candida albicans* (also the cause of yeast infections, diaper rash, and oral thrush; and varicella zoster (also the cause of chickenpox and shingles). Other factors include burns from hot liquids and other physical injuries to the throat area and the use of crack cocaine. In the past, Hib most frequently caused epiglottitis in children. However, because vaccination against this virus was started in children, it is now more prevalent among adults.

RISK FACTORS

Epiglottitis is a contagious disease. It is passed much like the common cold: through droplets released when sneezing and coughing. Anyone can develop epiglottitis; however, the following persons are at higher risk: children, ages three to seven years, who live in countries that do not offer vaccines; infants too young to receive vaccination (younger than two months of age); and, rarely, adults in their forties. Boys and men are more prone to the disease, and the disease is more common among African Americans and Hispanics. Other risk factors are living in close quarters, attending day care or school, working in an office, and wintertime.

SYMPTOMS

Persons experiencing any of the following symptoms should not assume they are caused by epiglottitis. These symptoms may be caused by other, less serious health conditions: cough, high fever (more than 103° Fahrenheit), sore throat and severe throat pain, difficulty swallowing, drooling, and muffled voice. Other symptoms are rapid breathing; increasingly difficult breathing; leaning forward and arching the neck backward to breathe; stridor (squeaky or raspy sounds while inhaling, caused by airway blockage); and symptoms associated with low oxygen levels, including cyanosis (bluish tint to skin or lips), sluggishness, confusion, and irritability. Symptoms will appear suddenly and worsen quickly.

One should not attempt to use a tongue depressor or any other utensil to look into the affected person's throat. A throat spasm could occur and cause the airway to close completely.

SCREENING AND DIAGNOSIS

Emergency care will determine, first, if the patient can breathe. Once this is affirmed, the doctor will begin a physical examination by asking about symptoms and medical history. If the patient is not having trouble breathing, the doctor may use a mirror to look down the patient's throat. Usually, initial diagnosis and testing are based on the reported symptoms. Tests include a neck X ray (a test that uses radiation to take a picture of the neck, so the doctor can check for a swollen epiglottis); a blood culture to screen for bacteria; a blood count to document the presence of a bacterial infection; a nasolaryngoscopy (a tiny, lighted tube inserted through the nose to look at structures such as the epiglottitis); and a throat culture, in which a cotton swab is used to collect cells from the infected tissue. The cells are plated on a nutrient-rich medium and are left to grow. The cells are then identified, and the results are given to the doctor.

TREATMENT AND THERAPY

The doctor will first stabilize the patient's airway and then give proper medication depending on the cause. The patient may also have secondary illnesses that need to be treated, depending on the cause of the epiglottitis (for example, blood infections caused by *Streptococcus*).

If the patient can breathe, he or she will be closely monitored in an intensive care unit. If the patient cannot breathe, the options include endotracheal intubation, in which a breathing tube is inserted through the nose or mouth and fed into the airway. This can be done only if the airway is not swollen shut. Another option is tracheotomy, in which a breathing tube is inserted directly into the trachea. This is done if the airway is swollen shut, or if the airway is too swollen to do an endotracheal intubation.

After the airway is stabilized, the patient will be monitored and started on medications, including antibiotics. Antibiotics that are given through the veins help kill the organism causing the infection and swelling. Initially, a variety of antibiotics may be given if the identity of the germ is not yet known. Once the laboratory test results are known, the doctor may prescribe a specific antibiotic. Once swelling decreases, the breathing tube can be removed. Most often, there are no lasting side effects of epiglottitis, and the outlook for the patient is good.

PREVENTION AND OUTCOMES

Vaccination is the only way to prevent epiglottitis. There are three different vaccines that can be given (HbOC, PRP-OMP, and PRP-T). Infants born in the United States are given one of these three vaccines at two months of age. Since vaccination began, adults have been at even lower risk of developing epiglottitis. However, if a person is immune compromised or on medications that may make him or her more susceptible to illness, the doctor should be consulted about vaccination. An antibiotic (such as rifampin) may be prescribed for postexposure coverage for household members and others who have spent time in the previous five out of seven days with an affected individual; the antibiotic is also available for day-care staff.

Jen Rymaruk;
reviewed by Elie Edmond Rebeiz, M.D., FACS

FURTHER READING

EBSCO Publishing. *DynaMed: Acute Epiglottitis.* Available through http://www.ebscohost.com/dynamed.

Ferrari, Mario. *PDxMD Ear, Nose, and Throat Disorders.* Philadelphia: PDxMD, 2003.

Levitzky, Michael G. *Pulmonary Physiology.* 7th ed. New York: McGraw-Hill Medical, 2007.

PM Medical Health News. *Twenty-first Century Complete Medical Guide to Throat and Pharynx Disorders: Authoritative Government Documents, Clinical References, and Practical Information for Patients and Physicians.* Mount Laurel, N.J.: Progressive Management, 2004.

Sack, J. L., and C. D. Brock. "Identifying Acute Epiglottitis in Adults." *Postgraduate Medicine* 112, no. 1 (2002).

World Health Organization. "Epiglottitis." Available at http://www.who.int.

WEB SITES OF INTEREST

American College of Emergency Physicians
http://www.acep.org

Centers for Disease Control and Prevention
http://www.cdc.gov

See also: Airborne illness and disease; Bacterial infections; Bronchiolitis; Bronchitis; *Candida*; Contagious diseases; Diphtheria; *Haemophilus influenzae* infection; Laryngitis; Mononucleosis; Nasopharyngeal infections; Pharyngitis and tonsillopharyngitis; Pneumonia;

Streptococcus; Thrush; Tuberculosis (TB); Vaccines: Types; Viral infections; Viral pharyngitis; Viral upper respiratory infections.

Epstein-Barr virus infection

CATEGORY: Diseases and conditions
ANATOMY OR SYSTEM AFFECTED: All

DEFINITION

Epstein-Barr virus (EBV) is a herpesvirus that was first isolated in 1964. It is best known as the cause of one of the most common viruses in humans, infectious mononucleosis, which is usually benign. In a few cases, EBV can cause more serious illnesses, such as autoimmune disorders or cancer.

CAUSES

As one of the most prevalent viruses, EBV has been present in the nasopharyngeal secretions of up to 95 percent of people around the world, although most people experience no symptoms. The route of transmission is through oral and nasal secretions. While the virus is infectious for four to six weeks, it remains dormant in all who have been infected, giving each person the lifelong potential for excreting and spreading EBV.

In developing countries, in which children are typically exposed to more infections, EBV usually strikes by the age of three years, causing no symptoms. In industrialized countries, in which young people are typically more protected from infection, EBV is usually delayed, striking in the teenage to young adult years and causing infectious mononucleosis in 35 to 69 percent of infected persons.

RISK FACTORS

In its most common form, mononucleosis, EBV can be spread by kissing; by sharing drinking glasses, eating utensils, toothbrushes, or similar personal items; or by touching items close to the nose or mouth of an infected person.

A severe manifestation of EBV, Burkitt's lymphoma, a tumor common to African children, is also associated with malaria. Non-Hodgkin's and Hodgkin's lymphomas are often tied to EBV. Immunocompromised persons carry special risks. For example, EBV may be fatal to persons with Duncan syndrome, a disease of

excess lymphocytes. Persons with ataxia-telangiectasia (a rare neurodegenerative disease), Chédiak-Higashi syndrome (autosomal recessive disorder), Wiskott-Aldrich syndrome (recessive disease), common variable immunodeficiency, post-transplant lymphoproliferative disorder, and immunodeficiencies related to cancer treatments are all at increased risk for being infected by EBV and for being further debilitated.

EBV also can cause systemic lupus erythematosus, rheumatoid arthritis, Sjögren's syndrome (inflammation of the glands), salivary gland tumors, thymomas (tumors of the epithelial cells of the thymus), and nasopharyngeal carcinomas. In persons with acquired immunodeficiency syndrome (AIDS), complications such as hairy leukoplakia, leiomyosarcoma, central nervous system lymphoma, and lymphoid interstitial pneumonitis are related to EBV, but EBV is not implicated in all cases.

SYMPTOMS

A person with EBV may notice swollen lymph nodes of the neck, armpits, and groin, and a persistent fever. Other common symptoms include fatigue and discomfort. Enlarged tonsils can cause dehydration, difficulty swallowing, or airway obstruction.

Certain people may experience complications of the liver (mild hepatitis), respiratory system (upper airway obstruction or pneumonitis), or spleen (rupture). Rarely occurring neurological complications include encephalitis (brain inflammation), aseptic meningitis (viral infection of the central nervous system), Guillain-Barré syndrome (autoimmune disorder of the peripheral nervous system), and transverse myelitis (inflammation of the spinal cord). Complications affecting the heart are unusual. EBV can cause rare cancers, such as Burkitt's lymphoma or nasopharyngeal carcinoma, in a limited group of persons.

SCREENING AND DIAGNOSIS

Diagnosis of infectious mononucleosis from EBV is first indicated by the person's age and by clinical symptoms such as fever, sore throat, and swollen lymph glands. A physical examination may show an enlargement of the liver or spleen, with tenderness. Typically, laboratory tests are done for confirmation, and, if the person is infected with EBV, the tests will show an elevated white blood cell count with increased atypical white blood cells and a positive reaction to a monospot test, a form of the heterophil antibody test.

Polymerase chain reaction is used to diagnose persons who are immunocompromised. Most persons with acute infectious mononucleosis will have elevated liver function tests. Additional screening tests are available for the rare conditions such as cancers and disorders of the immune system.

TREATMENT AND THERAPY

For persons with mononucleosis that was transmitted by EBV, physicians typically recommend supportive measures such as bed rest and increased fluids. Sore throat, fever, and myalgia (pain) may be treated with over-the-counter remedies such as saline gargles, acetaminophen, or ibuprofen. Antibiotics have no effect on the virus. Acyclovir can reduce virus production in the throat, but it does not shorten the duration of the disease.

In cases where mononucleosis occurs with a streptococcal throat infection, antibiotics may be prescribed. In severe cases with swelling, corticosteroid drugs may be used. Burkitt's lymphoma is sensitive to chemotherapy. Physicians do not agree on strategies for persons with post-transplant lymphoproliferative disorder (PTLD), which may respond to treatments such as antiviral therapy, chemotherapy, or surgery, or by reducing immunosuppression.

PREVENTION AND OUTCOMES

The spread of EBV can be curtailed by limited contact with saliva, such as avoiding kissing children on the mouth. Other commonsense measures include monitoring young children for drooling and hand-to-mouth actions, maintaining cleanliness in settings such as day care, and restricting children from sharing toys. Teens and adults should avoid all activities that could transmit oral and nasal secretions.

Researchers are investigating new therapies, including interferon alpha and cytotoxic T cells that are specific to EBV. Additionally, investigation is underway to develop a vaccine that would block primary infection with EBV. In clinical trials, scientists are also trying a peptide-based vaccine. A vaccine remedy also has the potential to block persons with PTLD from contracting EBV. In addition, researchers are looking for ways to use vaccines to limit symptoms that occur after infection.

Merrill Evans, M.A.

FURTHER READING

Cohen, J. I. "Epstein-Barr Virus Infections, Including Infectious Mononucleosis." In *Harrison's Principles of Internal Medicine*, edited by Joan Butterton. 17th ed. New York: McGraw-Hill, 2008.

National Center for Infectious Diseases. "Epstein-Barr Virus and Infectious Mononucleosis." Available at http://www.cdc.gov/ncidod/diseases/ebv .htm.

Pollard, Andrew J., and Adam Finn, eds. *Hot Topics in Infection and Immunity in Children II*. New York: Springer, 2005.

Rickinson, Alan B. "Human Cytotoxic T Lymphocyte Responses to Epstein-Barr Virus Infection." *Annual Review of Immunology* 15 (April, 1997): 405-431.

Robertson, Erle S., ed. *Epstein-Barr Virus*. Wymondham, England: Caister Academic Press, 2005.

Tselis, Alex C., and Hal B. Jenson, eds. *Epstein-Barr Virus*. New York: Taylor & Francis, 2006.

Umar, Constantine S., ed. *New Developments in Epstein-Barr Virus Research*. New York: Nova Science, 2006.

Wilson, Joanna B., and Gerhard H. W. May, eds. *Epstein-Barr Virus Protocols*. Totowa, N.J.: Humana Press, 2001.

Zuckerman, Arie J., et al., eds. *Principles and Practice of Clinical Virology*. Hoboken, N.J.: Wiley, 2004.

WEB SITES OF INTEREST

About Kids Health
http://www.aboutkidshealth.ca

American Academy of Family Physicians
http://familydoctor.org

Centers for Disease Control and Prevention
http://www.cdc.gov

National Institute of Allergy and Infectious Diseases
http://www.niaid.nih.gov

See also: Cancer and infectious disease; Children and infectious disease; Chronic fatigue syndrome; Encephalitis; Epstein-Barr virus vaccine; Herpesviridae; Herpesvirus infections; Immunodeficiency; Lymphadenitis; Mononucleosis; Nasopharyngeal infections; Parotitis; Pharyngitis and tonsillopharyngitis; Saliva and infectious disease; Strep throat; Viral infections; Viral pharyngitis; Viral upper respiratory infections.

Epstein-Barr virus vaccine

CATEGORY: Prevention

DEFINITION

No commercially available vaccine exists for the Epstein-Barr virus (EBV), a common virus that is spread through the exchange of saliva. EBV is a member of the herpes family of viruses. Other notable herpesviruses include herpes simplex-1, herpes simplex-2, varicella zoster virus, and cytomegalovirus.

EBV can cause infectious mononucleosis, although most infections are asymptomatic, with fewer than one-half of infected persons developing the disease. Mononucleosis initially manifests with general symptoms that may include fever, sore throat, and swollen lymph glands. Fatigue is a common sequelae and can persist for months. Regardless of the presence or absence of an initial infection, EBV remains in the host in a dormant state in some immune cells.

Research suggests that although rare, persons infected with EBV have an increased likelihood of developing Epstein-Barr-related cancers, including Burkitt's lymphoma and nasopharyngeal carcinoma, later in life.

GLYCOPROTEIN 350

Glycoprotein 350 (gp350) is a promising target for an EBV vaccine and has progressed through phase 1 and 2 studies for use in healthy adults and young adults for the prevention of mononucleosis. GP350 is an envelope glycoprotein that facilitates entry of EBV into human cells through interactions with the CD21 antigen receptors, and it is an important target of the host's antibody immune response. Additional research has indicated that gp350 may also be a target for antibody-dependent cellular cytotoxicity and cytotoxic T-lymphocyte-mediated cytotoxicity.

ONGOING RESEARCH

Ongoing studies are investigating EBV for the treatments of nasopharyngeal cancer and for EBV-positive persons with gastric, head and neck cancer; lymphoma; lymphoproliferative disorder; and nonneoplastic condition.

IMPACT

The Centers for Disease Control and Prevention estimates that among adults between the age of twenty-five and forty years, up to 95 percent may be infected with EBV. When the virus infects hosts at a younger age (childhood through adolescence), infected persons are more apt to develop mononucleosis. Clinical presentation may include nonspecific symptoms such as fever, sore throat, and cervical lymphadenopathy. The resulting illness can leave the infected person feeling fatigued and generally unwell for up to four months or longer. The need to develop an EBV vaccine is evident because of the high rate of EBV infection in the general population and because of the increased likelihood of developing certain EBV-associated cancers later in life.

Allison C. Bennett, Pharm.D.

FURTHER READING

Centers for Disease Control and Prevention. "Epstein-Barr Virus and Infectious Mononucleosis." Available at http://www.cdc.gov/ncidod/diseases/ebv.htm.

Cohen, J. I. "Epstein-Barr Virus Infections, Including Infectious Mononucleosis." In *Harrison's Principles of Internal Medicine*, edited by Joan Butterton. 17th ed. New York: McGraw-Hill, 2008.

Moutschen, Michael, et al. "Phase I/II Studies to Evaluate Safety and Immunogenicity of a Recombinant gp350 Epstein-Barr Virus Vaccine in Healthy Adults." *Vaccine* 25 (2007): 4697-4705.

Sokal, Etienne, et al. "Recombinant gp350 Vaccine for Infectious Mononucleosis: A Phase 2, Randomized, Double-Blind Placebo-Controlled Trial to Evaluate the Safety, Immunogenicity, and Efficacy of an Epstein-Barr Virus Vaccine in Healthy Young Adults." *Journal of Infectious Diseases* 196 (2007): 1749-1753.

WEB SITES OF INTEREST

Centers for Disease Control and Prevention
http://www.cdc.gov

National Institute of Allergy and Infectious Diseases
http://www.niaid.nih.gov

See also: Cancer and infectious disease; Children and infectious disease; Chronic fatigue syndrome; Encephalitis; Epstein-Barr virus infection; Herpes simplex infection; Herpesviridae; Immunodeficiency; Lymphadenitis; Mononucleosis; Nasopharyngeal infections; Parotitis; Pharyngitis and tonsillopharyngitis; Saliva and infectious disease; Strep throat; Vaccines:

Experimental; Viral infections; Viral pharyngitis; Viral upper respiratory infections.

Erysipelas

CATEGORY: Diseases and conditions
ANATOMY OR SYSTEM AFFECTED: Skin, upper respiratory tract
ALSO KNOWN AS: St. Anthony's fire

DEFINITION

Erysipelas is a common type of cellulitis, or skin infection, that appears on either the face or the lower extremities. The condition can affect anyone, but it is especially common in children and the elderly.

CAUSES

Erysipelas is typically caused by exposure to the bacterium *Streptococcus pyogenes*, but other microbial organisms can also cause erysipelas. The bacteria enter the body through the upper respiratory tract (nose and mouth) or through an area of broken skin such as a scratch, puncture wound, or bug bite, where they spread throughout the upper layers of the skin (epidermis) and into the nearby lymphatic system.

RISK FACTORS

Young children and the elderly are at increased risk for erysipelas because their immune systems are more vulnerable. Other risk factors include poor health and malnutrition, having had a recent upper respiratory tract infection, and having a chronic condition, such as lymphedema, that affects the skin, lymph, or the vascular system. Frequency of erysipelas infection is higher in developing countries than in industrialized countries, likely because of poorer sanitation and a lack of access to antibiotics.

SYMPTOMS

The first symptoms of erysipelas are fatigue, swollen lymph nodes, fever, and chills. Next, the skin infection appears rapidly, usually on the face or leg. The infected area becomes inflamed, bright red, and painful, and it is well-defined from the surrounding healthy skin. In some cases, blisters form at the site of infection or the infection spreads into the deeper layers of skin.

SCREENING AND DIAGNOSIS

Erysipelas is diagnosed by its symptoms. A doctor will take bacterial cultures of the affected area of skin and of any drainage.

TREATMENT AND THERAPY

Oral penicillin is the preferred treatment for erysipelas; if the patient is allergic to penicillin, erythromycin or another alternative antibiotic may be prescribed. The patient also will be instructed to rest, clean and apply dressing to areas where the skin is broken, and take aspirin or acetaminophen for fever or pain. Hospitalization for a few days may be necessary if the patient is very young or old, is extremely ill, or appears to have a more serious infection.

PREVENTION AND OUTCOMES

Risk for erysipelas can be reduced by avoiding injury, especially injury to the lower legs. However, some people will remain at risk because of their age or pre-existing-condition status.

Carita Caple, M.S.H.S., R.N.

FURTHER READING

Chong, F. Y., and T. Thirumoorthy. "Blistering Erysipelas: Not a Rare Entity." *Singapore Medical Journal* 49 (2008): 809-813.

Marquardt, William C., ed. *Biology of Disease Vectors*. 2d ed. New York: Academic Press/Elsevier, 2005.

Stevens, Dennis L. "Infections of the Skin, Muscle, and Soft Tissues." In *Harrison's Principles of Internal Medicine*, edited by Joan Butterton. 17th ed. New York: McGraw-Hill, 2008.

Van Tonder, Reinier J. "Erysipelas." In *The Five-Minute Clinical Consult 2010*, edited by Frank J. Domino. 18th ed. Philadelphia: Wolters Kluwer Health/Lippincott Williams & Wilkins, 2010.

Weedon, David. *Skin Pathology*. 3d ed. New York: Churchill Livingstone/Elsevier, 2010.

WEB SITE OF INTEREST

New Zealand Dermatological Society
http://dermnetnz.org

See also: Acne; Bacterial infections; Cellulitis; Respiratory route of transmission; Skin infections; Streptococcal infections; *Streptococcus*; Wound infections.

Erysipelothrix infection

CATEGORY: Diseases and conditions
ANATOMY OR SYSTEM AFFECTED: Skin
ALSO KNOWN AS: Erysipeloid

DEFINITION

The bacterium *Erysipelothrix rhusiopathiae*, found as a commensal organism in animals, birds, and fish, causes an occupational disease of food workers who come into contact with infected animals or animal products.

CAUSES

E. rhusiopathiae is a nonmotile, nonencapsulated, gram-positive bacillus that grows aerobically or as a facultative anaerobe. In most cases, infection occurs through abrasions or puncture wounds in the skin. The organism is found in many animals, especially swine, and in fish, shellfish, and decaying matter. In animals, transmission may be facilitated by mites. No human-to-human transmission occurs.

RISK FACTORS

Infection is common in fish and seafood handlers, particularly those who handle crabs. Immunocompromised persons or persons with chronic alcoholism may be more likely to have the infection enter the bloodstream, resulting in serious and even life-threatening illness.

SYMPTOMS

In most cases, the infection results in a localized skin lesion. Because the organism enters through a break in the skin, lesions on the fingers predominate. After an incubation period of two to seven days, a discrete, violaceous lesion develops on the finger or other part of the hand. The lesion is painful and slightly raised, and the affected finger or hand is usually swollen. An associated fever is sometimes present.

Less common is a more diffuse skin lesion, which spreads to other areas. When this occurs, fever is more often noted, but there is no bloodstream invasion. Systemic infection, though the most severe form of the disease, is much less common. Bacteremia, often with endocarditis, can occur with alcoholics. Bacteremia spreads the infection to other organs, causing sepsis; this occurs primarily in immunocompromised persons.

SCREENING AND DIAGNOSIS

In the usual case of *Erysipelothrix* infection, diagnosis is made based on epidemiological and clinical information. A definitive diagnosis can be made by culturing the organism from a skin biopsy or from blood or other sterile body fluids when systemic infection occurs. The organism, however, may be challenging to grow and identify in a laboratory. Polymerase chain reaction can be used to make a specific diagnosis, but is not widely available.

TREATMENT AND THERAPY

The organism is highly susceptible to penicillin and several other antibiotics. *Erysipelothrix* infection will usually resolve without treatment, but antibiotic therapy will shorten the recovery time. Endocarditis and other types of systemic infection require four to six weeks of treatment with an effective antibiotic.

PREVENTION AND OUTCOMES

Protection from skin abrasions and punctures is important for those persons engaged in risky occupational or recreational activities. Wearing gloves is one form of prevention. Other methods include handwashing and disinfection of contaminated surfaces. A vaccine is available for swine, but not for humans.

H. Bradford Hawley, M.D.

FURTHER READING

Reboli, Annette C. "*Erysipelothrix rhusiopathiae.*" In *Mandell, Douglas, and Bennett's Principles and Practice of Infectious Diseases*, edited by Gerald L. Mandell, John F. Bennett, and Raphael Dolin. 7th ed. New York: Churchill Livingstone/Elsevier, 2010.

Reboli, Annette C., and W. Edmund Farrar. "*Erysipelothrix rhusiopathiae*: An Occupational Pathogen." *Clinical Microbiology Reviews* 2 (1989): 354-359.

Stevens, Dennis L. "Infections of the Skin, Muscle, and Soft Tissues." In *Harrison's Principles of Internal Medicine*, edited by Joan Butterton. 17th ed. New York: McGraw-Hill, 2008.

Woods, Gail L., et al. *Diagnostic Pathology of Infectious Diseases*. Philadelphia: Lea & Febiger, 1993.

WEB SITES OF INTEREST

Centers for Disease Control and Prevention
http://www.cdc.gov

National Center for Biotechnology Information
http://www.ncbi.nlm.nih.gov

National Institutes of Health
http://www.nih.gov

See also: Bacterial infections; Fever; Pigs and infectious disease; Skin infections; Zoonotic diseases.

Erythema infectiosum

CATEGORY: Diseases and conditions
ANATOMY OR SYSTEM AFFECTED: Skin
ALSO KNOWN AS: Fifth disease, slapped-cheek disease

DEFINITION

Erythema infectiosum, commonly known as fifth disease, is an infection that results in a mild rash on the face, trunk, and limbs. In healthy people, fifth disease usually disappears without medical treatment, but pregnant women and persons who have an impaired immune system or have sickle cell anemia or other blood disorders may need to consult a physician.

CAUSES

Fifth disease is caused by a parvovirus B19 infection. This is not the same parvovirus that infects dogs and cats; parvovirus B19 only infects humans. It is estimated that about one-half of all adults have been infected with parvovirus B19 at some time. Because parvovirus is found in respiratory secretions (such as saliva, sputum, and nasal mucus), it is usually spread from person to person through direct contact with these secretions.

RISK FACTORS

The factors that increase one's chance of developing fifth disease are age (the disease is most common in children) and contact with someone infected with parvovirus B19.

SYMPTOMS

The symptoms of fifth disease may be caused by other, less serious health conditions, but if a person experiences any of these symptoms, he or she should consult a doctor. The first signs of fifth disease usually occur within four to fourteen days of becoming infected with parvovirus B19. These symptoms include a low-grade fever, headache, and a stuffy or runny nose. A few days after these symptoms pass, a bright red rash begins to develop on the face (known as a slapped-cheek rash). Several days later, this rash spreads as a lighter red, blotchy rash down the trunk and limbs. The rash usually resolves within seven to ten days. In previously uninfected adults, there may be no initial symptoms or development of a typical rash. Some adults also may have joint pain and swelling.

SCREENING AND DIAGNOSIS

A doctor will ask about symptoms and medical history and will perform a physical exam. Tests may include an examination of the rash and a blood test to identify antibodies to parvovirus.

TREATMENT AND THERAPY

Because fifth disease is caused by a virus, antibiotics are ineffective in treating it, and no antiviral medications exist that will treat the disease. Usually, fifth disease does not require any treatment other than rest. Medications such as acetaminophen may be used to relieve joint pain and reduce fever. Anti-itch medications may be used to relieve itching associated with the rash.

In people with sickle cell disease or other types of chronic anemia, parvovirus B19 can sometimes cause acute, severe anemia. In this case, the anemia will require treatment, which may include hospitalization and blood transfusion. People with immune problems may need special medical care, such as treatment with antibodies, to help cure the infection. Sometimes, a parvovirus B19 infection in pregnant women will cause severe anemia in the fetus or possibly cause miscarriage. This is infrequent (less than 5 percent of the time). Usually, there are no serious complications; however, pregnant women who believe they may have parvovirus B19 infection or believe they may have been exposed to someone with parvovirus B19 infection should consult an obstetrician for evaluation.

PREVENTION AND OUTCOMES

It is difficult to prevent the spread of fifth disease because the virus is most contagious before the rash appears. To help reduce the chance of getting fifth disease, one should practice good hygiene, especially handwashing, which can help prevent the spread of many infections.

Krisha McCoy, M.S.; reviewed by Kari Kassir, M.D.

FURTHER READING

Behrman, Richard E., Robert M. Kliegman, and Hal B. Jenson, eds. *Nelson Textbook of Pediatrics*. 18th ed. Philadelphia: Saunders/Elsevier, 2007.

Centers for Disease Control and Prevention. "Parvovirus B19 (Fifth Disease)." Available at http://www.cdc.gov/ncidod/dvrd/revb/respiratory/parvo_b19.htm.

_____. "Parvovirus B19 Infection and Pregnancy." Available at http://www.cdc.gov/ncidod/dvrd/revb/respiratory/B19&preg.htm.

"Fifth Disease." In *Ferri's Clinical Advisor 2011: Instant Diagnosis and Treatment*, edited by Fred F. Ferri. Philadelphia: Mosby/Elsevier, 2011.

Kemper, Kathi J. *The Holistic Pediatrician: A Pediatrician's Comprehensive Guide to Safe and Effective Therapies for the Twenty-five Most Common Ailments of Infants, Children, and Adolescents*. Rev. ed. New York: Quill, 2002.

Martin, Richard J., Avroy A. Fanaroff, and Michele C. Walsh, eds. *Fanaroff and Martin's Neonatal-Perinatal Medicine: Diseases of the Fetus and Infant*. 2 vols. 8th ed. Philadelphia: Mosby/Elsevier, 2006.

Turkington, Carol, and Jeffrey S. Dover. *The Encyclopedia of Skin and Skin Disorders*. 3d ed. New York: Facts On File, 2007.

Weedon, David. *Skin Pathology*. 3d ed. New York: Churchill Livingstone/Elsevier, 2010.

Weir, Erica. "Parvovirus B19 Infection: Fifth Disease and More." *Canadian Medical Association Journal* 172, no. 6 (March, 2005): 743.

Young, N. S., and K. E. Brown. "Parvovirus B19." *New England Journal of Medicine* 350 (2004): 586-597.

WEB SITES OF INTEREST

About Kids Health
http://www.aboutkidshealth.ca

American Academy of Dermatology
http://www.aad.org

American Academy of Family Physicians
http://familydoctor.org

Centers for Disease Control and Prevention
http://www.cdc.gov

FifthDisease.org
http:///www.fifthdisease.org

KidsHealth
http://www.kidshealth.org

See also: Airborne illness and disease; Chickenpox; Childbirth and infectious disease; Children and infectious disease; Contagious diseases; Erythema nodosum; Impetigo; Measles; Molluscum contagiosum; Parvoviridae; Parvovirus infections; Pityriasis rosea; Roseola; Rubella; Scarlet fever; Schools and infectious disease; Skin infections; Viral infections.

Erythema nodosum

CATEGORY: Diseases and conditions
ANATOMY OR SYSTEM AFFECTED: Skin, tissue

DEFINITION

Erythema nodosum (EN) is an inflammation of subcutaneous fat tissue characterized by nodules beneath the skin. EN is considered a nonspecific immune-related skin reaction with an incidence of 1 to 5 per 100,000 persons each year. EN is more common in women than in men. The predominant age of those infected is between fifteen and forty years.

CAUSES

Although the cause of about 50 percent of EN cases is unknown, the most common cause is streptococcal pharyngitis (up to 44 percent in adults and 48 percent in children). The most common bacterial agent for streptococcal pharyngitis in children and adolescents is *Streptococcus pyogenes* (group A *Streptococcus*, or GAS). Other causes of EN include gastrointestinal disorders (Crohn's disease, ulcerative colitis, bacterial gastroenteritis); diseases with large lymph nodes (hilar adenopathy) in the middle part of the chest (sarcoidosis, tuberculosis); diseases caused by various infectious agents (other bacteria, syphilis, cat scratch fever, leprosy); fungi (histoplasmosis, coccidiomycosis, blastomycosis); viruses (human immunodeficiency virus, hepatitis B, cytomegalovirus); protozoa (giardiasis, toxoplasmosis, amebiasis); medications (sulfonamides, amoxicillin, oral contraceptives); rheumatologic, inflammatory, and autoimmune disorders (systemic lupus erythematosus, rheumatoid arthritis, scleroderma); cancers (leukemia, lymphoma, colon cancer); and pregnancy.

RISK FACTORS

Persons with conditions noted in the foregoing section are at risk for developing EN.

SYMPTOMS

EN starts as a red, hot, flat, firm, palpable, and painful nodule or lump, most commonly in the shins, but it may affect other parts of the body (such as the forearms, arms, trunk, thighs, and ankles). The nodule is usually one inch in diameter but can be up to four inches in diameter. The nodules change color from purplish (in days) to brownish patches (in weeks). Other symptoms may occur one to three weeks before the appearance of the nodule, These symptoms include fever, malaise, and joint aches, and inflammation or swelling of the affected areas.

SCREENING AND DIAGNOSIS

A physician will perform a thorough medical history evaluation and a physical examination, considering the wide spectrum of conditions that can cause EN. Diagnosis is based on the clinical features of EN. To establish the most probable cause, studies may include blood tests (complete blood count with differential, erythrocyte sedimentation rate, C-reactive protein, liver enzymes and products, and basic metabolic panel), determining streptococcal infection (antistreptolysin-O level, throat culture, and polymerase chain reaction), chest radiograph to evaluate hilar adenopathy, tuberculin skin test for tuberculosis, and stool cultures to evaluate gastrointestinal causes. Excisional biopsy of the skin lesion may be needed, if EN diagnosis is uncertain.

TREATMENT AND THERAPY

EN usually resolves, and treatment focuses on managing the underlying cause. Pain relief can be provided with nonsteroidal anti-inflammatory drugs (such as naproxen or ibuprofen). A solution of potassium iodide taken for one month is another treatment and is most effective when taken during the early manifestation of EN. Thyroid function should be monitored if potassium iodide will be used long-term because it can cause hyperthyroidism. If infection and malignancy have been ruled out, oral steroid is another therapeutic option.

PREVENTION AND OUTCOMES

There is no vaccination or medication that can prevent EN. One should practice basic hygiene measures that help prevent infections. Recommended cancer screenings should be followed, such as colonoscopy for colon cancer screening, based on clinical guidelines. Finally, one should adhere to medication regimens for the causative diseases.

Miriam E. Schwartz, M.D., Ph.D.,
and Colm A. O'Morain, M.D., D.Sc.

FURTHER READING

Ferri, Fred F. "Erythema Nodosum." In *Ferri's Clinical Advisor 2011: Instant Diagnosis and Treatment*, edited by Fred F. Ferri. Philadelphia: Mosby/Elsevier, 2011.

Requena, Luis, and Evaristo Sanchez Yus. "Erythema Nodosum." *Dermatologic Clinics* 26 (2008): 425-438.

Schwartz, Robert A., and Stephen J. Nervi. "Erythema Nodosum: A Sign of Systemic Disease." *American Family Physician* 75 (2007): 695-700.

WEB SITES OF INTEREST

American Academy of Dermatology
http://www.aad.org

Dermatology Online Journal: "Erythema Nodosum"
http://dermatology-s10.cdlib.org/dojvol8num1

See also: Bacterial infections; Cellulitis; Erythema infectiosum; Inflammation; Leprosy; Molluscum contagiosum; Pharyngitis and tonsillopharyngitis; Roseola; Scarlet fever; Skin infections; Streptococcal infections; *Streptococcus*; Viral infections.

Escherichia

CATEGORY: Pathogen
TRANSMISSION ROUTE: Direct contact, ingestion

DEFINITION

Escherichia are gram-negative, facultative anaerobic bacteria that ferment lactose and other sugars. *Escherichia* is found in humans and animals, and some *Escherichia* species can cause mild to serious infections.

NATURAL HABITAT AND FEATURES

Escherichia is found in the intestines of warm-blooded animals, particularly cattle and humans.

Taxonomic Classification for *Escherichia*

Domain: Bacteria
Kingdom: Bacteria
Phylum: Protobacteria
Class: Gamma proteobacteria
Order: Coccidioides
Family: Enterobacteriaceae
Genus: *Escherichia*
Species:
E. coli
E. albertii
E. aurescens
E. blattae
E. communior
E. ellingeri
E. fergunsonii
E. freundii
E. hermannii
E. metacoli
E. noctuarii
E. sphingidis
E. vulneris

They are also found in soil, sand, and water. *E. coli* has been found in some marine animals. Different species are identified by their similarities to *Shigella*, *Salmonella*, and *Klebsiella* (O), motility by flagella (H), capsular antigens (K), and enterotoxin strains (CFAII, CRAIII). They are also differentiated by the sugars they do or do not ferment, by whether or not they produce toxins, and by how their disease mechanisms work to cause illness. Deoxyribonucleic acid (DNA) sequencing of *E. coli* has been extensive, and several subtypes of the species have been identified.

Microscopically, *Escherichia* appear as straight rods either nonmotile or motile with flagella. *E. coli* can be grown in a nutrient-rich Luria or Lennox broth at a temperature of 37° Fahrenheit (2.8° Celsius) or higher for twenty-four hours. A cloudy, fecal-smelling mix will result, which can be plated on clear agar; this will produce visible white colonies. Clinically, tests for *Escherichia* infections are cultured on a sorbital-MacConkey medium with a typing antiserum to check for the appearance of gram-negative rods. DNA analysis using the polymerase chain reaction method is also used to differentiate *Escherichia* species.

PATHOGENICITY AND CLINICAL SIGNIFICANCE

There are six main strains of *E. coli*, for example, that attack the human gut, each strain with distinct qualities. Enterohemorrhagic *E. coli* (EHEC) includes the most lethal strain of *E. coli* (that is, strain 0157:17), which produces a Shiga-toxin. EHEC is extremely virulent and can cause hemolytic-uremic syndrome in children and postdiarrheal thrombotic purpura in the elderly. Infantile diarrhea in developing countries can be caused by, primarily, three main species of *E. coli*: enteropathogenic *E. coli* (EPEC), enterotogenic *E. coli* (ETAC), and enteroaggregative *E. coli* (EAEC). ETEC is a major cause of travelers' diarrhea. Enteroinvasive *E. coli* (EIEC), also seen in developing countries, causes a type of mucus-filled diarrhea called bacillary dysentery.

Uropathogenic *E. coli* (UPEC) causes 90 percent of all urinary tract infections. Women are fourteen times more likely than men to get a UPEC infection. Gram-negative neonatal meningitis or sepsis caused by cross-contamination of maternal genital *E. coli* during birth can develop in neonates.

E. albertii has five strains and has been identified as a cause of diarrhea in Bangladeshi children. *E. albertii* is believed to act like the attaching and effacing gene that is typical of enterpathogenic *E. coli*.

E. fergusonii is an emerging pathogen and little is known about its natural habitat. It has been found in wound infections, urinary tract infections, diarrhea, and pleural infections. Naturally found in water and soil, *E. hermanii* acts as an infectious agent in wounds, sputum, and stool. *E. hermanii* is never the primary cause of an infection; for example, in an infected wound, a culture may show five bacteria present, two of which might be *E. hermanii* and *C. botulinum*. Treatment will focus on the virulent *C. botulinum* because the rest of the bacteria are secondary. Another species of *Escherichia*, *E. vulneris* (*vulneris* is Latin for "to wound") is also found in wounds, often with other bacteria present.

In 1988, Richard Lenski began long-term evolution experiments using *E. coli* by directly observing a major evolutionary shift of the organism in the laboratory. He observed one population of *E. coli* unexpectedly evolve the ability to aerobically metabolize citrate, a capacity that is extremely rare in *E. coli*. The inability to grow aerobically is normally used as a diagnostic criterion to differentiate *E. coli* from other, closely related bacteria such as *Salmonella*.

E. coli has continued to have significant clinical relevance in the laboratory for biochemists and geneticists and is frequently used as a model organism in microbiology studies. The ability to use plasmids and restriction enzymes to create recombinant DNA was instrumental in creating the field of biotechnology. *E. coli* is considered to be one of the most versatile organisms, enabling researchers to facilitate these procedures. Researchers manipulate the genes of *E. coli* to change its nature, leading to the creation of biotech products such as human insulin and vaccines. Cultivated strains of *E. coli* such as *E. coli* K12, which is used in the laboratory, are no longer pathogenic.

DRUG SUSCEPTIBILITY

Antibiotic resistance is a major issue for all species of *Escherichia*; however some infections are still susceptible to certain kinds of antibiotics. EIEC and ETAC are usually treated with trimethoprim-sultramethoxazole or flouroquinolones. Urinary tract infections are treated with a three-day course of trimethoprim-sulfamethoxazole or a fluoroquinoline. Treatment for neonatal meningitis and sepsis is antibiotic therapy with ampicillin and an aminoglycoside, or with an expanded-spectrum cephalosporin.

E. fergusononii is a multi-drug-resistant pathogen. Both *E. hermanii* and *E. vulneris* are more resistant to antibiotics than the majority of community acquired *E. coli* infections.

S. M. Willis, M.S., M.A.

FURTHER READING

Abbott, S. L., et al. "Biochemical Properties of Newly Described *Escherichia* Species *Escherichia albertii*." *Journal of Clinical Microbiology* 41 (2003): 4852-4854.

Donnenberg, Michael S., ed. *"Escherichia coli": Virulence Mechanisms of a Versatile Pathogen.* Boston: Academic Press, 2002.

Pien, F. D., et al. "Colonization of Human Wounds by *Escherichia vulneris* and *Escherichia hermannii*." *Journal of Clinical Microbiology* 22 (1985): 283-285.

Savini, V., et al. "Multi-drug resistant *Escherichia fergusonii*: A Case of Acute Cystitis." *Journal of Clinical Microbiology* 46 (2008): 1551-1552.

Snyder, Larry, and Wendy Champness. *Molecular Genetics of Bacteria.* 3d ed. Washington, D.C.: ASM Press, 2007.

Thielman, N. M., et al. "Acute Infectious Diarrhea." *New England Journal of Medicine* 350 (2004): 38-47.

Zimmer, C. *Microcosm: "E. coli" and the New Science of Life.* New York: Pantheon, 2008.

WEB SITES OF INTEREST

Bacteriome.org
http://www.compsysbio.org/bacteriome

Centers for Disease Control and Prevention, Division of Foodborne, Bacterial, and Mycotic Diseases
http://www.cdc.gov/nczved/divisions/dfbmd

coliBASE
http://xbase.bham.ac.uk/colibase

EcoliHub
http://ecolihub.org

See also: Amebic dysentery; Bacteria: Classification and types; Bacterial infections; *Enterobacter*, *Escherichia coli* infection; Fecal-oral route of transmission; Foodborne illness and disease; Infection; Intestinal and stomach infections; Pathogens; *Salmonella*; Sepsis; *Shigella*; Travelers' diarrhea; Waterborne illness and disease; Wound infections.

Escherichia coli infection

CATEGORY: Diseases and conditions
ANATOMY OR SYSTEM AFFECTED: Gastrointestinal system, intestines, urinary system
ALSO KNOWN AS: *E. coli* infection, *E. coli* O157:H7

DEFINITION

There are six main strains of the *Escherichia coli* bacterium that affect the human gastrointestinal tract, each with distinct qualities. Enterohemorrhagic *E. coli* (EHEC) includes the most lethal strain of *E. coli*, 0157:17, which releases a Shiga-toxin. EHEC is extremely virulent and can cause the potentially fatal hemolytic-uremic syndrome in children and can cause postdiarrheal thrombotic purpura in the elderly. Enteropathogenic *E. coli* (EPEC), enterotogenic *E. coli* (ETAC), and enteroaggregative *E. coli* (EAEC) are all causes of infantile diarrhea in developing countries. ETEC is a major cause of travelers' diarrhea. Entero-invasive *E. coli* (EIEC) causes bacillary dysentery.

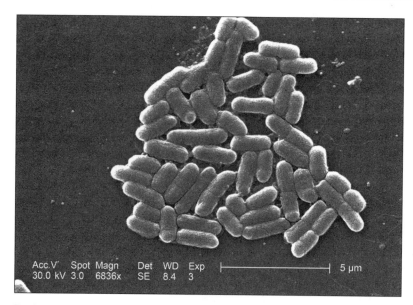

Escherichia coli *bacteria, which cause* E. coli *infections* (CDC)

Uropathogenic *E. coli* (UPEC) is the cause of 90 percent of all urinary tract infections. Gram-negative neonatal meningitis or sepsis caused by *E. coli* can develop in neonates.

CAUSES

In an EHEC infection, cytotoxins (or verotoxins) are secreted into the large intestine and absorbed into the circulatory system, creating an intense inflammatory response. During an infection of EPEC, lesions on the small bowel secrete bacterial proteins leading to inflammation of the bowels. ETEC causes two types of toxins to be secreted in the small intestine (ST), both of which cause watery diarrhea. In cases of EIEC, plasmid-mediated tissue invasion and epithelial cell destruction cause inflammation in the large intestine (LT). EAEC is characterized by "stacked brick" aggregated cells that release Shiga-toxins and hemolysins that damage intestinal walls.

Most urinary tract infections are caused by the colonization of *E. coli* from the rectal area in the urethra, leading to an infection of the urethra, kidneys, or prostate. Neonatal meningitis and sepsis are caused by *E. coli* contamination from the maternal genital area during birth or by fecal-contaminated persons or equipment, such as respiratory therapy machines in the neonatal nursery.

E. coli is primarily transmitted through the fecal-oral route. It is found in the intestines of cattle and humans. Unsanitary practices at slaughterhouses can cause beef (particularly ground beef) to become infected with fecal matter. Fecal contamination also occurs during milking. *E. coli* can also be transmitted from person to person. *E. coli* can live in water, including water for drinking and bathing and water for swimming.

RISK FACTORS

Children younger than five years of age and the elderly are most at risk of developing serious complications from *E. coli* infections; these infections include hemolytic-uremic syndrome and postdiarrhea thrombotic purpura. Those who suffer from malnutrition are also vulnerable to *E. coli* infections.

Women are fourteen times more likely than men to get a UPEC infection. Conditions predisposing women to urinary tract infections include urinary incontinence, post-void residual urine, sexual intercourse, menopause, diabetes mellitus, catheterization, and pregnancy. Risk factors for neonatal meningitis or sepsis include less than thirty-seven weeks gestation, low birth weight, and metabolic abnormalities.

SYMPTOMS

The symptoms of EHEC are a sudden onset of nonbloody diarrhea that develops into bloody stool, severe abdominal cramps and a low-grade fever. EPEC manifests as severe, chronic diarrhea with dehydration. Symptoms of ETEC are watery diarrhea, cramps, and a low fever. EIEC usually manifests with diarrhea with blood or mucus (or both), abdominal cramps, vomiting, chills, high fever, and malaise. Symptoms of EAEC are mucoid and watery diarrhea without fever or vomiting, often lasting more than fourteen days.

Symptoms of a urinary tract infection include pain with urination, urgency, back pain, cloudy urine, and chills. Neonatal meningitis and sepsis present with fever, grunting respirations, cyanosis, and apnea.

SCREENING AND DIAGNOSIS

E. coli is a gram-negative bacterium and will culture on a sorbital-MacConkey medium and typing antiserum. However, that test is not specific for strains of *E. coli*, which may be epidemiologically significant. Public health authorities recommend that all stool specimens be cultured for 0157:H7 and then reported. Enzyme-linked immunosorbent assay (ELISA) test kits are commonly used for rapid screening of fecal specimens. Cytotoxic assays are considered the gold standard because of their high specificity and sensitivity; however, they are slow and require special lab facilities. Deoxyribonucleic acid (DNA) based assays, such as polymerase chain reaction (PCR), are commonly used.

Treatment and Therapy

For most healthy persons, *E. coli* infections are self-limiting and do not require treatment other than for dehydration. In cases of EHEC, antibiotics should not be used; the antibiotic kills the bacteria, causing the toxin to be released into the bloodstream and thereby increasing the chance of HUS. Persons with HUS may require dialysis and transfusions. Antimotility agents and opiates should not be used because they prolong the time the toxin remains in the body. EIEC and ETAC are usually treated with trimethoprim-sultramethoxazole or fluoroquinolones for nonresistant strains, and with rehydration and electrolyte replacement therapy.

Some urinary tract infections may resolve without antibiotics; however, a three-day course of trimethoprim-sulfamethoxazole or a fluoroquinolone is standard. Treatment for neonatal meningitis and sepsis is antibiotic therapy with ampicillin and an aminoglycoside, or the use of an expanded-spectrum cephalosporin.

Prevention and Outcomes

General prevention for food-borne transmission of any of the *E. coli* infections includes cooking meat and poultry until juices run clear (162° Fahrenheit, or 72° Celsius). One should cook hamburger meat until the meat is no longer pink; avoid consuming raw milk or unpasteurized dairy products and juices; wash all fruits and vegetables; wash one's hands after using the toilet, after changing a diaper, and before touching and eating food. Travelers should drink only bottled water; avoid ice, unpeeled fruits, and salad; and eat only foods that are served steaming hot. Taking daily doses of a bismuth subsalicylate preparation can help protect against ETEC. In developing countries, mothers are encouraged to breast-feed their infants to prevent several infantile diarrheas. Cranberry juice has been

found to be effective in preventing recurring urinary tract infections. Neonates infected with meningitis or sepsis should be isolated to prevent cluster infections.

Rapid diagnosis and reporting of outbreaks enables epidemiological investigation and control measures. Vaccines for individual strains of *E. coli* are being developed for cattle and for humans.

S. M. Willis, M.S., M.A.

Further Reading

Donnenberg, Michael S., ed. *"Escherichia coli": Virulence Mechanisms of a Versatile Pathogen.* Boston: Academic Press, 2002. Provides a comprehensive analysis of the biology and molecular mechanisms that enable *E. coli* to cause human disease.

Parker, James N., and Philip M. Parker, eds. *The Official Patient's Sourcebook on "E. Coli."* San Diego, Calif.: Icon Health, 2002. An introductory work written especially for nonspecialists.

Perez-Lopez, F. R., et al. *"Vaccinnium macrocarpon:* An Interesting Option for Women with Recurring Urinary Tract Infections and Other Health Benefits." *Japan Society of Obstetrics and Gynecology* 35 (2009): 630-639. Insights into the preventive medical use of cranberries.

Thielman, N. M., et al. "Acute Infectious Diarrhea." *New England Journal of Medicine* 350 (2004): 38-47. Overview of causes, symptoms and treatments of infectious diarrhea.

U.S. Environmental Protection Agency. "Basic Information About *E. coli* O157:H7 in Drinking Water." Available at http://www.epa.gov/safewater/contaminants/ecoli.html. An introductory, federal government overview of drinking water and *E. coli* contamination.

Wong, C. S., et al. "The Risk of the Hemolytic-Uremic Syndrome After Antibiotic Treatment of *Escherichia coli* 0157:H7 Infections." *New England Journal of Medicine* 342 (2000): 1930-1936. Cases studies comparing use and nonuse of antibiotics in 0157:H7 infections.

Zimmer, C. *Microcosm: "E. coli" and the New Science of Life.* New York: Pantheon Books, 2008. Examines the persistence of *E. coli* in human history.

Web Sites of Interest

Canadian Food Inspection Agency
http://www.inspection.gc.ca

Centers for Disease Control and Prevention, Division of
Foodborne, Bacterial, and Mycotic Diseases
http://www.cdc.gov/nczved/divisions/dfbmd

World Health Organization
http://www.who.int/topics/escherichia_coli_
infections

See also: Amebic dysentery; Bacteria: Classification
and types; Bacterial infections; Enteritis; *Enterobacter*;
Escherichia; Fecal-oral route of transmission; Food-
borne illness and disease; Infection; Inflammation;
Intestinal and stomach infections; Pathogens; Sepsis;
Waterborne illness and disease.

Eye infections

CATEGORY: Diseases and conditions
ANATOMY OR SYSTEM AFFECTED: Eyes, vision

DEFINITION

Eyes are made up of different structures, and all are
at risk of an attack from a range of bacteria, viruses,
parasites, or fungi that can lead to inflammation and
infection. Eye infections are usually diagnosed and described by the specific part of the eye involved or by
the mechanism causing the infection. Mismanaged
or unresolved eye infections are among the leading
causes of blindness around the world. The most frequently occurring eye infection is infectious conjunctivitis, often called pinkeye, which is an inflammation
of the conjunctiva, the mucous membrane that lines
the eyelids. Conjunctivitis can be further classified as
bacterial, viral, or fungal.

The eye is made up of a series of complex structures. Some common infections of the eye structures
are blepharitis, an inflammation of the eyelid margins; scleritis, an infection of the sclera, the white out-
side-covering of the eye ball; iritis, inflammation of
the iris, the colored part of the eye; keratitis, inflammation of the cornea, the transparent part of the
sclera at the very front of the eye that covers the lens
and iris; vitritis, an infection of the liquid inside the
eye; chorioretinitis, an inflammation of the retina and
its blood vessels; and endophthalmitis, serious inflammation of the inside of the eye.

Anatomy of the Eye

- *Cornea.* The transparent structure forming the
  anterior part of the fibrous tunic of the eye; light
  must pass through this structure to reach the retina

- *Crystalline lens.* The transparent focusing mechanism of the eye; it is a biconvex structure situated
  between the posterior chamber and the vitreous
  body of the eye

- *Iris.* The circular pigmented membrane behind
  the cornea, perforated by the pupil; the most
  anterior portion of the vascular tunic of the eye

- *Optic nerve.* A nerve that carries impulses from the
  photoreceptors to the brain

- *Photoreceptor.* A light-responsive nerve cell or receptor that is located in the retina of the eye

- *Pupil.* The opening at the center of the iris through
  which light passes

- *Retina.* The innermost of the three tunics of the
  eyeball, which is situated around the vitreous body
  and is continuous posteriorly with the optic nerve;
  it contains the photoreceptors

- *Sclera.* The tough outer coat or fibrous tunic of
  the eyeball, which covers the posterior five-sixths
  of its surface and is continuous anteriorly with
  the cornea

- *Tunic.* Tissue of the eye

- *Vitreous body.* A clear, jellylike substance that fills
  the cavity containing the eyeball (the globe)

CAUSES

No specific pathogen is responsible for infecting
the eyes. The human body includes a normal amount
of bacteria and is exposed daily to viruses, fungi, and
parasites that can cause eye infection and irritation.
The most common eye infection is conjunctivitis,
caused by adenovirus, a virus of the common cold.
There are also more than sixty types of fungus that
can lead to eye infection. Leading eye infections are
described in the following sections.

Keratitis. Injury to the eye, a weakened immune
system, or a lack of oxygen from contact lens wear allows bacteria, fungi or parasites to penetrate the
cornea, causing keratitis. Most cases of bacterial kera-

titis are caused by *Staphylococcus*, which is found in the normal bacteria in the eyelids, skin, mouth, and nose of more than 20 percent of humans, or by *Streptococcus*, which is the same bacteria that causes strep throat and is normally found in the mouth, skin, intestine, and upper respiratory tract. This type of corneal infection can occur when the eye comes in contact with a contaminated object or person or if a person is already a carrier of *Staphylococcus* or *Streptococcus* and self-infects by touching his or her own eye.

Conjunctivitis. Chlamydia and gonorrhea are common sexually transmitted infections that can cause conjunctivitis. The infection can be transmitted to the eyes through direct contact with genital fluids or through people touching or rubbing their eyes after touching infected genital areas. These infections usually result in conjunctivitis; however, some bacteria such as *Neisseria gonorrhoeae* can penetrate the protective layers of the eye and cause inner eye infection and serious damage. Newborn babies whose mothers have chlamydia or gonorrhea are at high risk for developing severe eye infection.

Herpes simplex virus infection. The herpes simplex virus, which causes cold sores, can also infect the eye, leading to ulcers on the cornea. Recurring herpes infection in the eye can cause major destruction of retinal vessels, leading to vision damage. Chronic herpes simplex infections in the eye will cause some vision loss in approximately 15 percent of people who have the virus.

Herpes zoster virus infection. Herpes zoster is a virus that causes chickenpox and can be reactivated, causing shingles later in life. Eye infections often occur when the eyes are touched after a chickenpox or shingles lesion has been touched. Like ocular infection by the herpes simplex virus, herpes zoster can also cause corneal ulcers and can lead to retinal tissue damage.

Histoplasmosis. Histoplasmosis is a fungal infection of the lungs, which is caused by the inhalation of spores. These fungal spores can travel through the body to the inside of the eyes, causing ocular histoplasmosis syndrome. This migration may take years or even decades. The fungal infection can cause damage to the retina and, more specifically, to the macula, leading to reduced central vision, similar to macular degeneration. Histoplasmosis frequently occurs in river valleys around the world, and it has affected more than 90 percent of people in the southeastern United States. Most people infected with histoplasmosis have no symptoms, and only some develop ocular histoplasmosis syndrome. However, histoplasmosis remains a significant infectious cause of legal blindness for twenty to forty year olds in the United States.

Endophthalmitis. Endophthalmitis is a serious infection of the inside of the eye that could lead to blindness. All intraocular eye surgeries, such as cataract surgery or injectable treatments for age-related macular degeneration, carry a risk for endophthalmitis. Typically, the microbial organisms normally found on the patient's skin or conjunctiva are transferred into the eye cavity during the surgical procedure; contaminated surgical instruments may also be a cause. Once the organisms are inside the eye cavity, inflammation starts to occur, usually reaching serious levels within about six weeks of the original surgical procedure. Other causes may be trauma or be bloodstream-related because of an infection in another part of the body.

Acanthamoeba infection. Acanthamoeba is a single-celled ameba that is commonly found in water and soil. Before contact lens use was common, infection from Acanthamoeba was quite rare. Washing contact lenses with tap water or using a homemade saline solution allows the ameba to adhere to the lens and wait for an opportunity to invade the eye. A tiny scratch or abrasion on the surface of the eye will provide ample opportunity for the ameba to get inside the cornea, multiply, and cause a painful destructive infection called acanthamoeba keratitis.

Trachoma. Trachoma is a chronic and extremely contagious form of conjunctivitis caused by the microorganism *Chlamydia trachomatis*. It is a leading cause of blindness around the world, most prevalent in developing countries or in disadvantaged populations. If the inflammation persists and is left untreated, the eyelid may turn inward, causing the eyelashes to rub on the surface of the eye and leading to the formation of painful scar tissue, resulting in irreversible blindness.

Cellulitis. Cellulitis is a serious skin infection that can affect the tissues surrounding the eye. It is caused most usually by a spread of infection from an adjacent facial wound, eyelid trauma, insect bite, sinusitis, or tooth infection.

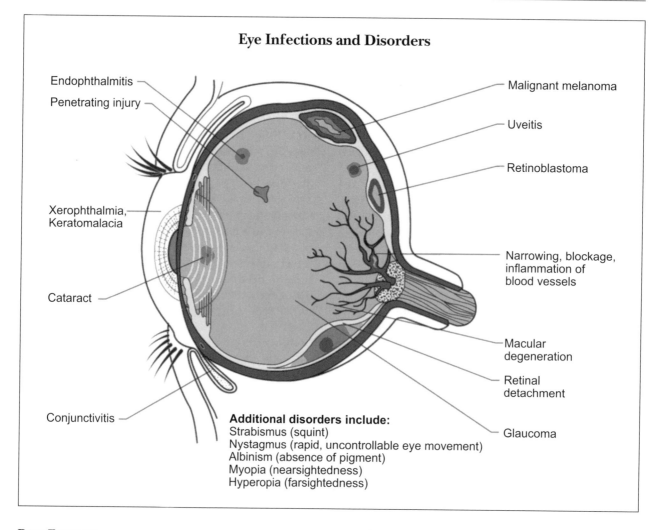

Eye Infections and Disorders

Endophthalmitis
Penetrating injury
Xerophthalmia, Keratomalacia
Cataract
Conjunctivitis

Malignant melanoma
Uveitis
Retinoblastoma
Narrowing, blockage, inflammation of blood vessels
Macular degeneration
Retinal detachment
Glaucoma

Additional disorders include:
Strabismus (squint)
Nystagmus (rapid, uncontrollable eye movement)
Albinism (absence of pigment)
Myopia (nearsightedness)
Hyperopia (farsightedness)

RISK FACTORS

Eyes are frequently exposed to potential pathogens, therefore making them vulnerable to infection. Certain diseases, behaviors, and environments can increase the risk for these infections. Quite often, an eye infection accompanies another infection, disease, or health condition in the body.

One of the greatest risk factors for eye infection is contact lens wear. Normal contact lens wear that carefully follows the recommendations for care and cleaning does not pose a significant risk. Prolonged wear and inadequate cleaning limit oxygen exposure to the eye and expose the eye to harmful bacteria for extended periods. Smoking when wearing contact lenses increases this risk, as the smoke dries and irritates the surface of the eye. Studies have shown that prolonged lens wear and sleeping with lenses in the

eyes increase the risk of infection more than fivefold and can potentially cause permanent vision loss. If an eye infection does occur, contact lenses must not be worn until the infection has completely resolved because the contact lens can cause reinfection.

Contact lens wearers can lower their risk of contracting acanthamoeba keratitis by never allowing their lenses or cases to come in contact with tap water and never wearing contacts when showering or swimming, even in chlorinated pools.

Exposure to ultraviolet light can damage the surface of the eye, making it more susceptible to infection, so proper eye wear outdoors or in tanning facilities is strongly recommended.

A weakened or compromised immune system can lead to increased risk of infection in the eye and elsewhere in the body.

Patients having any type of intraocular surgery are at an increased risk for endophthalmitis or other infection inside the eye. Common intraocular procedures include cataract surgery and injectable treatments for age-related macular degeneration.

Previous skin wounds or infections, or a sinus or tooth infection, may put patients at an increased risk for orbital cellulitis.

SYMPTOMS

Symptoms that occur when an infection is present on one of the outer surfaces of the eye, such as the conjunctiva or cornea, include redness and itching, excessive tear production, light sensitivity, mucuslike discharge, eyelid swelling, pain, and involuntary blinking. A symptom of a serious infection, such as cellulitis, includes proptosis, which is the displacement of the eyeball as the infection or abscess pushes the eye in an unnatural direction. Most of these symptoms are easily visible to others and can be quite uncomfortable.

Infections of structures of the inner eye cavity, such as the retina, optic nerve, vitreous fluid, or the blood vessels that feed them, are much more difficult to detect and often cause no pain. Normally, the first symptom for these eye infections is deteriorating vision, which can often be stopped but not reversed. A potential symptom of damage to the inner structures of the eye may be a sudden increase in the amount of floaters, which appear as small bubbles, strands, or dark spots or specks that slowly fall across the line of vision.

SCREENING AND DIAGNOSIS

The majority of eye infections are diagnosed by clinical evaluation and observation, although a computed tomography (CT) scan or a magnetic resonance imaging (MRI) scan may be used to confirm or detect infections at the back of the eye or in the surrounding tissues. The mucus, or discharge, from the eye can be collected on a swab and analyzed in a laboratory to determine what organism is causing the infection.

One should have regular eye examinations, during which a doctor will check for the presence of any infections or damage to the inner or outer structures of the eye. General practitioners can often easily diagnose many common eye infections; however, eye care professionals, such as ophthalmologists and optometrists, have specialized equipment that can carefully examine the structures of the eye. They can recognize various eye infections by the appearance of the eye and by the patient's medical history, because eye infections frequently accompany a disease or infection (such as a cold) in another part of the body.

TREATMENT AND THERAPY

Bacterial eye infections (conjunctivitis or keratitis) are often treated with broad spectrum antibiotic drops, but more specific antibiotics are used for infections caused by chlamydia or gonorrhea. More serious infections such as cellulitis or endophthalmitis may require intravenous antibiotics and a hospital stay.

Most cases of viral conjunctivitis will improve within a few days without treatment. Viruses such as herpes simplex remain in the body, and ocular flare-ups may recur; they can be managed with antiviral medications.

The majority of fungal infections can be treated with medication; however, infections such as histoplasmosis, which cause damage to the retina and macula, require surgical laser treatments to slow the deterioration of the macula in an attempt to preserve deteriorating vision.

Eye infections that are manifestations of systemic disease, such as tuberculosis or syphilis, will normally clear up when the entire body is being treated for the systemic infection. Parasitic infection to the eye structures can be destructive and requires aggressive treatment with antimicrobial agents or combinations of topical treatments. Serious cases of keratitis may require surgical debridement. In some cases, the damage to the cornea requires a corneal transplant.

PREVENTION AND OUTCOMES

To prevent many bacterial or viral eye infections, one should practice good hygiene and safer sex. Washing hands frequently can prevent the spread of organisms that cause infection. Persons with open sores because of shingles, cold sores, or chickenpox, for example, should not touch or treat these sores and then touch their eyes. Children are especially susceptible and should be watched carefully and kept from touching sores, mucus from their nose or mouth, and their eyes. Items such as towels, pillow cases, and cosmetics, which come in contact with eyes, should not be shared. If a family member is known to have an eye infection, it is advised that he or she use separate wash cloths, towels, and bed linens.

Contact lens wearers are particularly susceptible to eye infections and need to wash their hands before they insert or remove their lenses. It is very important that contact lenses are cleaned and cared for as per the manufacturer's instructions and are not worn longer than advised. Tap water should never come in contact with contact lenses.

Smoking and unprotected exposure to ultraviolet light, such as that from direct sunlight or from tanning beds, can damage the protective layers of the eyes, making them more susceptible to infection.

A person who has had many eye infections could have a sexually transmitted disease, which is highly contagious and is not easily detectable until infection is visible. Safer sexual practices, such as condom use, will reduce the risk of infection; also, one should always keep hands clean and keep them far from the eyes.

Trauma or scratches make the eye more vulnerable to infection because of damage to the protective layer, making it easier for contaminated foreign bodies to enter the eye. One should take steps to prevent eye injuries by using safety glasses or goggles.

April Ingram, B.S.

FURTHER READING

American Academy of Ophthalmology. "Eye Infections." Provides descriptions and diagrams of typical eye infections. Available at http://www.aao.org/eyesmart/infections.

Bartlett, Jimmy D., and Siret D. Jaanus, eds. *Clinical Ocular Pharmacology.* 5th ed. Boston: Butterworth-Heinemann/Elsevier, 2008. A well-illustrated and descriptive account of diseases of the eye and of surgical and pharmacological treatments. Though aimed at medical professionals, the book is a valuable reference for any interested reader.

Cronau, H., R. Kankanala, and T. Mauger. "Diagnosis and Management of Red Eye in Primary Care." *American Family Physician* 81, no. 2 (January, 2010): 137-144. This review article discusses the causes, symptoms, and treatment and referral requirements for patients presenting with red eyes, the cardinal sign of ocular inflammation.

Higgins, Jeffrey. *Eye Infections, Blindness, and Myopia.* Hauppauge, N.Y.: Nova Biomedical Books, 2009. A description of antibiotic-resistant infections and the treatments for and outcomes of serious ocular infections.

Johnson, Gordon J., et al., eds. *The Epidemiology of Eye Disease.* 2d ed. New York: Oxford University Press, 2003. A university-level text concerning eye disease. Descriptive, well referenced, and richly illustrated with color images.

Mandell, Gerald, and Thomas Bleck, eds. *Central Nervous System and Eye Infections.* Vol. 3 in *Atlas of Infectious Diseases.* New York: Churchill Livingstone, 1995. Provides a collection of clinical images and illustrations for many infectious diseases throughout stages of development and treatment.

Panjwani, Noorjahan. "Pathogenesis of Acanthamoeba Keratitis." *Ocular Surface* 8, no. 2 (April, 2010): 70-79. This review article discusses trends in understandings of acanthamoeba keratitis, the mechanism of infection by this parasite, and treatment options.

Riordan-Eva, Paul, and John P. Whitcher. *Vaughan and Asbury's General Ophthalmology.* 17th ed. New York: Lange Medical Books/McGraw-Hill, 2008. This well-illustrated textbook is an excellent reference for the serious student who desires detailed information on any aspect of the eye or its diseases.

Seal, David, and Uwe Pleyer. *Ocular Infection: Management and Treatment in Practice.* 2d ed. New York: Informa Healthcare, 2007. This book is an update of the first edition, published in 1998. Discusses the basic science of ocular infections and the diagnosis and management of ocular disease.

WEB SITES OF INTEREST

American Academy of Ophthalmology
http://www.aao.org

American Optometric Association
http://www.aoanet.org

Canadian Ophthalmological Society
http://www.eyesite.ca

National Foundation for Eye Research
http://www.nfer.org

See also: Acanthamoeba infection; Adenovirus infections; Bacterial infections; Cellulitis; Children and infectious disease; Chlamydia; Conjunctivitis; Contagious diseases; Dacryocystitis; Herpes simplex infection; Herpes zoster infection; Histoplasmosis; Hordeola; Hospitals and infectious disease; Keratitis; Neisserial infections; Ophthalmia neonatorum; Staphylococcal infections; Streptococcal infections; Trachoma; Viral infections; Wound infections.